INSTRUCTIONS FOR SURGERY PATIENTS

INSTRUCTIONS FOR SURGERY PATIENTS

Steven G. Economou, M.D.

Professor of Surgery

Rush Medical College of Rush University

Chairman Emeritus and Senior Attending Surgeon

Department of General Surgery

Rush–Presbyterian–St. Luke's Medical Center

Chicago, Illinois

Tasia S. Economou, M.D.

Department of Otolaryngology–Head and Neck Surgery

Kaiser Foundation Hospital–West Los Angeles

Los Angeles, California

W.B. Saunders Company

A Division of Harcourt Brace & Company

Philadelphia London Montreal Sydney Tokyo

W.B. SAUNDERS COMPANY
A Division of Harcourt Brace & Company

The Curtis Center
Independence Square West
Philadelphia, Pennsylvania 19106

Library of Congress Cataloging-in-Publication Data

Economou, Steven G.
Instructions for surgery patients / Steven G. Economou, Tasia S. Economou.—
1st ed.

p. cm.

ISBN 0–7216–7188–8

1. Surgery—Psychological aspects. 2. Preoperative care. 3. Patient education.
I. Economou, Tasia S. II. Title. [DNLM: 1. Surgery, Operative.
2. Patient Education. WO 500 E19i 1999]

RD31.5.E285 1999 617′.91′0071—dc21

DNLM/DLC

97–36789

INSTRUCTIONS FOR SURGERY PATIENTS

ISBN 0–7216–7188–8

Printed in the United States of America.

Last digit is the print number: 9 8 7 6 5 4 3 2 1

To

George and Helen Economou

and

George and Anastasia Dotska,

who were the essence

of lifelong encouragement,

perseverance, and sacrifice.

CONSULTANTS

The intent of this book is to serve the needs of many different surgeons who perform a spectrum of operations on patients with wide differences in understanding of their illnesses or of the surgical treatments needed.

A basic requirement, of course, is that the information in the various chapters be appropriately inclusive and totally accurate. In addition, this information has to read in a manner that an average layperson can understand. These goals could not have been reached without the involvement of our talented colleagues who readily—even enthusiastically—accepted our invitation to be consultants. We chose them with care, not for their knowledge alone but also for their skill and experience in communicating with patients. We are deeply grateful to them for their authoritative and insightful contributions.

Amjad Ali, M.D.
Professor of Radiology and Nuclear Medicine
Rush Medical College of Rush University
Senior Attending Physician
Department of Diagnostic Radiology and Nuclear Medicine
Rush–Presbyterian–St. Luke's Medical Center
Chicago, Illinois

Gunnar B. J. Andersson, M.D., Ph.D.
William A. Hark, M.D.–Susanne G. Swift Professor of Surgery
Rush Medical College of Rush University
Chairman, Department of Orthopedic Surgery
Senior Attending Surgeon
Rush–Presbyterian–St. Luke's Medical Center
Chicago, Illinois

Julian T. Archie, M.D.
West Suburban Hospital
Loyola University Medical Center
Maywood, Illinois

Bernard Bach, Jr., M.D.
Professor of Orthopedic Surgery
Rush Medical College of Rush University
Director, Section of Sports Medicine
Senior Attending Surgeon
Rush–Presbyterian–St. Luke's Medical Center
Chicago, Illinois

Shyamala K. Badrinath, M.D.
Associate Professor of Anesthesiology
Rush Medical College of Rush University
Medical Director, Rush Surgicenter
Senior Attending Physician
Rush–Presbyterian–St. Luke's Medical Center
Chicago, Illinois

Roger A. Billhardt, M.D.
Assistant Professor of Medicine
Rush Medical College of Rush University
Associate Attending Physician
Rush–Presbyterian–St. Luke's Medical Center
Chicago, Illinois

Zvi Binor, M.D.
Associate Professor of Obstetrics and Gynecology
Rush Medical College of Rush University
Associate Attending Surgeon
Rush–Presbyterian–St. Luke's Medical Center
Director of Assisted Reproduction Program at Rush–Presbyterian–St. Luke's Medical Center and Copley Memorial Hospital
Director, Reproductive Endocrinology, Rush North Shore Medical Center
Chicago, Illinois

Steven L. Blum, M.D.
Assistant Professor of Anesthesiology and Family Medicine
Rush Medical College of Rush University
Assistant Attending Physician, Department of Anesthesiology
Rush North Shore Medical Center
Skokie, Illinois

John Bojchuk, M.S., A.T.C.L.
Certified and Licensed Athletic Trainer
Sports Medicine Practice Coordinator
Midwest Orthopaedics
Rush–Presbyterian–St. Luke's Medical Center
Chicago, Illinois

Douglas V. Brown, M.D.
Assistant Professor of Anesthesiology
Rush Medical College of Rush University
Assistant Attending Physician, Department of Anesthesiology
Rush–Presbyterian–St. Luke's Medical Center
Chicago, Illinois

Richard G. Caldwell, M.D.
Clinical Associate Professor
University of Chicago
Senior Attending Surgeon, Department of General Surgery
Rush–Presbyterian–St. Luke's Medical Center
Attending Surgeon, Department of General Surgery
Lutheran General Hospital
Park Ridge, Illinois

Antonio H. Chaviano, M.D.
Assistant Professor of Urology and Pediatrics
Rush Medical College of Rush University
Assistant Attending Surgeon, Department of Urology and Department of Pediatrics
Director, Pediatric Urology
Rush–Presbyterian–St. Luke's Medical Center
Chicago, Illinois

James G. Clark, M.D.
Associate Professor of Cardiology
Rush Medical College of Rush University
Senior Attending Physician
Rush–Presbyterian–St. Luke's Medical Center
Chicago, Illinois

Mark S. Cohen, M.D.
Assistant Professor of Orthopedic Surgery
Rush Medical College of Rush University
Assistant Attending Surgeon
Director, Hand and Elbow Program
Director, Orthopedic Education
Department of Orthopedic Surgery
Rush–Presbyterian–St. Luke's Medical Center
Chicago, Illinois

Christopher L. Coogan, M.D.
Instructor, Rush Medical College of Rush University
Adjunct Attending Surgeon, Department of Urology
Rush–Presbyterian–St. Luke's Medical Center
Chicago, Illinois

John Q. Cook, M.D.
Instructor, Rush Medical College of Rush University
Assistant Attending Surgeon
Department of Plastic and Reconstructive Surgery
Rush–Presbyterian–St. Luke's Medical Center
Chicago, Illinois

Andrew M. Davidoff, M.D.
Assistant Professor of Surgery
Assistant Attending Surgeon
Department of General Surgery
St. Jude Children's Research Hospital
Memphis, Tennessee

Koen De Geest, M.D.
Assistant Professor of Obstetrics and Gynecology
Rush Medical College of Rush University
Assistant Attending Surgeon
Director, Section of Gynecologic Oncology
Department of Obstetrics and Gynecology
Rush–Presbyterian–St. Luke's Medical Center
Chicago, Illinois

Daniel J. Deziel, M.D.
Associate Professor of Surgery
Rush Medical College of Rush University
Associate Attending Surgeon
Associate Coordinator, Resident Clinical Activities
Department of General Surgery
Rush–Presbyterian–St. Luke's Medical Center
Chicago, Illinois

Edward J. Donahue, M.D., F.A.C.S.
Chief, Division of General Surgery
St. Joseph's Hospital and Medical Center
Phoenix, Arizona

Alexander Doolas, M.D.
Professor of Surgery
Rush Medical College of Rush University
Senior Attending Surgeon and Associate Chairman
Department of General Surgery
Rush–Presbyterian–St. Luke's Medical Center
Chicago, Illinois

Kambiz Dowlatshahi, M.D.
Associate Professor of Surgery
Rush Medical College of Rush University
Associate Attending Surgeon
Department of General Surgery
Rush–Presbyterian–St. Luke's Medical Center
Chicago, Illinois

R. Renée Edwards, M.D.
Assistant Professor of Obstetrics and Gynecology
Rush Medical College of Rush University
Assistant Attending Surgeon
Department of Obstetrics and Gynecology, Section of Urogynecology and Reconstructive Pelvic Surgery
Rush–Presbyterian–St. Luke's Medical Center
Chicago, Illinois

Shahid Ekbal, M.D.
Assistant Professor of Urology
Rush Medical College of Rush University
Associate Attending Surgeon
Rush–Presbyterian–St. Luke's Medical Center
Chicago, Illinois

L. Penfield Faber, M.D.
Professor of Cardiovascular and Thoracic Surgery
Rush Medical College of Rush University
Senior Attending Surgeon
Director, Section of Thoracic Surgery
Rush–Presbyterian–St. Luke's Medical Center
Chicago, Illinois

James C. Ferlmann, M.D.
Instructor, Department of Plastic and Reconstructive Surgery
Rush Medical College of Rush University
Adjunct Attending Surgeon
Rush–Presbyterian–St. Luke's Medical Center
Chicago, Illinois

Richard E. Fine, M.D., F.A.C.S.
Co-Director, The Breast Center
Atlanta, Georgia

Preston F. Foster, M.D.
Associate Professor of Surgery
Rush Medical College of Rush University
Associate Attending Surgeon
Department of General Surgery
Section of Transplantation
Rush–Presbyterian–St. Luke's Medical Center
Chicago, Illinois

James L. Franklin, M.D.
Associate Professor of Internal Medicine
Rush Medical College of Rush University
Senior Attending Physician
Department of Internal Medicine, Section of Digestive Diseases
Rush–Presbyterian–St. Luke's Medical Center
Chicago, Illinois

Constantine V. Godellas, M.D.
Assistant Professor of Surgery
Rush Medical College of Rush University
Assistant Attending Surgeon
Department of General Surgery
Rush–Presbyterian–St. Luke's Medical Center
Attending Surgeon, Division of Surgical Oncology
Cook County Hospital
Chicago, Illinois

Marshall D. Goldin, M.D.
Associate Professor of Cardiovascular-Thoracic Surgery
Rush Medical College of Rush University
Senior Attending Surgeon
Department of Cardiovascular-Thoracic Surgery
Director of Surgical Intensive Care Unit
Rush–Presbyterian–St. Luke's Medical Center
Chicago, Illinois

Wafik A. Hanna, M.D.
Assistant Professor of Surgery
Rush Medical College of Rush University
Assistant Attending Surgeon
Department of Otolaryngology and Bronchoesophagology
Rush–Presbyterian–St. Luke's Medical Center
Chicago, Illinois

Jerome Hoeksema, M.D.
Assistant Professor of Urology
Rush Medical College of Rush University
Associate Attending Surgeon
Director, Urologic Education
Department of Urology
Rush–Presbyterian–St. Luke's Medical Center
Chicago, Illinois

Anthony D. Ivankovich, M.D.
The William Gottschalk, M.D., Professor of Anesthesiology
Rush Medical College of Rush University
Senior Attending Physician and Chairman
Department of Anesthesiology
Rush–Presbyterian–St. Luke's Medical Center
Chicago, Illinois

Stephen C. Jensik, M.D., Ph.D.
Assistant Professor of Surgery
Rush Medical College of Rush University
Associate Attending Surgeon
Department of General Surgery, Section of Transplantation
Rush–Presbyterian–St. Luke's Medical Center
Chicago, Illinois

Peter M. Jokich, M.D.
Associate Professor of Radiology
Rush Medical College of Rush University
Associate Attending Radiologist
Department of Diagnostic Radiology and Nuclear Medicine
Director, Section of Breast Imaging
Rush–Presbyterian–St. Luke's Medical Center
Chicago, Illinois

John P. Kerchberger, M.D.
Assistant Professor of Anesthesiology
Rush Medical College of Rush University
Assistant Attending Physician
Rush–Presbyterian–St. Luke's Medical Center
Chicago, Illinois

Ken N. Kuo, M.D.
Professor of Orthopedic Surgery
Associate Chairman of Education
Rush Medical College of Rush University
Senior Attending Surgeon
Department of Orthopedic Surgery
Rush–Presbyterian–St. Luke's Medical Center
Chicago, Illinois

Stanley R. Levine, M.D.
Assistant Professor of Urology
Rush Medical College of Rush University
Assistant Attending Urologist
Department of Urology
Rush–Presbyterian–St. Luke's Medical Center
Chicago, Illinois

Eugene G. Lipov, M.D.
Assistant Professor of Anesthesiology
Rush Medical College of Rush University
Assistant Attending Physician
Rush–Presbyterian–St. Luke's Medical Center
Chicago, Illinois

Deborah Loeff, M.D.
Assistant Professor of Surgery
Rush Medical College of Rush University
Assistant Attending Surgeon
Head, Section of Pediatric Surgery
Rush–Presbyterian–St. Luke's Medical Center
Chicago, Illinois

Timothy R. Lubenow, M.D.
Associate Professor of Anesthesiology
Rush Medical College of Rush University
Associate Attending Physician
Director, Section of Pain Management
Rush–Presbyterian–St. Luke's Medical Center
Chicago, Illinois

Robert A. March, M.D.
Assistant Professor of Cardiovascular-Thoracic Surgery
Rush Medical College of Rush University
Assistant Attending Surgeon
Department of Cardiovascular-Thoracic Surgery
Rush–Presbyterian–St. Luke's Medical Center
Chicago, Illinois

Terence A. Matalon, M.D.
Associate Professor of Medicine
Rush Medical College of Rush University
Associate Attending Physician
Director of Interventional Radiology
Department of Diagnostic Radiology
Rush–Presbyterian–St. Luke's Medical Center
Chicago, Illinois

Lawrence P. McChesney, M.D.
Assistant Professor of Surgery
Rush Medical College of Rush University
Assistant Attending Surgeon, Department of General Surgery, Section of Transplantation
Director, Pancreas Transplant Program
Rush–Presbyterian–St. Luke's Medical Center
Chicago, Illinois

Bruce C. McLeod, M.D.
Professor of Medicine and Pathology
Rush Medical College of Rush University
Senior Attending Physician, Department of Internal Medicine and Pathology
Associate Medical Director, Blood Center
Rush–Presbyterian–St. Luke's Medical Center
Chicago, Illinois

Janet Millikan, M.S., R.D., L.D.
Formerly Clinical Dietician
Food and Nutrition Services
Department of Nutrition
Rush–Presbyterian–St. Luke's Medical Center
Chicago, Illinois

Keith W. Millikan, M.D.
Associate Professor of Surgery
Rush Medical College of Rush University
Associate Attending Surgeon
Director, Undergraduate Surgical Education
Department of General Surgery
Rush–Presbyterian–St. Luke's Medical Center
Chicago, Illinois

Heather A. Nath, M.D.
Assistant Professor of Anesthesiology
Rush Medical College of Rush University
Assistant Attending Physician
Department of Anesthesiology
Rush–Presbyterian–St. Luke's Medical Center
Chicago, Illinois

L. Michael Newman, M.D., Ph.D.
Associate Professor of Anesthesiology and Obstetrics and Gynecology
Rush Medical College of Rush University
Senior Attending Anesthesiologist and Director of Obstetric Anesthesia
Department of Anesthesiology
Rush–Presbyterian–St. Luke's Medical Center
Chicago, Illinois

Christopher O'Connor, M.D.
Assistant Professor
Rush Medical College of Rush University
Assistant Attending Anesthesiologist
Director, Cardiothoracic Anesthesia
Department of Anesthesiology
Rush–Presbyterian–St. Luke's Medical Center
Chicago, Illinois

Suresh K. Patel, M.D.
Professor of Radiology
Rush Medical College of Rush University
Senior Attending Physician
Department of Diagnostic Radiology and Nuclear Medicine
Rush–Presbyterian–St. Luke's Medical Center
Chicago, Illinois

Dennis A. Pessis, M.D.
Associate Professor of Urology
Rush Medical College of Rush University
Associate Attending Urologist
Associate Chairman, Department of Urology
Rush–Presbyterian–St. Luke's Medical Center
Chicago, Illinois

Richard A. Prinz, M.D.
Helen Shedd Keith Professor
Rush Medical College of Rush University
Senior Attending Surgeon
Chairman, Department of General Surgery
Rush–Presbyterian–St. Luke's Medical Center
Chicago, Illinois

Chadwick C. Prodromos, M.D.
Assistant Professor of Orthopedic Surgery
Rush Medical College of Rush University
Assistant Attending Surgeon
Department of Orthopedic Surgery
Rush–Presbyterian–St. Luke's Medical Center
Chicago, Illinois

Anthony A. Romeo, M.D.
Assistant Professor of Orthopedic Surgery
Rush Medical College of Rush University
Assistant Attending Surgeon
Department of Orthopedic Surgery
Rush–Presbyterian–St. Luke's Medical Center
Chicago, Illinois

Aaron G. Rosenberg, M.D.
Professor of Orthopedic Surgery
Rush Medical College of Rush University
Senior Attending Surgeon
Director, Section of Adult Joint Reconstruction
Department of Orthopedic Surgery
Rush–Presbyterian–St. Luke's Medical Center
Chicago, Illinois

Theodore J. Saclarides, M.D.
Professor of Surgery
Rush Medical College of Rush University
Associate Attending Surgeon
Head, Section of Colon and Rectal Surgery
Department of General Surgery
Rush–Presbyterian–St. Luke's Medical Center
Chicago, Illinois

Howard N. Sankary, M.D.
Associate Professor of Surgery
Rush Medical College of Rush University
Associate Attending Surgeon, Department of General Surgery, Section of Transplantation
Rush–Presbyterian–St. Luke's Medical Center
Chicago, Illinois

Cyrus Serry, M.D.
Associate Professor of Surgery
Rush Medical College of Rush University
Senior Attending Surgeon
Department of Cardiovascular-Thoracic Surgery
Rush–Presbyterian–St. Luke's Medical Center
Chairman, Division of Cardiothoracic Surgery
Department of Surgery, Cook County Hospital;
Chief, Section of Cardiac Surgery
Department of Surgery, Elmhurst Memorial Hospital
Elmhurst, Illinois

Mitchell Ben Sheinkop, M.D.
Associate Professor of Surgery
Associate Attending Surgeon
Department of Orthopedic Surgery
Rush–Presbyterian–St. Luke's Medical Center
Chicago, Illinois

Morton Shulman, M.D.
Professor of Anesthesiology
Rush Medical College of Rush University
Senior Attending Physician
Rush–Presbyterian–St. Luke's Medical Center
Chicago, Illinois

Claire S. Smith, M.D.
Professor of Radiology
Rush Medical College of Rush University
Senior Attending Physician
Director of Residency Training Program
Director, Gastrointestinal Radiology
Department of Diagnostic Radiology and Nuclear Medicine
Rush–Presbyterian–St. Luke's Medical Center
Chicago, Illinois

Timothy W. Starck, M.D.
Assistant Professor of Anesthesiology
Director, Medical Student Education
Rush Medical College of Rush University
Assistant Attending Physician
Department of Anesthesiology
Rush–Presbyterian–St. Luke's Medical Center
Chicago, Illinois

Edgar Staren, M.D., Ph.D.
Professor of Surgery
Associate Dean, Medical Student Programs
Rush Medical College of Rush University
Associate Attending Surgeon
Rush–Presbyterian–St. Luke's Medical Center
Chicago, Illinois

Wayne M. Swenson, M.D.
Professor and Regional Assistant to the Chairman
Department of Surgery
University of North Dakota School of Medicine
Bismarck, North Dakota

David A. Turner, M.D.
Robert R. McCormick Professor
Rush Medical College of Rush University
Senior Attending Radiologist
Director, MRI
Department of Diagnostic Radiology and Nuclear Medicine
Rush–Presbyterian–St. Luke's Medical Center
Chicago, Illinois

José Velasco, M.D.
Professor of Surgery
Rush Medical College of Rush University
Senior Attending Surgeon
Department of General Surgery
Rush–Presbyterian–St. Luke's Medical Center
Chairman, Department of Surgery
Rush North Shore Medical Center
Chicago, Illinois

Thomas R. Witt, M.D.
Associate Professor of Surgery
Rush Medical College of Rush University
Associate Attending Surgeon
Department of General Surgery
Rush–Presbyterian–St. Luke's Medical Center
Chicago, Illinois

Norman Wool, M.D.
Assistant Professor of Surgery
Rush Medical College of Rush University
Director, Resident Clinical Activities
Associate Attending Surgeon
Rush–Presbyterian–St. Luke's Medical Center
Chicago, Illinois

PREFACE

Most surgeons who are in practice today relate to their patients in ways that were thought quite unnecessary not too long ago. Generally, patients needing an operation were not told by the surgeon too much about the particulars. Most patients did not think to ask questions, or even know which questions to ask, relative to their operation, and many were intimidated from doing so by the aura of the surgeon. Usually, the need for an operation was announced, the patient and family acknowledged or accepted it, and a date was set.

Except for the most minor problems, surgical patients were admitted to the hospital at least the afternoon before the planned operation. Oftentimes, they would be admitted several days before surgery if preoperative tests were required. During this period, patients came to learn more about what was planned for them, albeit commonly in a paternalistic atmosphere.

The period of postoperative care in the hospital was likewise much longer, often measured in weeks. There was ample nursing help to take care of the patient's needs. Actually, the patients did not need to do much for themselves, and when sent home they were almost totally self-sufficient. Accordingly, few instructions were necessary on home care. This no longer is the case.

The swiftly tightening constraints of managed health care, the scientific advances, and the evolving social climate all have changed the practice of surgery significantly. The time the surgeon and patient can spend with each other preparing for what is often a major event in that patient's life has been abbreviated drastically. Diagnostic tests—some of them daunting—are done on an outpatient basis. Patients undergo major elective operations just hours after registering in the hospital. The postoperative hospital stay has been shortened severely so that recovery from surgery has become increasingly an outpatient experience. Add to these considerations the appropriate and increasing expectation by patients that they be told more about their illnesses and the recommended options for therapy and it becomes obvious that both the patient and the surgeon need assistance to manage all this.

Instructions for Surgical Patients is a response to that need. It is an attempt to support and supplement rather than to supplant instructions and other information given by the surgeon to the patient. It is hoped that such assistance will reduce the burden on the surgeon. Also, it can help reduce the anxiety of the patients and, importantly, help provide them with information they want and to which they are entitled.

Most of the operations included are those that are done commonly, and they were chosen with minimal regard to the specialty in which they fell. We included some operations that are not done commonly but that deserve exposition. Some frequently performed operations (example: ophthalmologic procedures) were not included simply because they are so narrowly specialized or because many of the surgeons performing them have their own specifically tailored instructions. Certain operations (example: liver transplant) were felt to be too complex and varied to describe in the format we used. Some of the operations included are frequenty done on an urgent or emergency basis. We included them for the times they can be of value to the patient or to the relatives who often act as surrogates in such circumstances.

We have been diligent throughout to avoid words that might intimidate a patient or might simply not be understood. As much as possible we favored conversational, informal English and avoided medical lingo. And although we avoided expressions such as "pit of the stomach" because they were not refined, we likewise avoided "epigastrium" because it would not be understood. The narrative strives to avoid talking down to the informed patient, but we were more concerned about how best to inform the less sophisticated patient. Stated differently, we chose to possibly annoy patients who already know a lot about the proposed operation rather than to have patients remain in the dark because they either know nothing about the procedure or are slow at understanding explanations.

As part of our aim to inform the patient, treatment options (and their advantages and disadvantages) are mentioned when appropriate, with attention focused primarily on the recommended treatment. We tried to omit fine details of an operation because they rarely truly inform and most often produce anxiety. When it seemed to be appropriate, simple line drawings were included.

We assiduously avoided making judgmental statements about therapy or its worth, because these are for the surgeon to consider and explain. We also were mindful not to undercut the surgeon or to confuse the patient by making dogmatic statements on issues of diagnosis or therapy when omission or inclusion of something could be equally justified.

Properly and adequately informing patients about something as important as an operation is essential to the practice of good surgery in the fullest sense. To do so in a wide variety of circumstances is not an easy matter. Nonetheless, surgeons should strive for such a goal in the best interests of all concerned. We sincerely hope that *Instructions for Surgical Patients* can help the reader come closer to that goal.

STEVEN G. ECONOMOU, M.D.
TASIA S. ECONOMOU, M.D.

USERS' GUIDE

A variety of the more common operations in almost all surgical specialties are described here. A number of diagnostic procedures relevant to these operations are also described. Some points to keep in mind:

- These patient instructions are designed to be copied to be given to patients as additional help in understanding the recommended operation. Alternately, they may be printed from the enclosed disks. Each entry is either one or two pages long.
- All procedures are listed alphabetically. When different names are used for the same procedures, these alternative names are also listed or may be listed in the index.
- An Appendix in the back of the book contains a number of full-page illustrations of various parts of the body. These illustrations are meant to be used by the surgeon to explain the procedure to the patient.
- Notice that occasionally, more than one topic may be appropriate for a patient's use. An example might be the description of "ultra-sound," which would be helpful for a patient having a breast mass evaluated.
- Each procedure includes space at the end for your telephone number, should you wish to include it, as well as additional instructions you may wish to give the patient.

ACKNOWLEDGMENTS

A work such as this, with so many small parts, all of which need to be written, reworded, evaluated by consultants, rechurned again, and then sent to the editor, can become a logistical nightmare. Jan Nunnally did not let this happen. Multitalented as a superb typist, juggler of manuscripts, follower of a nearly impossibly hectic schedule, and meeter of firm deadlines, she was a wonder to behold. She has our sincerest appreciation. We also thank Halina Lubonski, who saw to it that the generation of what seemed like a paper blizzard still resulted in an unfailing availability of whatever was necessary for an orderly completion of this book.

Lisette Bralow, who broached the idea of this book originally and then, in a low-key but effective style, guided it all to completion, truly exemplifies the title of Editor-in-Chief.

Every book needs someone to read and reread everything carefully to keep convoluted syntax and embarrassing errors from making it into print. Lee Ann Draud did just that and much more, for which we are truly grateful.

Finally, Kathryn Dotska Economou played important roles in this book. If she didn't adequately understand the narrative or if the illustrations didn't clarify the text, she made cogent suggestions—and she was listened to, usually most attentively. After all, as wife and mother, who else could be so direct and totally focused in her advice? And as usual, she was a master at accepting manuscripts lying about and illustrations positioned on the table or the mantle as a normal part of household decor. For these and a number of similar contributions, a significant part to this book belongs to her.

STEVEN G. ECONOMOU, M.D.
TASIA S. ECONOMOU, M.D.

CONTENTS

△ GENERAL INFORMATION

An *abscess* is one type of infection. Many people think all infections are the same, but they are not. This is important to remember because different types of infection often need to be treated differently.

Below is a list of some types of infection that occur in the body.

- *Cellulitis* is inflamed tissue that is red, swollen, and painful, but no liquid pus is present.
- *Lymphangitis* is inflammation along the lymph channels; they commonly show as red streaks.
- *Erysipelas* is a combination of both of the above that comes on suddenly, spreads swiftly, and causes pain, chills, and fever.
- *Abscess* (boil) is a local collection of pus.
- *Furuncle* is a tiny pus pocket of the sweat gland or hair follicle.
- *Carbuncle* is a number of furuncles together.
- *Bacteremia*: Bacteria are in the blood but do not cause any symptoms.
- *Septicemia*: Bacteria are in the blood stream and produce severe symptoms of infection.

○ TREATMENT: Nonsurgical

When antibiotics are used to treat an infection, the following should be considered:

- *Choosing an antibiotic to kill the responsible bacteria*: Whenever possible and useful, some of the pus will be obtained for testing to see which antibiotic is most likely to kill the bacteria found in it. When it is not possible to get some pus from the area, the doctor will use the antibiotic most often effective against the bacteria that usually causes such infections.
- *Knowing if the antibiotic can reach the infection*: The doctor has information regarding which kinds of infection block the antibiotics from reaching them.
- *Does the selected antibiotic itself have any harmful side effects*: Some antibiotics are good at fighting the infection but can have harmful side effects. The antibiotic will have to be chosen with this in mind.
- *How to help the body boost its own defenses*: Increasing the flow of blood to the area brings in white blood cells, whose important job is to fight infection. One way is to place warm, moist packs over the area as follows:
  - Dissolve 1 tablespoon of ordinary table salt in a quart of warm—*not hot*—tap water.
  - Dip a clean washcloth into this fluid and squeeze out the excess.
  - Place the washcloth over the area to be treated.
  - Over this, place a thin sheet of plastic.
  - Over this place a dry towel.
  - Over this place a heating pad on *low* (not medium or high, but low).
  - Make yourself comfortable and keep the warm packs on for 20 minutes, three times a day, or as often as you are instructed. You do not have to change the moist towels during a session.
  - For each new session, you should change the washcloth, but you can keep the same plastic and dry towel (Fig. 1).

○ TREATMENT: Surgical

If pus is present, it is necessary to let it out. Usually, this is done by an operation.

PREOPERATIVE PREPARATION

- You may be given antibiotics even before the pus is drained so that they can have a head start in your blood stream.
- Do not eat or drink anything for 8 hours before the operation.
- You will be given medicine that will make you feel drowsy before you are brought to the operating room.

□ OPERATION

- The type of operation performed on you and whether it is done under local or general anesthesia will depend on your special circumstances. This will be explained to you beforehand.
- If the operation is to be done under local anesthesia, the skin over the area of the abscess will be made numb and draped with towels.
- Generally, an incision is made over the area of the pus to let it out.
- A soft rubber drain may be left in the incision for a while to make certain the incision doesn't heal over before all the pus is out.

POSTOPERATIVE CARE

- When your blood pressure, pulse, and breathing are stable, a decision will be made regarding when you can go home.
  - For most surface abscesses, you should be able to go home that same day.
  - If yours is a deep abscess requiring more than just making an incision on your skin you may need to stay in the hospital.
- When you are ready to go home, arrangements will be made for the following:
  - A prescription for antibiotics and pain medicine.
  - Instructions on how to change the dressing, if this is necessary.

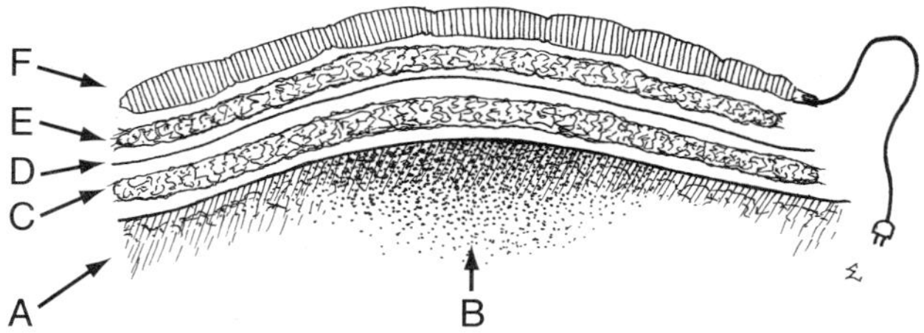

Figure 1. A, Flesh; B, inflamed area; C, moist towel, D, thin sheet of plastic; E, Dry towel; F, heating pad.

- Directions on whether you should continue with warm, moist packs.

HOME CARE

- You may walk about as you wish. You may eat as you wish.
- Increase your diet as tolerated.
- Speak with a doctor on the best way for you to shower or bathe.
- The treatment and aftercare of an abscess can vary widely for each patient. There may be detailed discussions with you on what you may do and how to help take care of yourself.

CALL OUR OFFICE IF

- You develop any unusual symptoms.
- You develop a temperature higher than 100°F.
- You have any questions.

△ GENERAL INFORMATION

Doctors sometimes need an easier and less painful way to put medicine or fluids into a vein, or they may need to draw blood repeatedly for laboratory examination. An access catheter is a good way to do a number of these important things. The following are some examples:

- A patient needs to have medicine given continuously over a number of days as an outpatient. There may be a rest period for a week or so, and then more medicine needs to be given for a few weeks. This routine may need to be repeated.
- Some medicines are so irritating to tissue that they clot the small vessels in the hand and elbow usually used for this purpose.
- A patient needs to be fed a special concentrated liquid diet by vein for a period of time. Using the veins in the back of the hand won't do because they clot when such fluids go through them.

In the above and similar situations, a large vessel with a lot of blood flowing through it is needed. The large amount of blood in such a large vein can dilute the irritating medicine quickly. The solution is to place a catheter the size of skinny macaroni into a large vein that empties directly into the heart. This is called an *access catheter*.

You are in need of such a catheter so that your condition can be treated in a way that is more predictable and more comfortable for you. This is done by a surgeon in the operating room and usually is an outpatient procedure.

METHODS

There are two main methods of placing such an access catheter:

- **Hickman:** In this method, the end of the catheter is placed in a big vein in the neck and advanced down to the heart. It then is "tunneled" under the skin, and the other end is brought out through the skin, 4 to 6 inches below the clavicle (collarbone). Medicine can be given through it, fluids connected to it, or blood drawn through it (Fig. 1).

  The advantages to this method are as follows:
  - The tube comes straight to the outside, and it's easy to connect fluids to it.
  - When the tube is no longer needed, the stitch that holds it in place is cut and the tube is pulled out.

  The disadvantages to this method are as follows:
  - The bandages that cover the place where the catheter comes out through the skin need to be changed very carefully so that the area around the incision and the catheter itself do not become infected.
  - The tube that dangles may interfere with some activities (e.g., swimming) or the wearing of some clothing.
- **Port-A-Cath:** In this method, the tip of the catheter is in the big vein in the neck and goes to just inside the heart; the other end is under the skin just below the clavicle. The end under the skin has a special gadget attached to it that is the size of three stacked silver dollars and hollow (a *chamber*). The special rubber wall on one side of the chamber is placed so that the rubber wall faces the skin.

When medicine, fluids, or nourishment need to be given, or blood drawn, an anesthetic ointment is placed on the skin over the gadget to make the skin numb. A needle is placed through the numb skin, then through the rubber wall to reach the chamber that is connected to the tube in the large vein. When it is not needed for a while, some blood thinner (heparin) is placed in the chamber and the needle is pulled out. The port-A-Cath remains in place, ready to be used again later.

The advantages to this method are as follows:

- There is nothing hanging from the body, and no maintenance is necessary.
- The catheter site is less likely to become infected.

The disadvantages are as follows:

- A nurse or technician is needed to connect fluids to the port-A-Cath.

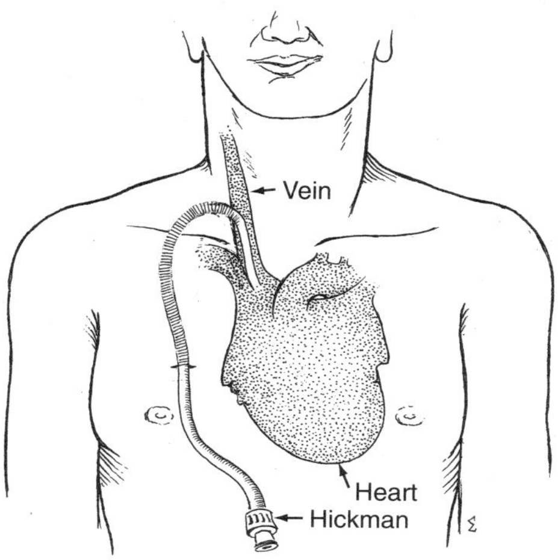

Figure 1. In performing an access procedure using a Hickman catheter, an incision is made in the neck, a large vein is located, and the plain end of the catheter is inserted into it. The other end of the catheter is then tunneled under the skin and brought to the outside at a convenient spot several inches below the clavicle. This end is used to introduce medications or nourishment.

- When the port-A-Cath is not being used, it has to be flushed with a blood thinner solution every week or so to prevent clotting of the catheter.

After careful consideration of all factors, the recommendation is that you have a Hickman catheter.

PREOPERATIVE PREPARATION

- Do not eat or drink anything for 8 hours before the operation.
- Shower or bathe on the morning of the operation.
- You may be given medicine that will make you feel drowsy before you are brought to the operating room.

☐ OPERATION

- Medical reasons will determine the type of anesthesia you will have. Generally, however, the operation is done under local anesthesia along with medicine to keep you drowsy during the operation.
- The area in front of one side of your neck and your chest will be swabbed with an antiseptic solution and surrounded with sterile drapes.
- An area just below the collarbone and in the lower neck will be made numb.
- One incision will be just above the inner side of the clavicle and another in an area 4 to 6 inches below this.
- During the operation, you may feel some tugging but not pain.
- X-rays will be used to check that the catheter is in the correct area.
- The operation generally takes 1 hour.
- The incision where the catheter comes through the skin to the outside will have a dressing over it. The catheter will hang free but will be taped securely in place.

POSTOPERATIVE CARE

- You will be taken to a recovery room and observed. When your blood pressure, pulse, and breathing are stable and you are completely alert, you should be able to go home accompanied by a responsible adult.
- Pain will be controlled with medicine.
- Arrangements will be made for your medicine, office follow-up visit, and stitch removal.

✚ HOME CARE

- Resume your usual activities.
- You may walk about as you wish, even climb stairs.
- You may eat as you did before the operation.
- You may shower if you wish, but do not get the dressings or the wound wet. Covering the area with a sheet of plastic and sealing the edges usually is satisfactory.
- You will be given instructions on how to take care of your incisions.
- You probably will be able to feel the catheter under your skin, especially in the area of the clavicle.
- You may return to work when you feel up to it.

✆ CALL OUR OFFICE IF

- The incisions become red or swollen or there is any drainage from them.
- You develop a temperature higher than 100°F.
- You have any questions.

△ GENERAL INFORMATION

Doctors sometimes need an easier and less painful way to put medicine or fluids into a vein, or they may need to draw blood repeatedly for laboratory examination. An access catheter is a good way to do a number of these important things. The following are some examples:

- A patient needs to have medicine given continuously over a number of days as an outpatient. There may be a rest period for a week or so, and then more medicine needs to be given for a few weeks. This routine may need to be repeated.
- Some medicines are so irritating to tissue that they clot the small vessels in the hand and elbow usually used for this purpose.
- A patient needs to be fed a special concentrated liquid diet by vein for a period of time. Using the veins in the back of the hand won't do because they clot when such fluids go through them.

In the above and similar situations, a large vessel with a lot of blood flowing through it is needed. The large amount of blood in such a large vein can dilute the irritating medicine quickly. The solution is to place a catheter the size of skinny macaroni into a large vein that empties directly into the heart. This is called an *access catheter*.

You are in need of such a catheter so that your condition can be treated in a way that is more predictable and more comfortable for you. This is done by a surgeon in the operating room and usually is an outpatient procedure.

METHODS

There are two main methods of placing such an access catheter:

- **Hickman:** In this method, the end of the catheter is placed in a big vein in the neck and advanced down to the heart. It then is "tunneled" under the skin, and the other end is brought out through the skin, 4 to 6 inches below the clavicle (collarbone). Medicine can be given through it, fluids connected to it, or blood drawn through it (Fig. 1).

  The advantages to this method are as follows:
- The tube comes straight to the outside and it's easy to connect fluids to it.
- When the tube is no longer needed, the stitch that holds it in place is cut and the tube pulled out.

  The disadvantages to this method are as follows:
- The bandages that cover the place where the catheter comes out through the skin need to be changed very carefully so that the area around the incision and the catheter itself do not become infected.
- The tube that dangles may interfere with some activities (e.g., swimming) or in the wearing of some clothing.
- **Port-A-Cath:** In this method, the tip of the catheter is in the big vein in the neck and goes to just inside the heart; the other end is under the skin just below the clavicle. The end under the skin has a special gadget attached to it that is the size of three stacked silver dollars and hollow (a *chamber*). The special rubber wall on one side of the chamber is placed so that the rubber wall faces the skin.

When medicine, fluids, or nourishment needs to be given, or blood drawn, an anesthetic ointment is placed on the skin over the gadget to make the skin numb. A needle is placed through the numb skin, then through the rubber wall to reach the chamber that is connected to the tube in the large vein. When it is not needed for a while, some blood thinner (heparin) is placed in the chamber and the needle is pulled out. The port-A-Cath remains in place, ready to be used again later.

The advantages to this method are as follows:

- There is nothing hanging from the body, and no maintenance is necessary.
- The catheter site is less likely to become infected.

The disadvantages are as follows:

- A nurse or technician is needed to connect fluids to the port-A-Cath.

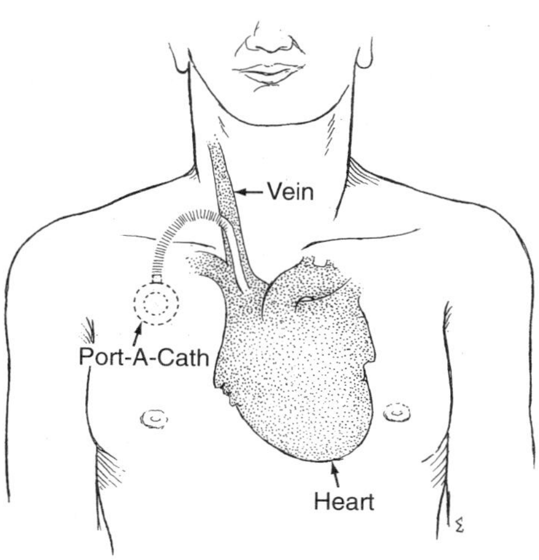

Figure 1. The plain end of a port-A-Cath is inserted into a large vein either in the neck or into a vein just below the clavicle (collarbone) near the shoulder. The other end, containing the gadget through which the medicine is injected, is positioned several inches lower. Whether all this is done through one or two incisions depends on which vein is used. When the operation is completed, the entire port-A-Cath is under the skin.

- When the port-A-Cath is not being used, it has to be flushed with a blood thinner solution every week or so to prevent clotting of the catheter.

After careful consideration of all factors, the recommendation is that you have a port-A-Cath.

PREOPERATIVE PREPARATION

- Do not eat or drink anything for 8 hours before the operation.
- Shower or bathe on the morning of the operation.
- You may be given medicine that will make you feel drowsy before you are brought to the operating room.

□ OPERATION

- Medical reasons will determine the type of anesthesia you will have. Generally, however, the operation is done under local anesthesia along with medicine to keep you drowsy during the operation.
- The area in front of one side of your neck will be swabbed with an antiseptic solution and surrounded with sterile drapes.
- An area just below the collarbone and in the lower neck will be made numb.
- One incision will be just above the inner side of the clavicle and another in an area 4 to 6 inches below this.
- During the operation, you may feel some tugging but not pain.
- X-rays will be used to check that the catheter is in the correct area.
- The operation generally takes 1 hour.

POSTOPERATIVE CARE

- You will be taken to a recovery room and observed. When your blood pressure, pulse, and breathing are stable and you are completely alert, you should be able to go home accompanied by a responsible adult.
- Pain will be controlled with medicine.
- Arrangements will be made for your medicine, office follow-up visit, and stitch removal.

✣ HOME CARE

- Resume your usual activities.
- You may walk about as you wish, even climb stairs.
- You may eat as you did before the operation.
- You may shower if you wish, but do not get the dressings or the wound wet before the stitches are removed. Covering the area with a sheet of plastic and sealing the edges usually is satisfactory.
- You will be given instructions on how to take care of your incisions.
- You probably will be able to feel the catheter under your skin, especially in the area of the clavicle.
- You may return to work when you feel up to it.
- You may drive if you wish but not if you are taking medicines that reduce your alertness.

✆ CALL OUR OFFICE IF

- The incisions become red or swollen or there is any drainage from them.
- You develop a temperature higher than 100°F.
- You have any questions.

△ GENERAL INFORMATION

Achalasia is a nerve condition of the *esophagus*, the tube through which the food you eat is pushed, as well as drops, down into the stomach.

- There are at least two problems present: The esophagus doesn't help push along the food you swallow, and when the food reaches the end of the esophagus the *sphincter* (a valve) there does not relax properly to let the food enter the stomach.
- This condition occurs in women and men of any age but mostly in those 30 to 50 years of age.
- Cancer of the esophagus is several times more common in a person with achalasia than in one without this condition.

COMMON SIGNS AND SYMPTOMS

The most frequent problem is an increasing difficulty with swallowing.

- At first, this difficulty comes and goes, but later it is present at all times.
- Cold foods are more difficult to swallow than warm foods.
- Early on, solid foods seem to go down more easily than do liquids.
- The food tends to come up, especially at night when a person is lying flat during sleep (because the food has not moved out of the esophagus). Lung infections can occur because small amounts of this fluid in the esophagus can trickle up into the throat and then go down into the *trachea* (windpipe).

DIAGNOSIS

- Anyone with the above history or symptoms should be concerned about achalasia.
- **Esophagogram:** You will be given liquid barium (it looks and flows like buttermilk) to swallow, and x-rays will be taken as it goes down the esophagus. The x-rays may show the following:
  - The esophagus may be of normal size. At a later stage, it can be enlarged—sometimes in a dramatic way.
  - At its bottom end, the esophagus narrows, and very little is seen to go into the stomach.

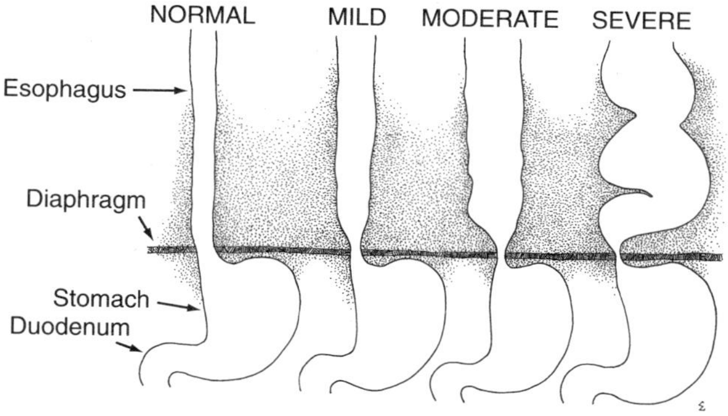

Figure 1.

  - The esophagus may be seen to work but in fits and spurts, and it does not work in a smooth way to push the food along (Fig. 1).
- **Esophagoscopy:** This is done with an optical instrument with a light at its tip that is smooth, flexible, and as big around as the tip of your little finger. Your mouth and throat will be sprayed with an anesthetic to make them numb, and you will be given medicine to make you feel drowsy. The instrument then will be placed gently down your esophagus so that it can be examined thoroughly. This is to be certain not to miss some other cause for your swallowing difficulty. The instrument will then be passed into your stomach as well as into the duodenum, which is just past the stomach, and both of these areas will also be examined carefully.
- **Manometry:** This is done with a thin tube that has pressure sensors built in it. The tiny tube is swallowed so that the sensor can be placed along the entire length of your esophagus. The sensors will record how well your esophagus muscle squeezes down or relaxes.

○ TREATMENT

- Diets and medicines are not helpful for this condition. The aim of treatment is to cut the muscle fibers that surround and squeeze down on the lower part of the esophagus to allow food to pass freely by gravity from the esophagus into the stomach.

  The treatment options are as follows:

Open Chest: The chest is opened through an incision and the esophagus worked on directly with the hands.

Thoracoscopy: It is done with a long instrument called a *thoracoscope*. It is as big around as the tip of your little finger, has lenses and a light, and has the ability to cut tissue. The instrument is placed in your chest through a tiny incision.

Through the Abdomen: This method is used when both the lower esophagus and the upper stomach need some repair and it cannot be done through the chest.

Balloon Dilation: This is done with a long, thin tube that has a deflated balloon at its end. The tube with the deflated balloon is passed down the esophagus so that the balloon sits inside the narrow area. The balloon is then inflated to stretch the narrow area. There is some benefit from this technique, but it doesn't last too long.

After careful consideration of all factors, the recommendation is that you have an operation through the abdomen to correct your problem.

PREOPERATIVE PREPARATION

- In addition to the tests already mentioned, you will have an examination of your blood, urine, heart (EKG), and lungs (chest x-ray).
- You may be given medicine that will make you feel drowsy before you are brought to the operating room.

☐ OPERATION

- You will be asleep for the operation.
- The operation usually takes 2 to 3 hours.

POSTOPERATIVE CARE

- You will be taken to a recovery room and observed. When your blood pressure, pulse, and breathing are stable, you will be taken to a regular hospital room.
- You will have a thin plastic tube in your nose for a few days.
- That evening you will be helped to sit up in bed and on the next day to get out of bed.
- Pain will be controlled with medicine.
- After the tube in your nose is removed, you will be started on a carefully outlined diet and instructed on how to manage your diet when you go home.
- You should be able to go home in 3 to 6 days.
- As with any operation, complications are always possible. With this operation, they can include injury to the esophagus or spleen, bleeding, infection, peritonitis, and possibly others.
- Arrangements will be made for your medicine, follow-up office visit, and stitch removal.

✚ HOME CARE

- You may walk about as you wish, even climb stairs, but don't overdo things.
- Follow the diet outlined for you while you were in the hospital.
- Unless instructed otherwise, you may shower as you wish and with any dressings on or off. After you dry yourself, replace any dressings with clean, dry ones.
- Do not drive until we talk about it during your follow-up office visit.
- You may return to work when you feel up to it.

✆ CALL OUR OFFICE IF

- Your food sticks or won't go down, or if you vomit the food.
- The incision becomes red or swollen or there is drainage from it.
- You develop a temperature higher than 100°F.
- You have any questions.

ACHALASIA: Balloon Dilation

△ GENERAL INFORMATION

Achalasia is a nerve condition of the *esophagus*, the tube through which the food you eat is pushed down into the stomach.

- There are at least two problems present: The esophagus doesn't help push along the food you swallow, and when the food reaches the end of the esophagus the *sphincter* (a valve) there does not relax properly to let the food enter the stomach.
- This condition occurs in women and men of any age but mostly in those 30 to 50 years of age.
- Cancer of the esophagus is several times more common in a person with achalasia than in one without this condition.

COMMON SIGNS AND SYMPTOMS

The most frequent problem is an increasing difficulty with swallowing.

- At first, this difficulty comes and goes, but later it is present at all times.
- Cold foods are more difficult to swallow than warm foods.
- Early on, solid foods seem to go down more easily than do liquids.
- The food tends to come up, especially at night when a person is lying flat during sleep (because the food has not moved out of the esophagus). Lung infections can occur because small amounts of this fluid in the esophagus can trickle up into the throat and then go down into the *trachea* (windpipe).

DIAGNOSIS

- Anyone with the above history or symptoms should be concerned about achalasia.
- **Esophagogram:** You will be given liquid barium (it looks and flows like buttermilk) to swallow, and x-rays will be taken as it goes down the esophagus. The x-rays may show the following:
  - The esophagus may be of normal size. At a later stage, it can be enlarged—sometimes in a dramatic way.
  - At its bottom end, the esophagus narrows, and very little is seen to go into the stomach.
  - The esophagus may be seen to work but in fits and spurts, and it does not work in a smooth way to push the food along (Fig. 1).
- **Esophagoscopy:** This is done with an optical instrument with a light at its tip that is smooth, flexible, and as big around as the tip of your little finger. Your mouth and throat will be sprayed with an anesthetic to make them numb, and you will be given medicine to make you feel drowsy. The instrument then will be placed gently down your esophagus so that it can be examined thoroughly. This is to be certain not to miss some other cause for your swallowing difficulty. The instrument will then be passed into your stomach as well as into the duodenum, which is just past the stomach, and both these areas will be examined carefully.
- **Manometry:** This is done with a thin tube that has pressure sensors built in it. The tiny tube is swallowed so that the sensors can be placed along the entire length of your esophagus. The sensors will record how well your esophagus muscle squeezes down or relaxes.

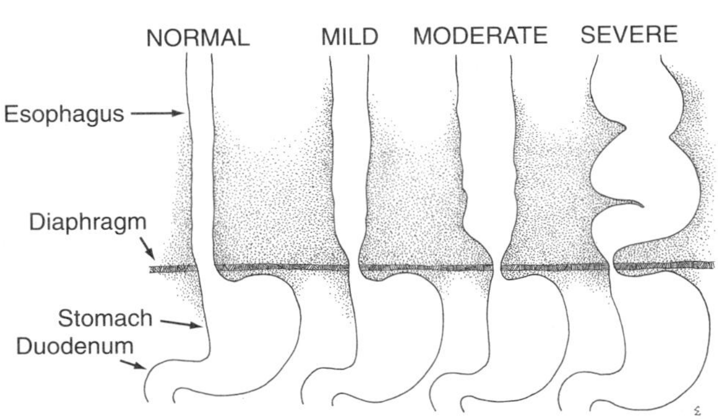

Figure 1.

○ TREATMENT

- Diets and medicines are not helpful for this condition. The aim of treatment is to cut the muscle fibers that surround and squeeze down on the lower part of the esophagus to allow food to pass freely by gravity from the esophagus into the stomach.

  The treatment options are as follows:

Open Chest: The chest is opened and the esophagus worked on directly with the hands.

Thoracoscopy: It is done with a long instrument called a *thoracoscope*. It is as big around as the tip of your little finger, has lenses and a light, and has the ability to cut tissue. The instrument is placed in your chest through a tiny incision.

Through the Abdomen: This method is used when both the lower esophagus and the upper stomach need some repair and it cannot be done through the chest.

Balloon Dilation: This is done with a long, thin tube that has a deflated balloon at its end. The tube with the deflated balloon is passed down the esophagus so that the balloon sits inside the narrow area. The balloon is then inflated to stretch the narrow area. There is some benefit from this technique, but it doesn't last too long.

After careful consideration of all factors, the recommendation is that your achalasia be treated with balloon stretching.

PREOPERATIVE PREPARATION

- In addition to the tests already mentioned, you will have an examination of your blood, urine, heart (EKG), and lungs (chest x-ray).

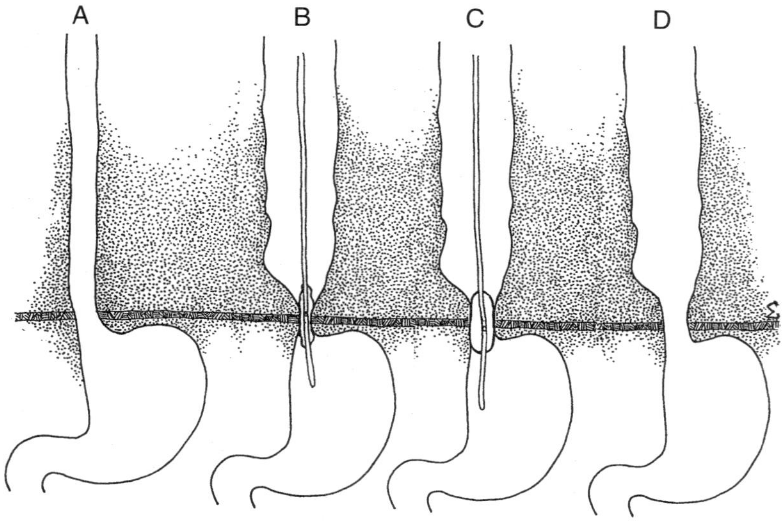

Figure 2. *A*, Normal esophagus. *B*, Esophagus with moderate achalasia and deflated balloon in narrowed area. *C*, Balloon distended. *D*, Appearance of esophagus following dilation.

□ OPERATION

- During the procedure you will be given medicine to keep you drowsy.
- The procedure usually takes about 1 hour.

POSTOPERATIVE CARE

- You will be taken to a recovery room and observed for any unusual development. Commonly, a patient is able to go home the same day or the following day.
- You will be given a carefully outlined diet and instructed on how to manage it when you go home.
- As with any operation, complications are always possible. With this operation, they can include injury to the esophagus, bleeding, infection, and possibly others.
- Arrangements will be made for your medicine and follow-up office visit.

✙ HOME CARE

- You may walk about as you wish, even climb stairs, but don't overdo things.
- Follow the program and diet outlined for you.
- You may return to work when you feel up to it.

✆ CALL OUR OFFICE IF

- You feel faint, vomit blood, have pain in your chest, or pass stool that is very dark.
- Your food sticks or won't go down, or you vomit the food.
- You develop any unusual signs or symptoms.
- The incision becomes red or swollen or there is drainage from it.
- You develop a temperature higher than 100°F.
- You have any questions.

△ GENERAL INFORMATION

Achalasia is a nerve condition of the *esophagus*, the tube through which the food you eat is pushed down into the stomach.

- There are at least two problems present: The esophagus doesn't help push along the food you swallow, and when the food reaches the end of the esophagus the *sphincter* (a valve) there does not relax properly to let the food enter the stomach.
- This condition occurs in women and men of any age but mostly in those 30 to 50 years of age.
- Cancer of the esophagus is several times more common in a person with achalasia than in one without this condition.

COMMON SIGNS AND SYMPTOMS

The most frequent problem is an increasing difficulty with swallowing.

- At first, this difficulty comes and goes, but later it is present at all times.
- Cold foods are more difficult to swallow than warm foods.
- Early on, solid foods seem to go down more easily than do liquids.
- The food tends to come up, especially at night when a person is lying flat during sleep (because the food has not moved out of the esophagus). Lung infections can occur because small amounts of this fluid in the esophagus can trickle up into the throat and then go down into the *trachea* (windpipe).

DIAGNOSIS

- Anyone with the above history or symptoms should be concerned about achalasia.
- **Esophagogram:** You will be given liquid barium (it looks and flows like buttermilk) to swallow, and x-rays will be taken as it goes down the esophagus. The x-rays may show the following:
  - The esophagus may be of normal size. At a later stage, it can be enlarged—sometimes in a very dramatic way.
  - At its bottom end, the esophagus narrows, and very little is seen to go into the stomach.
  - The esophagus may be seen to work but in fits and spurts, and it does not work in a smooth way to push the food along (Fig. 1).

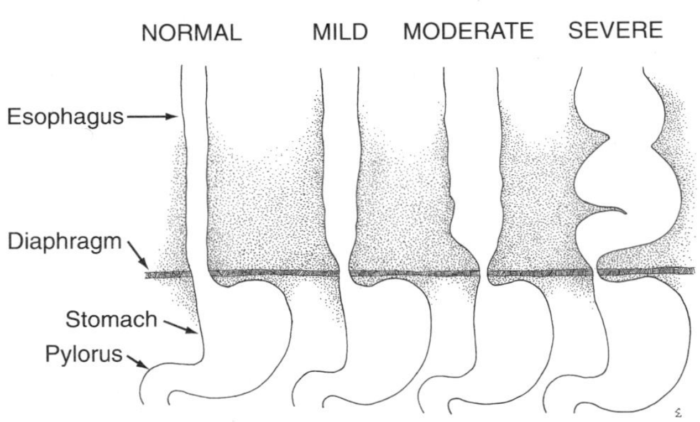

Figure 1.

- **Esophagoscopy:** This is done with an optical instrument with a light at its tip that is smooth, flexible, and as big around as the tip of your little finger. Your mouth and throat will be sprayed with an anesthetic to make them numb, and you will be given medicine to make you feel drowsy. The instrument then will be placed gently down your esophagus so that it can be examined thoroughly. This is to be certain not to miss some other cause for your swallowing difficulty. The instrument will then be passed into your stomach as well as into the duodenum, which is just past the stomach, and both of these areas will be examined carefully.
- **Manometry:** This is done with a thin tube that has pressure sensors built in it. The tiny tube is swallowed so that the sensors can be placed along the entire length of your esophagus. The sensors will record how well your esophagus muscle squeezes down or relaxes.

○ TREATMENT

- Diets and medicines are not helpful for this condition. The aim of treatment is to cut the muscle fibers that surround and squeeze down on the lower part of the esophagus to allow food to pass freely by gravity from the esophagus into the stomach.

The treatment options are as follows:

Open Chest: The chest is opened through an incision and the esophagus worked on directly with the hands.

Thoracoscopy: It is done with a long instrument called a *thoracoscope*. It is as big around as the tip of your little finger, has lenses and a light, and has the ability to cut tissue. The instrument is placed in your chest through a tiny incision.

Through the Abdomen: This method is used when both the lower esophagus and the upper stomach need some repair and it cannot be done through the chest.

Balloon Dilation: This is done with a long, thin tube that has a deflated balloon at its end. The tube with the deflated balloon is passed down the esophagus so that the balloon sits inside the narrow area. The balloon is then inflated to stretch the narrow area. There is some benefit from this technique, but it doesn't last too long.

After careful consideration of all factors, the recommendation is that your achalasia be treated through an incision in your chest.

PREOPERATIVE PREPARATION

- In addition to the tests already mentioned, you will have an examination of your blood, urine, heart (EKG), and lungs (chest x-ray).

- Shower (and shave) as usual on the morning of the operation.
- You will be given medicine that will make you feel drowsy before you are brought to the operating room.

☐ OPERATION

- You will be asleep for the operation.
- The operation usually takes 2 to 3 hours.

POSTOPERATIVE CARE

- You will be taken to the Surgical Care Unit, where the doctors and nurses are very experienced in taking care of patients like yourself. As soon as you are coming along well enough, you will be transferred to a regular hospital room.
- There will be a plastic tube coming out of your chest for a few days.
- You will have a thin plastic tube in your nose for a few days.
- That evening you will be helped to sit up in bed and on the next day to get out of bed.
- Pain will be controlled with medicine.
- You may be given an incentive spirometer. Breathing into this as you are instructed will help expand your lungs and reduce the risk of developing pneumonia.
- After the tube in your nose is removed, you will be started on a carefully outlined diet and instructed on how to manage your diet when you go home.
- You should be able to go home in several days.
- As with any operation, complications are always possible. With this operation, they can include injury to the esophagus or lung, bleeding, infection, and possibly others.
- Arrangements will be made for your medicine, follow-up office visit, and stitch removal.

✚ HOME CARE

- You may walk about as you wish, even climb stairs, but don't overdo things.
- Follow the program and diet outlined for you while you were in the hospital.
- Unless instructed otherwise, you may shower as you wish and with any dressings on or off. After you dry yourself, replace any dressings with clean, dry ones.
- Do not drive until we talk about it during your follow-up office visit.
- You may return to work when you feel up to it.

✆ CALL OUR OFFICE IF

- Your food sticks or won't go down, or if you vomit the food.
- The incision becomes red or swollen or there is drainage from it.
- You develop a temperature higher than 100°F.
- You have any questions.

ACHALASIA: Thoracoscopic Repair

△ GENERAL INFORMATION

Achalasia is a nerve condition of the *esophagus*, the tube through which the food you eat is pushed down into the stomach.

- There are at least two problems present: The esophagus doesn't help push along the food you swallow, and when the food reaches the end of the esophagus the *sphincter* (a valve) there does not relax properly to let the food enter the stomach.
- This condition occurs in women and men of any age but mostly in those 30 to 50 years of age.
- Cancer of the esophagus is several times more common in a person with achalasia than in one without this condition.

COMMON SIGNS AND SYMPTOMS

The most frequent problem is an increasing difficulty with swallowing.

- At first, this difficulty comes and goes, but later it is present at all times.
- Cold foods are more difficult to swallow than warm foods.
- Early on, solid foods seem to go down more easily than do liquids.
- The food tends to come up, especially at night when a person is lying flat during sleep (because the food has not moved out of the esophagus). Lung infections can occur because small amounts of this fluid in the esophagus can trickle up into the throat and then go down into the *trachea* (windpipe).

DIAGNOSIS

- Anyone with the above history or symptoms should be concerned about achalasia.
- **Esophagogram:** You will be given liquid barium (it looks and flows like buttermilk) to swallow, and x-rays will be taken as it goes down the esophagus. The x-rays may show the following:
  - The esophagus may be of normal size. At a later stage, it can be enlarged—sometimes in a dramatic way.
  - At its bottom end, the esophagus narrows, and very little is seen to go into the stomach.

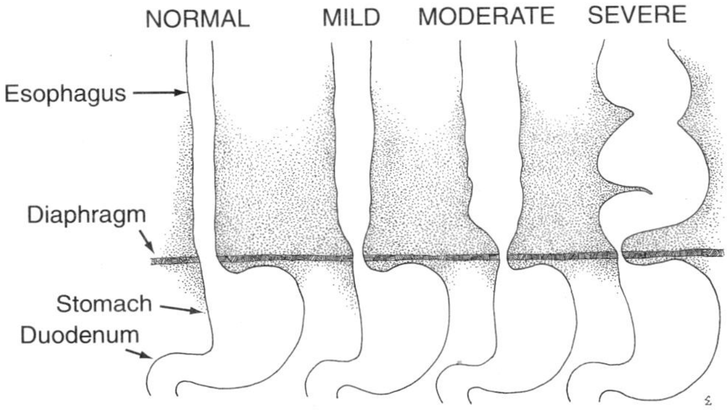

Figure 1.

  - The esophagus may be seen to work but in fits and spurts, and it does not work in a smooth way to push the food along (Fig. 1).
- **Esophagoscopy:** This is done with an optical instrument with a light at its tip that is smooth, flexible, and as big around as the tip of your little finger. Your mouth and throat will be sprayed with an anesthetic to make them numb, and you will be given medicine to make you feel drowsy. The instrument then will be placed gently down your esophagus so that it can be examined thoroughly. This is to be certain not to miss some other cause for your swallowing difficulty. The instrument will then be passed into your stomach as well as into the duodenum, which is just past the stomach, and both of these areas examined carefully.
- **Manometry:** This is done with a thin tube that has pressure sensors built in it. The tiny tube is swallowed so that the sensors can be placed along the entire length of your esophagus. The sensors can record how well your esophagus muscle squeezes down or relaxes.

○ TREATMENT

- Diets and medicines are not helpful for this condition. The aim of treatment is to cut the muscle fibers that surround and squeeze down on the lower part of the esophagus to allow food to pass freely by gravity from the esophagus into the stomach.

The treatment options are as follows:

Open Chest: The chest is opened and the esophagus worked on directly.

Thoracoscopy: It is done with a long instrument called a *thoracoscope*. It is as big around as the tip of your little finger, has lenses and a light, and has the ability to cut tissue. The instrument is placed in your chest through a tiny incision.

Through the Abdomen: This method is used when both the lower esophagus and the upper stomach need some repair and it cannot be done through the chest.

Balloon Dilation: This is done with a long, thin tube that has a deflated balloon at its end. The tube with the deflated balloon is passed down the esophagus so that the balloon sits inside the narrow area. The balloon is then inflated to stretch the narrow area. There is some benefit from this technique, but it doesn't last too long.

After careful consideration of all factors, the recommendation is that your achalasia be treated with the use of a thoracoscope. Once in a while, when the thoracoscope is placed inside the chest and everything is examined, the conditions are such that the operation cannot be done with a thoracoscope. If that happens in your case, an incision will have to be made in your chest.

PREOPERATIVE PREPARATION

- In addition to the tests already mentioned, you will have an examination of your blood, urine, heart (EKG), and lungs (chest x-ray).

☐ OPERATION

- You will be asleep for the operation.
- The operation usually takes 2 to 3 hours.

POSTOPERATIVE CARE

- You will be taken to a recovery room and observed. When your blood pressure, pulse, and breathing are stable, you will be taken to a regular hospital room.
- You will have a thin plastic tube in your nose for several days.
- That evening you will be helped to sit up in bed and on the next day to get out of bed.
- Pain will be controlled with medicine.
- After the tube in your nose is removed, you will be started on a carefully outlined diet and instructed on how to manage your diet when you go home.
- You should be able to go home in 2 or 3 days.
- As with any operation, complications are always possible. With this operation, they can include injury to the esophagus or lung, bleeding, infection, and possibly others.
- Arrangements will be made for your medicine, follow-up office visit, and stitch removal.

✚ HOME CARE

- You may walk about as you wish, even climb stairs, but don't overdo things.
- Follow the program and diet outlined for you while you were in the hospital.
- You may shower as you wish and with any dressings on or off. After you dry yourself, replace any dressings with clean, dry ones.
- You may return to work when you feel up to it.

✆ CALL OUR OFFICE IF

- Your food sticks or won't go down, or if you vomit the food.
- The incision becomes red or swollen or there is drainage from it.
- You develop a temperature higher than 100°F.
- You have any questions.

△ GENERAL INFORMATION

Fibrous adhesions are normal in tissue that has been disturbed. They can be troublesome in the abdominal cavity, especially when they affect the small intestine. Adhesions usually are strands of scar tissue. They can be thin and stringy or thick like rubberbands, long or short, a few or in the hundreds, and in one area or all over the abdomen. A good description of the appearance of adhesions is to imagine a gob of sticky chewing gum that you slowly stretch into many strands as you pull it apart (Fig. 1).

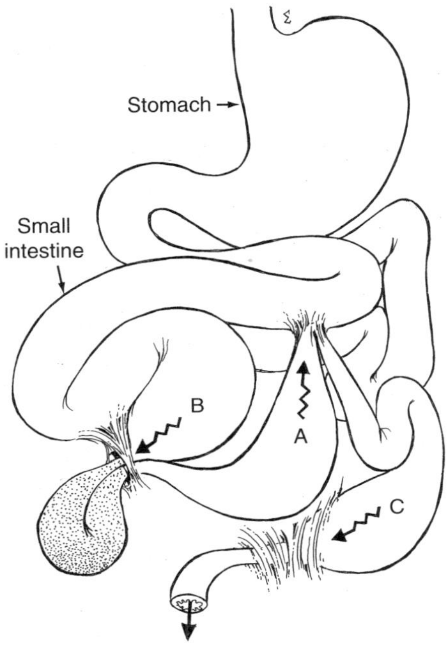

Figure 1. *A*, A portion of intestine is stuck to another area and becomes kinked. *B*, A loop of intestine has slipped through an opening between adhesions, is stuck, and becomes blocked. It can also become twisted (and possibly gangrenous), requiring an emergency operation. *C*, Multiple adhesions lay across a length of bowel and block it.

CAUSE

- Of the many causes, the most common is dissection from a previous operation. Other causes can be repeated or severe infections in the abdomen that cause peritonitis.
- Most of the adhesions following an operation are dissolved by the body in a few weeks. Usually, those that remain do not cause any trouble. Some, however, can cause problems because small bowel (as big around as a jumbo hot dog) can get partly or completely blocked or twisted.

COMMON SIGNS AND SYMPTOMS

- These depend on how serious the blockage or twisting is at any particular time.
- If the blockage is minimal and in one spot only, there may be an occasional cramp or bloating as the food tries to pass through the narrowed area.
- If the blockage is more severe, the cramping occurs more frequently, is worse, and lasts longer. The backed-up bowel distends the abdomen. Vomiting is common.
- If the blockage is complete, then all the above signs and symptoms are more severe.
- If the intestine becomes trapped and twisted among the adhesions, it can develop gangrene and die. This is a very serious matter requiring an emergency operation.

DIAGNOSIS

- A careful taking of the history of your past medical or surgical problems and of your symptoms, along with an examination of your abdomen, can often determine the cause of the problem.
- X-rays of the abdomen can show whether the bowel is blocked and how seriously it is blocked. They are useful in deciding whether to operate.
- Laboratory tests and your blood pressure and pulse measurements, along with the physical examination, will help determine whether your blocked intestine is at risk of dying.

○ TREATMENT

- A tube passed through your nose and down into the stomach will let the swallowed air come back out through the tube, because you will feel worse if it is allowed to go past your stomach and down to the blocked area.
- You will be given fluids by vein to make up for what you have vomited or not been able to eat or drink.
- Antibiotics will be given to help treat or ward off infection.

An operation is advisable and actually safer if

- Your signs and symptoms, although not serious now, continue without letup for longer than 36 hours.
- Your signs and symptoms, the laboratory findings, and how you feel are obviously getting worse, and something more serious will happen if the problem is not corrected promptly.

This is evidence that you have gangrene of the intestine (an immediate operation is necessary).

PREOPERATIVE PREPARATION

- Your condition will be improved as much as possible, with special attention given to your heart, lungs, and kidneys.
- Intravenous fluids will be given to meet the needs of your body.
- You will be given some medicine that will make you feel drowsy before you are brought into the operating room.

□ OPERATION

- You will be completely asleep during the operation.
- The exact type of operation will depend on the

particular way the adhesions caused the blockage and how much needs to be done to correct it.
  - Sometimes just cutting an adhesion or two is all that is necessary.
  - Often, a large number of adhesions may need to be cut.
  - Occasionally, a length of intestine may need to be removed. The cut ends will be reconnected.
- You will not receive a blood transfusion unless it is absolutely necessary.

POSTOPERATIVE CARE

- You will wake up in a recovery room, and when your blood pressure, pulse, and breathing are stable you will be transferred to a regular hospital room.
- You will have a thin plastic tube in your nose. It goes down to your stomach to suck up the air you swallow. It will be removed when your bowels start working.
- Pain will be controlled with medicine.
- You will have a catheter in your bladder to make it easier for you to urinate and for the nurses to measure how much urine you make.
- You will be given fluids by vein until you can start drinking and eating.
- As with any operation, complications are always possible, some of them serious. With this operation, they can include bleeding, peritonitis, blood clots, wound infection, repeat obstruction, heart problems, and possibly others.
- You will be discharged from the hospital when you can safely eat again.
- Arrangements will be made for your medicines, follow-up office visit, and stitch removal.

✚ HOME CARE

- You may walk about as you wish, even climb stairs.
- Follow any diet instructions given to you.
- You may shower if you wish and with any dressings on or off.
  - There may be narrow strips of tape across the incision. It's all right if they get wet. They will be removed in the doctor's office.
  - After you dry yourself, replace any dressings with clean, dry ones.
- Your incision and the muscles of the abdomen may ache, especially at the end of the day and after you have been standing for a long period. You can support them by wearing a girdle or similar garment that is snug (but not too tight). Wearing it over a cotton undergarment is easier on your incision and the stitches.
- Don't lift anything heavier than 5 pounds. Ask someone to do it for you. Inactivity is not good for you but neither is overdoing it. Don't try to do too much too soon.
- Driving a car with an automatic shift is not too demanding. But if you suddenly have to slam on the brakes or twist to turn a wheel, you may strain the sutures or tear something. During your follow-up visit, let's discuss when you can resume driving.
- You may resume sexual activity whenever you choose.
- You may return to work when you feel up to it, but let's first talk about it during your follow-up visit.

✆ CALL OUR OFFICE IF

- Any of your original symptoms come back or new ones appear.
- You develop constipation or your bowels otherwise don't move for 36 hours.
- The incision becomes red or swollen or there is drainage from it.
- You develop a temperature higher than 100°F.
- You have any questions.

△ GENERAL INFORMATION

The two adrenal glands regulate minerals and hormones in your body. Each gland is about 1½ inches long and wide and ½ inch thick, and one sits on top of either kidney (Fig. 1). The cause of adrenal tumors is not known.

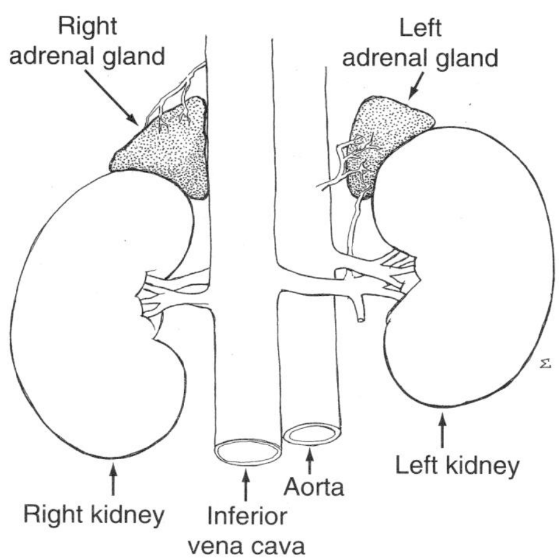

Figure 1.

COMMON SIGNS AND SYMPTOMS

Because the adrenal glands have a number of different functions, the symptoms the tumors produce depend a lot on which of these functions is disturbed. The types of tumors are as follows:

- **Adenoma:** These often do not produce any symptoms.
- **Aldosteronoma:** These are not cancerous but can cause high blood pressure and serious changes in the chemicals in your body.
- **Pheochromocytoma:** These mostly are benign tumors that are dangerous because they can produce very severe blood pressure problems as follows: a constant high blood pressure; a sudden attack of very high blood pressure that may last for just a few minutes or for several hours; "pounding" headache; sweating; fast pulse; severe nervousness; trembling; nausea; weakness, even death; or stroke.
- **Cancer:** The adrenal mass can be cancerous.

DIAGNOSIS

- A detailed history will be taken, and a thorough physical examination will be done.

You will have some, and possibly all, of the following tests:

- Measurements of hormones and chemicals in your blood and urine to determine the exact nature of the mass.
- CT scan (computed tomography scan): These special x-rays are taken by a machine that is shaped like a huge doughnut. You will lie on a table inside the hole in the "doughnut." The x-rays are taken as very thin slices through the upper abdomen. This makes it possible to see the size and shape of the adrenal glands and surrounding tissues.
- MRI (magnetic resonance imaging): No x-rays are used with this technique. Instead, it is done with harmless magnetic fields and radio waves. A computer develops the pictures to show organs from several angles.
- Adrenal scintigraphy: This is a special way to locate masses in the adrenal glands.

○ TREATMENT

Some conditions of the adrenal glands can be treated with medicine, and others require an operation. An operation can be the main treatment for the following:

- **Adenoma:** Many adenomas do not cause any problems and are not dangerous. They can be observed carefully as long as they remain smaller than a walnut and show no signs of being cancerous.
- **Aldosteronoma:** The symptoms can be cured by removing the tumor.
- **Pheochromocytoma:** Removal by an operation is the only treatment. If these tumors are not removed, practically all patients die from the complications caused by heart and blood pressure problems.
- **Cancer:** The best chance for cure is to remove the tumor completely by performing an operation.

PREOPERATIVE PREPARATION

- Any associated problems will be corrected as much as possible before the operation.
- Do not eat or drink anything for 8 hours before your operation.
- If you are taking medicine to control blood pressure, be certain the doctors know about this.
- You may be given medicine that will make you feel drowsy before you are brought into the operating room.

□ OPERATION

- You will be asleep during this operation.
- A number of wires will be taped to your skin so that your heart rate and other functions can be followed during the operation.
- The adrenal gland can be removed through an incision on the abdomen, the flank, or the back. The type of incision is determined by the size and type of tumor that is to be removed, the build and condition of the patient, and the surgeon's preference. This will be discussed with you before the operation.
- Some adrenal glands can be removed with laparoscopy. The operation is done with instruments about as big around as your little finger. They are placed in the abdomen through small puncture holes.
- It may be absolutely necessary that you receive blood transfusions.
- The operation generally takes about 3 hours.

POSTOPERATIVE CARE

- You will be taken to the Surgical Care Unit, where the doctors and nurses are very experienced in taking care of patients like yourself. When you are doing well enough, you will be transferred to a regular hospital room.
- That evening you will be able to get out of bed with assistance.
- Pain will be controlled with medicine.
- Your diet will be as you tolerate it.
- Your length of stay in the hospital will depend on where the incision was made and what type of tumor was removed.
- As with any operation, complications are always possible. Although they are uncommon with this type of operation, they can include bleeding, infection, lung problems, or continued blood pressure problems.
- Arrangements will be made for your pain medicine, office visit, and stitch or clip removal.

✣ HOME CARE

- You may walk about as you wish, even climb stairs, but don't overdo it; take frequent rests.
- You may eat as you wish.
- Take medicine as prescribed for your pain.
- You may shower if you wish, with any dressings on or off. There may be narrow strips of tape across the incision. It's all right if they get wet; they will be removed in the doctor's office. After you dry yourself, replace any dressings with clean, dry ones.
- Do not drive if you cannot move freely or are taking medicines that decrease your alertness.
- You may resume sexual activity whenever you choose.
- You may return to work when you feel up to it.

✆ CALL OUR OFFICE IF

- You suddenly feel weak or lightheaded.
- You have new or unusual symptoms.
- The incision becomes red or swollen, or there is drainage from it.
- You develop a temperature higher than 101°F.
- You have any questions.

△ GENERAL INFORMATION

When part of the stomach needs to be removed for whatever reason, there are several parts to the operation.

Figure 1*A* shows the stomach, which empties into the duodenum. The bile and the pancreas ducts also empty into the duodenum. The duodenum enters the jejunum (the upper part of the small intestine). The stippled area shows the part of the stomach that is commonly removed.

The problem, shown in Figure 1*B*, is that sometimes the jejunum swells or kinks at the point where food leaves the stomach to empty into it *(asterisk)*. Because of this swelling or kinking, the bile and pancreas juices (about 1 quart per day) can enter the stomach but a lot of this liquid can't leave it. The same happens with fluid made by the stomach itself and with food and water that you might take by mouth.

Because the food and fluids in the stomach cannot go out, the stomach swells. The part of the intestine coming from the bile duct and pancreas duct to the stomach (called the *afferent* loop) also swells.

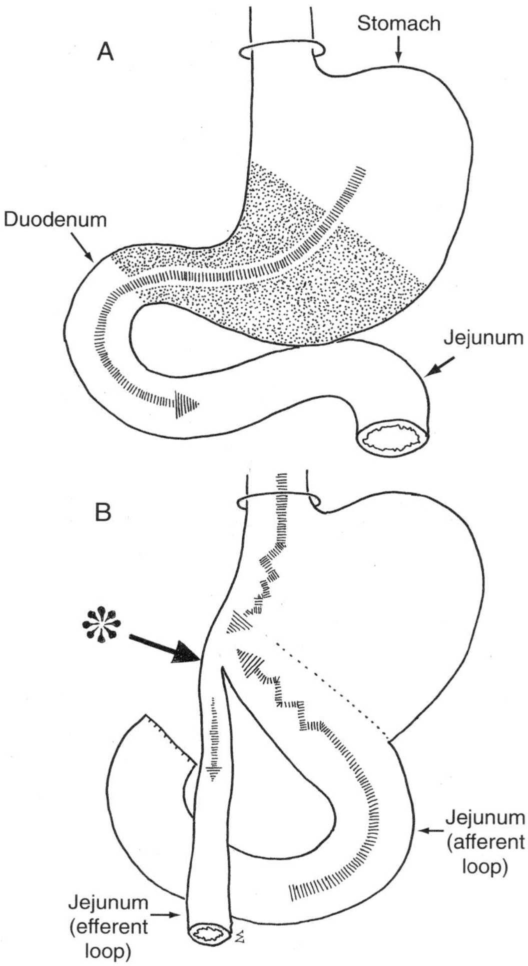

Figure 1. When part of the stomach is removed *(stippled area)*, the remaining stomach is reconnected to the small intestine as shown *(A* and *B)*.

COMMON SIGNS AND SYMPTOMS

- If there is only partial blockage, the symptoms may be some burping (as mouthfuls of bile juice), usually an hour or so after eating.
- Later, there is a feeling of fullness in the stomach and maybe some pain in the upper part of the abdomen, which is followed by vomiting.
- The stools become bulky and gray, because there is no bile or pancreas juice in them.
- Even later, the liver and pancreas become affected.

DIAGNOSIS

- Usually the diagnosis can be suggested by taking a careful history. It can be confirmed by several tests:
- Stomach x-rays: Barium is swallowed, and x-ray pictures are taken as it goes down the esophagus and into the stomach. With the afferent loop syndrome, the barium leaves the stomach very slowly and through a narrow opening.
- Gastroscopy: This is done with an optical instrument with a light at its tip that is smooth, flexible, and as big around as the tip of your little finger. Your throat will be sprayed with an anesthetic to make it numb. Also, you will be given some medicine to make you feel drowsy. The lubricated instrument will be placed gently down your esophagus and into your stomach, and the openings into the stomach (the *afferent* loop) and out of it (the *efferent* loop) will be examined.

○ TREATMENT

- Most problems with the *afferent loop syndrome* happen the first week after the operation to remove part of the stomach.
- Most of the time there actually is some opening, and eventually some liquid does manage to get through.
- Usually, the blockage is from swelling of the tissue in this area because it is cut and sewn during the operation. Fortunately, most of the time the swelling goes down in a few days or a week and then the opening lets food through as expected. Once in a while, however, the opening is just not big enough to let enough food and fluid go through for you to lead a normal life.
- After careful consideration of all factors, the opinion is that you have been in this situation too long, that you are losing ground, and that an operation is necessary to correct the problem before your condition gets even worse.

PREOPERATIVE PREPARATION

- Every effort will be made to get you in the best possible condition so that the operation can be done in the safest way and with the best chance for success. The choice of the operation that is likely to be used to correct the problem will be explained to you.

- You will have an examination of your blood, urine, heart (EKG), and lungs (chest x-ray).

☐ OPERATION

- You will be asleep for the operation.
- The operation usually takes about 2 to 3 hours.

POSTOPERATIVE CARE

- You will be taken to a recovery room and observed. When your blood pressure, pulse, and breathing are stable, you will be taken to a regular hospital room.
- You will have a thin plastic tube in your nose. It goes down to your stomach to suck up the air you swallow. It will be removed when your stomach again empties properly and your bowels start working.
- That evening you will be helped to sit up in bed and on the next day to get out of bed.
- Pain will be controlled with medicine.
- When your intestines start working and the tube in your nose is removed, you will be started on a liquid diet that will be increased to more solid food as you tolerate it.
- As with any operation, complications are always possible. With this type of operation, they can include bleeding, pneumonia, infection, and possibly others.
- Arrangements will be made for your medicines, follow-up office visit, and stitch or clip removal.

✚ HOME CARE

- Continue with the program started while you were in the hospital.
- You may walk about as you wish, even climb stairs, but don't overdo things.
- You will be given an appropriate diet to follow during your convalescence.
- You will be given instructions on bathing or taking a shower.
- Take the medicines as prescribed for you.
- Do not drive your car or return to work until we first talk about it during your follow-up office visit.
- You may resume sexual activity whenever you choose.

✆ CALL OUR OFFICE IF

- You vomit or develop any unusual signs or symptoms.
- The incision becomes red or swollen, or there is drainage from it.
- You develop a temperature higher than 100°F.
- You have any questions.

△ GENERAL INFORMATION

Amputation of the leg is done mostly because of poor circulation caused by narrowing of the arteries *(atherosclerosis)*, sometimes because of diabetes. This narrowing decreases blood flow to the tissues of the leg. Although medical treatments can help with the circulation problem, an amputation is eventually necessary for some individuals. There have been so many advances with prostheses in recent years that many people who have had an amputation can get back to a reasonably normal life.

COMMON SIGNS AND SYMPTOMS

- Early, there may be cramping of the leg muscles during long walks, but in time, this happens even with short walks.
- Later, there is cramping of the leg muscles at night, when the leg is at rest; it occurs more often, lasts longer, and is more severe.
- Finally, the pain may be almost constant.
- Gangrene of the toes or foot can be the final stage.

DIAGNOSIS

- Usually, the diagnosis can be made by taking a detailed history, doing a thorough physical examination, and considering the laboratory report.
- Several tests can be done to see how the blood flows to the tissue. Of course, if gangrene already is present, nothing can be done to bring life back to the tissue. If a person is seen before gangrene sets in, tests can be done to determine whether an amputation can be avoided.
- Ultrasound: Harmless sound waves are aimed at the blood vessels of the leg. The sound waves bouncing back (the echoes) from this area are seen as a picture on a screen. This is a convenient, painless, and harmless way to examine the blood vessels to see where they are seriously blocked.
- Arteriography: Dye is injected into the artery, and x-ray pictures are taken of it as it flows through the artery and its branches. This makes it possible to see accurately the location and seriousness of the blockage.

○ TREATMENT

If gangrene has not set in, medicines are used to try to keep the vessels open so that enough blood can flow through them. This is not possible in your case.

- The leg is too far gone to be saved.
- After careful consideration of your condition and the test results, an amputation of your leg above the knee is recommended. The reasons for this have been explained to you.

PREOPERATIVE PREPARATION

- You will have an examination of your blood, urine, heart (EKG), and lungs (chest x-ray). Particular attention will be given to your other arteries, especially those to your brain, heart, and lungs. Your aorta will also be evaluated carefully.
- Do not eat or drink anything for 8 hours before the operation.
- You will be given medicine that will make you feel drowsy before you are brought to the operating room.
- The aim of the operation is as follows:
  - To do the safest operation for your condition.
  - To amputate the shortest amount of leg yet have the tissue left behind be healthy.
  - To give you the best chance of being able to wear a prosthesis that will help you walk.
  - To do the operation in such a manner that the prosthesis can be fitted as soon as possible.

□ OPERATION

- You will be asleep for the operation, or you may be given a spinal type of anesthesia.
- You will not need a blood transfusion.
- The operation usually takes about 2 hours.
- You will wake up in a recovery room. When your blood pressure, pulse, and breathing are stable, you will be taken to a regular hospital room.
- There will be a snug bandage around the amputated leg.
- That evening you will be helped to sit up in bed and on the next day to get out of bed and into a chair.
- Pain can be controlled with medicine.
- Specialists in making and fitting you with a prosthesis and helping you learn how to walk on it will be working with you very closely and very early. The earlier you start using the prosthesis, the better.
- Thousands of people like you have had an amputation and are now up and about living a good life.
- You will leave the hospital when the healing is going well enough and you can take care of yourself with help.
- As with any operation, complications are possible. With your type of operation, they can include infection in the leg stump, poor wound healing, blood clots, and possibly others.
- Arrangements will be made for your medicine, follow-up office visit, and stitch removal.
- Arrangements can be made for a home visiting nurse if one is needed.

✚ HOME CARE

- Continue with the program started while you were in the hospital.
- Take medicine as prescribed for your pain.
- You may eat as you did before the operation.

- Be careful that you do not become constipated.
  - Include enough roughage and liquid in your diet.
  - You may need a mild laxative (example: milk of magnesia).
- You will be helped by all of the people involved with your care to learn how to get back to a relatively normal life.

✆ CALL OUR OFFICE IF

- There are any unusual new signs or symptoms.
- The wound becomes red or swollen, or there is drainage from it.
- You develop a temperature higher than 100°F.
- You have any questions.

AMPUTATION: Below Knee

△ GENERAL INFORMATION

Amputation of the leg is done mostly because of poor circulation caused by narrowing of the arteries *(atherosclerosis)*, sometimes because of diabetes. This narrowing decreases the blood flow to the tissues of the leg. Although medical treatments can help with the circulation problem, an amputation is eventually necessary for some individuals. There have been so many advances with prostheses in recent years that many people who have had an amputation can get back to a reasonably normal life.

COMMON SIGNS AND SYMPTOMS

- Early there may be cramping of the leg muscles during long walks, but in time, this happens even with short walks.
- Later, there is cramping of the leg muscles at night, when the leg is at rest; it occurs more often, lasts longer, and is more severe.
- Finally, the pain may be almost constant.
- Gangrene of the toes or feet can be the final stage.

DIAGNOSIS

- Usually, the diagnosis can be made by taking a detailed history, doing a thorough physical examination, and considering the laboratory report.
- Several tests can be done to see how the blood flows to the tissue. Of course, if gangrene already is present, nothing can be done to bring life back to the tissue. If a person is seen before gangrene sets in, tests can be done to determine whether an amputation can be avoided.
- Ultrasound: Harmless sound waves are aimed at the blood vessels of the leg. The sound waves bouncing back (the echoes) from this area are seen as a picture on a screen. Ultrasound is a convenient, painless, and harmless way to examine the blood vessels and see how seriously they are blocked.
- Arteriography: Dye is injected into the artery, and x-ray pictures are taken of it as it flows through the artery and its branches. The location and seriousness of the blockage can be seen accurately in this way.

○ TREATMENT

If gangrene has not set in, medicines are used to try to keep the vessels open so that enough blood can flow through them. This is not possible in your case.

- The leg is too far gone to be saved.
- After careful consideration of your condition and the test results, an amputation of your leg below the knee is recommended. The reasons for this have been explained to you.

PREOPERATIVE PREPARATION

- You will have an examination of your blood, urine, heart (EKG), and lungs (chest x-ray). Particular attention will be given to your other arteries, especially those to your brain, heart, and lungs. Your aorta will also be evaluated carefully.
- Do not eat or drink anything for 8 hours before the operation.
- You will be given medicine that will make you feel drowsy before you are brought to the operating room.
- The aim of the operation is as follows:
  - To do the safest operation for your condition.
  - To amputate the shortest amount of leg, yet have the tissue left behind be healthy.
  - To give you the best chance of being able to wear a prosthesis that will help you walk.
  - To do the operation in such a manner that the prosthesis can be fitted as soon as possible.

□ OPERATION

- You will be asleep for the operation, or you may be given a spinal type of anesthesia.
- You will not need a blood transfusion.
- The operation usually takes about 2 hours.
- You will wake up in a recovery room. When your blood pressure, pulse, and breathing are stable, you will be taken to a regular hospital room.
- There will be a snug bandage around the amputated leg.
- That evening you will be helped to sit up in bed and on the next day to get out of bed and into a chair.
- Pain can be controlled with medicine.
- Specialists in making and fitting you with a prosthesis and helping you learn how to walk on it will be working with you very closely and very early. The earlier you start using the prosthesis, the better.
- Thousands of people like you have had an amputation and are now up and about living a good life.
- You will leave the hospital when the healing is going well enough and you can take care of yourself with help.
- As with any operation, complications are possible. With your type of operation, they can include infection in the leg stump, poor wound healing, and blood clots, among others.
- Arrangements will be made for your medicine, follow-up office visit, and stitch removal.
- Arrangements can be made for a home visiting nurse if one is needed.

✣ HOME CARE

- Continue with the program started while you were in the hospital.
- Take medicine as prescribed for your pain.
- You may eat as you did before the operation.

- Be careful that you do not become constipated.
  - Include enough roughage and liquid in your diet.
  - You may need a mild laxative (example: milk of magnesia).
- You will be helped by all of the people involved with your care to learn how to get back to a relatively normal life.

✆ CALL OUR OFFICE IF

- There are any unusual new signs or symptoms.
- The wound becomes red or swollen, or there is drainage from it.
- You develop a temperature higher than 100°F.
- You have any questions.

△ GENERAL INFORMATION

The metatarsal area is the long bones from just back of your toes to about halfway to the heel. A transmetatarsal amputation cuts across this area (Fig. 1).

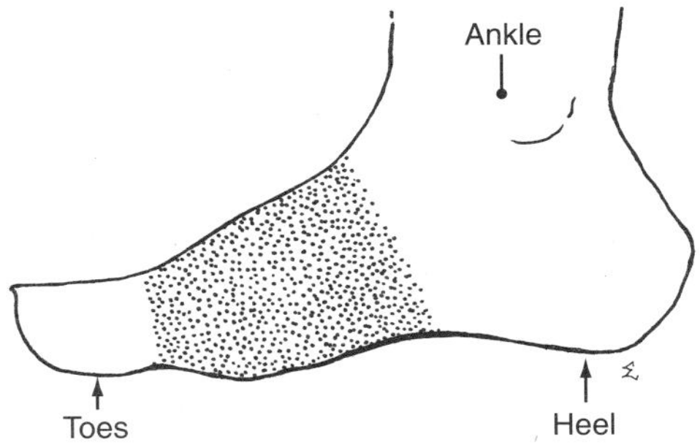

Figure 1. The transmetatarsal amputation usually is done within the stippled area.

COMMON SIGNS AND SYMPTOMS

- The usual symptom is that of pain. This is most commonly the result of decreased circulation that can be caused by diabetes or hardening of the arteries *(atherosclerosis)*.
- There may be a change in color of the toes.

DIAGNOSIS

- The diagnosis usually can be made by taking a detailed history and doing a thorough physical examination with particular attention to the color, pulses, sensation, and overall appearance of the toes.
- Plethysmography: This test measures the blood flow to the toes. It is helpful in determining the extent of the problem and at what level the amputation should be carried out.

PREOPERATIVE PREPARATION

- You will have an examination of your blood, urine, heart (EKG), and lungs (chest x-ray).
- Do not eat or drink anything for 8 hours before the operation.
- Shower as usual on the morning of the operation.
- You may be given medicine that will make you feel drowsy before you are brought to the operating room.

□ OPERATION

- The goal of treatment is to establish a foot that can bear your weight, that will allow you to walk without a limp, and, at the same time, that will make it possible for you to wear "essentially" normal shoes without a prosthesis.
- The amputation level is what one would consider the midfoot.
- The operation usually takes about 1 to 2 hours.

POSTOPERATIVE CARE

- You will be taken to a recovery room and observed. When your blood pressure, pulse, and breathing are stable, you will be taken to a regular hospital room.
- On the affected foot, you may have one of the following: a bulky dressing, a plaster cast, a brace, or a dressing that will allow you to wear a firm shoe. The choice will depend on the exact nature of the operation.
- That evening you will be helped to sit up in bed and on the next day to get out of bed.
- Pain can be controlled with medicine.
- Your diet will be as you tolerate it.
- You should be able to go home in 1 to 2 days.
- Arrangements will be made for your medicines, crutches, follow-up office visit, and stitch removal.
- As with any operation, complications are always possible. With your type of operation, they can include infection or the need to reoperate at a higher level because your circulation is not good enough for the wound to heal or because the disease has progressed.

✚ HOME CARE

- For the first several days you will need to sit as much as possible with your foot level with your hip. This will help reduce the pain and any swelling and help with healing.
- During this time, get up (on crutches) only as necessary for your personal needs, such as using the bathroom.
- How the wound is cared for varies quite a bit and depends on your special circumstances. You will be given detailed instructions on how to do this.
- Arrangements can be made for a home visiting nurse if one is needed.
- Either sponge bathe or sit in the tub with your operated leg hanging out.
- Take medicine as prescribed for your pain.
- Be careful that you do not become constipated.
  - Include enough roughage and plenty of liquids in your diet.
  - You may need some help with a mild laxative (example: milk of magnesia).
- As your healing progresses, you will be advanced to a brace and ultimately to a specially constructed support shoe with a toe filler in the front of the shoe.
- Do not drive a car or go to work before we discuss this during your follow-up visit.

✆ CALL OUR OFFICE IF

- The incision becomes red or swollen, or there is drainage from it.
- You develop a temperature higher than 100°F.
- You have any questions.

△ GENERAL INFORMATION

The anus is the opening of the large intestine through which stool comes to the outside. Squamous cell cancer of the anus is not common. Also, it is a different type of cancer than is found in the rest of the colon and rectum.

COMMON SIGNS AND SYMPTOMS

- Squamous cell cancer of the anus often is slow growing.
- There can be a slightly raised lump in the anal area. Sometimes, there is a raw area in this mass that may or may not bleed or hurt too much.

For the above reasons, such a lump may be mistaken for something unimportant and may be ignored.

DIAGNOSIS

Any lesion of the anus that is persistent, painful, or bleeding should be investigated to be certain of its nature.

- A first step is looking at the lesion carefully if some of it is on the outside.
- Next, feeling it with a lubricated, gloved finger can give valuable information as to its nature.
- Anoscopy: This is done with a short, hollow instrument called an *anoscope,* which is about as thick and as long as your finger. The anoscope is lubricated and gently inserted into the anal opening, which is thoroughly examined. If any abnormality is seen, a small piece of it is removed (a *biopsy*) for examination in the laboratory. This examination establishes the diagnosis and also provides information on whether it is a fast- or a slow-growing cancer.
- Barium enema: Liquid barium (it has the appearance and consistency of buttermilk) is given as an enema (just like a regular enema). As the barium flows throughout the colon, x-ray pictures are taken to look for any other unsuspected tumors.
- CT scan (computed tomography scan): These special x-rays are taken by a machine that is shaped like a huge doughnut. You will lie on a table inside the hole in the "doughnut." The x-rays are taken as very thin slices through the pelvis. This helps find lymph nodes in the pelvis that are involved with cancer spread from the anal area.
- Intraluminal ultrasound: This is done with an instrument called a *probe* that is as big around as your little finger. It is lubricated and gently inserted into the anus. From the tip of the probe, harmless, painless sound waves come out in all directions. The waves bouncing back (the echoes) are seen as pictures on a screen. This is an effective way to see how deeply the cancer has penetrated the anal wall and the associated sphincter (valve) muscles.

After these tests and examinations are done, important information will be available. *All* of this information will be considered in deciding on the treatment that has the best chance to bring about a cure. For example:

- **Size of the Cancer:** If the cancer is small, it may be possible to remove it locally adequately, yet leave enough of the opening and the anal sphincter muscles intact so that stools can be expelled in the normal manner.
- **Exact Location of the Cancer:** Whether the cancer is exactly over the sphincters or one-half or 1 inch away can make a significant difference in determining whether it can be treated without having to remove the anal sphincter and the need for a colostomy.
- **Growth Rate:** The microscopic examination of the biopsy will show whether it is a fast-growing and spreading tumor or a less aggressive one. This information helps determine how widely the tumor may need to be removed; which drug might be best for chemotherapy if it is to be used; whether any x-ray therapy needs to be given; and the likelihood that the therapy will be effective.

All of the above information—not just parts of it—will be considered in arriving at a decision on the recommended therapy. The most important part of the decision is to give you the best chance for a cure and, if at all possible, to leave the anal sphincter muscle in place rather than removing it and performing a colostomy.

After the most careful consideration of all factors, the recommendation is that your treatment should attempt to save the anal sphincter. There will be extensive consultations with the radiotherapist (x-ray doctor) and a medical oncologist.

Radiotherapy: This involves a determination of at least the following:

- Exactly where to give the x-ray (radiation) treatment. It must be wide enough to include all of the cancer but not so wide that too much uninvolved tissue is treated and scarred.
- The dose of radiation. It must be a dose that is enough to kill the cancer. However, an excessive amount of radiation can also scar down or possibly destroy the sphincter muscle itself.
- Over what period the radiation should be given. Giving all the radiation in too short a period of time can cause unnecessary blistering and an acute type of damage to the treated tissue; giving it too slowly may reduce its effectiveness.

Chemotherapy: There will be a decision on whether to give chemotherapy and, if so, what drug is to be used, the dose of it, and whether it will be given before or after the radiation therapy.

When any x-ray treatment or chemotherapy is completed, the anal area will again be examined carefully and a biopsy will be performed of the area to determine as accurately as possible whether the cancer has been eliminated with the above treatments. Following this evaluation, a decision will be made regarding whether further chemotherapy or radiation is necessary or only a very limited resection needs to be done. In the event that the cancer has not been completely eliminated and still affects the sphincter area, a more radical operation may need to be performed.

In your particular instance, the cancer has responded sufficiently well that only a limited operation can be done locally and your sphincter muscle can be spared. The recommendation, therefore, is that this operation be performed on you.

PREOPERATIVE PREPARATION

- Do not eat or drink anything for 8 hours before the operation.
- On the day before the operation, drink only liquids.
- Shower or bathe on the morning of the operation.
- You will be given medicine that will make you feel drowsy before you are brought to the operating room.

☐ OPERATION

- You will be asleep for the operation.
- The operation will focus on removing the cancer entirely but sparing your anal sphincter muscle.
- The operation usually takes about 2 to 3 hours.

POSTOPERATIVE CARE

- You will be taken to a recovery room and observed. When your blood pressure, pulse, and breathing are stable, you will be taken to a regular hospital room.
- You may have a catheter in your bladder for a day or two.
- That evening you will be helped to get out of bed.
- Pain can be controlled with medicine.
- You will be placed on an appropriate soft diet.
- Your condition can be cured. An estimate of your chances can be made only after all the test results are back.
- Arrangements will be made for your medicine and follow-up office visit.

✚ HOME CARE

- Resume your usual activities.
- You may walk about as you wish, even climb stairs, but don't overdo things.
- You may shower in the usual manner.
- At the beginning, your sphincter may not work as well as you would like. You will be helped to improve this.
- Be careful that you do not become constipated.
  - Include enough roughage and plenty of liquids in your diet.
  - You may need some help with a mild laxative (example: milk of magnesia).
- You may drive as you wish but not if you are taking medicines that may decrease your alertness.
- You may resume sexual activity whenever you choose.
- You may return to work when you feel up to it.

✆ CALL OUR OFFICE IF

- You develop any unusual signs or symptoms.
- You develop a temperature higher than 100°F.
- You do not have a bowel movement in 36 hours.
- You have any questions.

△ GENERAL INFORMATION

Anal fissure is a tear in the skin of the anus, the opening through which the bowel movements pass to the outside. This tear most often is caused by a large, hard bowel movement as it passes through the anus. There are other causes of anal fissure, but they don't apply to you.

COMMON SIGNS AND SYMPTOMS

At the beginning, there is a little burning and some pain in the anus while having a bowel movement.

- With repeated tearing, the pain during and for a short while after the bowel movement can be very severe. Some describe it as like a "hot poker."
- There may be bright red blood on the toilet tissue, on the surface of the stool, or in the toilet bowl.
- Persons with an anal fissure often become afraid of the pain that will follow a bowel movement, so they tend to hold back the bowel movement. This lets the stool become dry and even harder; as it finally passes, it reopens the fissure.

DIAGNOSIS

- Anyone with the above signs and symptoms should be checked for an anal fissure.
- Usually, the diagnosis can be made by taking a detailed history and doing a thorough physical examination of the area.
- Often careful separation of the buttocks will show the lower part of the fissure. It usually is located on the back side of the anus. Sometimes there is a small tag of scar tissue at the lower end of the fissure.
- A gloved lubricated finger is inserted gently through the anus. It may reproduce the pain when the fissure is touched.
- Anoscopy: This is done with a hollow instrument as thick and as long as your thumb (called an *anoscope*). You will lie on your side on the examining table as the lubricated anoscope is inserted gently into the anus and the area examined.

○ TREATMENT

- About one third of anal fissures will heal if the following are used:
  - A diet that has enough roughage and plenty of liquids in it so that the stools are soft.
  - Stool softener (example: Colace) or a mild laxative (example: milk of magnesia), if necessary.
  - Sitz baths: This involves sitting in a bathtub filled with enough warm (*not* hot) water to cover your anal area for 15 minutes three times a day and, if possible, after each bowel movement.
- If the fissure does not respond to the above treatment after a month or so, then a very effective operation can be done to help the fissure heal.

After consideration of all the factors, the recommendation is that you have an operation to help the tissue heal.

PREOPERATIVE PREPARATION

- You will have an examination of your blood and urine and possibly of your heart (EKG).
- Do not eat or drink anything for 8 hours before the operation.
- Shower or bathe as usual on the morning of the operation.
- You may be given medicine that will make you feel drowsy before you are brought to the operating room.

□ OPERATION

- The operation usually is done by using a fine needle to inject an anesthetic in the area to make it numb. In addition, medicine is given to make you feel drowsy. Sometimes, the operation is done under general anesthesia.
- The operation generally takes 30 minutes or less.

POSTOPERATIVE CARE

- You will be taken to a recovery room and observed. When your blood pressure, pulse, and breathing are stable and you are completely alert, you should be able to go home that same day with a responsible adult.
- Arrangements will be made for your medicines and follow-up office visit.

✣ HOME CARE

- Resume your usual activities.
- Take medicine as prescribed for your pain.
- Continue with the sitz baths if they make you feel more comfortable.
- Be careful that you do not become constipated.
  - Include enough roughage and plenty of liquids in your diet.
  - You may need some help with a mild laxative (example: milk of magnesia).
- You may return to work when you feel up to it.

✆ CALL OUR OFFICE IF

- You do not have a bowel movement in a 36-hour period.
- You develop a temperature higher than 100°F.
- You have any questions.

△ GENERAL INFORMATION

The spinal cord is as big around as the tip of your little finger. It travels inside a tunnel within your spine from the head down to the waist. Along the way it gives off nerves right and left to all parts of the body.

In the neck area, it gives off a bundle of nerves to the shoulder and arm. This is called the *brachial plexus* (Fig. 1). These nerves carry signals from the brain to the muscles of the shoulder and arm to make them move. They also carry all types of sensation (including pain) back from the arm and shoulder to the brain.

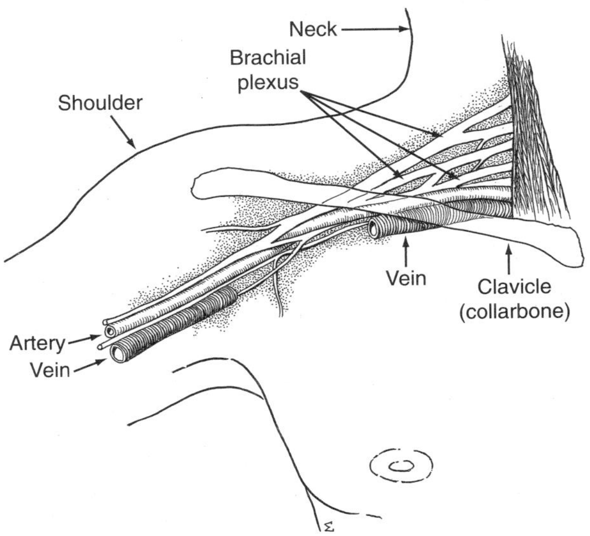

Figure 1. The brachial plexus is a group of nerves that branch off separate areas of the spinal cord in the neck area. The nerves travel primarily in the direction of the arm and affect mostly motion and sensation of the arm. These nerves can be anesthetized as a group or sometimes singly.

The nerves in the brachial plexus travel outward just under the skin in the lower side of the neck. They then pass under the skin in the axilla (armpit) to go to the various muscles of the shoulder and arm.

THE ANESTHETIC

The location of the nerves that make up the brachial plexus in the neck and the axilla makes it possible for the anesthesiologist to inject a local anesthetic around the nerves of the brachial plexus in one of these areas. This local anesthetic interrupts pain sensations that start in your arm and shoulder and keeps them from reaching the brain. Also while this anesthetic is working, you cannot move the arm.

This type of anesthesia given alone is often called a *block* anesthesia (it "blocks" sensation from traveling along the nerves). Or, sometimes it is called a *regional* anesthesia (because only one "region" of the body is anesthetized).

This type of anesthesia can be given along with medicine to make you feel drowsy.

Sometimes it is combined with general anesthesia (you are asleep). This makes it possible for you to be free of pain after the operation and until the anesthetic around the nerves wears off. Usually, this is from 6 to up to 18 hours.

USES OF BRACHIAL PLEXUS ANESTHESIA

- This technique is especially useful for patients who are sensitive to medicines by mouth or by vein.
- Operations that are most appropriate for brachial plexus anesthesia include the following:
  - Operation on the shoulder joint.
  - Operations on the bones in the arm.
  - Operations on the elbow.
  - Operations on the wrist or hand.

PREPARATION

- Your blood and urine will be checked, and other tests will be done as determined by the surgeon and anesthesiologist.
- Unless you have been directed otherwise, do not eat or drink anything for 8 hours before the operation.
- Shower or bathe on the morning of the operation.
- You may be given medicine that will make you feel drowsy before you are brought to the operating room.

THE PROCEDURE

- You will be placed on an operating table.
- Some fluids will be started in your vein.

There are two ways to reach the brachial plexus: through the neck skin or through the armpit *(axilla)*.

Lower Neck Approach

- This approach is used primarily for an operation on the shoulder and upper arm.
- The side of your neck will be swabbed with an antiseptic solution and the area surrounded with sterile towels.
- A very fine short needle will be used to inject a local anesthetic in the skin to make it numb.
- A different needle will be introduced into the neck to locate the nerves. A special nerve stimulator may be used to do this. This causes a mild twitching sensation of the shoulder or arm but is not painful.
- At this point, the local anesthetic will be injected near the nerves. Sometimes this causes a feeling of pressure or fullness.

Axillary Approach

- This approach is used primarily for operations on the elbow, forearm, and hand.
- You will be on your back with your arm behind your head.
- The underarm area will be swabbed with antiseptic solution and the area surrounded with sterile towels.
- A short, thin needle will be used to place an anesthetic in the skin to make it numb.
- A separate needle will be inserted deeper in the area to locate the nerves. You may feel a tingling

sensation in your forearm or hand. Also, the anesthesiologist may use a nerve stimulator to help locate the nerves. This causes a mild twitching sensation but is not painful.

When everything is ready, the local anesthetic will be injected around the nerves. This sometimes causes a sensation of pressure or fullness.

FOLLOWING THE PROCEDURE

- You may notice a warm, heavy, or tingling sensation in your arm. This will continue over 10 to 20 minutes, so don't be alarmed if your arm is not completely numb immediately following the injection of the anesthetic.
- It is important to avoid moving the arm after the injection because your muscles will be weak and not coordinated for several hours.

☐ OPERATION

- During the operation, you may feel some tugging but not pain.

POSTOPERATIVE CARE

- You will be taken to a recovery room and observed. When your blood pressure, pulse, and breathing are stable and you are completely alert, you will be examined to see that you can move your arm properly before you are permitted to go home with a responsible adult. Remember that you will be able to move your arm before all of the numbness is gone.
- As with all procedures, complications are always possible. Although they are very uncommon with both techniques of brachial plexus anesthesia, they may include the following: bleeding, infection, nerve injury, and possibly others. Temporary loss of consciousness or seizure is a side effect that can occur whenever local anesthetics are used.

✚ HOME CARE

- Follow the surgeon's directions carefully on what to do after the operation.

For the First 24 Hours

- Do not in any way handle power equipment with the arm that had the anesthetic.
- Do not use any hot utensils. Remember, your hand may still be numb enough so that you can burn yourself without realizing it.
- Do not drive your automobile.

✆ CALL OUR OFFICE IF

- You do not begin to have sensation in your arm within 12 hours.
- You develop any unusual signs or symptoms.
- You have any questions.

△ GENERAL INFORMATION

General anesthesia is the use of medication to cause you to become unconscious while an operation takes place. During this time you cannot feel pain, are not aware of the operation, and usually do not dream.

General anesthesia is given by specially trained physicians (anesthesiologists) or by a team consisting of an anesthesiologist supervising a nurse anesthetist (nurses with additional training in anesthesia). The anesthesiology team is very important in your care. After all, it is the anesthesiology team who "puts you to sleep" and who brings you back from that sleep. During the operation the anesthesiologist must watch both you and the surgeon. Keeping you asleep properly and safely makes it easier for the surgeon to perform a successful operation—all to your benefit.

It is important that the person administering your anesthetic has skill and experience and is caring. This person needs to know a number of ways to anesthetize a patient and which methods to use for a specific problem with a particular patient. Before, during, and after the operation, the anesthesiologist or anesthetist will be concerned about a number of things.

BEFORE COMING TO THE OPERATING ROOM

- You may have an examination of your blood and urine and possibly of your heart (EKG) and lungs (chest x-ray) and other tests requested by the surgeon and anesthesiologist.
- Do not eat or drink anything for 8 hours before the operation.
- You may take your usual oral medications on schedule with a sip of water. The only medication you should not take the day of surgery is a diuretic (a water pill). If you take medicine for diabetes or depression, your doctor will give you instructions on whether to take them.
- The anesthesiologist will review your medical record to learn some things:
  - The nature of your present problem: The methods to anesthetize you safely can vary according to the reason you require the procedure.
  - The nature of other medical problems you may have: A history of a heart attack, breathing problems, and other medical illnesses can make a significant difference in how you are put to sleep and what to watch for when you are asleep.
  - Results of the laboratory tests: Abnormalities can give important clues about possible problems (example: abnormal EKG or abnormal chest x-ray results).
  - Medicines you are taking: It is necessary to know what medicines you are taking. Also, it is vital that you tell the anesthesiologist of reactions to drugs or to previous anesthetics so that these can be avoided.
- Interview: There will be an interview regarding your health in general and a brief physical examination. The anesthesiologist will also ask to look in your mouth.
- The anesthesiologist will decide whether any special arrangements need to be made (example: special monitoring equipment or infrequently used medications) based on the nature of the operation.

You will be informed of the type of anesthesia planned and the reasons for it. The considerations are as follows:

- **Local Anesthesia:** A fine needle is used to inject an anesthetic in the area to make it numb. In addition, you may be given medicine that will make you feel drowsy.
- **Regional (Nerve) Anesthesia:** This can be done by anesthetizing the nerves to a specific area being operated on or by giving a spinal anesthetic, which covers the abdomen and legs.
- **General Anesthesia:** You can be put to sleep by having an anesthetic injected into your vein or by breathing an anesthetic vapor.

You will be informed of the important things that will take place before you are brought to the operating room.

- You will have some intravenous fluids started in one of your veins. Medicines and anesthetics will be given through this small plastic tube.
- You may be given medicine that will make you feel drowsy before you are brought to the operating room.

IN THE OPERATING ROOM

- When you enter the operating room, you will be moved onto a narrow bed—the operating table.
- The operating room staff will make certain that your position on the table is correct. Your arms may be placed by your side and a belt placed across your lap.
- A blood pressure cuff will be placed around your upper arm, EKG stickers will be placed on your chest, and an oxygen probe will be placed on a finger. In this way you will be monitored closely during the operation, allowing the anesthesiologist to watch your heart rate, blood pressure, and breathing continuously while you are under the anesthetic.
- Before "going to sleep," you will be given extra oxygen to breathe through an anesthesia mask for a few minutes.
- The anesthesiologist will inject an anesthetic medication into the intravenous solution; you will fall asleep in about 30 seconds.

DURING THE OPERATION

During the operation, the anesthesia team will be looking after a number of things including monitoring the different parts of your body to see how well they are working during the operation and making adjustments as necessary.

- Breathing: This is vital because it is how you get oxygen into your body. How you breathe while you are asleep is influenced by the anesthetic used, the operation being done, and any medical conditions you might have.

- Heart and circulation: The heart rate, rhythm, and blood pressure are recorded continuously.
- Kidneys: For an operation expected to last longer than about 2 hours, a catheter may be placed into the bladder to see how much urine you are producing and how to adjust the intravenous fluids to help your kidneys make urine at the proper rate.
- Temperature: The body temperature can rise or fall, and this can be corrected as needed.

IN THE RECOVERY ROOM

- The anesthesiology team will accompany you to the recovery room. They will have a short conference with the recovery room nurses about what occurred in the operating room and what special precautions may need to be taken regarding your immediate condition.
- In the recovery room, you will have monitoring of your blood pressure and heart as well as the oxygen level of your blood stream.
- You should be able to leave the recovery room when your blood pressure, pulse, and breathing are stable and any pain is under control. If you are going home that same day you will need to be quite alert, be able to walk (with a little help), be able to drink some fluids, and finally, be able to urinate before you leave.
- You will be permitted to leave only if you are accompanied by a responsible adult.

✣ HOME CARE ON THE DAY OF THE OPERATION

- Take it easy for the day; follow the surgeon's instructions.
- Don't drive a car, operate any machinery (no cooking), or make any important decisions the day of the operation.
- Avoid spicy or greasy foods.
- Have a member of the family or a friend stay with you overnight.
- The anesthetic should wear off completely in about 24 hours.

△ GENERAL INFORMATION

Spinal anesthesia involves a single injection of a local anesthetic medicine into your back that produces numbness and muscle relaxation of the region of your body from about your waist down to your toes. For this reason, it is called a "regional" anesthetic.

Spinal anesthesia is most commonly used for operations on the legs, groin, organs in the pelvis, and buttocks.

It is important that the person giving you anesthesia has skill and experience and is caring. This person needs to know a number of ways to anesthetize a patient and which method to use for a specific patient with a particular problem. Before, during, and after the operation, the anesthesiologist or anesthetist will be concerned about a number of things.

BEFORE COMING TO THE OPERATING ROOM

- You will have an examination of your blood and urine and possibly of your heart (EKG) and lungs (chest x-ray) as well as other tests as requested by the surgeon and anesthesiologist.
- You may take your usual medications on schedule with a sip of water. The only medications you should not take the day of surgery are diuretics (water pills). If you take medicine for diabetes or depression, your doctor will give you instructions on whether to take them.
- The anesthesiologist will review your medical record to learn some things:
  - The nature of your present problem: The anesthesiologist knows which operations are best suited for spinal anesthesia.
  - The nature of other medical problems you might have: A history of heart attack, breathing problems, and other medical problems can make a significant difference in the type of anesthetic you should have and what to watch for during the operation.
  - Results of laboratory tests: Abnormalities can give important clues to the severity of medical illnesses and the precautions to be taken.
  - Medicines you are taking: This is important information to know. Also, it is vital that you tell the anesthesiologist of reactions to drugs or to a previous anesthetic so that these can be avoided.
  - Interview: There will be an interview of your health in general and a brief physical examination.
  - The anesthesiologist will examine your backbone to assess the ease of doing a spinal anesthetic, if this is the anesthetic choice.
- The anesthesiologist will determine whether any special arrangements (for anesthesia equipment and medications) should be made based on the nature of the operation to be performed.

You will be informed of the type of anesthesia planned and the reasons for it. The considerations are as follows:

- **Local Anesthesia:** A fine needle is used to inject an anesthetic in the area to make it numb. Also, you may be given medicine to make you feel drowsy.
- **Regional (Nerve) Anesthesia:** This can be done by anesthetizing a bundle of nerves, producing numbness to your legs or arms as needed for the surgery.
- **General Anesthesia:** You might be anesthetized by having an anesthetic medicine injected into your intravenous fluids or by breathing an anesthetic vapor.

In your instance, the recommendation is that you have a spinal anesthetic.

SPINAL ANESTHESIA

The spinal column has a tunnel on its back part that runs through its entire length. Inside this tunnel runs the spinal cord (it's a little thicker than a pencil) from the bottom of your skull to just below your waist. Nerves come from and go to the spinal cord all along its length. They carry all the sensations (including pain) from the body to the brain. In return, signals from the brain come down the cord and travel along these nerves to make your body move as necessary.

A "spinal" involves giving a local anesthetic next to the nerves that leave the spinal cord (Fig. 1). When this anesthetic touches a nerve coming off the spinal cord, the sensation of pain and the ability to move the muscles

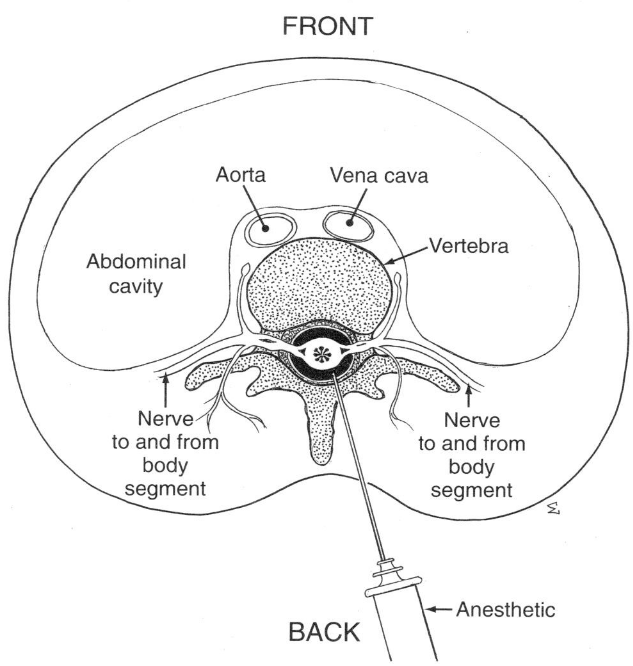

Figure 1. One vertebra as seen from the top. The needle connected to the anesthetic solution is inserted so that it is in the spinal fluid *(black area)* that surrounds the spinal cord *(asterisk)*. The anesthetic solution is now injected into this area. The nerves that go to and from that area of the body are bathed by the solution. That segment now is paralyzed and has no sensation.

below that area are no longer present. The anesthesiologist can control how long this will last by using drugs that wear off after different lengths of time.

When the operation is over and the anesthesia wears off, your sensation and movement will gradually return to normal.

IN THE OPERATING ROOM

- You may be given some medication that will make you feel slightly drowsy.
- You will have some fluids started in your vein. Also, you will have a blood pressure cuff placed around your upper arm that will measure your blood pressure frequently. Some EKG wires will be taped to your skin. They will record your heart rate and rhythm.
- You will then be asked to sit on the operating table or to lie on your side. In either case, once in position, you will be asked to bend forward as much as possible. This position is just temporary; it helps the anesthesiologist to perform the spinal anesthetic.
- Your lower back will be swabbed with an antiseptic solution and the area surrounded with sterile towels.
- A very thin, tiny needle will be used to inject an anesthetic into the skin to make it numb.
- The anesthesiologist will then use an extremely thin needle to inject less than half a teaspoon of local anesthetic right next to the spinal nerves.
- In about 5 minutes, your feet and buttocks will begin to feel warm, then tingle, and finally "fall asleep."
- The operating room staff will then get you in the appropriate position for the operation.

DURING THE OPERATION

- The part of your body being operated on will remain numb during the operation. Also, you will not be able to move that part of your body during the operation.
- You will be awake and be able to talk. However, medicine is available if you want to feel very drowsy or be in a "twilight sleep" during the operation.

AT THE END OF THE OPERATION

- The anesthesia team will accompany you to the recovery room where they will inform the recovery room nurses about what took place in the operating room. The recovery room nurses will also be informed about your spinal anesthetic and will follow the instructions for routine care of patients who have had a spinal.
- Your heart rate, blood pressure, and breathing will be monitored closely. After they are stable and you are alert, a decision will be made about discharging you from the recovery area. You will need to be able to walk (with a little help), be able to drink some fluids, and finally be able to urinate before you can go home.
- You will be permitted to go home that same day only if you are accompanied by a responsible adult.

✣ HOME CARE ON THE DAY OF THE OPERATION

- Take it easy for the day; do not engage in any physical activity; follow the surgeon's instructions.
- Eat a bland diet.
- Have a member of the family or a friend stay with you overnight.

✆ CALL OUR OFFICE IF

- You develop a headache.
- You develop any backache, stiff neck, or fever.
- You develop a temperature higher than 100°F.
- You have any questions.

ANESTHESIA FOR LABOR AND DELIVERY

△ GENERAL INFORMATION

Epidural, *spinal*, or combined *spinal-epidural* anesthesia may be used either to relieve labor pains or to provide the anesthetic for delivery by cesarean section.

SOME ANATOMY

The spine extends from the head down to the pelvis. In the back part of the spine, there is a tunnel (about as big as your little finger). The spinal cord goes down this tunnel. The spinal cord is the big nerve that comes down from the brain, and as it travels down toward the pelvis it gives off nerves to the left and right and then finally splits into many nerves that go into the pelvis. These nerves carry sensation (including pain) to the spinal cord and then up to the brain. They also carry sensation down the cord and in through the nerves that stimulate your muscles to move.

The spinal cord is surrounded by a sleeve (called the *dura*). Inside the dura is the spinal cord and some fluid (the *spinal fluid*).

WHAT IS EPIDURAL, SPINAL, OR COMBINED SPINAL-EPIDURAL ANESTHESIA?

All three techniques are somewhat similar.

Spinal: The medication is placed in the spinal fluid *inside* the dura (the sleeve).

Epidural: The medication is placed *outside* the dura, where the nerves come through to get to the various parts of the body.

Combined Spinal-Epidural: The medication is placed in both locations.

Walking Epidural: The medication is placed so that you can be up and walking in your room but feel very little of the labor pain.

WHAT MEDICINES ARE USED

Local Anesthetics

A number of local anesthetics are available. The anesthesiologist will choose the anesthetic and the dose of the anesthetic best suited to your special needs. Considerations on which drug or drugs to use and how much include the following:

- Whether you will have a spinal or an epidural anesthetic.
- How quickly anesthesia is needed.
- How long the anesthesia is to last.
- Whether the anesthetic is for relief of labor pain or for a cesarean section.

There is no evidence that these drugs have any short- or long-term effect on the baby, including the ability to nurse.

Narcotics

Often, very small doses of these drugs are used or combined with the local anesthetic when this is appropriate.

- To give a boost to the local anesthetic.
- During a routine vaginal delivery.
- To provide pain relief after a cesarean section.
- To provide relief after a vaginal delivery with repair of a laceration.

In the last two situations, the anesthetic may be continued after the cesarean section or to complete a vaginal delivery repair.

Again, there is no evidence that these drugs have any short- or long-term effect on the baby, including the ability to nurse.

Epinephrine

Epinephrine keeps the anesthetic in place longer so that it does not wear out too soon, and it has pain-killing effects of its own.

PREPARATION

No special preparation is necessary on your part. You will be consulted, and an explanation will be given of any anesthetic administration before it is done.

THE PROCEDURE

Spinal

You will be seated on a table with your feet over the side and your back bent forward as much as possible.

- Your lower back will be swabbed with an antiseptic solution and surrounded with sterile towels.
- A fine, short needle will be used to inject an anesthetic in the skin to make it numb.
- A special thin needle will then be used to go between the bones of your spine down through the dura surrounding the spinal cord and into the spinal fluid.
- Once inside the area where the spinal fluid is located, the anesthetic is injected, the needle removed, and a bandage applied over the needle puncture site. *Note*: The tip of the needle is below the spinal cord itself so there cannot be an injection into the cord.
- You will now be placed on your back on the table.

Advantages to this method:

- The anesthetic takes effect in several minutes.
- It is more reliable than an epidural anesthetic.

Disadvantages to this method:

- The single dose of anesthetic lasts up to 2 hours, so it needs to be timed correctly. If it is given too soon, it will wear off and not be available when pain is still present.

Epidural

Your are prepared in the same way as for the spinal anesthetic except for the following differences:

- The needle is placed just outside the dura and just where the nerves come through it.
- A tiny plastic catheter (tube) is placed through the needle up to its tip. The needle itself is removed, but

the catheter is left there. The other end is taped to your back and shoulder.

- Medicine now can be given into the catheter as needed.

Advantages to this technique:

- The medicine can be dripped in as necessary for relief of pain, even after the cesarean section or vaginal delivery is over.
- Headache is rare with this technique.

Disadvantages to this technique:

- The anesthetic is slower to take effect; sometimes it takes 15 minutes or so.
- It is less reliable than a spinal anesthetic.

Combined Spinal-Epidural

It uses both techniques described. It is useful in the following situations:

- When quick anesthesia is needed.
- When it is desirable to be able to walk around during labor yet not have pain.
- When you must have a cesarean section.
- When you need pain relief after the delivery or a cesarean section.

EFFECTS OF SPINAL OR EPIDURAL ANESTHESIA ON LABOR

- There are no unfavorable side effects on the fetus, mother, or newborn.
- These anesthetic drugs may increase uterine blood flow (and thus oxygen to the fetus) during labor.
- The labor may be longer.
- When done properly when you are in active labor, epidural anesthesia does not increase the chance that you will need a cesarean section.
- When administered properly, these drugs should not interfere with your ability to push or to focus on where to push during labor and delivery.

POSSIBLE COMPLICATIONS

Backache

Backache is common in women before and after delivery. There may be a number of reasons for this, including the following:

- During pregnancy, a hormone is secreted, called *relaxin*, that relaxes the ligaments of the pelvis. This is supposed to help the baby come out through the vagina.
- The above hormone also relaxes the ligaments along the spine. This is combined with the added weight on the spine by the pregnancy.
- The mother spends a lot of time bending over, lifting, and other such back-straining movements while taking care of the baby.

In summary, there appears to be no relationship between the use of spinal or epidural anesthesia for labor or delivery by cesarean section and any backache after delivery.

Headache

This can occur in about one out of 100 patients. In most cases it is mild, does not progress, and is easily treated with a pain reliever such as Tylenol. A cure is accomplished in more than 99% of cases.

Nerve Damage

This can occur in one out of 10,000 to 20,000 patients and is rarely associated with the anesthesia. The most common cause is the position of the patient and how long she stays in that position during delivery.

Death or Paralysis

This can occur in one out of 500,000 patients. The risk is less than that of being struck by lightning.

As you can see, spinal, epidural, or combined spinal-epidural anesthesia is a safe and rapid way to provide pain relief in obstetrics.

ANKLE FRACTURE

△ GENERAL INFORMATION

The ankle contains a number of bones. An ankle fracture is a partial or complete break of one or more of these bones. The usual cause of an ankle fracture is a fall, a twist, or a direct blow.

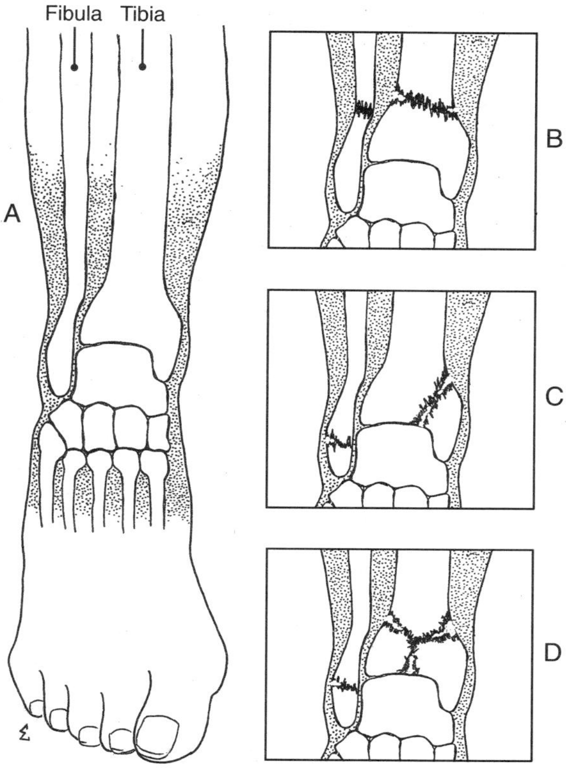

Figure 1. *A,* Normal ankle. *B, C,* and *D,* Three types of possible fractures of the ankle. Each fracture may require treatment that is very different from the others. Also, the chance for long-term success of the repair of each of these fractures varies considerably.

COMMON SIGNS AND SYMPTOMS

In some instances, the signs and symptoms of an ankle fracture are similar to those of an ankle sprain.

- There is pain and swelling of the ankle, mostly over the injured area.
- The ankle cannot be moved freely because of the pain and swelling.
- Bleeding in the deeper tissue causes the skin over this area to become black, blue, or purple.

DIAGNOSIS

- The diagnosis of a fracture can often be made by taking a detailed history of how the injury occurred and by doing a thorough physical examination.
- X-rays of an ankle are necessary to know whether a fracture is present and precisely the location and nature of the fracture of one or more bones.
- The patient often reports experiencing or hearing a "pop" at the time of the injury.
- On examination, the ankle may not be stable.
- The ability or inability of the patient to walk after the injury often has little bearing on whether there is a fracture or a sprain of the ankle.

○ TREATMENT

The treatment of a fracture depends on a number of factors: whether it involves one bone or several bones; which bones are involved; whether these bones are broken but not out of place; whether a bone is fractured and is in a number of pieces; and the age and general physical condition of the individual.

Some simple ankle fractures can be treated with a cast or a brace. After the cast or brace is applied, you will need to lie down on a couch or chair with your ankle elevated on two pillows for a day or two. You can be out of this position only for your essential needs, such as going to the bathroom.

- When you do need to get up, you will be required to use crutches or a walker so that you don't put weight on your fractured ankle.
- You will be instructed on how to use the crutches or walker properly.

More complicated fractures may require an operation to reposition the broken bone fragments and keep them in the correct position until they heal.

If an operation is required, the extent and nature of such an operation depends on which ankle bones are involved and how they are fractured. The surgeon may choose to use metal rods applied to the lower leg and ankle from the outside to keep the bones steady and in proper position until they heal. Other fractures may require an incision through which the surgeon lines up the bones correctly and then holds them in this correct alignment with screws, plates, pins, staples, or rods. Some of these devices remain in place permanently; others are removed after a year or two.

After careful consideration of all factors, the recommendation is that you have an operation for your ankle fracture.

PREOPERATIVE PREPARATION

- You will have an examination of your blood, urine, heart (EKG), and lungs (chest x-ray).
- Do not eat or drink anything for 8 hours before the operation.

□ OPERATION

- You may either be asleep for the operation or have a spinal type of anesthesia in which you will be numb from the waist down. In addition, you will be given some medicine to make you feel drowsy.
- The duration of the operation depends on what is found and what needs to be done.

POSTOPERATIVE CARE

- You will be taken to a recovery room and observed. When your blood pressure, pulse, and breathing are stable, you will be taken to a regular hospital room.
- Your leg will be in a cast or a brace and be elevated on several pillows.
- Pain will be controlled with medicine.
- Your diet will be as you tolerate it.
- The doctors and nurses or technicians will work with you so that you can get out of bed and use crutches or a walker as soon as possible. Please remember that you will not be allowed to bear weight on your foot or ankle for a number of weeks.
- You will be discharged from the hospital at the earliest time it is safe to do so.
- Arrangements will be made for your medicine and follow-up office visit.
- As with any operation, complications are always possible, some of them serious. With this type of operation, they can include the fracture slipping out of the correct position; the skin incision being slow to heal; infection; numbness around the area of the incision; arthritis, particularly with fractures that affect the ankle joint itself; and possibly others.

HOME CARE

- You will need some help at home.
- The emphasis at home will be on rest and on keeping the fractured leg elevated on two pillows.
- You should not place weight on your injured leg until you are specifically permitted to do so.
- Take the medicines prescribed for you.
- Include plenty of roughage and liquids in your diet to help prevent constipation.
- At the appropriate time, you may have home or outpatient physical therapy prescribed for you.
- Initially, you will need to sponge bathe. The advisability of when to start taking a bath and how to do it without getting the cast wet will be discussed with you if you wish.

CALL OUR OFFICE IF

- You develop numbness of the toes or cannot move them without pain.
- You have uncontrollable pain.
- You develop fever or chills.
- You have any questions.

△ GENERAL INFORMATION

A ligament is a strong cord-like material that goes between two bones across a joint to keep that joint stable (Fig. 1). A sprain of the ankle is a partial or complete tear of one or more of these ligaments. Usually, it is the result of a twisting injury.

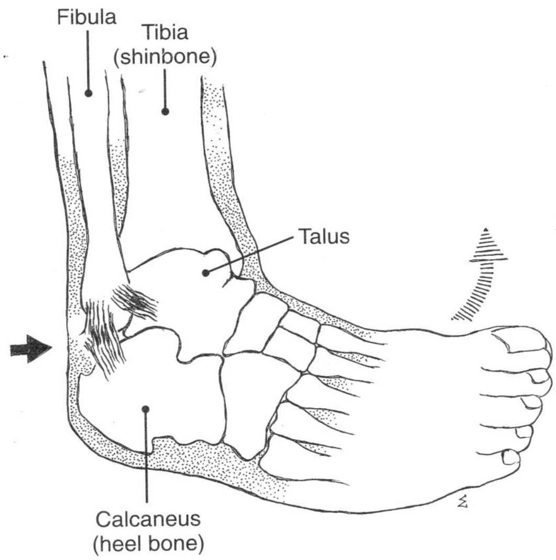

Figure 1. A number of ligaments hold together the bones of the ankle. A common injury occurs when the ankle is forcibly "turned in" and results in a "sprain" of the ankle. The two ligaments shown are often affected.

COMMON SIGNS AND SYMPTOMS

- There is pain and swelling of the ankle, mostly over the torn ligament.
- The ankle cannot be moved freely because of the pain and swelling.
- The bleeding in the deeper tissue causes the skin over the injured area to become black, blue, or purple.

DIAGNOSIS

The diagnosis usually can be made by taking a detailed history of how the injury occurred and then doing a thorough physical examination.

- The patient often reports experiencing or hearing a "pop" at the time of the injury.
- Demonstrating the specific location of the pain and swelling helps establish the correct diagnosis.
- In some instances, it may be possible by maneuvering the ankle to demonstrate that the ankle is not stable.
- An x-ray of the ankle can demonstrate that the injury is a sprain rather than a fracture.

○ TREATMENT

In general, practically all sprains are treated initially by using four things: Remember the acronym RICE.

Rest: You should rest your ankle. Normally, you will not be permitted to bear weight on it, or you will have protected weight bearing by supporting the ankle with a cast or a brace. Crutches may be used for a week or two.

Ice: Cold should be applied over the bruised area for 20 minutes every hour during the daytime for the first 24 to 48 hours unless you are instructed to do otherwise. A plastic bag filled with ice cubes is suitable for this or even a bag of frozen peas (it drapes well over the curved areas).

Compression: Compression dressings such as an elastic bandage help keep the swelling down and reduce some of the pain.

Elevation: Lie down or sit on a couch or chair with your leg resting on one or two pillows. Do this for at least the first 24 to 48 hours except when you need to attend to your personal needs such as going to the bathroom.

- You will be given medicine for pain and to help you sleep more comfortably at night.
- Include plenty of roughage and liquids in your diet to help prevent constipation.
- After the early phase of swelling, pain, and inflammation improves, you may be started on a home or outpatient program of physical therapy.
- The goals of treatment are to reestablish strength and balance of your ankle.

POSSIBLE COMPLICATIONS

As with any injury or treatment, complications are always possible. With an ankle sprain, these can include the following:

- Skin blisters over the swollen area. If this occurs, you will be instructed on how to take care of the skin so that it does not become infected.
- Long-term instability of the ankle. You may experience repeated sprains of the ankle for some time after the first accident.
- Chronic pain and swelling of the ankle.
- In some instances, the x-ray results at the time of the accident may appear normal. However, an x-ray repeated a few days or weeks later may show a hairline or stress fracture. This is the reason you may be asked to return for a follow-up visit within 1 to 3 weeks after your injury.

✆ CALL OUR OFFICE IMMEDIATELY IF

- You develop numbness of the toes or cannot move them without pain.
- You have uncontrollable pain.
- You develop fever or chills.

ANORECTAL ABSCESS

△ GENERAL INFORMATION

Anorectal abscess is an infection with pus in it that is located in the area of the anus or lower rectum.

An anorectal abscess usually begins when bacteria enter through a tear in the lining of the rectum or anus. The bacteria develop into an abscess that may appear next to the anus (this is the most common) or some distance from the anus. Or, the abscess may remain inside, causing destruction of tissue before the pus is released or comes to the surface and breaks out on its own. Sometimes, the abscess may affect the sphincters (the valves) that open and close the anus during a bowel movement (Fig. 1).

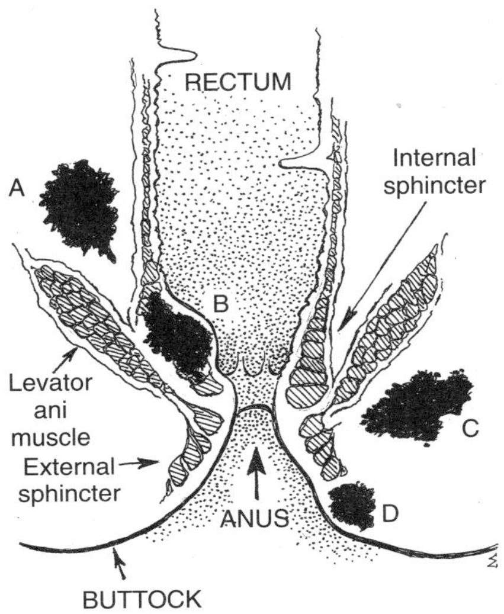

Figure 1. Types of anorectal abscess: supralevator (A); intersphincteric (B); ischiorectal (C); perineal (D).

COMMON SIGNS AND SYMPTOMS

The symptoms depend on whether the abscess is trapped inside or has come to the outside next to the anus. These symptoms may be as follows:

- Redness, swelling, and pain in an area around the anus.
- Deep, throbbing pain for an abscess that has remained on the inside. It is not easy to point to the specific tender area.
- Pain with bowel movements.
- Fever and chills.

DIAGNOSIS

- Usually, the diagnosis can be made by taking a detailed history, doing a thorough physical examination, and considering the laboratory reports.
- Anoscopy: This is done with a hollow instrument (called an *anoscope*) that is as long and as thick as your thumb. The anoscope is lubricated and gently inserted into the anus to examine the entire area, looking for an internal cause of the abscess.
- Flexible sigmoidoscopy: This is done with an instrument that is pliable, smooth, and as thick as the tip of your little finger. It has lenses in it and a light at the tip. The flexible sigmoidoscope is inserted through the anus, and the entire lower rectum is examined carefully.

○ TREATMENT

The treatment for an anorectal abscess is to perform an operation to drain the pus. This not only makes you more comfortable, but also helps to prevent unnecessary damage to the tissue by the pus left standing there.

Another aim of the operation is to determine the cause of the abscess and to treat the cause at the same time as the abscess, or, if this is not possible, to make plans to treat the cause later, after the abscess has been drained and the infection has quieted down.

Sometimes the abscess affects the sphincters of the anus so that the entire operation cannot be done at one setting. There is too much risk of damage to the sphincters. If the sphincters were to be damaged, you might not be able to close your anus tightly after the operation. The solution is to do the operation in two stages. Often, the second operation is done several weeks later on an outpatient basis.

It is clear after examining you and taking all factors into consideration that you need a prompt operation to drain the abscess.

PREOPERATIVE PREPARATION

- You will have an examination of your blood, urine, heart (EKG), and lungs (chest x-ray).
- You may be given medicine that will make you feel drowsy before you are brought to the operating room.

□ OPERATION

- The operation will be done under general anesthesia.
- The operation usually takes about an hour, depending on what needs to be done.

POSTOPERATIVE CARE

- You will be taken to a recovery room and observed until your blood pressure, pulse, and breathing are stable and you are fully alert. If the decision is that you go home that day, it will have to be with a responsible adult.
- If the necessary operation was more complicated, you will need to remain in the hospital for a day or two.
- The evening of your operation you will be helped to get out of bed.
- Very likely, you will have a small, soft rubber drain in your anal area. The purpose of it and how it will be handled will be explained to you in detail.

- Arrangements will be made for your medicine and follow-up office visit.
- As with any operation, complications are always possible. With this type of operation, they can include continued infection, weakness of your sphincter, and possibly others.

✙ HOME CARE

- You may walk about as you wish, even climb stairs, but don't overdo things.
- You will be given a suggested diet to follow during your convalescence.
- You will be instructed on taking sitz baths for 10 to 15 minutes three times a day. This involves sitting in a bathtub that has enough warm (*not* hot) water in it to completely cover your anal area. Sitz baths help speed up healing, keep the area cleaner, and also make you more comfortable.
- Be careful that you do not become constipated.
  - Include enough roughage and plenty of liquids in your diet.
  - You may need some help with a mild laxative (example: milk of magnesia).
- You may resume sexual activity whenever you choose.
- You may return to work when you feel up to it, but let's talk about it first during a follow-up office visit.

✆ CALL OUR OFFICE IF

- You develop any unusual signs or symptoms.
- The pain in the operated area becomes worse than before, or you have increasing discharge from the incision.
- You develop a temperature higher than 100°F.
- You have not had a bowel movement in any 36-hour period.
- You have any questions.

△ GENERAL INFORMATION

The lining just inside the anus is puckered, the same as the skin around the anus on the outside. Sometimes a tiny piece of stool gets stuck in one of the puckered areas on the inside, causing an infection. This can develop into an abscess deep to the surface. The abscess inside the anus can work its way toward the outside of the anus. Next, the abscess breaks to the surface or needs to be opened to relieve the pus. Now a tunnel exists between the inside and the outside. The tunnel connecting the inside usually comes to the outside very close to the anus. This is called an *anal fistula* (Fig. 1).

- Most persons present with a history of previous abscess that either drained by itself or needed to be drained by the surgeon.
- There is a history of a recurring abscess or drainage from an opening right next to the anus or a short distance from it.

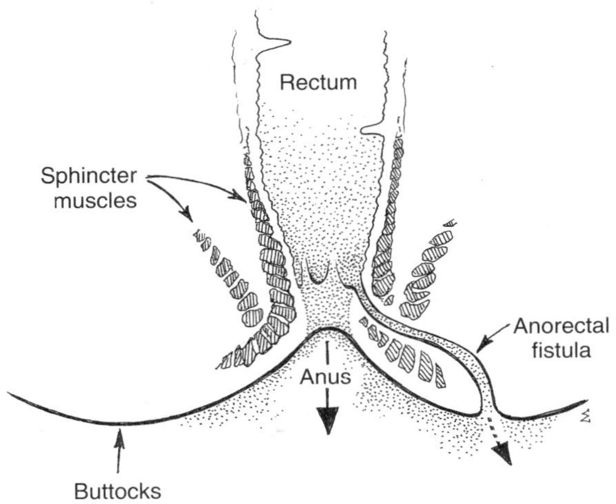

Figure 1. An anorectal abscess can find its way to the outside in various way. A typical way is illustrated.

COMMON SIGNS AND SYMPTOMS

- A slightly red opening to the side of the anus draining infected fluid.
- Sometimes, the tract comes from the inside to the outside and can be felt under the skin. At other times the outside opening is seen with no clue as to where it started on the inside.

DIAGNOSIS

- The ways to establish a diagnosis are not always the same for each person, even though the same disease or condition is suspected. A test is done, and if the results don't make the diagnosis clear enough, then the next test is done. That's why the necessary tests on you will include at least some and possibly all of the following:
- Anoscopy: This is done with a hollow instrument as long and as thick as your thumb called an *anoscope.* It is lubricated and gently inserted inside the anus to search for an internal opening.
- Flexible sigmoidoscopy: A *sigmoidoscope* is an optical instrument that is about as thick as your little finger and is smooth, flexible, and has a light at its tip. While you lie on your side, it is inserted gently in your anus and into the rectum. The lower one-third of the large bowel can be examined for an internal opening as well as for any other abnormality.
- Small bowel x-ray: You will be given some liquid barium to swallow. The barium will be watched as it travels through your entire small intestine. This examination is done to see if the fistula might have its beginning in the small intestine.

○ TREATMENT

- The best treatment for an anal fistula is to remove it.
- A fistula may travel through several areas of tissue before coming to the outside. Some of this tissue may be the muscles (the *sphincters*) that close and open your anus. For this reason, a number of operations are available for each situation. In all the available operations, the most important precaution is *not* to damage the sphincter muscles. To protect these very important muscles, sometimes it is necessary to do the operation in two stages a few weeks apart.

After careful consideration of all factors, the recommendation is that you have an operation to remove your fistula.

PREOPERATIVE PREPARATION

- You will have an examination of your blood and urine and possibly of your heart (EKG) and lungs (chest x-ray).
- Do not eat or drink anything for 8 hours before the operation.
- Shower or bathe on the morning of the operation.
- You may be given medicine that will make you feel drowsy before you are brought to the operating room.

□ OPERATION

- The operation usually is done under general anesthesia or a spinal type of anesthesia. The choice will be discussed with you beforehand.
- Most of the time the fistula is removed and the tissue permitted to heal in a routine fashion. On occasion, however, the internal opening may be quite a distance high in the rectum. It is this circumstance that may require the operation to be done in two stages.
- The operation usually takes about 1 hour.

POSTOPERATIVE CARE

- You will be taken to a recovery room and observed. When your blood pressure, pulse, and breathing are stable and you are completely alert and if the operation was not extensive, you might be able to go

home that same day with a responsible adult. Otherwise, you will need to stay in the hospital for a day or two.
- Arrangements will be made for your medicine and follow-up office visit.

✚ HOME CARE

- Resume your usual activities.
- Take medicine as prescribed for your pain.
- Be careful that you do not become constipated.
  - Include enough roughage and plenty of liquids in your diet.
  - You may need some help with a mild laxative (example: milk of magnesia).
- Take sitz baths for 15 minutes two times a day and following a bowel movement, if possible. This involves sitting in a bathtub filled with enough warm (*not* hot) water to cover your bottom. This will make you feel more comfortable, and it helps keep the area clean and helps with the healing.
- You may resume sexual activity whenever you choose.
- You may return to work when you feel up to it.

✆ CALL OUR OFFICE IF

- You do not have a bowel movement in any 36-hour period.
- You develop a temperature higher than 100°F.
- You have any questions.

△ GENERAL INFORMATION

Anorectal fistula *(fistula-in-ano)* is a condition in which there is a connection (or tract) between the distal-most part of the rectum and the skin of the buttocks surrounding the anus (Fig. 1). It usually begins as an infection in some folds (called *crypts*) at the distal rectum just inside the anus. This infection forms a tract that stays deep to the surface of the rectum until it finally breaks to the outside—usually next to the anus. The tract sometimes remains open, and infection comes back again. In an adolescent, fistula-in-ano may occur in association with Crohn's disease. Such a fistula requires entirely different treatment than that discussed here.

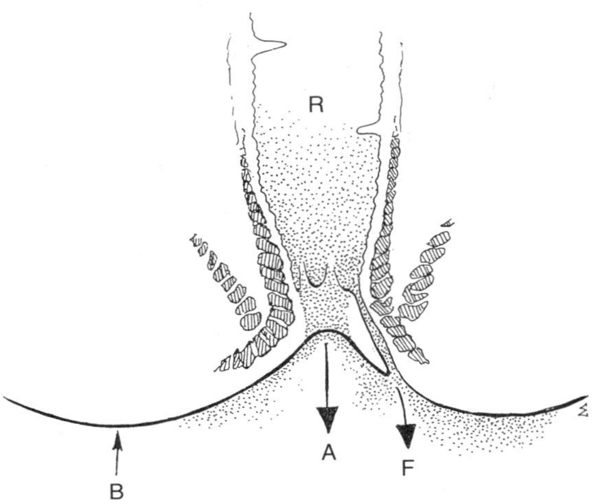

Figure 1. An anorectal abscess may find its way to the outside (and thus create an anorectal fistula) in a variety of ways. A typical one is illustrated. R, rectum; B, buttock; A, anus; F, fistula.

COMMON SIGNS AND SYMPTOMS

- Typically, the infant is healthy with a pustule (abscess) in the skin next to the anus.
- On occasion, the area of infection is fairly broad. This causes the area to be quite tender.
- At times the fistula may open and drain by itself.
- A fistula-in-ano typically has a cycle of opening, healing, and then opening again.

DIAGNOSIS

- This can be made by taking a detailed history and doing a thorough physical examination.
- If there is an abscess present, it's usually too painful to palpate the area. If there is chronic drainage, however, the area can be examined gently to feel for the tract.

○ TREATMENT

- An intial abscess around the anus in infants is best treated with incision and drainage of the pus. Antibiotics may also be given for extensive infection.
- If an abscess comes back at the same site, this suggests that a fistula-in-ano is present, namely, that a tract (a tunnel) is present between the inside (the rectum) and the outside (the skin around the anus).
- In such a situation, an operation is necessary to correct the problem.

PREOPERATIVE PREPARATION

- Do not give your child anything to eat or drink for 4 hours before the operation.

□ OPERATION

- The operation will be done under a general anesthesia and on an outpatient basis.
- The fistula will be removed, and the wound will be left open. It will heal by itself in about 1 week. The operation generally takes 1 hour.

POSTOPERATIVE CARE

- Resume the usual activities and diet.
- Bathe the child in the usual manner. If there is no bowel movement in 2 days, a mild laxative may be necessary (example: milk of magnesia).

✆ CALL OUR OFFICE IF

- There are any unusual signs or symptoms.
- The incision becomes red and swollen again.
- There is persistent constipation.
- The child develops a temperature higher than 101°F.
- You have any questions.

AORTA: Abdominal Aneurysm

△ GENERAL INFORMATION

An *aortic aneurysm* is a bulge in the aorta (Fig. 1), the main vessel that comes from the heart. The aorta (Fig. 1) passes through the abdomen, gives off branches to various organs along the way, and then divides into the vessels going to the legs. Normally, it is about as big as a broomstick (Fig. 2). Aortic aneurysms occur mostly in older people and are 10 times more common in men. The usual cause is hardening of the arteries *(atherosclerosis)*.

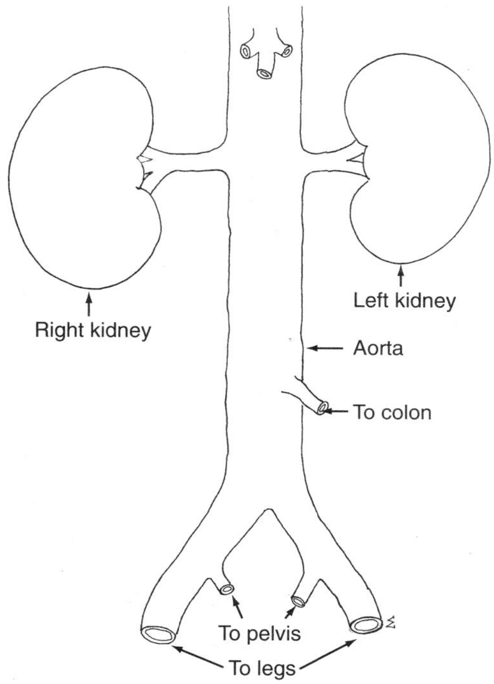

Figure 1. Normal aorta.

COMMON SIGNS AND SYMPTOMS

- Most aneurysms do not produce symptoms; they are found by the doctor during a routine examination.
- If there are symptoms, usually it is discomfort to pain in the middle of the abdomen. Later, the pain can be severe and can be in the back or on the side.
- An aortic aneurysm has a strong tendency to get larger. If it has reached a size of 2 inches and is not treated—even though it produces no symptoms—there is a good chance it will rupture within 1 year.
- If the aneurysm already has produced symptoms and is not removed, there is about a 75% chance that it will rupture and kill the person.

DIAGNOSIS

- An aneurysm usually can be felt during a physical examination of the abdomen if it has bulged up to 2 inches. Obesity can make detection very difficult.
- Often, an x-ray of the abdomen can be most helpful in showing the calcium in the wall of the aneurysm.
- Ultrasound: Harmless sound waves are aimed at the abdomen. The sound waves bouncing back (the echoes) from this area are seen as a picture on a screen. This is a convenient, painless, and harmless way to examine the aorta to see how wide it is and to see the blood vessels coming from it. Also, other organs and tissues in the abdomen can be seen.
- CT scan (computed tomography scan): These special x-rays are taken as very thin slices through the abdominal organs to include the aorta. This makes it possible to see the fine details in the aorta and the vessels coming from it.

○ TREATMENT

- If an aortic aneurysm is smaller than 2 inches and does not produce symptoms, it may be reasonable just to follow it closely.
- If the aneurysm is producing symptoms or is larger than 2 inches, it must be removed because of the high risk that it will rupture. If this happens, the probability is high that the rupture will be fatal. After careful consideration of all factors, the recommendation is that you have an operation to remove the aneurysm.

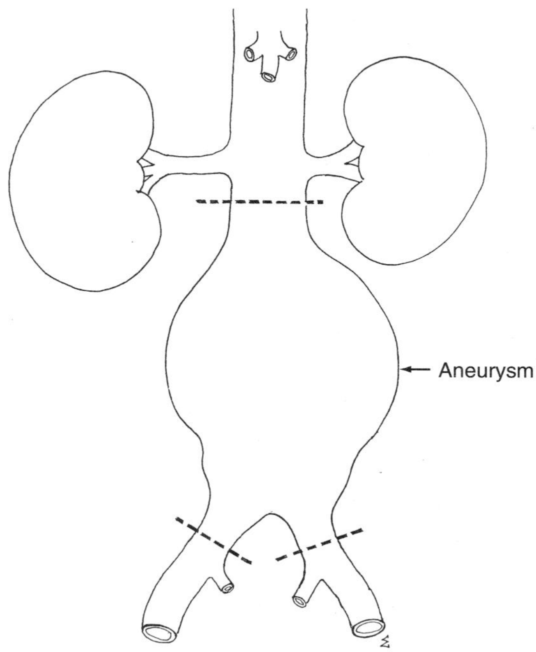

Figure 2. Aneurysm of aorta. Dashed lines indicate where it will be resected and replaced with a graft.

PREOPERATIVE PREPARATION

- You will be checked very carefully for other possible problems, especially those caused by hardening of the arteries. The arteries to your brain, your heart, your kidneys, and your legs will receive special attention.

- The kidneys also will be examined carefully.
- Do not eat or drink anything for 8 hours before the operation.

☐ OPERATION

- You will be asleep for the operation.
- During the operation, the aneurysm will be removed and replaced by a tube graft made of strong synthetic material (Fig. 3).
- You will not receive a blood transfusion unless it is absolutely necessary.
- The operation usually takes 4 hours.

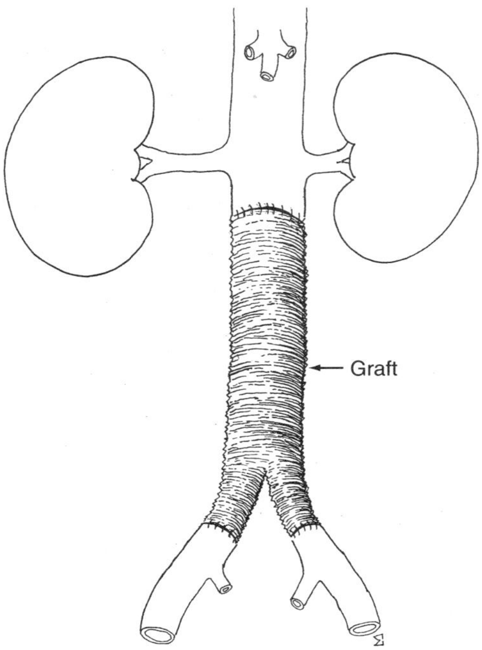

Figure 3. Appearance after aneurysm is removed and replaced with a graft.

POSTOPERATIVE

- You will be taken to the Surgical Care Unit, where the doctors and nurses are very experienced in taking care of patients who have had this operation. As soon as you are coming along well enough, you will be transferred to a regular hospital room.
- You will have a thin plastic tube in your nose for a few days until your bowels start working.
- Pain will be controlled with medicine.
- That evening you will be helped to sit up in bed and on the next day to get out of bed.
- After the thin plastic tube in your nose is removed, you will start on a liquid diet and then eat more solid food as you tolerate it.
- As with any operation, complications are always possible. With your type of operation they can include heart attack, infection, blood clots, and possibly others.
- There is about a 35% chance that your sexual potency will be lowered following this operation. If you wish we can discuss this further.
- You should be able to go home in 1 week.
- Arrangements will be made for your medicines and follow-up office visit.

✙ HOME CARE

- Continue with the program started while you were in the hospital.
- You may walk about as you wish, even climb stairs, but don't overdo things.
- Unless advised otherwise, you may shower as you wish and with any dressings on or off. After you dry yourself, replace any dressings with clean, dry ones.
- Take the medicines prescribed for you.
- You may eat as you wish.
- Include plenty of roughage and liquids in your diet to help prevent constipation.
- Do not drive a car or return to work until we first talk about it during your follow-up visit.

✆ CALL OUR OFFICE IF

- You develop abdominal swelling, diarrhea, or a change in the appearance of your feet.
- The incision becomes red or swollen, or there is drainage from it.
- You develop a temperature higher than 100°F.
- You have any questions.

△ GENERAL INFORMATION

The aorta is the large artery (about the size of a broomstick) that comes off the heart and goes down through the chest and into the abdomen, giving off branches along the way. At about the level of the umbilicus, it divides into two arteries that supply blood to the organs in the pelvis and to the legs (Fig. 1).

Sometimes the aorta becomes narrow because of cholesterol deposits *(atheromas)* on its wall (called *atherosclerosis*). This narrowing prevents enough blood from getting to the organs in the pelvis and, finally, the legs.

This condition affects mostly men between the ages of 45 and 60 years.

COMMON SIGNS AND SYMPTOMS

- There is extreme tiredness of the legs and painful buttocks.
- There can be some thinning of the legs, loss of hair, or breakdown of the skin.
- The legs and feet are pale.
- Sometimes a man cannot maintain an erection of the penis during sexual intercourse.
- The pulses in the legs are weak.

DIAGNOSIS

- Usually, the diagnosis can be made by taking a detailed history, doing a thorough physical examination, and considering the laboratory report.
- Ultrasound: Harmless sound waves are aimed at the area of your abdominal aorta and its branches. The sound waves bouncing back (the echoes) from this area are seen as a picture on a screen. Ultrasound is a quick, easy, and harmless way to examine the arteries in this area of your body.
- The pressures of the arm arteries will be compared with those of the ankle arteries. Normally, they are equal. Usually, with the problem you have, the ankle pressures are lower.
- Arteriography: Contrast dye is injected into the aorta, and x-ray pictures are taken of it as it travels through the abdominal aorta and its branches to your legs. This makes it possible to see the location of the blockage and how serious it may be and to determine where to connect the artificial artery (the graft) to get the best results.

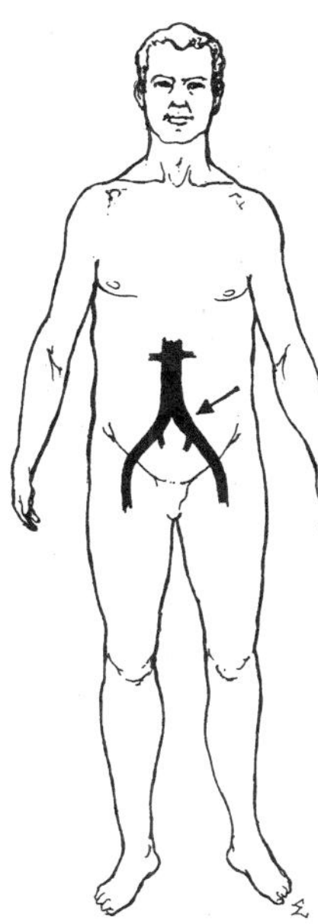

Figure 1. Arrow indicates a common site of blockage of the aorta.

○ TREATMENT

- This condition usually does not come on suddenly. It may take 5 to 10 years to reach the point described above.
- When a person's condition reaches a certain point, however, a new connection needs to be made to get blood to the legs and to relieve pain.

PREOPERATIVE PREPARATION

- Your blood, urine, heart (EKG), lungs (chest x-ray), and arteries to the brain will be examined with special care.
- Do not eat or drink anything for 8 hours before the operation.
- You may be asked to take a cathartic to clean out your bowels the day before the operation.
- Shower (and shave) as usual on the morning of the operation.
- You will be given medicine that will make you feel drowsy before you are brought to the operating room.

□ OPERATION

- All of your abdomen and both of your legs will be painted with an antiseptic solution and covered with sterile drapes.
- The abdomen will be opened and the aorta examined to locate a spot on it that is *above* the blockage.
- An incision will be made over the *femoral* artery in both groins to locate a spot *past* the blocked area.
- When the spots on the aorta and the femoral artery are found, a synthetic tube (a graft) will be used to make a new connection from the aorta to the femoral arteries. In this way, the flow of blood to the pelvis and the legs will be improved (Fig. 2). Occasionally, both femoral arteries may be narrowed and need to have more blood brought to them.
- You will not receive a blood transfusion unless it is absolutely necessary.
- The operation generally takes about 3 hours.

POSTOPERATIVE CARE

- You will be taken to the Surgical Care Unit, where the doctors and nurses are very experienced in taking

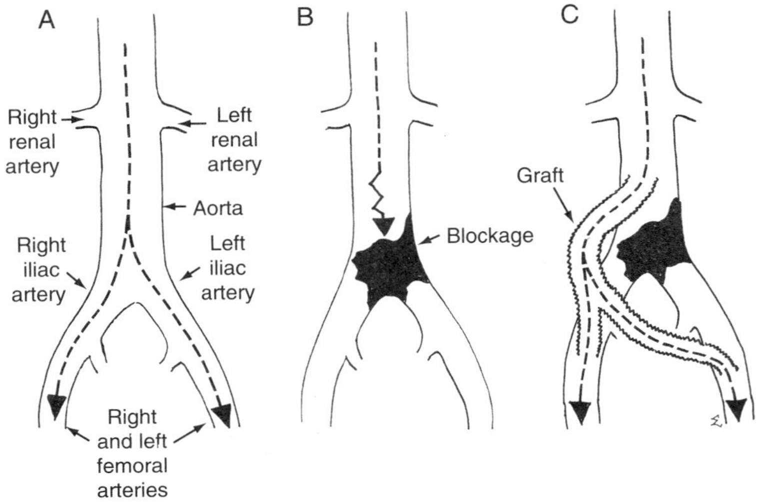

Figure 2. There are a number of ways to bypass a blocked area in the artery to get better blood flow to the leg. A common method is shown. *A*, normal aorta; *B*, blocked aorta; *C*, blockage bypassed with a graft.

care of patients like yourself. As soon as you are coming along well enough, you will be transferred to a regular hospital room.

- You will have a thin, plastic tube in your nose. It was placed there while you were asleep. The tube will be removed as soon as your bowels start working.
- Pain can be controlled with medicine. The nurse will give it to you, or you can give yourself a preset amount of pain medicine when you feel you need it. This is done using patient-controlled analgesia (PCA) that is connected to the tubing giving you intravenous fluids.
- That evening you will be helped to sit up in bed and on the next day to get out of bed.
- You may be given an incentive spirometer. Breathing into this as you are instructed will help expand your lungs and reduce the risk of developing pneumonia.
- You should be able to go home in about 5 to 7 days.
- As with any operation, complications are always possible. With your type of operation, they can include wound infection, blood clots, pneumonia, and clot forming in the graft, among others.
- Arrangements will be made for your medicine, follow-up office visit, and stitch or clip removal.

✚ HOME CARE

- Continue with the program started while you were in the hospital.
- You may walk about as you wish, even climb stairs, but don't overdo things.
- Don't lift anything. Ask someone to do it for you.
- You may shower as you wish and with any dressings on or off.
  - There may be narrow strips of tape across the incision. It's all right if they get wet. They will be removed in the doctor's office.
  - After you dry yourself, replace any dressings with clean, dry ones.
- You may eat as you did before the operation.
- Be careful that you do not become constipated.
  - Include enough roughage and liquids in your diet.
  - You may need a mild laxative (example: milk of magnesia).
- Your incision and the muscles of the abdomen may ache, especially at the end of the day and after you have been standing for a long period. You can support them by wearing a girdle or similar garment that is snug (but not too tight). Wearing it over a cotton undergarment is easier on your incision and the stitches.
- Driving a car with an automatic shift is not too demanding. But if you suddenly have to slam on the brakes or twist to turn a wheel, you may strain the sutures or tear something. Remind me during the follow-up visit to discuss with you when you can resume driving.
- You may return to work when you are certain you are up to it. This should not be before 1 month, and you should begin on a part-time basis.
- You may resume sexual activity whenever you choose.
- The "graft" that was placed is durable, and you can expect it to be safe for the rest of your life.

✆ CALL OUR OFFICE IF

- You develop severe pain in your legs.
- The incisions become red or swollen, or there is drainage from them.
- You develop a temperature higher than 100°F.
- You have any questions.

△ GENERAL INFORMATION

The end of your small intestine empties into the beginning of your large bowel that is located in the right part of your lower abdomen. From this beginning part of your large bowel hangs the appendix. It is a tube about 5 inches long and a little thicker than a pencil (Fig. 1). If this tube becomes plugged and infected, appendicitis can develop. Acute appendicitis is the most common emergency surgical condition of the abdomen.

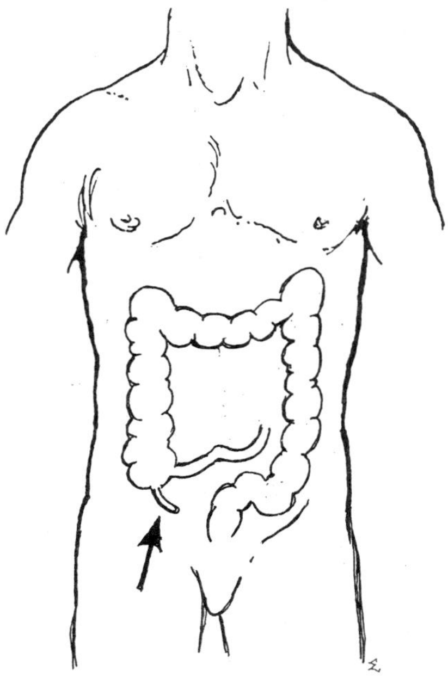

Figure 1.

Appendicitis occurs at all ages and in both sexes but is more common between the ages of 10 and 45 years. It is uncommon for appendicitis to get well by itself or with the use of antibiotics. Most of the time it continues to get worse and may even lead to gangrene and peritonitis.

COMMON SIGNS AND SYMPTOMS

- There usually is pain in the pit of your stomach.
- You may experience loss of appetite or nausea and even vomiting.
- In a few hours the pain shifts to your lower abdomen, usually the right side, and soon this area becomes tender when one presses down on it.
- In a later stage, the pain is severe and may spread to other areas of the abdomen.
- There is fever, but usually your temperature is not much higher than 100°F.

DIAGNOSIS

- If anyone has the above complaints, there should be concern about appendicitis. It is important to remember that *not all* cases of appendicitis follow the same pattern of signs and symptoms. Also, many conditions can look like appendicitis. Because appendicitis can become so serious if it is not treated properly, it is important for someone with these symptoms to be seen by a doctor early. Other possible conditions that look like appendicitis may become dangerous even faster than appendicitis.
- Taking a very careful history and performing a thorough physical examination are the most important ways to make a correct diagnosis.
- A blood analysis is ordered to see whether you have an infection or another organ in your body is the cause of your problem. Your urine will be examined for any pus or blood. A chest x-ray will be done (pneumonia in children can look like appendicitis).
- An x-ray of your abdomen may be done to see whether gallstones are present or your intestine might be perforated.
- A rectal examination will be done to determine whether any swelling can be felt with the tip of the finger, or there is tenderness in this area.
- An internal (pelvic) examination is done in women to see whether the female organs are inflamed.
- An ultrasound of your abdomen may be done. This consists of bouncing harmless sound waves off your abdomen to look for any abnormalities inside.
- By doing at least all of the above, other possible causes of your problem can be eliminated. They include gastroenteritis, swelling of the lymph nodes in this area (more often seen in children after a viral infection), infection of the tubes of the uterus, pregnancy in a tube, endometriosis (in women), inflammation of the small bowel (Crohn's disease), inflammation of the large bowel (diverticulitis), perforated ulcer, or inflammation of the gallbladder.
- The diagnosis can never be made with 100% certainty. If it is a close call, it is safer to operate than to risk having an infected appendix rupture.

○ TREATMENT

The treatment for appendicitis is an operation to remove the appendix. The appendix can be removed in one of two ways:

- **Open Technique:** Usually, a 2- to 3-inch incision is made over the appendix, the abdomen entered, and the appendix removed.
- **Laparoscopic Technique:** The *laparoscope* is an optical instrument that is as big around as your little finger and that has a light at its tip. Three or possibly four laparoscopes are inserted into the abdomen through incisions as wide as your fingernail. The infected appendix is dissected free and removed through one of the holes. The advantages to this method are less pain after the operation and less visible scars. Sometimes it is found at operation that your appendix cannot be removed safely by the laparoscope. In such an instance, a regular incision is made.

After considering all factors, the recommendation is

that you have your appendix removed by a laparoscope.

PREOPERATIVE PREPARATION

- You will also have an examination of your urine, heart (EKG), and lungs (chest x-ray).
- Fluids will be started through your vein to make up for what you didn't drink, or for what you lost before you came to the hospital.
- Be certain to tell the doctor or nurse of any allergies you have or medicines you are taking, including aspirin.
- Now that the diagnosis is made, you will be given pain medicine to make you comfortable.
- You must not take anything by mouth until after the operation.
- You may be given some medicine that will make you feel drowsy before you are brought into the operating room.

□ OPERATION

- You will be asleep for the operation.
- The operation usually takes about 1 hour.
- You will not need a blood transfusion.

POSTOPERATIVE CARE

- You will be taken to a recovery room. When you are awake and your blood pressure, pulse, and breathing are stable, you will be taken to a regular hospital room.
- Any pain can be controlled easily with medicines that you can ask the nurse for or even give to yourself.
- You might have a thin plastic tube in your nose. It goes down to your stomach to suck up the air you swallow. It will be removed when your bowels start working.
- That evening you will be helped to sit up in bed and on the next day to get out of bed.
- You should be able to go home in 1 to 2 days, depending on how seriously your appendix or surrounding tissue was infected.
- As with any operation, complications are always possible. With this type of operation, they can include wound infection, peritonitis, bowel obstruction, and possibly others.
- Arrangements will be made for your medicine, follow-up office visit, and stitch removal.

✚ HOME CARE

- You may walk about as you wish, even climb stairs, but don't overdo things.
- Take medicine as prescribed for your pain.
- You may eat as you did before the operation. Include enough roughage and plenty of fluids in your diet to help avoid constipation.
- You may shower if you wish and with any dressings on or off.
    - There may be narrow strips of tape across the incisions. It's all right if they get wet; they will be removed in the doctor's office.
    - After you dry yourself, replace any dressings with clean, dry ones.
- Your incision and the muscles of the abdomen may ache, especially at the end of the day and after you have been standing for a long period. This will get better soon.
- During your follow-up visit, let's talk about when you can resume driving.
- You may resume sexual activity whenever you choose.
- You may return to work when you feel up to it, but let's talk about it first during your follow-up office visit.

✆ CALL OUR OFFICE IF

- The incisions become more painful, red, or swollen, or there is drainage from them.
- You develop a temperature higher than 100°F.
- You do not have a bowel movement within 2 days.
- You have any questions.

△ GENERAL INFORMATION

The end of your small intestine empties into the beginning of your large bowel that is located in the right part of your lower abdomen. From this beginning part of your large bowel hangs the appendix. It is a tube about 5 inches long and a little thicker than a pencil (Fig. 1). If this tube becomes plugged and infected, appendicitis can develop. Acute appendicitis is the most common emergency surgical condition of the abdomen.

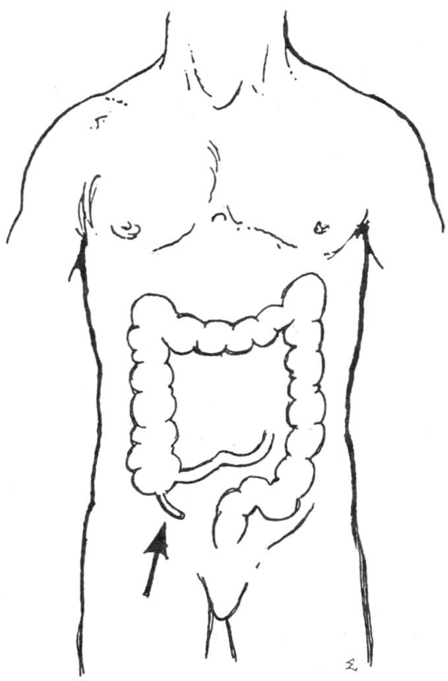

Figure 1. An infected appendix can be in a number of positions and locations in the right side of the lower abdomen. The most typical location is shown.

Appendicitis occurs at all ages and in both sexes but is more common between the ages of 10 and 45 years. It is uncommon for appendicitis to get well by itself or with the use of antibiotics. Most of the time it continues to get worse and may even lead to gangrene and peritonitis.

COMMON SIGNS AND SYMPTOMS

- There usually is pain in the pit of the stomach.
- You may experience loss of appetite or nausea and even vomiting.
- In a few hours the pain shifts to your lower abdomen, usually the right side, and soon this area becomes tender when one presses down on it.
- In a later stage, the pain is severe and may spread to other areas of the abdomen.
- There is fever, but usually your temperature is not much higher than 100°F.

DIAGNOSIS

- If anyone has the above complaints, there should be concern about appendicitis. It is important to remember that *not all* cases of appendicitis follow the same pattern of signs and symptoms. Also, many conditions can look like appendicitis. Because appendicitis can become so serious if it is not treated properly, it is important for someone with these symptoms to be seen by a doctor early. Other possible conditions that look like appendicitis may become dangerous even faster than appendicitis.
- Taking a very careful history and performing a thorough physical examination are the most important ways to make a correct diagnosis.
- A blood analysis is ordered to see whether you have an infection or another organ in your body is the cause of your problem. Your urine will be examined for any pus or blood. A chest x-ray will be done (pneumonia in children can look like appendicitis).
- An x-ray of your abdomen may be done to see whether gallstones are present or your intestine might be perforated.
- A rectal examination will be done to determine whether any swelling can be felt with the tip of the finger, or there is tenderness in this area.
- An internal (pelvic) examination is done in women to see whether the female organs are inflamed.
- An ultrasound of your abdomen may be done. This consists of bouncing harmless sound waves off your abdomen to look for any abnormalities inside.
- By doing at least all of the above, other possible causes of your problem can be eliminated. They include gastroenteritis, swelling of the lymph nodes in this area (more often seen in children after a viral infection), infection of the tubes of the uterus, pregnancy in a tube, endometriosis (in women), inflammation of the small bowel (Crohn's disease), inflammation of the large bowel (diverticulitis), perforated ulcer, or inflammation of the gallbladder.
- The diagnosis can never be made with 100% certainty. If it is a close call, it is safer to operate than to risk having an infected appendix rupture.

○ TREATMENT

The treatment for appendicitis is an operation to remove the appendix. The appendix can be removed in one of two ways:

- **Open Technique:** Usually, a 2- to 3-inch incision is made over the appendix, the abdomen entered, and the appendix removed.
- **Laparoscopic Technique:** The laparoscope is an optical instrument that is as big around as your little finger and that has a light at its tip. Three or possibly four laparoscopes are inserted into your abdomen through incisions as wide as your fingernail. The infected appendix is dissected free and removed through one of the holes. The advantages to this

method are less pain after the operation and a less visible scar.

Sometimes, it is found at operation that your appendix cannot be removed safely by the laparoscope. In such an instance, a regular incision is made.

After careful consideration of all factors, the recommendation is that your appendix should be removed through an incision that opens your abdomen.

PREOPERATIVE PREPARATION

- You will have an examination of your urine, heart (EKG), and lungs (chest x-ray).
- Fluids will be started through your vein to make up for what you didn't drink or for what you lost before you came to the hospital.
- Be certain to tell the doctor or nurse of any allergies you have or medicines you are taking, including aspirin.
- Now that the diagnosis is made, you will be given pain medicine to make you comfortable.
- You must not take anything by mouth until after the operation.
- You may be given some medicine that will make you feel drowsy before you are brought into the operating room.

□ OPERATION

- You will be asleep for the operation.
- Your incision will be in the right lower part of your abdomen.
- The operation usually takes about 1 hour.
- You will not need a blood transfusion.

POSTOPERATIVE CARE

- You will be taken to a recovery room. When you are awake and your blood pressure, pulse, and breathing are stable, you will be taken to a regular hospital room.
- Pain will be controlled with medicine. The nurse will give it to you, or you can give yourself a preset amount of pain medicine when you feel you need it. This is done with a device called patient-controlled analgesia (PCA) that is connected to the tubing giving you intravenous fluids.
- You might have a thin plastic tube in your nose. It goes down to your stomach to suck up the air you swallow. It will be removed when your bowels start working.
- That evening you will be helped to sit up in bed and on the next day to get out of bed.
- You should be able to go home in 2 to 4 days, depending on how seriously your appendix or surrounding tissue was infected.
- As with any operation, complications are always possible. With this type of operation, they can include wound infection, peritonitis, bowel obstruction, and possibly others.
- Arrangements will be made for your medicine, follow-up office visit, and stitch or clip removal.

✚ HOME CARE

- You may walk about as you wish, even climb stairs, but don't overdo things.
- Take medicine as prescribed for your pain.
- You may eat as you did before the operation. Include enough roughage and plenty of fluids in your diet to help avoid constipation.
- You may shower if you wish and with any dressings on or off.
  - There may be narrow strips of tape across the incision. It's all right if they get wet; they will be removed in the doctor's office.
  - After you dry yourself, replace any dressings with clean, dry ones.
- Your incision and the muscles of the abdomen may ache, especially at the end of the day and after you have been standing for a long period. This will get better soon.
- Driving a car with an automatic shift may not seem to be too demanding. However, you may have to slam on the brakes or twist to turn the steering wheel and may strain your sutures or tear something. During your follow-up visit let's talk about when you can resume driving.
- You may resume sexual activity whenever you choose.
- You may return to work when you feel up to it, but let's talk about it first during your follow-up office visit.

✆ CALL OUR OFFICE IF

- The incision becomes more painful, red, or swollen, or there is drainage from it.
- You develop a temperature higher than 100°F.
- You do not have a bowel movement within 2 days.
- You have any questions.

ARTERIAL CATHETERIZATION

△ GENERAL INFORMATION

Most patients are familiar with an intravenous (commonly referred to as IV) line, which is a needle connected to a tube that is placed in a vein. Arterial catheterization involves insertion of the catheter into an *artery*, whereas an IV line is placed in a *vein*. Arteries are blood vessels that transport blood *away* from the heart, and veins are vessels that *return* blood to the heart. Arteries have a pulse (you can feel it) and have a higher pressure in them than veins. When blood pressure is measured, it is the blood pressure in the artery that is being measured. Unlike IV lines, arterial catheters are not used for giving fluids or medication. Rather, arterial catheters are used for measurement of blood pressure and sometimes for withdrawing blood samples.

The blood pressure can be measured with a blood pressure cuff or an arterial catheter.

Measuring with a Pressure Cuff: The blood pressure cuff measures the blood pressure by inflating the arm cuff and squeezing the arm tightly enough so that no blood passes by it. The cuff is then deflated slowly, and when a sound can be heard over the artery, this is the *systolic* blood pressure. The pressure at which blood continually passes by the cuff completely freely (and so, no pulse is heard) is the *diastolic* blood pressure. Using a cuff takes 20 seconds or so to measure the blood pressure. Frequent use of a blood pressure cuff to measure the blood pressure places stress on the underlying tissue and can result in tissue and nerve injury. Also, the measurement of blood pressure with a cuff provides an indirect measure of blood pressure and is prone to inaccuracy.

Measuring Pressure with an Arterial Catheter: An arterial catheter is placed inside the artery. The catheter is then connected to what is called a *pressure transducer*, a piece of electronic equipment that measures the blood pressure directly and continually.

REASONS FOR ARTERIAL CATHETERIZATION

Continual Blood Pressure Measurement

- Continual blood pressure measurement is important when the blood pressure changes rapidly. This makes it possible to know immediately what the pressure is and to treat for low or high blood pressure if necessary.
- When anesthesia is administered and an operation performed, the patient's blood pressure may increase or decrease very suddenly. Most patients tolerate such changes in blood pressure well. Measuring the blood pressure using a cuff every 1 to 3 minutes usually is enough to manage the changes in blood pressure. However, if a patient has certain medical conditions that require strict blood pressure control, an arterial catheter is required for continual monitoring.
- Certain operations cause rapid changes in the blood pressure. Operations in which there is the potential for rapid blood loss (for example, liver resection) can quickly drop the blood pressure. Operations involving clamping and unclamping major arteries, such as aorta surgery, can increase or decrease blood pressure dramatically.

Unable to Use Blood Pressure Cuff

- In conditions of very low blood pressure, blood pressure cuff measurements are inaccurate; arterial catheterization is needed.
- Blood pressure cuff measurements in obese individuals may be inaccurate because the cuff must compress more tissue to compress the vessel deep inside this tissue.
- Blood pressure cuff measurements require the heart to be beating to measure the blood pressure. Operations in which a heart-lung machine is used (and the heart is stopped) require an arterial catheter to measure blood pressure.

Frequent Arterial Blood Sampling

- Blood can be withdrawn easily from an arterial catheter for blood analysis. These analyses may have to be repeated several times during an operation. Analysis of arterial blood provides important information about the ability of the lungs to oxygenate blood. Routine analysis of venous blood cannot provide this information.

PERFORMING THE CATHETERIZATION

In the arm there are four arteries that are used for arterial catheterization. The *radial* artery is used most commonly. The radial artery is in the wrist and is the artery that most people feel to take their pulse. It is on the side of the wrist closest to the thumb. The *ulnar* artery (on the side of the wrist farthest from the thumb), *brachial* artery (level of the elbow), and *axillary* artery (in the axilla) can be used for catheterization but usually only if attempts at catheterizing the radial artery are unsuccessful. In the legs, the *dorsalis pedis* and *posterior tibial* arteries can be catheterized in the foot. The *femoral* artery (in the region of the groin) is used frequently.

Placement of an arterial catheter is in many ways similar to placement of an IV line. The skin over the artery is swabbed with an antiseptic solution. A fine, short needle is used to inject an anesthetic in the skin over the artery to make the area numb. Insertion of the arterial catheter is usually performed easily. Occasionally, however, placement of the arterial catheter can be difficult and requires several attempts, using a different artery.

POSSIBLE COMPLICATIONS

Arterial catheterization is often described as a "low risk–high benefit procedure." Even so, as with any procedure, complications are always possible and can include the following:

- **Thrombosis in the Catheterized Artery:** *Thrombosis* (blood clot) formation in the cannulated artery occurs in at least 20% of patients. The arterial thrombosis usually produces no symptoms and resolves by itself within a month. Very rarely, the thrombosed artery prevents adequate blood supply to tissue and may cause permanent damage.

- **Air or Blood Clot Embolization:** Small air bubbles or blood clots may be injected into the arterial catheter unintentionally and travel into the small blood vessels in the hand (if the catheter is placed in the radial artery).
- **Nerve Injury:** Nerve injury during arterial cannulation is unlikely if the radial artery is used. Ulnar, brachial, axillary, and femoral arteries are much closer to nerves that might be injured directly by the needle during catheter placement, and their location is one of the reasons they usually are not the first choice.
- **Infection:** Infection resulting from the use of arterial catheters can occur but is rare.

As you can now appreciate, arterial catheters may have an important role in making some operations safer and more successful.

△ GENERAL INFORMATION

An *arterial* embolus is a blood clot that breaks off from where it formed (most often the heart) and travels to practically anywhere in the body. Most often, however, it gets stuck in the end of the aorta or one of the branches from there such as the femoral artery (Fig. 1). Most patients who have an embolus are elderly and have heart disease or other associated illnesses.

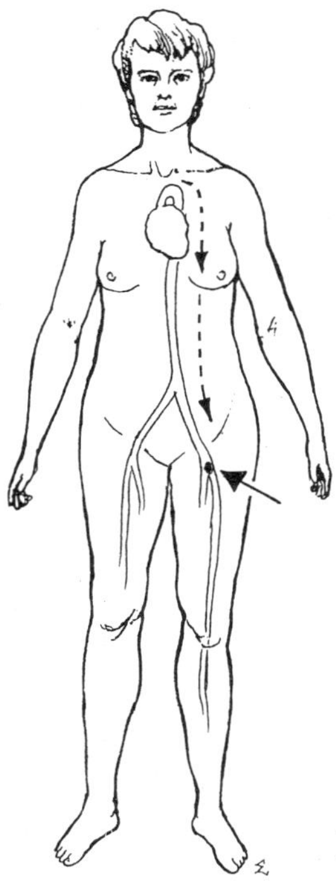

Figure 1. This illustration shows how a blood clot formed in the heart breaks off and travels as an embolus *(dashed line)* down the aorta and gets stuck in the femoral artery *(solid arrow)*.

COMMON SIGNS AND SYMPTOMS

Whatever the symptoms of acute blockage of an artery by an embolus, they are influenced by several factors:

- The exact site of the blockage.
- Whether detour vessels are available as an alternative way for the blood to get where it should go.
- Whether the blockage happens rapidly or slowly or how complete it is and how long it has been present.

The signs and symptoms can be remembered by the five Ps:

- ***Pain*** in the leg that is not receiving enough blood (and oxygen).
- ***Pallor:*** The leg is pale because it is not receiving enough blood.
- ***Paresthesias:*** Decreased sensation of the leg from damage to the nerves.
- ***Paralysis:*** Death of the nerves and muscles involved in moving the leg.
- ***Pulselessness:*** No pulse is felt in the blocked artery.

DIAGNOSIS

- A detailed history of past illnesses and present symptoms is important. This, along with a thorough examination of the entire patient with a focus on the blood vessels that lead to the leg will provide the diagnosis in at least 75% of the patients.
- A comprehensive examination of your blood.

Any or all of the following tests will be performed:

- Doppler ultrasound: Harmless, painless sound waves are directed toward the suspected blood vessels. The sound waves bouncing back (the echoes) are shown on a television screen and can demonstrate the condition inside the blood vessel.
- Arteriography: A contrast fluid is injected into the artery and x-rays taken of it as it flows throughout the artery. It can provide critical information on the location and extent of the blockage.
- Examination of the heart (EKG) and lungs (chest x-ray) will show the condition of these organs and can help demonstrate the source of the embolus.

○ TREATMENT

Most commonly, the treatment for embolus is an operation, but there are exceptions. Also, although an operation is the main treatment for the embolus, the related medical conditions often pose as great a risk as an operation.

After careful consideration of all factors, the recommendation is that you have an operation to try to correct your embolus problem.

- Most of the time, the sooner the operation is done, the better the chance for success. If at all possible, it should be done within 12 hours, but there are exceptions. If there is numbness or paralysis, the operation should be done within 4 to 6 hours for the best chance to save the leg.
- Time permitting, every effort will be made to correct any associated medical problems as much as possible.
- Fluids will be started in the vein.
- Anticoagulants (blood thinners) will be started.
- A very thin plastic tube will be placed in the vein that leads to the heart so that the workings of your heart and your lung can be observed carefully.
- A catheter will be placed in the bladder to measure and regulate the amount of urine being made. The kidneys can suffer greatly in this situation. The leg will be protected from heat, cold, and pressure, because the tissues are very vulnerable to damage in such situations.
- You will not receive anything by mouth before the operation.

□ OPERATION

- The aim of the operation is to remove all of the embolus.
- The type of anesthesia used will depend on the circumstances at that time.
- The operation to remove the embolus can be simple

and uncomplicated, or it can be difficult to remove all of the embolus without prolonged, tedious, and careful surgery. For this reason, the operation can take 1 to 2 hours or several times longer.

- Often, an arteriogram is performed on the operating table to document that the artery has been opened.

POSTOPERATIVE CARE

- You will be taken to the Surgical Care Unit, where the doctors and nurses are experienced in taking care of patients like yourself. As soon as you are coming along well enough, you will be transferred to a regular hospital room.
- The doctors and nurses will be checking the pulses of your leg at very short intervals to be certain the circulation (the blood flow) is adequate.
- Pain will be controlled with medicine.
- Your diet will be as you tolerate it.
- You will be helped to get out of bed as soon as possible.
- Your stay in the hospital will depend on the operation performed and how swiftly you recover from it.
- As with any operation, complications are always possible, some of them serious. With your type of operation, they can include reoperation because the artery has clotted again, infection, bleeding, heart problems, blood clots, and possibly others.

✣ HOME CARE

- Continue with the program started while you were in the hospital.
- Be certain to take the medicines prescribed for you.
- Your diet can be as you tolerate it.
- You will be instructed on bathing or showering.
- Arrangements can be made for a home visiting nurse if one is needed.
- Do not drive until we first discuss it during your postoperative office visit.

✆ CALL OUR OFFICE IF

- Any of the symptoms that caused you to see the doctor in the first place return.
- The incision becomes red or swollen, or there is drainage from it.
- You develop a temperature higher than 100°F.
- You have any questions.

△ GENERAL INFORMATION

The armpit *(axilla)* has many lymph nodes in it. These lymph nodes normally strain the fluid (called *lymph*) that passes through them as it comes from the arm, the breast, and the chest wall on that side. As part of their job, they also strain cancer cells from these same areas and begin to swell as they fill with these cells.

The purpose of dissecting out the lymph nodes in the axilla (the operation is called *axillary dissection*) is to remove lymph nodes that are suspected or are known to have cancer in them. Otherwise, the cancer cells may escape from the lymph node and spread to other areas of the body.

COMMON SIGNS AND SYMPTOMS

- There is no set number of lymph nodes in the axilla (or in any location in the body), just as there is no set number of hairs in your scalp.
- Most of the time, lymph nodes are small, but often a few can be felt (especially in a thin person) even though there is nothing wrong with them; they are normal.
- When a lymph node strains lymph that has infected material or cancer cells in it, the lymph node swells. It can swell to the size of an olive or larger. Often many lymph nodes in the area swell.

DIAGNOSIS

A detailed history and thorough physical examination will often provide the answer on the nature of lymph nodes that can be felt. However, swollen lymph nodes in the axilla might *not* contain cancer. The lymph nodes might be swollen because of a mild infection, or they might be responding to something else in the body. Also, lymph nodes may be small because the cancer in them is not yet large.

A decision often needs to be made on what is in an enlarged lymph node or what to do with lymph nodes that are not enlarged but are still likely to have cancer in them.

- The surest way to know about the nature of an enlarged lymph node is to remove a piece of it for microscopic examination. A common method of doing this is to place a needle in the suspicious lymph node and remove a tiny piece of it (called an *aspiration* biopsy). However, if such a tiny piece is negative for cancer, there is the risk that cancer actually is present in the lymph node but not in the area of the lymph node sampled by the needle.
- Before a decision is made to do an axillary dissection, tests will be done to be as certain as possible that cancer is not in other areas of your body such as the lungs, bones, liver, and others.

○ TREATMENT

After careful consideration of all factors in your case, it is recommended that you have an axillary dissection.

PREOPERATIVE PREPARATION

- You will have an examination of your blood, urine, heart (EKG), and lungs (chest x-ray), as well as other indicated tests.
- Do not eat or drink anything for 8 hours before the operation.

□ OPERATION

- You will be asleep for the operation.
- Tissue that contains lymph nodes will be removed from an area in your armpit that is bordered by specific muscles and blood vessels (Fig. 1).
- You will not need a blood transfusion.
- The operation usually takes about 1½ hours.

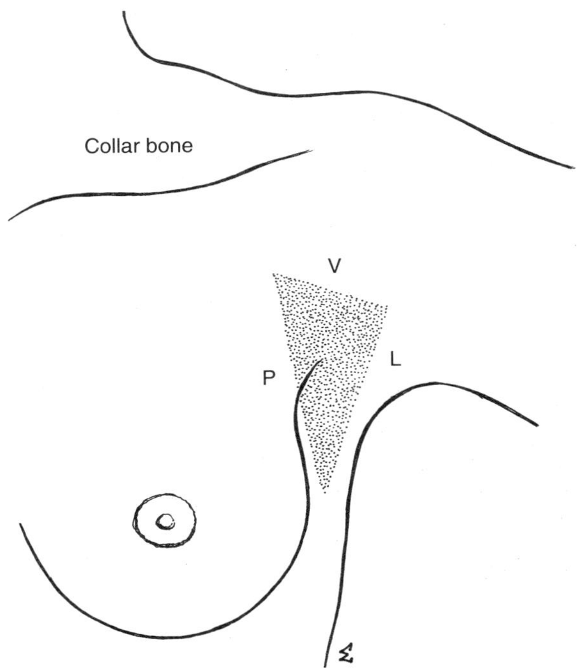

Figure 1. During an axillary dissection, it is not a specific number of lymph nodes that are removed but the lymph nodes within a specific area. Customarily, the area is bounded by the axillary vein (V) on the top, the pectoral muscles (P) on the middle side, and the latissimus muscle (L) on the outer side.

POSTOPERATIVE CARE

- You will be taken to a recovery room and observed. When your blood pressure, pulse, and breathing are stable and you are completely alert, you may be able to go home that same day. Otherwise, you will go home the following day.
- Pain will be controlled with medicine.
- A thin plastic tube may be coming out of the wound to drain any extra fluid in the area. You will be shown how to take care of it; it's not difficult.
- Arrangements will be made for your medicine, follow-up office visit, and drain and stitch removal.

- As with any operation, complications are always possible. With this type of operation, they can include bleeding, collection of fluid in the axilla, infection, and possibly others.

✚ HOME CARE

- Resume your usual activities except for those that require excessive use of the arm on the side of the operation.
- You may walk about as you wish, even climb stairs.
- Limit any activity that requires use of the arms on the operated side.
- Sponge bathe until after the drain is removed.
- Do not begin any arm exercises until you are shown how to do them by the surgeon.
- Even though all the lymph nodes were removed, there still are enough lymph channels in this area to drain your arm under normal conditions. Just the same, those that are left behind can be hurt by infection in the wound, x-ray therapy to the axilla, and repeated hard work for long periods with the affected arm (e.g., using that arm to pull weeds for 2 to 3 hours).
- Occasionally the hand or forearm will swell. There are treatments for this.
- You should not drive your car until you can move your arm freely and without pain.
- You may return to work when you feel up to it.

✆ CALL OUR OFFICE IF

- The axilla becomes swollen, or there is drainage from the incision.
- You develop a temperature higher than 100°F.
- You develop any swelling or redness of the hand or arm.
- You have any questions.

BARIUM ENEMA (LOWER GASTROINTESTINAL)

△ GENERAL INFORMATION

A barium enema (lower GI) is a valuable way to examine the large bowel (Fig. 1–1) for a number of things that may be wrong with it.

HOW A BARIUM ENEMA WORKS

- The barium used is the color and consistency of buttermilk.
- An x-ray picture of the colon without any preparation would simply look black because the x-rays would pass right through such soft tissue. Barium, however, does not let x-rays pass through it. For this reason, when any barium is placed in the large bowel, and x-rays are taken, the large bowel with barium in it will look white, and everything else around it will be black (Fig. 1–2).
- However, if some growth is in the large bowel (Fig. 1–3), and it keeps the barium from getting to the area occupied by the growth, this part of the large bowel will not appear white; x-rays will pass right through it, and it will appear black (Fig. 1–4).

Radiologists are experts at giving barium enemas and on reading the x-rays. They can pick up lesions as small as a pea.

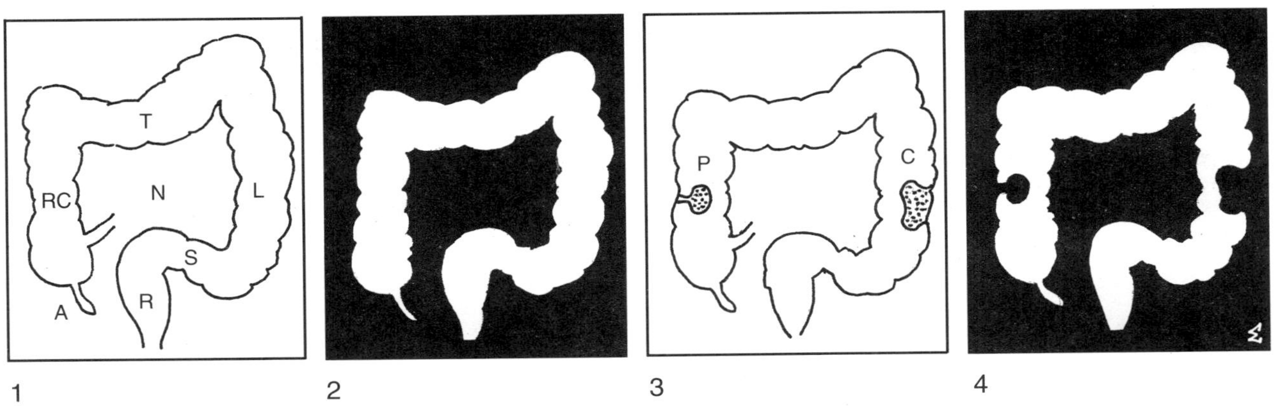

Figure 1. *1,* Anatomy of normal large bowel. A, Appendix; RC, right colon; T, transverse colon; L, left colon; S, sigmoid colon; R, rectum; N, navel. *2,* An x-ray of normal large bowel with barium in it. *3,* Anatomy of large bowel with polyp (P) and cancer (C) in it. *4,* An x-ray of large bowel shown in Part 3 after it has been filled with barium.

PREPARATION FOR A BARIUM ENEMA

The large bowel must be clean; otherwise pieces of stool in it may be mistaken for tumors. One of several ways to clean your bowel is as follows:

- Eat a clear liquid breakfast, lunch, and supper on the day before the examination. Do not drink milk or cream.
- Starting at 1 o'clock on the day before, drink an 8-ounce glass of water. At 6 o'clock, drink a cold, full (10-ounce) bottle of citrate of magnesia. At 7 o'clock swallow whole, four Dulcolax tablets and one full glass or more of water.
- On the morning of the examination:
  - Do not eat breakfast.
  - Use one Dulcolax rectal suppository according to the instructions supplied.
- There may be conditions that would make it advisable to use a different method to cleanse your bowel.
- Vital medications can be taken with a tiny sip of water. Talk with your doctor about taking any diabetic medications before the study.
- Let the doctor know if you are, or think you are, pregnant.

THE PROCEDURE

- You will lie on the x-ray table on your left side.
- A smooth enema tip with petroleum jelly (Vaseline) on it will be inserted in the anus gently and the barium allowed to flow in very much like a regular enema.
- As the radiologist watches the barium flow into your large bowel, x-ray pictures will be taken of important areas and of any suspicious lesions.
- During the examination, the x-ray machine and the x-ray table will move in several directions. Also, you will be asked to roll in various positions.
- You may feel the urge to have a bowel movement, but you should try to hold the barium in the colon.
- You may feel some bowel cramping. If necessary, medicine can be given to relax your bowel during the examination.
- When this part of the examination is completed, the barium will be let out through the same enema tip and tube already in place. If necessary, you also will be able to evacuate additional barium in the bathroom toilet right next to the x-ray room.
- You will be asked to get on the table again for more pictures after you have evacuated the barium. Most of the time a thin film of barium still sticks to the

bowel lining, making it possible to see even more and finer details.

- The entire procedure usually takes less than 1 hour.
- You are free to leave after the examination.
- You are free to eat as usual after the examination.
- Drink plenty of liquids to help you avoid constipation.
- You may be instructed to take a mild laxative.
- The first bowel movement or two will be white because of the barium.

The results of your examination will be reported to your doctor.

△ GENERAL INFORMATION

Bartholin's gland is located immediately outside of the entrance to the vagina. The gland produces a slippery liquid that travels through a very small tube (called a *duct*). This fluid helps keep the entrance to the vagina lubricated. One gland empties on the right side and the other on the left.

Sometimes this small duct gets plugged, and the fluid cannot get out. The duct forms a sac (called a *cyst*) filled with this fluid. This fluid can become infected, producing an *abscess*.

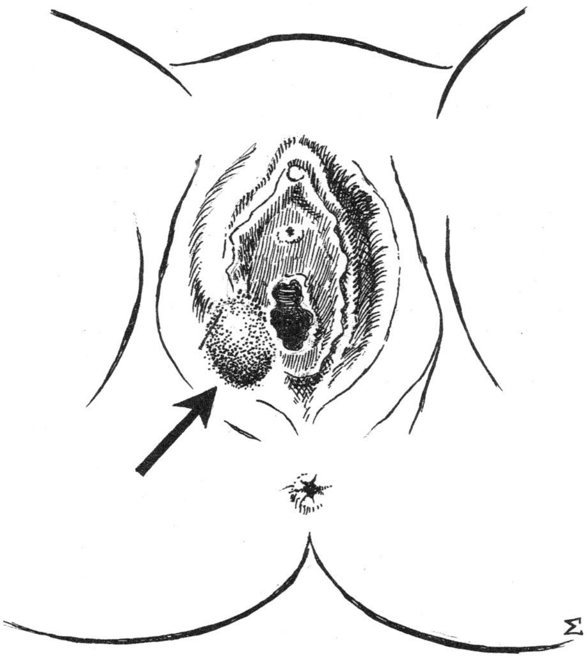

Figure 1. Typical location *(arrow)* of a Bartholin's cyst abscess.

COMMON SIGNS AND SYMPTOMS

- Early on, a Bartholin's gland cyst might not produce any symptoms at all. If it is small, many women don't even know it is there. If it gets larger, it can cause pain with sexual intercourse or with walking and sitting.
- If the cyst becomes infected, it becomes swollen and can be extremely painful to touch.

DIAGNOSIS

- Usually, the diagnosis can be made by taking a detailed history and doing a thorough physical examination.
- The cyst can be seen just next to the opening of the vagina. It can be felt easily with the fingers. It is not usually confused with anything more serious.

THERAPY

- Many Bartholin cysts may be treated conservatively with warm sitz baths. Often this helps the cyst to open and drain on its own.
- Cysts or abscesses that come back usually need an operation.
- The treatment for a Bartholin cyst abscess is to drain the pus in it, or to open it wide and purposely leave it that way (this is called *marsupialization*).
- If a symptomatic Bartholin cyst is not infected, then the treatment is to remove it entirely.
- Abscesses of the gland that come back even though they were drained properly need to be removed after the acute infection is treated.
- After careful consideration of all factors, the recommendation is that you have an operation to correct your problem.

PREOPERATIVE PREPARATION

- An examination of your blood, urine, heart (EKG), and lungs (chest x-ray) may be done.
- Do not eat or drink anything for 8 hours before the operation.
- You may be asked to douche on the morning of the operation.

□ OPERATION

For an Abscess of Bartholin's Cyst

- This may be performed in the doctor's office or as an outpatient procedure.
- You will be positioned on the table, the same as for a pelvic examination.
- The area around the abscess will be painted with an antiseptic solution and draped with sterile towels.
- A very fine short needle will be used to inject an anesthetic in the skin over the abscess. This will make the area numb.
- The abscess will be opened and drained. You should get pain relief very soon. If the abscess is marsupialized, the abscess edges will be sewn open to help prevent recurrence.
- You should be able to go home directly after the operation.
- Arrangements will be made for any antibiotics or pain medicine and for a follow-up office visit.
- The doctor will discuss with you the possibility of having this cyst removed entirely after things quiet down.

For a Noninfected Bartholin Cyst

- You will be given medicine that will make you feel drowsy before you are brought to the operating room.
- The operation will be done under general anesthesia or a spinal-epidural block.
- You will be positioned on the table the same as for a regular pelvic examination.
- The area around the cyst will be painted with an antiseptic solution and draped.
- The entire cyst will be removed and the skin closed with absorbable suture.

- You will wake up in a recovery room. When your blood pressure, pulse, and breathing are stable, you will be taken to a regular hospital room.
- You should be able to go home the next day.
- Arrangements will be made for any antibiotics or pain medicine and for the follow-up office visit.
- As with any operation, complications are always possible. With your type of operation they can include bleeding and infection and possibly others.

✣ HOME CARE

- Resume your usual activities.
- You may eat as you did before the operation.
- You may shower as you wish.
- You may wish to take sitz baths to relieve discomfort in the area.
- Be careful that you do not become constipated.
  - Include enough roughage and liquid in your diet.
  - You may need a mild laxative (example: milk of magnesia), a stool softener (Colace, Surfak), or a glycerine suppository.
- You may return to work when you feel up to it.
- Driving your car is all right, but do not do so if you are taking pain medicine that reduces your alertness.
- During your follow-up visit, let's discuss when you may resume sexual activity.

✆ CALL OUR OFFICE IF

- The area becomes red or swollen, and there is drainage from it.
- You develop a temperature higher than 100°F.
- You have any questions.

BILE DUCT STRICTURE

△ GENERAL INFORMATION

Bile is a fluid that helps to digest the fats you eat. Bile is made in the liver and passes down to your intestine through tubes called bile *ducts*. The main bile duct is about as big around as a pencil. Some of the bile is stored in the gallbladder, and some of it goes straight into the intestine through the main bile duct (Fig. 1).

Sometimes the duct becomes scarred, and it narrows down. This is called a *stricture*. The most common cause of a stricture is scarring of the duct from a previous operation in this area.

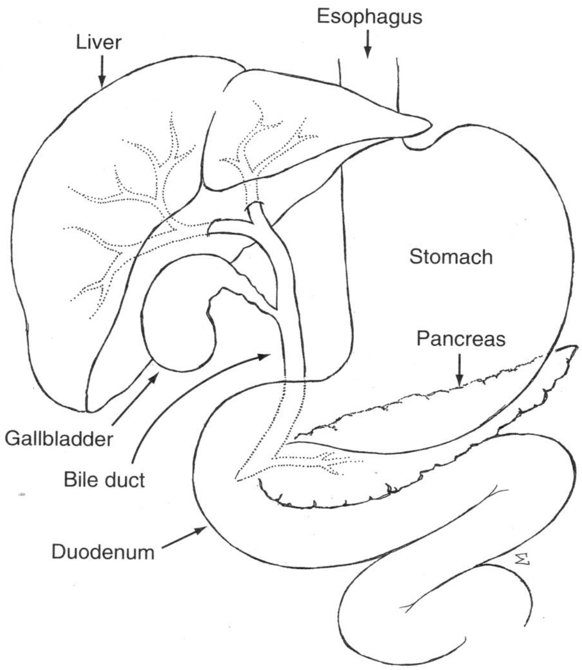

Figure 1.

COMMON SIGNS AND SYMPTOMS

- There may be pain in the upper part of the abdomen, shaking chills and fever, or loss of appetite and weight.
- Jaundice (yellow eyes and skin) occurs because the yellow bile is blocked; instead of being able to get to the intestine, it backs up into the tissues of the body.

DIAGNOSIS

You may have some or all of these tests:

- CT scan (computed tomography scan): These special x-rays are taken by a machine that is shaped like a huge doughnut. You will lie on the table inside the hole in the "doughnut." The x-rays are taken as very thin slices through the area of the liver and bile ducts. This makes it possible to see the fine details in the liver and bile ducts.
- ERC (endoscopic retrograde cholangiogram): This is a way to take pictures of the bile ducts. You will be given medicine into your vein that will make you drowsy, and your mouth and throat will be sprayed with numbing medicine. A narrow, flexible tube called an *endoscope* is then gently and painlessly passed through the mouth and stomach to the end of the bile duct. A liquid that can be seen on x-rays is then injected into the bile ducts and x-rays taken of the stricture (Fig. 2).
- Percutaneous cholangiography: This is another way to get pictures of the bile ducts. You will lie on an x-ray table and be given medicine to make you feel drowsy. The skin over the liver will be made numb. A very fine plastic tube will be passed through the numbed skin, into the liver, and then into a bile duct that is dilated because of the blockage. A special liquid will be placed into the ducts and x-rays taken of them. This can show where the stricture is located and how serious it is. Often, the plastic tube is left so that bile can drain to the outside through the skin to empty into a small plastic bag. This relieves the pressure until the problem can be corrected.

After very careful consideration of all factors, the recommendation is that you have an operation to correct the problem.

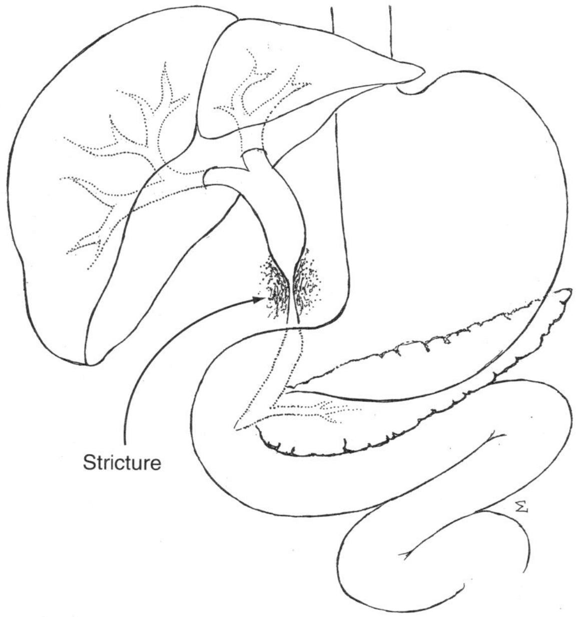

Figure 2. A stricture of the bile duct can vary in extent and location along the duct, so the way it is repaired varies.

PREOPERATIVE PREPARATION

- You will have an examination of at least your blood, urine, heart (EKG), and lungs (chest x-ray).

- Do not eat or drink anything for 8 hours before the operation.
- Shower or bathe as usual on the morning of the operation.
- You may be given medicine that will make you feel drowsy before you are brought to the operating room.
- You will be given antibiotics.

☐ OPERATION

- You will be asleep for the operation.
- The strictured area will be removed and a new connection made.
- You will not receive a blood transfusion unless it is absolutely necessary.
- The operation usually takes about 3 to 4 hours.

POSTOPERATIVE CARE

- You will be taken to the Surgical Care Unit for a few days, where the doctors and nurses are very experienced in taking care of patients like yourself.
- You will have a thin plastic tube in your nose until your bowels start working properly.
- There may be one or two plastic tubes coming out of the skin near the incision to drain local fluids to the outside.
- Pain can be controlled with medicine. The nurse will give it to you, or you can give yourself a preset amount of pain medicine when you feel you need it. This is done using patient-controlled analgesia (PCA) that is connected to the tubing giving you intravenous fluids.
- That evening you will be helped to sit up in bed and on the next day to get out of bed.
- After the tube in your nose is removed, you will be started on liquids that will be advanced to more solid food as you tolerate it.
- As with any operation, complications are always possible. With this type of operation they can include infection, pneumonia, heart problems, and blood clots, among others.
- You should be able to go home in 7 to 10 days.
- Arrangements will be made for your medicine, follow-up office visit, and stitch or clip removal.

✚ HOME CARE

- You may walk about as you wish, even climb stairs, but don't overdo things.
- Continue with the program started while you were in the hospital.
- Take medicine as prescribed for your pain.
- You will be given instructions on when and how you may take showers. In the meantime, take sponge baths.
- Arrangements can be made for a home visiting nurse if one is needed.
- Do not drive your car unless you can move freely without pain and are not taking medicines that reduce your alertness.
- You may resume sexual activity whenever you choose.
- You may return to work when you feel up to it.

✆ CALL OUR OFFICE IF

- The incision becomes red or swollen, or there is drainage from it.
- You develop a temperature higher than 101°F.
- You have any questions.

△ GENERAL INFORMATION

Cancer of the urinary bladder is a difficult challenge, for both the physician and the patient, because it may appear in a number of different ways and several different treatments are available. Also, what may work for one person may not work for another person, even though each has bladder cancer that looks the same. It is important that you realize there's not just one way to treat bladder cancer. Each patient needs to be treated on an individual basis. Cancer of the bladder is seen more often in men and between the ages of 50 and 70 years.

COMMON SIGNS AND SYMPTOMS

- There is blood in the urine.
- The bleeding comes and goes.
- There may be symptoms from irritation of the bladder: urinating frequently, an urge to urinate that must be satisfied without delay, burning or pain when passing urine.

DIAGNOSIS

- A person who has the above history or symptoms should be concerned about a bladder tumor.
- Blood seen in the urine one time must be investigated, even though there is a good chance that nothing serious is wrong.
- Examination of the urine under the microscope should be done to search for cancer cells.
- Intravenous pyelogram (IVP): You will lie on an x-ray table, and a special liquid will be injected into your vein. X-rays will be taken of it as it moves through your kidneys and the tubes *(ureters)* through which urine reaches your bladder. This helps the doctor pick up abnormalities in these areas.
- Cystoscopy: An anesthetic will be squirted into your urethra (the opening into the bladder) to make it numb. The cystoscope will be inserted gently into your urethra and passed into the bladder. If anything suspicious is seen, a small piece of it will be taken (a *biopsy*) for examination in the laboratory.
- There is a good chance that it will not be necessary to do much more than to look inside your bladder.
- You will be free to go home, accompanied by a responsible adult, directly after the cystoscopy.

If a deeper biopsy or a biopsy of more than one area needs to be done, you will need either to be asleep or to have a spinal type of anesthesia. Arrangements will be made to have this done as follows:

- You will have an examination of your blood, urine, heart (EKG), and lungs (chest x-ray).
- Do not eat or drink anything for 8 hours before the cystoscopy.
- Shower or bathe as usual on the morning of the operation.
- The cystoscope will be placed through the urethra and into the bladder, and several biopsies will be taken of areas as follows: the surface of the tumor, to see what type it is; the inside of the tumor, to see how deep it has gone; and the surrounding areas, to see if anything is there.
- All the removed tissue will be sent to the laboratory for thorough examination.

○ TREATMENT

The type of treatment for bladder cancer depends on several things:

- What type of cancer it is.
- Whether the cancer is slow or fast-growing.
- The size of the cancer and how far it has progressed.
- Your health in general.

Your bladder cancer affects the surface as well as the muscle of your bladder. Fortunately, it appears that the tumor is not too large. After considering all factors, it is recommended that part of the bladder wall be removed (Fig. 1).

- This means that your bladder will be smaller but you will be able to urinate in the normal way.
- In time, the bladder may stretch so that you might be able to hold as much urine as you did before the operation.

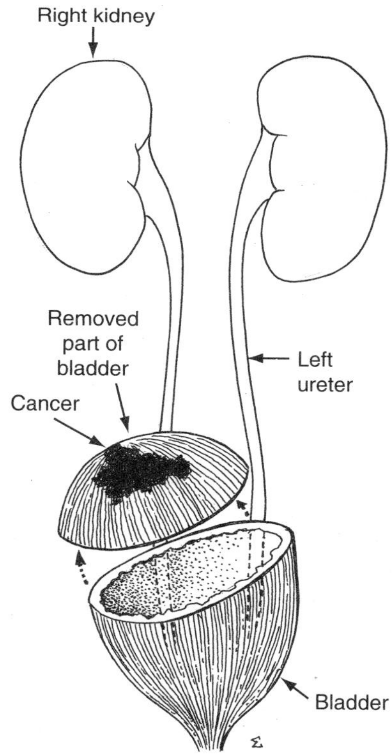

Figure 1.

PREOPERATIVE PREPARATION

- You will have an examination of your blood, urine, heart (EKG), and lungs (chest x-ray). Other tests may be done:

- CT scan (computed tomography scan): These special x-rays are taken as very thin slices through the area of the bladder. This makes it possible to see the fine details in the bladder and determine whether the tumor has spread to the lymph nodes outside the bladder.
- Bone scan: A solution with a tiny amount of a harmless radioactive material is injected in your vein. The solution circulates throughout your entire body and attaches itself to any part of a bone that has something wrong with it. You will lie on a table, and a special machine will pass over your entire body taking a photograph (a *scan*) of all the bones from your skull to your toes. A specialist then examines the scan, looking for any abnormalities in the bones.

- Do not eat or drink anything for 8 hours before the operation.
- Shower or bathe as usual on the morning of the operation.
- You may be given medicine that will make you feel drowsy before you are brought to the operating room.

☐ OPERATION

- A general or spinal anesthetic will be used.
- The incision will be in your lower abdomen. The cancerous part of the bladder will be removed and the hole securely stitched closed.
- The operation usually takes about 3 hours.

POSTOPERATIVE CARE

- You will be taken to a recovery room and observed. When your blood pressure, pulse, and breathing are stable, you will be taken to a regular hospital room.
- You may have a thin plastic tube in your nose. The tube will be removed as soon as your bowels start working.
- A catheter will be in your bladder that will continue to drain your urine.
- You may have a very strong sensation to urinate. This is because your bladder has sutures and a catheter in it. The sensation will lessen with time. If it persists, you will be given some medicine to limit the discomfort.
- Pain can be controlled with medicine.
- The catheter from your bladder will be removed in about 7 to 10 days.
- You should be able to go home in 1 week.
- As with any operation, complications are always possible. With your type of operation, they can include infection, heart attack, blood clots, leakage of urine, blockage of urine, and possibly others.
- Arrangements will be made for your medicine, follow-up visit, stitch removal, and discussion about any additional therapy that might increase your chances for cure.

✚ HOME CARE

- Continue the program started while you were in the hospital.
- You may walk about as you wish, even climb stairs.
- You may eat as you did before the operation.
- Unless instructed otherwise, you may shower as you wish and with any dressings on or off. After you dry yourself, replace any dressings with clean, dry ones.
- Include plenty of roughage and liquids in your diet to help prevent constipation.
- Do not drive a car until we first talk about it during your follow-up office visit.

✆ CALL OUR OFFICE IF

- The catheter in your bladder stops draining urine, or you feel your bladder getting distended.
- You develop a temperature higher than 101°F.
- The incision becomes red or swollen, or there is drainage from it.
- You have any questions.

△ GENERAL INFORMATION

Cancer of the urinary bladder is a difficult challenge because it shows up in a number of different ways and there are several different treatments for it. Also, what may work for one person may not work for another person even though each may have bladder cancer that looks the same. Each patient needs to be treated on an individual basis.

COMMON SIGNS AND SYMPTOMS

- There is blood in the urine; it may come and go.
- There may be frequent urination, an urgency to urinate, or a burning sensation with urination.

DIAGNOSIS

- Examination of the urine is done for blood and for cancer cells.
- Ultrasound: Harmless sound waves are aimed at the bladder. The sound waves bouncing back (the echoes) from this area are seen as a picture on a screen. This is a convenient and painless way to see if anything suspicious is in the bladder. It is an office procedure.
- Cystoscopy: The surest way to make a diagnosis is to examine the bladder with a hollow instrument called a *cystoscope*. It is as big around as a pencil with lenses in it and has a light at its tip.

PREPARATIONS FOR CYSTOSCOPY

If Nothing Suspicious Is Seen on Ultrasound

- Do not eat or drink anything for 4 hours before the cystoscopy.
- The cystoscopy is done in the office as an outpatient procedure.
- An anesthetic is squirted into the urethra to make it numb. The cystoscope will be inserted gently into your bladder. If anything suspicious is seen, a small piece will be taken (a *biopsy*) for examination in the laboratory.
- You will be free to go home after the cystoscopy.

If Something Suspicious Is Seen During the Ultrasound

- You will need to be asleep for this cystoscopy because a deeper biopsy or multiple biopsies may need to be done.
- An examination of your blood, urine, heart (EKG), and lungs (chest x-ray) will be done.
- Do not eat or drink anything for 8 hours before the operation.
- Sometimes, if the tumor is not too large, all of it can be removed through the cystoscope at this time.

○ TREATMENT

The type of treatment for bladder cancer depends on several things: The type of cancer, how fast it is growing, how widely it has spread, and your health in general.

The cancer in your bladder is at a serious stage because it is deep into the muscle of the bladder and affects practically all of the bladder. There is a chance that your bladder cancer can be cured, but this will require major therapy. Basically, two possible treatments have a chance for cure.

Choice Number One

- Your entire bladder and prostate will be removed, and a new bladder will be fashioned from your intestine. The new bladder will need to be emptied with a small tube every 4 to 6 hours or so (Figs. 1 and 2).

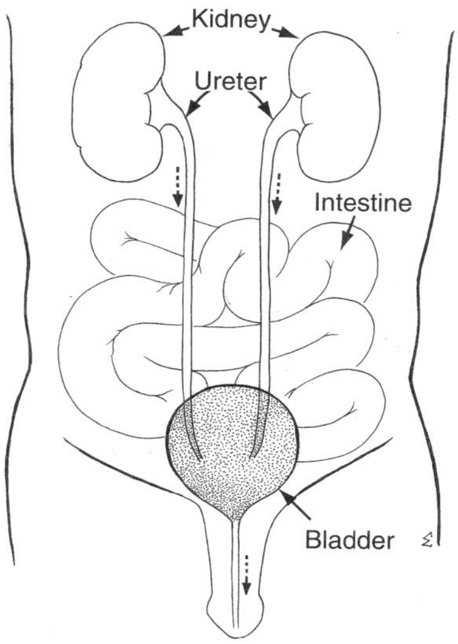

Figure 1. Normal anatomy of the kidneys, ureters, and bladder. Dashed arrows show flow of urine.

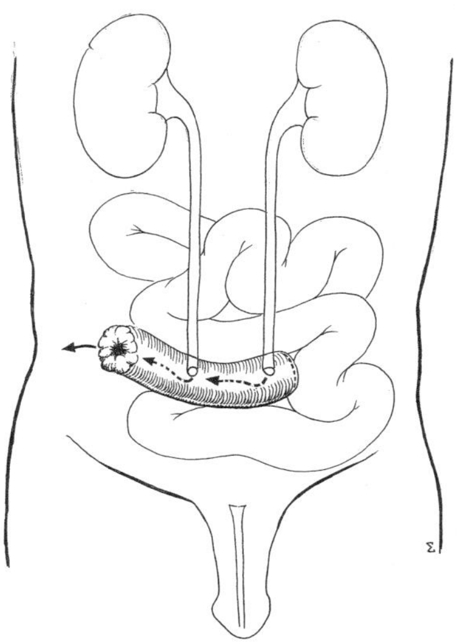

Figure 2. This is one of several ways for urine to reach the outside. The bladder has been removed. The ureters have been connected to a segment of small intestine that has been separated from the rest of the intestine. One end of this segment is closed, and the other is brought to the outside. The urine now flows out the side and is collected in a special receptacle.

- The ability to have sexual relations is severely limited following this operation, especially for men.

Choice Number Two

- The bladder is treated with x-rays for about a month to try to kill the cancer. This causes you to urinate very frequently for a few months until things quiet down.
- The x-ray therapy will be followed by strong chemotherapy.
- You will be followed closely.
- If the tumor does not go away, the only course at this point is to remove your bladder entirely as in Choice Number One. Removing your bladder at this point is more risky than if the x-ray therapy and the chemotherapy had not been given.

It has not been shown that Choice Number Two gives you as good a chance for cure as Choice Number One.

After the most careful consideration of all factors, the recommendation is that you have your bladder removed.

PREOPERATIVE PREPARATION

- You will have a thorough examination of your blood, function of your kidneys, heart (EKG), and lungs (chest x-ray).
- Bone scan: This test is done to look for any spread of the cancer to the bones in the body.
- CT scan (computed tomography scan): These special x-rays are taken as very thin slices through the bladder and surrounding tissue. This makes it possible to look for any spread of the cancer outside the bladder.
- Do not eat or drink anything for 8 hours before the operation.
- You will be instructed on how to cleanse your bowel.
- Shower or bathe as usual on the morning of the operation.
- You may be given medicine that will make you feel drowsy before you are brought to the operating room.

☐ OPERATION

- You will be asleep for the operation.
- The operation usually takes about 5 hours.

POSTOPERATIVE CARE

- You will first be taken to the Surgical Care Unit for a few days, where the doctors and nurses are very experienced in taking care of patients like yourself.
- You will have a thin, plastic tube in your nose for a few days.
- That evening you will be helped to sit up in bed and on the next day to get out of bed.
- Pain will be controlled with medicine.
- Your diet will be as you tolerate it.
- The hospital team of doctors and nurses will begin early to teach you how to manage your "new" bladder; it's not difficult.
- You should be able to go home in about 10 days.
- Arrangements will be made for your medicines, follow-up office visit, and stitch removal.
- Your condition can be cured. An estimate of your chances can be made only after all the test results are back.
- As with any operation, complications are always possible, some of them serious. With your type of operation, they can include bleeding, pneumonia, heart attack, blood clots, leakage of urine, blockage of urine, and possibly others.

✚ HOME CARE

- Continue with the program started while you were in the hospital.
- You will be instructed on showering and wound care.
- Take medicine as prescribed for your pain.
- Include plenty of roughage and liquids in your diet to help prevent constipation.
- Arrangements can be made for a home visiting nurse if one is needed.
- Do not drive a car or return to work until we discuss it during your follow-up office visit.

✆ CALL OUR OFFICE IF

- You develop any unusual signs or symptoms.
- There is no urine coming out the side of your abdomen.
- The incision becomes red or swollen, or there is drainage from it.
- You develop a temperature higher than 101°F.
- You have any questions.

△ GENERAL INFORMATION

Cancer of the urinary bladder is a difficult challenge, for both the physician and the patient, because it may appear in a number of different ways and several different treatments are available. Also, what may work for one person may not work for another person, even though each has bladder cancer that looks the same. It is important that you realize there's not just one way to treat bladder cancer. Each patient needs to be treated on an individual basis. Cancer of the bladder is seen more often in men and between the ages of 50 and 70 years.

COMMON SIGNS AND SYMPTOMS

- There is blood in the urine.
- The bleeding comes and goes.
- There may be symptoms from irritation of the bladder: urinating frequently, an urge to urinate that must be satisfied without delay, burning or pain when passing urine.

DIAGNOSIS

- A person who has the above history or symptoms should be concerned about a bladder tumor.
- Blood seen in the urine one time must be investigated, even though there is a good chance that nothing serious is wrong.
- Examination of the urine under the microscope should be done.
- Intravenous pyelogram (IVP): You will lie on an x-ray table, and a special liquid will be injected into your vein. X-rays will be taken of it as it moves through your kidneys and the tubes *(ureters)* through which urine reaches your bladder. This helps the doctor pick up any abnormalities in this area.
- Cystoscopy: An anesthetic will be squirted into your urethra (the opening into the bladder) to make it numb. The cystoscope will be inserted gently into your urethra and passed into the bladder. If anything suspicious is seen, a small piece of it will be taken (a *biopsy*) for examination in the laboratory.
- There is a good chance that it will not be necessary to do much more than to look inside your bladder.
- You will be free to go home, accompanied by a responsible adult, directly after the cystoscopy.

If a deeper biopsy or a biopsy of more than one area needs to be done, you will need either to be asleep or to have a spinal type of anesthesia. Arrangements will be made to have this done as follows:

- You will have an examination of your blood, urine, heart (EKG), and lungs (chest x-ray).
- Do not eat or drink anything for 8 hours before the cystoscopy.
- The cystoscope will be placed through the urethra and into the bladder, and several biopsies will be taken of areas as follows: the surface of the tumor, to see what type it is; the inside of the tumor, to see how deep it has gone; and the surrounding areas, to see if anything is there.
- All the removed tissue will be sent to the laboratory for thorough examination.

○ TREATMENT

The type of treatment for bladder cancer depends on several things:

- What type of cancer it is.
- Whether the cancer is slow or fast-growing.
- The size of the cancer and how far it has progressed.
- Your health in general.

After careful consideration of all factors, the recommendation is that your bladder cancer be treated by removing it through the cystoscope.

PREOPERATIVE PREPARATION

- You will have an examination of your blood, urine, heart (EKG), and lungs (chest x-ray).
- Shower or bathe as usual on the morning of the operation.
- Do not eat or drink anything for 8 hours before the operation.

□ OPERATION

- A general or spinal anesthetic will be used. This will be discussed with you beforehand.
- Removal of the cancer is done using an electrical current and a specially designed "resectoscope" that is inserted into your bladder through the urethra.
- The operation usually takes about 2 hours.

POSTOPERATIVE CARE

- You will be taken to a recovery room and observed. When your blood pressure, pulse, and breathing are stable, you will be taken to a regular hospital room.
- There will be a catheter (small rubber tube) in your bladder.
- You may feel as though you very urgently want to pass urine. This sensation is expected from the area where the tumor was resected. It will get better in a few days.
- You may be sent home with a catheter in the bladder that is connected to a collecting bag attached to your leg. You'll be shown how to take care of it; it's not difficult.
- As with any operation, complications are always possible. With this type of operation, they can include infection, heart attack, blood clots, leakage of urine, blockage of urine, and possibly others.
- Arrangements will be made for your medicines, follow-up office visit, catheter removal, and discussion of possible additional therapy.

✚ HOME CARE

- You may walk about as you wish, even climb stairs, but don't overdo things.
- You may eat as you did before the operation.
- You may shower as you wish.
- Do not drive a car until we first talk about it during your follow-up office visit.

✆ CALL OUR OFFICE IF

- The catheter in your bladder stops draining urine, or you feel your bladder getting distended.
- You develop a temperature higher than 101°F.
- You have any questions.

BLEPHAROPLASTY (EYELID PLASTY)

△ GENERAL INFORMATION

Blepharoplasty is derived from the Greek words *blepharon*, "eyelid," and *plassein*, "to mold or form." There are descriptions from many hundreds of years ago of removing skin in treating relaxed eyelids. This operation, however, has become very widely used only in the last 50 years.

With modern medical and technical advances, and a fuller appreciation of the complex functional anatomy of this area, a number of operations are available for conditions affecting the eyelids. When choosing a facial or general plastic surgeon for a blepharoplasty, it is wise to look for one who has a continuing interest, specific training, appropriate experience, and demonstrated skills in performing this cosmetic operation.

CANDIDATES FOR BLEPHAROPLASTY

By far, most persons have this procedure for cosmetic improvement. For this reason, you should have this operation because *you* want to rather than because someone else wants you to. Getting an opinion from two facial or general plastic surgeons is appropriate.

First, you and the surgeon should discuss at least the following:

- The problem as it is perceived by you. Also, to what degree the surgeon agrees with you.
- The planned operation.
- The expected (not guaranteed) results. Also, you should have a realistic expectation of the results.
- The fact that both your expectations and the surgeon's might not be realized.
- The possible complications that may accompany this operation.

○ TREATMENT

- There are a number of eyelid problems (Figs. 1–4 show some examples). Each problem requires a different operative technique to correct it.

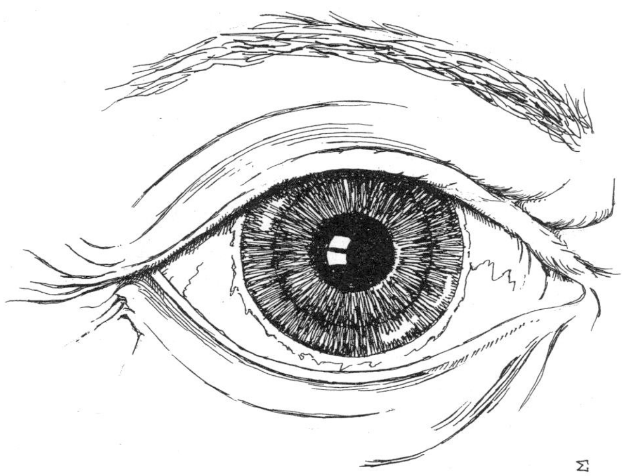

Figure 1. Crow's-feet.

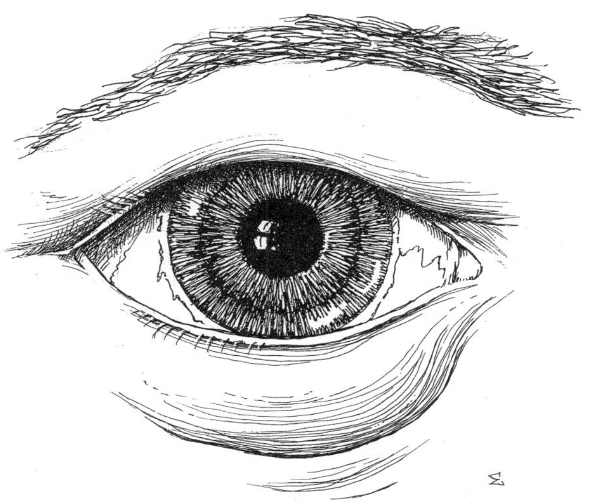

Figure 2. Sagging forehead as cause of sagging upper eyelid. Infraorbital fat.

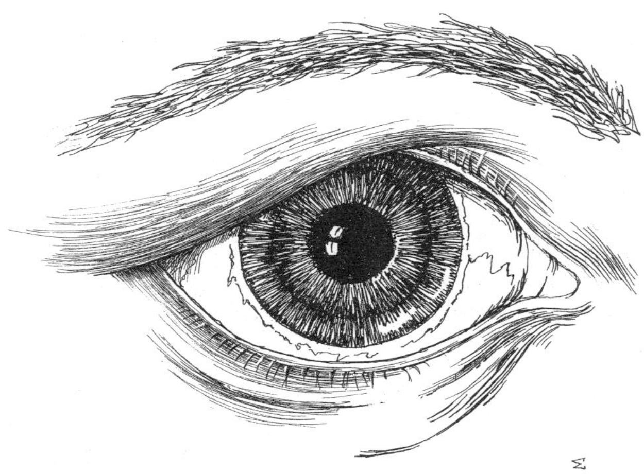

Figure 3. Sagging upper eyelid.

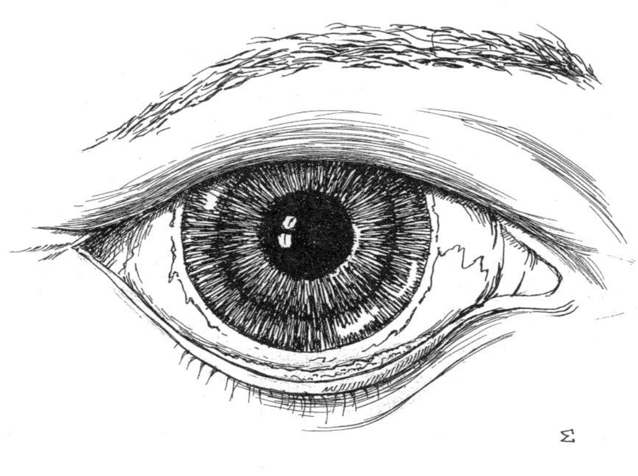

Figure 4. Ectropion (lower lid). Sagging upper eyelid.

• Your particular problem—or combination of problems—will be pointed out to you as well as the method necessary to correct it.

PREOPERATIVE PREPARATION

• You will have a detailed history and physical examination as it pertains to your face and neck, with emphasis on your eyelids.
• It will be necessary to have assurance that you are not troubled with any significant illness that might affect your ability to have the blepharoplasty safely.
• Some general medical conditions affect the eyelids and the tissue around them. Examples are thyroid and kidney disease. It will be necessary to have appropriate tests or documentation that you do not have such a condition.
• A number of photographs will be taken of you (with special attention to the eye) and from several angles.
• You may be shown a gallery of photos of other patients to give you an idea *(only)* of the possible results in your case.
• Do not take aspirin or aspirin-containing compounds, vitamin-E, or mood-altering drugs, and do not eat garlic, drink alcohol, or smoke for 1 week before the operation.
• Shower or bathe as usual the morning of the operation.
• Completely remove all facial makeup, especially mascara.
• You may want to bring a pair of dark glasses with you.

☐ OPERATION

• You will be given medicine that will make you feel drowsy before you are brought to the operating room.
• The operation will be done under local or general anesthesia. If it is done under local anesthesia, the affected area will be made numb by injecting an anesthetic into it with a fine needle. Also, during the operation you will be given medicine that will keep you drowsy.
• During the operation, you may feel some tugging but not pain.
• The operation usually takes about 1 to 2 hours.

POSTOPERATIVE CARE

• You will be taken to a recovery room. When your blood pressure, pulse, and breathing are stable and you are completely alert, you should be able to go home that same day with a responsible adult.
• Arrangements will be made for your medicine and follow-up office visit; the stitches are the type that dissolve.
• As with any operation, complications are always possible. Although they are uncommon with your type of operation, they can include bleeding, swelling, bruised areas, pulling downward of the lower eyelid, dry eyes, eyelids that do not close as tightly as before, and possibly others.

✣ HOME CARE

• Lie down with your head on two pillows as much as possible for the first 24 hours.
• "Ice is nice." Apply a cool pack over the eyes for 20 minutes every hour for the first day. After the third day, gentle local heat may be helpful.
• You may eat as you did before the operation.
• Do not rub your eyes.
• Do not try to pull down the lower lid to look at the suture line (if you had lower lid surgery).
• Driving a car with an automatic shift is not too demanding. But if you have to slam on the brakes suddenly or twist to turn the steering wheel, you may have an accident or you may strain the sutures or tear something. During your follow-up visit let's discuss when you can resume driving.
• You can wear contact lenses after the first week.
• You may resume sexual activity whenever you choose.
• You may return to work when you feel up to it, but let's first talk about it during a follow-up office visit.
• When washing your face, do not rub; use dabbing motions.

✆ CALL OUR OFFICE IF

• You develop any unusual signs or symptoms.
• Your eyes swell shut.
• The incision becomes red or swollen, or there is drainage from it.
• You develop a temperature higher than 100°F.
• You have any questions.

△ GENERAL INFORMATION

The ability to transfuse blood has been one of the important advances in surgery. It has made it possible to perform operations more safely. Some operations would not even be attempted without the availability and use of blood and its byproducts. Most of the time, however, blood is simply held in reserve in case it is truly needed.

Many patients who are told that they may—not *will*, just *may*—need a blood transfusion become anxious about the entire process and especially about how safe the transfusion may be.

BLOOD TRANSFUSION PROGRAMS IN THE UNITED STATES

Blood is considered a *drug*. For this reason, it comes under the regulation of the U.S. Food and Drug Administration (FDA) that imposes a number of requirements to safeguard the person donating the blood as well as the one receiving it. The American Association of Blood Banks is a voluntary, nonprofit organization that accredits blood banks. It has additional standard requirements.

In the United States, blood donations are obtained in several ways. There are large community blood centers, such as those run by the Red Cross and smaller hospital blood centers. A small amount of blood is imported. Around 14 million units of blood are donated each year by about 10 million donors.

Even though most blood is donated by volunteers and collected by agencies that are nonprofit, there is a considerable cost involved in collecting blood and then putting it through all the various steps before getting it to the patient. This cost is passed on to the patient.

The aims of this entire process are to ensure the safety of the donor and to obtain a high-quality blood component that is as safe as possible for the person who is to receive it. The steps include screening the donor, collecting the blood, testing it, getting it ready, and distributing it. Doing this involves at least the following:

DONOR SCREENING

Only volunteers are accepted as donors. For the safety of the person receiving donated blood, the donors are asked about the following:

- Their general health.
- Whether they are under the care of a physician.
- Whether there is anything wrong with their heart or lungs.
- Recent donations or major illness, unexplained weight loss, or unusual bleeding.
- Any bleeding disorder.
- Whether they are receiving growth hormones.
- Exposure to malaria and hepatitis or other liver diseases.
- Whether they are infected with acquired immunodeficiency syndrome (AIDS) or have symptoms of AIDS and other questions about sex-related diseases and behavior that might put them at risk for AIDS or hepatitis.

Sometimes, a family doctor's opinion may be that the donor is perfectly okay, but a number of conditions are not acceptable, according to FDA standards, and may cause a donor to be rejected.

PHYSICAL EXAMINATION AND LABORATORY TESTING

Screening of the donor includes the following:

- Blood count.
- Blood pressure, pulse, and respiration.
- A focused physical examination with special attention for any signs of illness, effects of drug abuse or alcohol, needle marks indicating intravenous drug abuse, AIDS or related diseases, and skin infection.
- Laboratory tests for two types of hepatitis, human immunodeficiency virus (HIV), and syphilis.

BLOOD COLLECTION

- Blood is collected in specially designed sterile containers that are licensed by the FDA and can be used only once.
- The skin over the donor's vein is examined with great care to be certain there is no skin disease in that area. The skin is washed with soap and water and then swabbed with an antiseptic solution.
- A one-time use sterile needle is used to puncture the vein to obtain the blood.
- The donation takes about 7 to 10 minutes.
- As the blood is being collected, a blood thinner *(anticoagulant)* is mixed with it to prevent it from clotting. Also, the blood is mixed with a special solution to keep it in the best possible condition until it is ready for use.

BLOOD TYPES

There are several different major blood types, and they are designated as A, B, O, and AB. They must be matched for all transfusions; otherwise, a serious reaction can result. In addition, a number of minor blood types may need to be taken into account.

In general, patients who get a blood transfusion do not necessarily receive the blood donated by their friends or relatives. They receive blood that best matches their own blood. There are some variations or exceptions to this as follows.

SPECIAL DONATIONS

Autologous Blood Transfusion

Individuals donate their *own* blood some days before the operation and expect to receive that blood during the operation. The rules for this practice are as follows:

- There is no age or weight restriction.
- Pregnant women are discouraged from doing it.
- The blood level of the donor must be high enough to begin with.
- A person can donate blood every 7 days for up to 3 donations before the operation.

Collecting blood from a patient so that it can be used later by that same patient can be harmful if the donor has any of the following:

- A blood infection *(bacteremia)*.
- Symptoms of coronary heart disease or disease of the heart valves.
- Recent seizures.

A person choosing to donate his or her own blood should be reasonably certain the blood will be needed. Such blood may be discarded if it does not meet FDA standards for transfusion to a person other than the donor.

Directed Donor Blood

Relatives and friends donate blood for the patient, believing that such blood is safer than blood from unknown donors. In fact, there is no evidence that this is true. Blood donated by friends or relatives must meet the same FDA requirements for routine blood donation because the blood will be used by others in the community if it is not used by the patient.

SAFETY OF A BLOOD TRANSFUSION

- The risk of developing hepatitis C (the more serious type of hepatitis) is one in 103,000 transfusions.
- The risk of developing HIV (that commonly leads to AIDS) is one in 490,000 transfusions.

So, although blood transfusion is very safe, it still is not risk free. It should be given after careful consideration of the patient's clinical situation and needs. Using these guidelines, the risks of a blood transfusion are far outweighed by the benefits that follow.

△ GENERAL INFORMATION

What Is a Bone Scan?

A bone scan is a test to see whether anything is "disturbing" your bones. A bone scan does not show only cancer in the bones; it can also show other things such as injury, arthritis, or infection.

The test uses a specific drug combined with a tiny amount of radioactive material. Such a combination is called a *radiopharmaceutical*. The radiopharmaceutical used for a bone scan has the special ability to attach itself to bone that has something disturbing it.

How Is a Bone Scan Done?

- A bone scan is done on an outpatient basis.
- A fine needle will be used to inject the radiopharmaceutical into your vein.
- You then can go about your business for 1 hour while the radiopharmaceutical circulates throughout your body and attaches itself to any disturbed bone.
- You will be asked to drink two to three glasses of water during this 1 hour, which will help wash away into the urine any of the radiopharmaceutical that was not taken up by the bones.
- After this 1 hour, you will lie on a padded table. A machine that can pick up the signals from the radiopharmaceutical will pass slowly over your entire body, taking a picture of all of your bones from your skull to your toes.
- Disturbed bones show up as darker spots (Fig. 1).
- This part of the examination takes 30 minutes.
- All of the radiopharmaceutical will pass out of your body through the urine in a few hours.
- After this you are free to leave.
- The pictures (scans) will be examined by specialists in this field to determine whether any bones are affected. Most important, a decision will be made on the nature of the lesions that might appear.
- The results will be reported to your doctor.

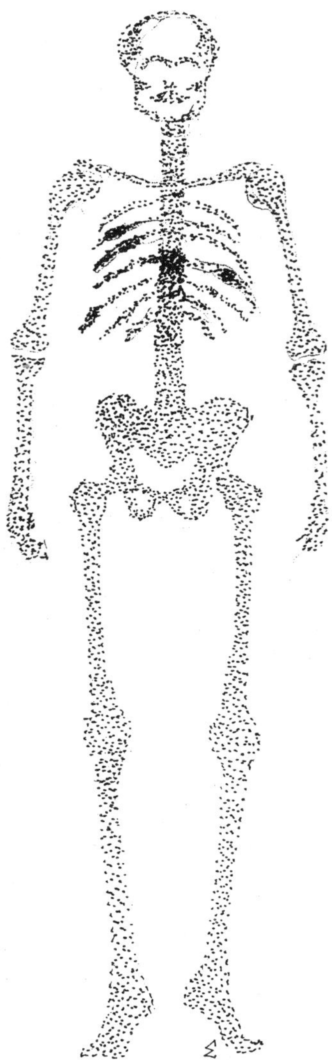

Figure 1. Example of a positive bone scan result in a woman who has had breast cancer treated by mastectomy 2 years previously. She has a new onset of persistent back pain. The dark areas in the three ribs on her right side and the one on the left side, as well as in the one vertebra, are highly suggestive of metastatic cancer.

HOW CAN A BONE SCAN HELP?

- A bone scan is valuable because sometimes it picks up problems in the bone even before there are any symptoms.
- Often, it can show something is wrong in the bones (not necessarily cancer) even before regular x-rays show it.
- If the scan results are normal, this is very reliable evidence that there is no cancer in the bone.
- If a bone scan shows something is wrong, it does *not* mean that it is cancer. It just means something is disturbing that bone. Many times it is just arthritis.
- Often, when the bone scan shows a dark spot, it may be necessary to do regular x-rays, special x-rays, a CT (computed tomography scan), or an MRI (magnetic resonance imaging). Sometimes they help clear up any questions.

With information collected as noted above, the bone scan helps the doctor know more about your problem. This helps the doctor plan your treatment more intelligently so that it will have the highest chance of success.

WHO USUALLY HAS A BONE SCAN?

- A person who has not been sick before but now is having vague, new, different, persistent, or unusual pains in the bones.
- Patients with certain types of cancer that appears to be localized and for whom treatment is about to begin. The doctor wants to be as certain as possible that the bones are not involved with cancer before treatment is started.
- Patients who have had treatment for certain types of cancer for whom a bone scan is part of the customary follow-up to check on the status of the bones.

△ GENERAL INFORMATION

Bowen's disease is a condition of the skin that has the characteristics of cancer except for one thing: it doesn't have "roots." It does not go deeper than the surface of the skin. For this reason, it cannot spread to other areas in the body. It occurs on any part of the skin, including the genital area in women and men.

COMMON SIGNS AND SYMPTOMS

Bowen's disease often looks like a crusting lesion with some areas of redness in it. It has a sharp but irregular border.

DIAGNOSIS

- Usually, the diagnosis can be made by taking a detailed history and doing a thorough physical examination.
- The only way to be certain of the diagnosis is to use a very short, thin needle to inject some anesthetic in the area around the lesion to make it numb. Then a piece of it is taken (a *biopsy*) for laboratory examination.

○ TREATMENT

- Often, a lesion of Bowen's disease will develop roots; it will invade the deep tissue. When it does this, it can behave aggressively and spread to other areas of the body.
- The safest and most reliable treatment is an operation to remove the lesion.

PREOPERATIVE PREPARATION

- Do not eat or drink anything for 4 hours before the operation.
- Shower (and shave) as usual on the morning of the operation.
- The involved skin and surrounding area will be washed with soap and water and surrounded with sterile drapes.
- The operation will be done under local anesthesia. A very fine needle will be used to inject the area of the lesion with an anesthetic. The affected area will be made numb. Also, you may be given medicine that will make you feel drowsy.
- During the operation you may feel some tugging but not pain.
- The operation usually takes 1 hour.

POSTOPERATIVE CARE

- You will be taken to a recovery room. When your blood pressure, pulse, and breathing are stable and you are completely alert, you should be able to go home that same day with a responsible adult.
- Arrangements will be made for your medicine, follow-up office visit, and stitch removal.

✚ HOME CARE

- Resume your usual activities.
- You may walk about as you wish, even climb stairs.
- You may eat as you did before the operation.
- Take medicine as prescribed for your pain.
- You may shower as you wish and with any dressings on or off.
  - There may be narrow strips of tape across the incision. It's all right if they get wet. They will be removed in the doctor's office.
  - After you dry yourself, replace any dressings with clean, dry ones.

✆ CALL OUR OFFICE IF

- You develop any unusual signs or symptoms.
- The incision becomes red or swollen, or there is drainage from it.
- You develop a temperature higher than 100°F.
- You have any questions.

BRANCHIAL CLEFT CYST

△ GENERAL INFORMATION

Branchial cleft cyst is a condition that has its beginning when the neck of the tiny embryo begins to take shape in the mother's womb. During this time of development, several deep grooves *(branchial clefts)* in the neck don't disappear as they should. As a result, a thin tube of tissue not much thicker than spaghetti remains under the skin of the neck. This tube usually runs from the middle or lower part of the neck upward and inward toward the throat on the side of the neck. Branchial cleft cyst is most commonly seen in children and young adults.

COMMON SIGNS AND SYMPTOMS

- Often, this tube does not cause a problem. At other times, it drains clear fluid to the outside through an opening in the skin, usually at the lower part of the side of the neck.
- Sometimes, the tube does not have an outside opening, and the fluid accumulates in the tube to create the swelling (a *cyst*) (Fig. 1).
- The cyst can be the size of a small olive or as large as a chicken egg.
- Most of the time, the cyst is not painful. However, if the fluid inside it becomes infected, it can be very painful.

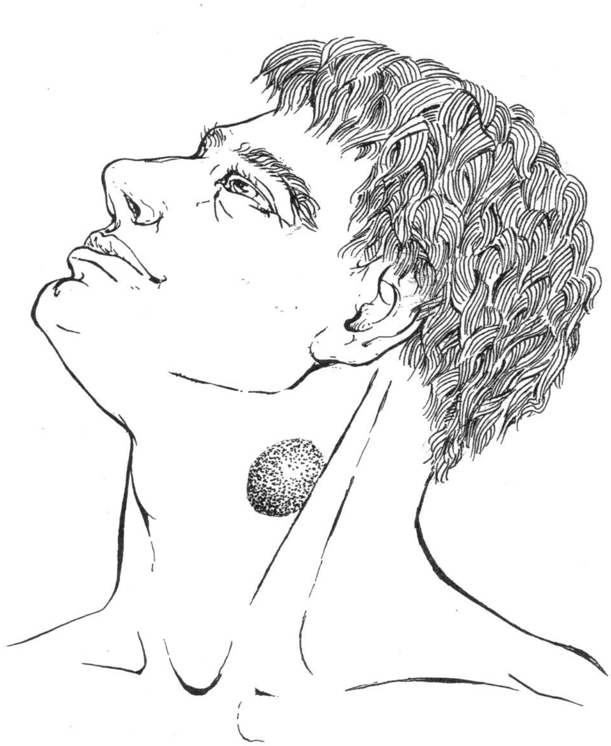

Figure 1. Most often the branchial cleft cyst is found in the location shown. However, it can be anywhere along a line from the bottom of the ear to the breast bone.

DIAGNOSIS

- Usually the diagnosis can be made by taking a detailed history and doing a careful physical examination. If there are questions about the diagnosis, ultrasound can help clear up any doubts.
- Ultrasound: Harmless sound waves are aimed at the area of your neck. The sound waves bouncing back (the echoes) from this area are seen as a picture on a screen. Ultrasound is a convenient, painless, and harmless way to examine organs and tissues inside the neck. It is especially useful to determine whether the "mass" is solid or filled with fluid.

○ TREATMENT

The appropriate treatment for a branchial cleft cyst or sinus is an operation to remove it. After consideration of all factors, the recommendation is that you have an operation to remove the branchial cleft cyst.

PREOPERATIVE PREPARATION

- There will be an examination of your blood and urine and possibly of your heart (EKG) and lungs (chest x-ray).
- Do not eat or drink anything for 8 hours before the operation.
- Shower or bathe as usual on the morning of the operation.
- You may be given medicine that will make you feel drowsy before you are brought to the operating room.

□ OPERATION

- You will be asleep for the operation.
- Careful consideration will be given to make a cosmetic incision in a natural crease in the neck.
- There will be a cosmetic closure.
- The operation usually takes about 1, sometimes 2, hours, depending on how much dissection is necessary.

POSTOPERATIVE CARE

- You will be taken to a recovery room and observed. When your blood pressure, pulse, and breathing are stable and you are completely alert, you may be able to go home that same day with a responsible adult. Otherwise, you will be taken to a regular hospital room.
- There will be a small bandage over the incision.
- Pain will be controlled with medicine.
- Your diet will be as you tolerate it.
- As with any operation, complications are always possible. Although they are uncommon with this type of operation, they can include bleeding, infection, temporary hoarseness, and possibly others.
- Arrangements will be made for your medicine, follow-up office visit, and stitch removal.

✚ HOME CARE

- Resume your usual activities.
- You may walk about as you wish, even climb stairs.
- You may eat as you did before the operation.
- Take medicine as prescribed for your pain.
- You may shower if you wish and with any dressings on or off.
  - There may be narrow strips of tape across the incision. It's all right if they get wet; they will be removed in the doctor's office.
  - After you dry yourself, replace any dressings with clean, dry ones.
- You may drive a car if you wish but not if you are taking any medicines that reduce your alertness.
- You may return to work when you feel up to it.

✆ CALL OUR OFFICE IF

- You develop any unusual signs or symptoms.
- The incision becomes red or swollen, or there is drainage from it.
- You develop a temperature higher than 100°F.
- You have any questions.

△ GENERAL INFORMATION

Sometimes a woman will have a bloody discharge from the nipple. Usually, this happens with no warning.

COMMON SIGNS AND SYMPTOMS

- A maroon-colored stain, usually no bigger than a quarter, is seen on the nightgown on awakening or on the bra at the end of the day.
- A drop of red or maroon-colored fluid may come out of the nipple while taking a shower.
- If the breast tissue close to the nipple is squeezed, maroon or blood-tinged fluid comes out.
- Occasionally, there is mild itching of the nipple before the fluid appears.
- The discharge is usually from one breast only, often from a single-duct opening on the nipple.

DIAGNOSIS

- A reliable history (by the woman) that the above has occurred.
- The assurance that the bleeding is not from trauma (sexual foreplay) or from injury to the breast.
- The history of bleeding is not enough to start thinking seriously about treatment (that is, an operation).
- Information on how often it happens.
- Sometimes the patient may bring in a bra or a nightgown with evidence of a blood stain.
- Usually the patient has squeezed the breast just before coming to see the doctor, so there is no fluid left to come out during the office visit. For this reason, do not squeeze the breast or take a shower on the day of the office visit, and do not wear a bra to your appointment (if this is reasonable).
- In the office, the breast will be squeezed, and, ideally, "bloody discharge" will come out. A small amount of this will be sent to the pathology laboratory for examination.
- If the squeeze does not produce any fluid, then you may need to be reevaluated in 6 to 8 weeks.
- Keep a record of how often you see bleeding and what you were doing when the bleeding occurred.
- A mammogram will be done to look for any abnormality.
- A *ductogram* may be ordered. You will lie on an x-ray table. The nipple will be painted with an antiseptic solution. A hollow tube, about the size of the lead in a wood pencil, will be placed in the opening of the nipple from where the blood is seen to come. Dye will be injected to fill the duct. X-rays of the breast will be taken. These can show where the lesion blocks the duct and prevents it from filling.
- *Ultrasound* may also be used to look at the ducts.

Some Causes of Nipple Discharge

- Nipple discharge can be found in 50 to 80% of women even when no disease is present.
- The breast ducts normally have a tiny bit of moisture in them. It is not abnormal to have a small amount of discharge. This fluid usually is straw colored, pale to dark green, or even blood tinged. Normal discharge is usually from both breasts and from several duct openings in the nipple.
- Rarely, it is cancer in the duct that is the cause of a bloody discharge.
- If the fluid from the breast is red and "bloody," the most common cause is a tiny growth called a *papilloma* that usually is not much bigger than a sesame seed. Most are benign, but some can show changes of early cancer.
- An imbalance of hormones and some medications may cause breast discharge. Usually, this is clear or slightly milky in appearance.
- Trauma: This can be from squeezing the nipple excessively during breast self-examination or from sexual foreplay.
- A pregnant woman may have discharge from both breasts during pregnancy, even blood-tinged discharge during the last 2 months of pregnancy.
- Delayed drying up of the breast following childbirth and nursing can cause discharge.

○ TREATMENT

- If the fluid is straw colored or greenish and the mammogram result is negative, the patient can be observed carefully at intervals of 3 to 4 months.
- The type of discharge that concerns the doctor is one that is persistent throughout the month, happens without squeezing the breast, is from one opening (in the nipple), and is "bloody" in color.
- If the fluid is bloody, an operation is necessary to remove the involved duct for the following reasons:
  - One cannot be certain it is not cancerous.
  - The exact diagnosis cannot be made unless the actual bleeding tissue is removed and examined in the pathology laboratory.
  - To stop the discharge.

After careful consideration of all factors, the recommendation is that you have an operation to try to solve your problem.

PREOPERATIVE PREPARATION

- Do not eat or drink anything for 8 hours before the operation.
- You may be given medicine that will make you feel drowsy before you are brought to the operating room.

□ OPERATION

- It is best if the operation is done with you asleep. Injecting a local anesthetic in this area of the breast to make it numb and do the operation with you awake is not advisable. Sometimes the injected anesthetic causes the tissue in this area to become

too watery, which makes it difficult to find something very small.
- The incision will be made in the dark part of your breast (the *areola*) because it will show the least in this location.
- The area under the nipple will be explored. Usually the affected duct will be swollen with fluid. The duct will be removed from the nipple down into the breast tissue (Fig. 1).
- How much tissue is removed depends on how easily the growth (usually a papilloma or involved duct) is found. Sometimes it is not possible to see the papilloma clearly; it is either small or not seen within the duct. If a dilated duct cannot be found with a papilloma, then the duct under the nipple will be removed down into the breast tissue.
- Of course, if the duct papilloma is seen, it will be removed and the operation will be over.
- The incision will be closed in a cosmetic fashion.

POSTOPERATIVE CARE

- You will wake up in a recovery room. When your blood pressure, pulse, and breathing are stable and you are completely alert, you should be able to go home that same day with a responsible adult.
- Arrangements will be made for your pain medicine, follow-up office visit, and stitch removal.
- As with any operation, complications are always possible. Although they are uncommon with this type of operation, they can include bleeding, infection, and possibly others.
- With any future pregnancy, it may not be possible for you to nurse with this breast.

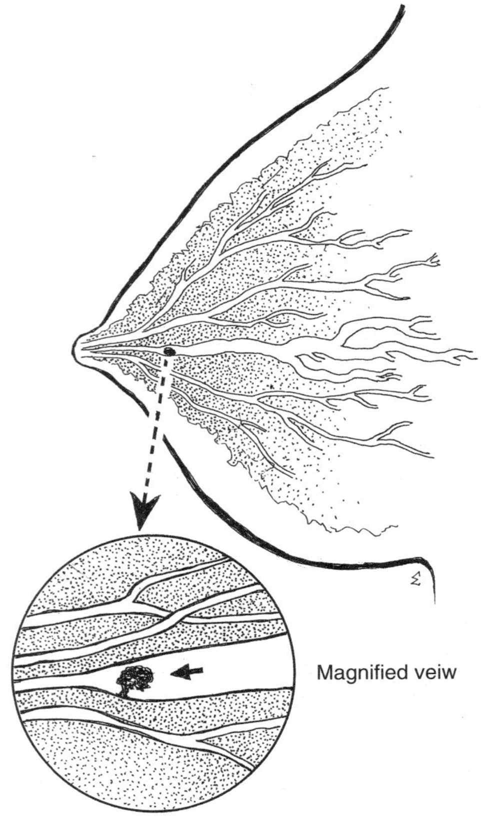

Figure 1. A papilloma is shown in a duct *(short arrow)*. The duct is blocked considerably, causing it to become distended above the point of obstruction.

HOME CARE

- Resume your usual activities.
- Unless you are advised to the contrary, you may shower beginning on the next day and with any dressings on or off.
  - There may be narrow strips of tape across the incision. It's all right if they get wet; they will be removed in the doctor's office.
  - After you dry yourself, replace any dressings with clean, dry ones.
  - You may return to work when you feel up to it.

CALL OUR OFFICE IF

- The incision becomes red or swollen, or there is drainage from it.
- You develop a temperature higher than 100°F.
- You have any questions.

△ GENERAL INFORMATION

There are a number of names for this very common problem, and "fibrocystic disease" is not one of the better ones because it is not a disease. It is a variation of the normal changes that occur in the breast with menstruation. As such, it is being referred to increasingly as *fibrocystic changes*.

Probably, some imbalance of hormones produces an exaggerated response in the breasts. It is seen most commonly in women aged 20 to 55 years.

COMMON SIGNS AND SYMPTOMS

- Usually fibrocystic change occurs in both breasts but not necessarily equally. Mostly, it appears in the upper outer part of the breast (Fig. 1).
- It may be characterized by pain or a lump in the breast or tenderness in many locations. The tenderness can be mild or very disabling. Many women can't sleep on their abdomen before their menstrual cycle. Some find even wearing a brassiere is too uncomfortable.
- The clear-cut lumps usually are large cysts.
- Sometimes the lump is made up of a number of small cysts bunched together (like a bunch of grapes).

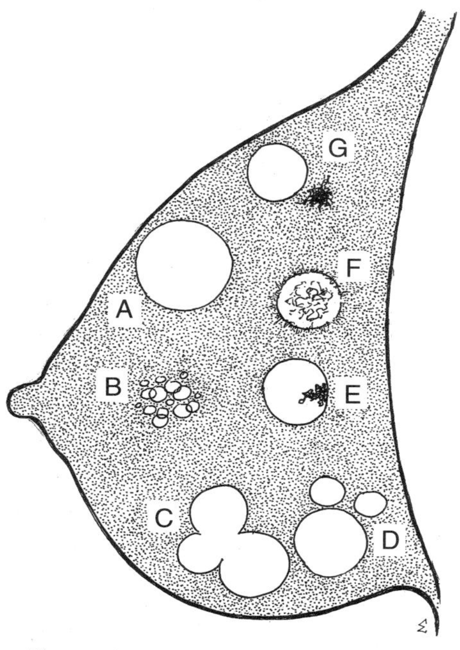

Figure 1. Fibrocystic changes in the breast can present in a number of ways. Some examples are as follows: Simple cyst (A) that could be drained easily with a needle. A grouping of small cysts ("soap bubbles") (B) that would be difficult to aspirate. Multiple cysts that connect with one another (C); a draining needle in one of them would drain all of them. Disconnected grouped cysts (D); help would be needed (for example, with ultrasound) to see them accurately and make a decision on drainage. A cyst with a growth (possibly cancer) in it (E). A cyst that is inflamed and has thick fluid in it, making it more difficult to drain (F). A cancer "hidden" by an innocent-feeling cyst over it (G).

- The cyst may appear somewhat suddenly and stay that way, or it may go away with the next menstrual cycle.

DIAGNOSIS

- It is necessary to remember that both fibrocystic change and cancer are common and that they can both occur in the same age group of patients before their menopause.
- The most important concern is not to mistake a cancer for fibrocystic disease; they both can appear as lumps.
- **Mammography:** This is a very valuable way to pick up a cancer even in a breast with fibrocystic change.
- **Ultrasound:** Harmless sound waves are aimed at the area of your breast. The sound waves bouncing back (the echoes) from this area are seen as a picture on a screen. Ultrasound is a convenient, painless, and harmless way to examine tissues inside your breast. It can do the following:
  - Demonstrate whether a lump is filled with fluid (called a *cyst*).
  - Help the surgeon guide a needle to a small cyst that cannot be felt so that the fluid inside it can be removed and examined in the laboratory.
- If the mass is solid, the nature of it can be determined in one of the following ways:
  - A fine needle is used to remove a few cells for examination (called *fine needle aspiration biopsy*).
  - The skin over the lump is made numb with an anesthetic. A larger needle is inserted through the numbed skin and down to the lump. A sliver of tissue, the size of the lead in a wood pencil, is removed (a *core biopsy*) for examination in the pathology laboratory.

○ TREATMENT

- A single lump that can be felt can be aspirated with a needle and syringe. If the fluid is clear, straw colored, or pale green, it is rarely cancer.
- A *biopsy* is advised if, with aspiration, a needle is placed in the mass and one or more of the following occur:
  - No fluid can be withdrawn.
  - The fluid is bloody.
  - The mass does not go away completely.
  - The mass goes away but comes right back. If this happens several times in close succession, it arouses concern that it might be a cancer causing the fluid to form.
- If there is any question about the diagnosis, then removing the lump (an *excision biopsy*) is wise.
- The biopsy may show only fibrocystic disease. There should be no regrets or apologies for this. This is the only way to be certain a suspicious mass is not cancer. If it is a cancer, an early diagnosis and treatment greatly improve the chances for cure.

PREOPERATIVE PREPARATION

- Usually the biopsy is performed under local anesthesia along with some medicine to make you feel drowsy.
- You may have a routine examination of your blood, urine, heart (EKG), and lungs (chest x-ray).
- Do not eat or drink anything for 8 hours before the operation.
- You may shower as usual the morning of the operation.

☐ OPERATION

- The breast will be painted with an antiseptic solution and draped with sterile towels.
- Local anesthesia: A very thin, short needle will be used to inject an anesthetic in the skin over the lump. The area will become numb.
- The incision will be selected carefully and made in a cosmetic fashion so that it will show as little as possible.
- During the operation, you may feel some tugging but not pain.
- The incision will be closed in a cosmetic fashion.
- Usually the operation takes about 1 hour.

POSTOPERATIVE CARE

- You will be taken to a recovery room. When your blood pressure, pulse, and breathing are stable and you are completely alert, you should be able to go home that same day with a responsible adult.
- Arrangements will be made for your medicine, follow-up office visit, stitch removal, and a discussion of the laboratory findings.
- As with any operation, complications are always possible. Although uncommon with this type of operation, they can include bleeding, infection, and possibly others.

✚ HOME CARE

- Resume your usual activities.
- Unless instructed otherwise, you may shower as you wish and with any dressings on or off.
  - There may be narrow strips of tape across the incision. It's all right if they get wet. They will be removed in the doctor's office.
  - After you dry yourself, replace any dressings with clean, dry ones.
- Take medicine as prescribed for your pain.
- Wearing a loose bra at bedtime—mostly to keep your breasts from moving around too much as you shift during sleep—will make you more comfortable.
- Do not drive a car if you cannot move your arm freely or are taking pain medicine that may decrease your alertness.
- You may return to work when you feel up to it.

✆ CALL OUR OFFICE IF

- You develop any unusual signs or symptoms.
- The incision becomes red or swollen, or there is drainage from it.
- You develop a temperature higher than 100°F.
- You have any questions.

△ GENERAL INFORMATION

Paget's disease of the breast is a serious problem that at first doesn't look like anything very important. It is a cancer but at first appears as a rash or crusted and oozing "eczema" of the nipple and surrounding tissue, and it is treated as such. Any rash or eczema of the nipple that does not heal completely in 2 weeks and stay healed after being treated with salves, ointments, or whatever must be seen by a doctor, especially if it occurs in older women.

This particular cancer starts in the lining of the tiny ducts of the nipple and slowly comes to the surface; also it creeps down deep into the breast tissue. Although most of the findings are on the surface of the nipple, this is just the tip of the volcano; most of the trouble is inside (Fig. 1).

Incidentally, there are other diseases called Paget's; they are different from this one.

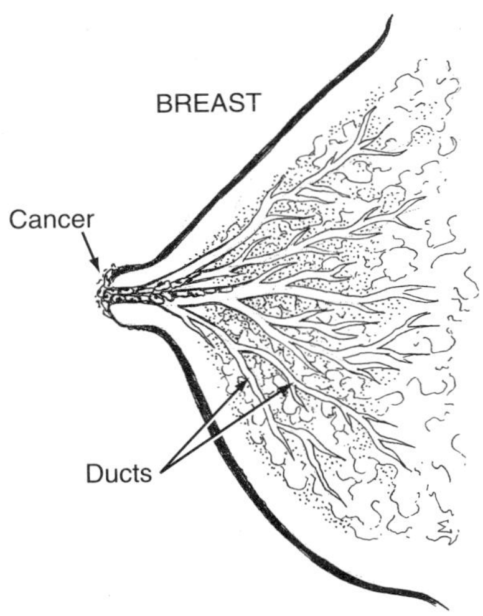

Figure 1. In Paget's disease most of the external findings are in the nipple and areola (the dark tissue around the nipple). Often the findings are not too significant because Paget's disease does not begin on the surface; it begins in the ducts deep to the nipple and gradually works its way to the outside to affect the nipple and areola. Sometimes a mass is present in the breast.

COMMON SIGNS AND SYMPTOMS

- A rash or eczema of the nipple that persists for longer than 2 weeks, even after treatment.

DIAGNOSIS

- A detailed history of the behavior of the rash, a careful physical examination, and a high suspicion for this disease are the first steps in making the diagnosis.
- A mammogram is done, looking for anything deep in the breast. It is important to remember that many times, the mammogram results are negative. This does not mean that Paget's is not a possible diagnosis.
- The surest way to establish the diagnosis is to examine some tissue under the microscope. The nipple is painted with an antiseptic solution and surrounded with sterile towels. A fine, short needle is used to inject an anesthetic into the nipple tissue to make it numb. Then, a small piece is removed (a *biopsy*) for laboratory examination.

○ TREATMENT

- Modified radical mastectomy (removal of the entire breast and the lymph nodes under the armpit but not the muscle) is the proper and best treatment because the cancer can be anywhere along the ducts of the breast. Paget's disease of the breast is not something to be treated by lumpectomy; often there is no lump.
- If treated early and aggressively, there is a good chance for a cure, usually better than that for the common variety of breast cancer.
- It has been established that you have Paget's disease. After careful consideration of all factors, it is recommended that you have a modified radical mastectomy.

PREOPERATIVE CARE

- You will have an examination of your blood, urine, heart (EKG), and lungs (chest x-ray).
- Do not eat or drink anything for 8 hours before the operation.
- Shower or bathe as usual on the morning of the operation.
- You may be given medicine that will make you feel drowsy before you are brought to the operating room.

□ OPERATION

- You will be totally asleep for the operation.
- Usually the operation takes about 2 hours.
- You will not need any blood transfusion.

POSTOPERATIVE CARE

- You will be taken to a recovery room and observed. When your blood pressure, pulse, and breathing are stable, you will be taken to a regular hospital room.
- That evening you will be helped to sit up in bed and the next morning to get out of bed.
- Pain will be controlled with medicine.
- There may be a small plastic tube coming from your incision. It was placed there to drain any extra fluid.
- You should be able to go home in about 3 or 4 days.
- Arrangements will be made for your medicines, follow-up office visit, stitch or clip removal, and discussion of the laboratory findings.

✣ HOME CARE

- You may walk about if you wish, even climb stairs, but don't overdo things.
- Take medicine as prescribed for your pain.

- Unless instructed otherwise, after the first change of dressings in the doctor's office, you may shower if you wish and with any dressings on or off.
  - There may be narrow strips of tape across the incision. It's all right if they get wet; they will be removed in the doctor's office.
  - After you dry yourself, replace any dressings with clean, dry ones.
- Favor the arm on the operated side except for essential activities.
- Do not start any arm exercises until you are instructed by the surgeon.
- You may resume sexual activity whenever you choose.
- You may return to work when you feel up to it, but let's talk about it during a follow-up office visit.

✆ CALL OUR OFFICE IF

- You develop any unusual signs or symptoms.
- The incision becomes red or swollen, or there is drainage from it.
- You develop a temperature higher than 100°F.
- You have any questions.

BREAST ABSCESS

△ GENERAL INFORMATION

Breast abscess is a collection of pus in the breast. Although most of the time it is localized, it can spread to affect separate areas away from the main abscess.

Breast abscess is seen most commonly in women who are breast-feeding their infants. Abscesses in such patients can occur in any part of the breast. Breast abscesses are also seen in women who are not breast-feeding. These abscesses usually are under the nipple and *areola* (the dark skin around the nipple).

COMMON SIGNS AND SYMPTOMS

- Usually there is a tender lump in the breast.
- Often there is redness and swelling of the skin over the infected area.
- The abscess may already be draining through either the nipple or the skin.
- There is fever.
- Lymph nodes in the *axilla* (armpit) may be swollen.

DIAGNOSIS

- Taking a careful history and doing a thorough physical examination often are enough to make the diagnosis of breast abscess.
- Aspiration: Placing a needle into the swollen area (sometimes under ultrasound guidance) to obtain pus for examination in the laboratory is an available technique. Finding pus is proof of an abscess.
- Ultrasound: Harmless sound waves are aimed at the area of the breast. The sound waves bouncing back (the echoes) from this area are seen as a picture on a screen. Ultrasound is a convenient, painless, and harmless way to examine the tissue inside the breast, as well as to see if the mass is solid or filled with liquid.
- Mammogram: This is another way to examine the inside of the breast (without cutting into it) for evidence of cancer. The x-rays that must pass through the breast to take the mammogram have no effect on the milk in your breast and are not a risk to your infant if you are breast-feeding. However, a mammogram is of limited value in women immediately after childbirth or when breast-feeding because the breasts are swollen with milk and thus severely restrict the ability of the mammogram to demonstrate abnormalities.
- The most common cause of breast infection is the inflammation sometimes seen in the breast of a nursing mother that develops into an abscess.

  Other causes must be considered, however.
- Inflammatory cancer: The breast in this condition is red and swollen but usually is not painful. Fever is not common. The lymph nodes in the axilla may be swollen. If the signs of infection do not go away with antibiotics, then the breast must be evaluated for inflammatory breast cancer, which can look like an infection.
- Irradiation: A patient who has had a breast cancer treated by a lumpectomy with x-ray therapy after the operation can have a red and tender breast.
- A silicone implant that has leaked can produce redness, drainage, and firm areas in the breast.
- An infected sebaceous cyst (oil gland) can produce redness of the skin, a tender mass (usually in the skin itself), and even enlarged lymph nodes in the axilla.
- An ordinary cancer can lead to the death of tissue at its center that becomes infected. Although it is true that an abscess is present, one must not miss a cancer that also may be present.

○ TREATMENT

- Making the correct diagnosis is critical not only to providing relief by releasing the pus, but also to ensuring that a cancer with an abscess in it is not overlooked.
- Antibiotics will be started that are effective against the bacteria identified if pus was removed with a needle. If the type of bacteria causing the abscess is unknown, the antibiotic that is effective against the most likely type of bacteria will be given.
- Aspiration of abscess: The skin over the inflamed area is swabbed with an antiseptic solution. A very fine, short needle is used to inject an anesthetic at a spot in the skin to make it numb. A large-bore needle is used to remove all the pus. Ultrasound can be used to guide the needle as well as to check that all the free-flowing pus was removed. Aspiration of a tiny bit of tissue at this time to see if cancer is present is not reliable.
- Insertion of a drain: The preparation for this is the same as that for aspiration. A small plastic tube is placed into the abscess with ultrasound guidance. The tube is connected to a suction bulb to collect additional pus. The abscess is irrigated with saline (salt water) several times a day until it heals.
- An open incision to drain the abscess is often necessary for several reasons:
  - The abscess and infection do not go away with antibiotics or aspiration.
  - The abscess may have several pockets *(loculations)*, all of which might not be seen or drained if the drainage is performed with a needle. In such a situation, the abscess process would continue and destroy more breast tissue.
  - The abscess may have made tunnels to several areas of the breast that must be identified and cleaned out. This usually is an abscess in a woman who is not breast-feeding and is found under the area of the nipple and areola.
  - If the abscess does not go away completely within a reasonable period of time, small pieces of tissue *(biopsy specimens)* may need to be taken from the wall of the abscess to be certain not to miss an associated cancer that may be present.

The recommendation is that you have an open drainage of the abscess and possibly biopsies of the surrounding tissue.

PREOPERATIVE PREPARATION

- You will have an examination of your blood and possibly of your heart (EKG) and lungs (chest x-ray), depending on your age and general health.
- If you are nursing an infant, there will be a discussion on the advisability of your taking medicines to "dry" your breasts. The decision will be influenced by your special circumstances.
- Do not eat or drink anything for 8 hours before the operation.
- Shower or bathe as usual on the morning of the operation.
- You may be given medicine that will make you feel drowsy before you are brought to the operating room.

□ OPERATION

- The operation will be done under quick-acting general anesthesia.
- The incisions will be made in as cosmetic a fashion as possible.
- The operation usually takes less than an hour.
- A drain may be brought from the abscess cavity to the outside.
- The abscess cavity may be packed with gauze, leaving it to heal from the inside out.

POSTOPERATIVE CARE

- You will be taken to a recovery room and observed. When your blood pressure, pulse, and breathing are stable and you are completely alert, you should be able to go home that same day with a responsible adult.
- Arrangements will be made for your antibiotics, follow-up office visit, stitch removal, and discussion of any laboratory results and plans for continued treatment.
- As with any operation, complications are always possible. With this type of operation, they can include missed infected pockets that need to be cleansed, breakdown of the incision, and possibly others.

✣ HOME CARE

- You may walk about as you wish, even climb stairs, but don't overdo things.
- Continue taking any antibiotics prescribed for you.
- Take medicine as prescribed for your pain.
- Eat as you wish.
- Wearing a loose bra at bedtime—mostly to keep your breasts from moving around too much as you shift during sleep—will make you more comfortable.
- You may sponge bathe as you wish. Otherwise, you will be instructed on when and how to shower and to take care of your dressings.
- Don't drive if you are taking medicines that may reduce your alertness.
- You may return to work when you feel up to it.

✆ CALL OUR OFFICE IF

- You develop any unusual signs or symptoms.
- The incision becomes red or swollen, or there is new or increased drainage from it, or the drainage continues in the same way for longer than 1 week.
- You develop new lumps or areas of tenderness.
- You develop a temperature higher than 100°F.
- You have any questions.

△ GENERAL INFORMATION

Generally, breast agumentation is done to make breasts larger or to correct volume loss after pregnancy but still have them be normal in appearance and function.

○ TREATMENT

- Most commonly, the implant is positioned *behind* the *pectoralis muscle* (the "pecs"), which lies under the breast tissue. In some instances, the implant is placed behind the breast and on top of the muscles. This pushes the breast tissue, skin, nipple, and areola forward, making the breast larger. In most patients the implant does not interfere with sensation in the breast or its functioning, including the ability to nurse.
- The prosthesis is a silicone plastic bag shaped like a breast. It is filled with a *saline* (salt water) solution.
- The prosthesis comes in various sizes. The proper size will be selected, and this will be discussed with you.

PREOPERATIVE PREPARATION

- You will have an examination of your blood and urine. Other tests may be done based on your age and medical history.
- Do not drink or eat anything for 8 hours before the operation.
- You may shower as usual on the morning of the operation.
- You will be given medicine that will make you feel drowsy before you are brought to the operating room.

□ OPERATION

- The entire front of your chest will be painted with an antiseptic solution and surrounded with sterile drapes.
- The operation can be done under general anesthesia or under local anesthesia while you also are given medicine to make you feel drowsy. The choice will be discussed with you.
- The most common location for the incision (about 2 inches long) is in the crease under each of your breasts. Sometimes the incision is made along the border of the *areola* (the dark skin around your nipple) or in the armpit. The breast tissue and muscle are lifted away from the chest wall just enough to make room for the prosthesis to fit. The prosthesis is positioned so that it pushes your own breast tissue forward in the most pleasing cosmetic fashion. The incision will be closed in a cosmetic fashion (Fig. 1).
- The operation generally takes about 2 hours.
- You will not need a blood transfusion.

POSTOPERATIVE CARE

- You will be taken to a recovery room and observed. When your blood pressure, pulse, and breathing are stable and you are completely alert, you should be able to go home on the same day with a responsible adult. On occasion, it is necessary to remain in the hospital overnight.
- There will be a snug elastic bandage across both your

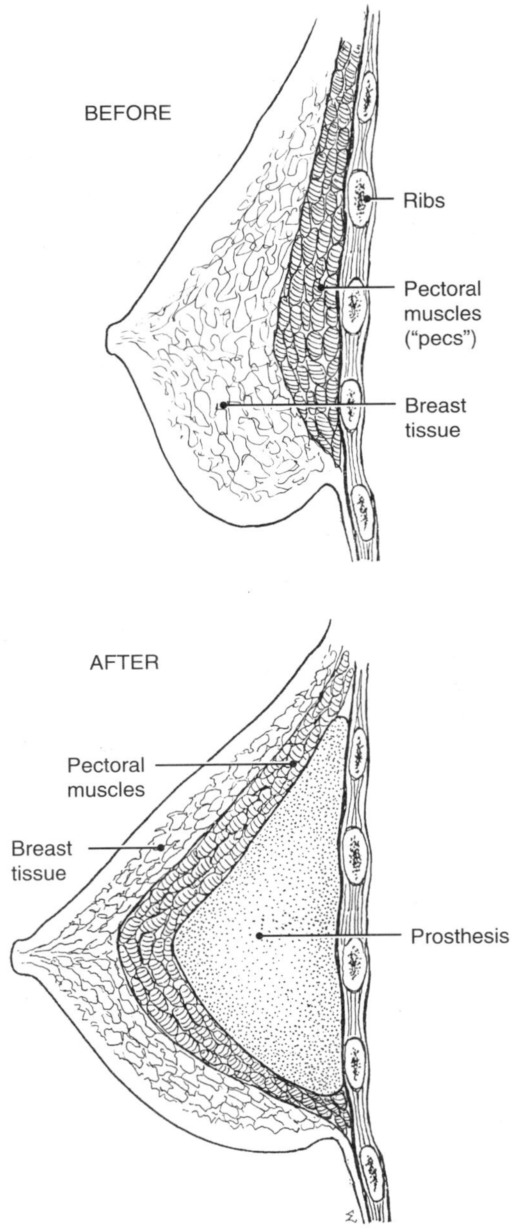

Figure 1. Several types of incision can be used to insert the prosthesis for breast augmentation. The most common is a short incision at the crease below the breast. Notice that the prosthesis is placed deep to the pectoral muscles.

breasts. This dressing will remain in place until your first follow-up office visit.

- Pain can be controlled with medicine.
- Antibiotics must be taken to protect the prosthesis.
- Arrangements will be made for your medicine and follow-up office visit.
- As with any operation, complications are always possible. Although they are uncommon with this type of operation, they can include bleeding, infection, breakage of the prosthesis, formation of excess scar tissue around the prosthesis, numbness of the nipple, and possibly others.

✣ HOME CARE

- You may walk about as you wish, even climb stairs, but until you feel stronger, don't overdo things. Avoid exercise for about a month.
- Unless instructed otherwise, you may shower after the dressings are removed on your first follow-up visit.
    - There may be narrow strips of tape across the incision. It's all right if they get wet; they will be removed in the doctor's office.
- After your dressings are removed, you will need to wear a support bra for about a month. Bring this bra with you on your first follow-up visit.
- Most patients can resume driving within 1 week of the operation.
- You should wear your support bra both during the day and when you sleep.
- Most patients in nonphysical occupations may return to work about a month after the operation.
- Some months after the operation, a few patients develop a thick *capsule* (scar) around the prosthesis. This makes the breasts lose some of their softness. This will be explained to you further, as well as ways to try to prevent it or treat it.

✆ CALL OUR OFFICE IF

- The incisions become red or swollen, or there is drainage from them.
- You develop a temperature higher than 100°F.
- You have any questions.

△ GENERAL INFORMATION

Many thousands of women have breast abnormalities that may cause some concern. These lumps can be smaller than a pea or as large as an orange. There may be one lump or many lumps. They can be solid or filled with fluid *(cysts)*. Some are benign, and others are likely to be cancerous; a few of them are in between. Some lumps can be felt, whereas some are seen only on mammography. Some abnormalities in the breast are as small as grains of sand. These are referred to as *microcalcifications*. Because not all lumps are the same, they do not all need to have a sample taken of them *(biopsy)* in the same way.

DIAGNOSIS

The majority (75%) of these breast lumps are not cancerous. In a woman whose mammogram indicates a risk of cancer of less than 2%, it is usually reasonable that she be observed carefully by her physician and have another mammogram in 4 months. Generally, if the risk of cancer is thought to be greater than 2%, removing some of the suspicious tissue for testing (a *biopsy*) is recommended. The biopsy can be done in one of several ways as follows:

Fine-Needle Aspiration Biopsy: The skin of the breast over the suspicious area is swabbed with an antiseptic solution. A fine needle is used to inject an anesthetic into the skin to make the area numb. Using x-ray or ultrasound as a guide, a fine needle is placed through the numbed skin and down into the suspicious mass, and some cells are removed.

Needle Core Biopsy: Sometimes, a larger needle is used so that several *cores* (that are about as thick as the lead in a pencil) of the suspicious area are removed.

In both instances, the specimens are sent to the pathology laboratory for examination.

Open Biopsy: Generally, if the risk of the mass being a cancer is substantially higher than 2%, removal of the entire lump by an operation is advised.

○ TREATMENT

Your lump can be seen on a mammogram, but it cannot be felt. The mammogram tells the surgeon fairly accurately how far to the left, right, and up and down the mass is but not how deep it is. The surgeon will need some help to be absolutely certain that the biopsy is performed on the suspicious mass and not on something else.

Imagine you are looking at an airplane in the distance. You can estimate fairly well how far to the left or right or how far up and down in the sky it may be, but it's very difficult to know how far away it is. It is much easier if you can look at the airplane from two different angles at the same time. This is called *stereotactic* vision. Stereotactic localization does just that: The mammograms are taken the *same distance* from the breast but from *two different angles*.

After careful consideration of all factors, the recommendation is that you have a core biopsy done with the help of stereotactic x-ray.

PREOPERATIVE PREPARATION

- Shower as usual on the morning of the operation.

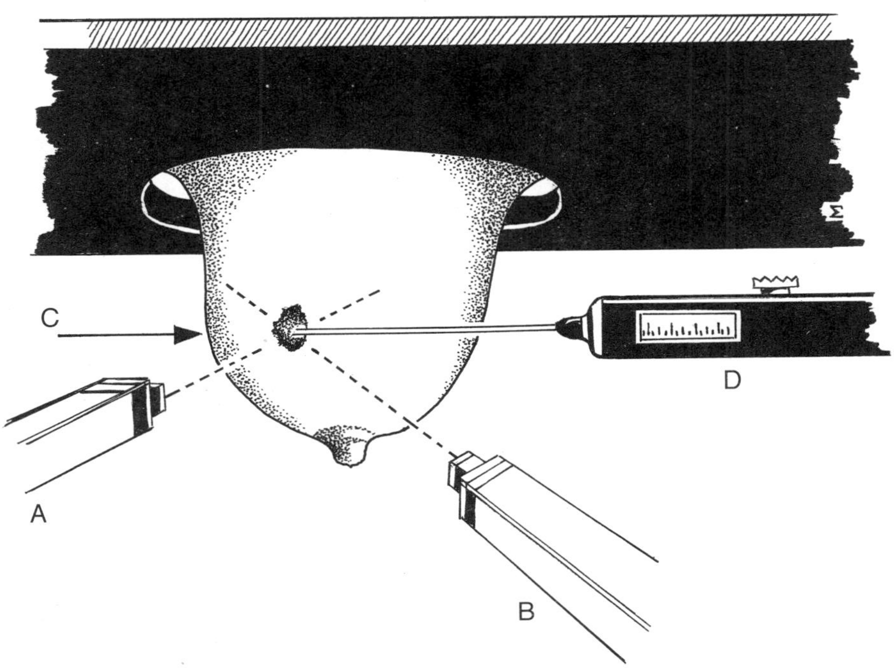

Figure 1.

PROCEDURE

- You'll be asked to lie face down on a special table with an opening in it. You will be positioned so that your breast falls through the opening (Fig. 1). In this position, gravity will pull the breast away from the chest so that more of it can be x-rayed.
- Your breast will be held in place gently by two plates. The front plate has a 2-inch by 2-inch window. The position of the breast will be adjusted so that the abnormal area will be in the center of the window.
- The x-ray machine will take pictures, each from a different angle (A and B). A computer will help determine the exact location of the lump (along the line of arrow C).
- A spot on the breast that is over the lump will be painted with an antiseptic solution.
- A very thin, short needle will be used to inject the skin in the painted area with an anesthetic to make it completely numb.
- Using the measurement developed by the computer that is part of the machine, a special needle will then be placed through the numbed area and down to the lump (D).
- A double-check x-ray will be taken to be certain the needle is in the lump.
- Several pieces of tissue the size of the lead in a wood pencil and about one-half inch long will be taken from different areas of the lump for examination in the pathology laboratory. You will hear clicking sounds during the biopsy but should not feel any pain.
- Quick processing (frozen section) that takes 15 minutes or so usually is not done because these small fragments are too fragile for the most reliable testing.
- The results from the pathology laboratory will be known in 2 to 3 days. You will be notified of the results as soon as possible.
- After the biopsy is completed, a small bandage will be applied over the needle puncture site and you will be free to leave.
- You should expect a small bruise around the needle puncture site and minimal tenderness.
- Resume your usual activities.
- You may shower as you wish and with the dressings in place. After you dry yourself, replace the dressing with a clean dry one.
- Wearing a loose bra at bedtime—mostly to keep your breasts from moving around too much as you shift during sleep—will make you more comfortable.

△ GENERAL INFORMATION

Thousands of women have breast masses that may cause them concern. These masses can be smaller than a pea or as large as an orange. There may be one mass or many masses. They can be solid or filled with fluid *(cysts)*. Some are benign, and others are likely to be cancerous; a lot of them are in between. Some masses can be felt, whereas some are seen only on mammography. Because not all masses are the same, they all do not need to have a sample (a *biopsy*) taken of them in the same way.

DIAGNOSIS

The majority (75%) of these breast lumps are not cancerous. In a woman whose mammogram indicates a risk of cancer of less than 2%, it is usually reasonable that she be observed carefully by her physician and have another mammogram in 4 months. Generally, if the risk of cancer is thought to be greater than 2%, removing some of the suspicious tissue for testing (a *biopsy*) is recommended. The biopsy can be done in one of several ways as follows:

Fine-Needle Aspiration Biopsy: The skin of the breast over the suspicious area is swabbed with an antiseptic solution. A fine needle is used to inject an anesthetic into the skin to make the area numb. Using x-ray or ultrasound as a guide, a fine needle is placed through the numbed skin and down into the suspicious mass, and some cells are removed.

Needle Core Biopsy: Sometimes, a larger needle is used so that several *cores* (that are about as thick as the lead in a pencil) of the suspicious area are removed.

In both instances, the specimens are sent to the pathology laboratory for examination.

Open Biopsy: Generally, if the risk of the mass being a cancer is substantially higher than 2%, removal of the entire lump by an operation is advised.

○ TREATMENT

After careful consideration of all the factors, it is recommended that you have a biopsy of the abnormal appearing tissue in your breast and that this be done through a standard (open) incision.

PREOPERATIVE CARE

- Customarily, the biopsy is done under local anesthesia with sedation. Usually preoperative tests are not necessary.
- If the biopsy is to be done under general anesthesia, you may have an examination of your blood, urine, heart (EKG), and lungs (chest x-ray).
- Do not eat or drink anything for 8 hours before the operation.
- Shower or bathe as usual on the morning of the operation.
- You may be given medicine that will make you feel drowsy before you are brought to the operating room.

□ OPERATION

- Your breast will be examined under a bright light to see the direction of the skin creases (Fig. 1).

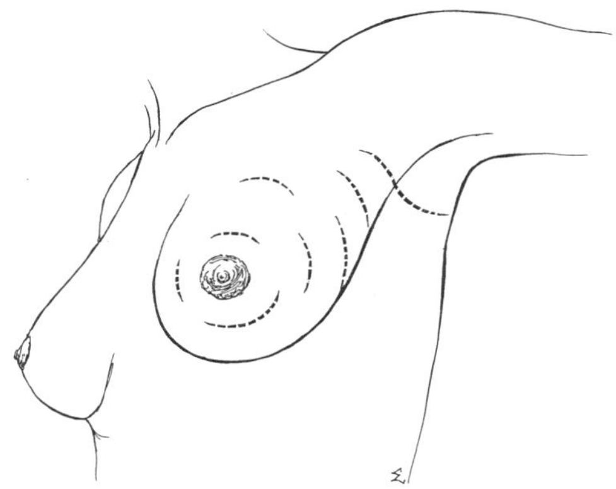

Figure 1. Placement and handling of the incision for a breast biopsy are important. One that is unobtrusive is always desirable. Whenever possible, the incision should be placed along natural skin creases. Some examples are shown.

- The breast will be swabbed with an antiseptic solution and surrounded with sterile drapes.
- A cosmetic incision will be made in a crease that is near the mass.
- A fine needle will be used to inject an anesthetic into the skin and surrounding tissue to make the entire area numb. You may also be given a medication to make you feel drowsy.
- During the operation, you may feel some tugging but not pain.
- The removed tissue will be sent to the pathology laboratory for examination.
- The wound will be examined carefully to be sure there is no bleeding.
- The skin will be closed in a cosmetic fashion.

POSTOPERATIVE CARE

- You will be taken to a recovery room and observed. When your blood pressure, pulse, and breathing are stable and you are completely alert, you should be able to go home that same day with a responsible adult.
- Arrangements will be made for your medicine, follow-up office visit, stitch removal, and discussion of laboratory findings.
- As with any operation, complications are always possible. Although they are uncommon with this type of operation, they can include bleeding and infection.

✚ HOME CARE

- Resume your usual activities.
- Take medicine as prescribed for your pain.
- Wearing a loose bra at bedtime—mostly to keep your breasts from moving around too much as you sleep—will make you more comfortable.
- Unless instructed otherwise, you may shower as you wish and with any dressings on or off.

- There may be narrow strips of tape across the incision. It's all right if they get wet; they will be removed in the doctor's office.
- After you dry yourself, replace any dressings with clean, dry ones.

- You may drive your car as long as you are not taking any medicine that may reduce your alertness.
- You may return to work when you feel up to it.

✆ CALL OUR OFFICE IF

- You develop any unusual signs or symptoms.
- The incision becomes red or swollen, or there is drainage from it.
- You develop a temperature higher than 100°F.
- You have any questions.

BREAST BIOPSY: Open, Stereotactic-Guided

△ GENERAL INFORMATION

Thousands of women have breast lumps that may cause some concern. These lumps can be smaller than a pea or as large as an orange. There may be one lump or many lumps. They can be solid or filled with fluid *(cysts)*. Some are benign, and others are likely to be cancerous; a few of them are in between. Some lumps can be felt, whereas some are seen only on mammography. Some abnormalities in the breast are as small as grains of sand. These are referred to as *microcalcifications*. Because not all lumps are the same, they do not all need to have a sample (a *biopsy*) taken of them in the same way.

DIAGNOSIS

The majority (75%) of these breast lumps are not cancerous. In a woman whose mammogram indicates a risk of cancer of less than 2%, it is usually reasonable that she be observed carefully by her physician and have another mammogram in 4 months. Generally, if the risk of cancer is thought to be greater than 2%, removing some of the suspicious tissue for testing (a *biopsy*) is recommended. The biopsy can be done in one of several ways as follows:

Fine-Needle Aspiration Biopsy: The skin of the breast over the suspicious area is swabbed with an antiseptic solution. A fine needle is used to inject an anesthetic into the skin to make the area numb. Using x-ray or ultrasound as a guide, a fine needle is placed through the numbed skin and down into the suspicious mass, and some cells are removed.

Needle Core Biopsy: Sometimes, a larger needle is used so that several *cores* (that are about as thick as the lead in a pencil) of the suspicious area are removed.

In both instances, the specimens are sent to the pathology laboratory for examination.

Open Biopsy: Generally, if the risk of the mass being a cancer is substantially higher than 2%, removal of the entire lump by an operation is advised.

○ TREATMENT

Your lump can be seen on a mammogram, but it cannot be felt. The mammogram tells the surgeon fairly accurately how far to the left, right, and up and down the mass is but not how deep it is. The surgeon will need some help to be absolutely certain that the biopsy is performed on the suspicious mass and not on something else. This is done with *stereotactic* localization. Imagine you are looking at an airplane in the distance. You can estimate fairly well how far to the left or right or how far up and down in the sky it may be, but it's very difficult to know how far away it is. It is much easier if you can look at the airplane from two different angles at the same time. Stereotactic localization does just that: The mammograms are taken the same distance from the breast but from two different angles.

After careful consideration of all factors, it is recommended that you have a biopsy of the abnormal tissue in your breast with the help of stereotactic x-rays as described above.

PREOPERATIVE PREPARATION

- Shower as usual on the morning of the operation.

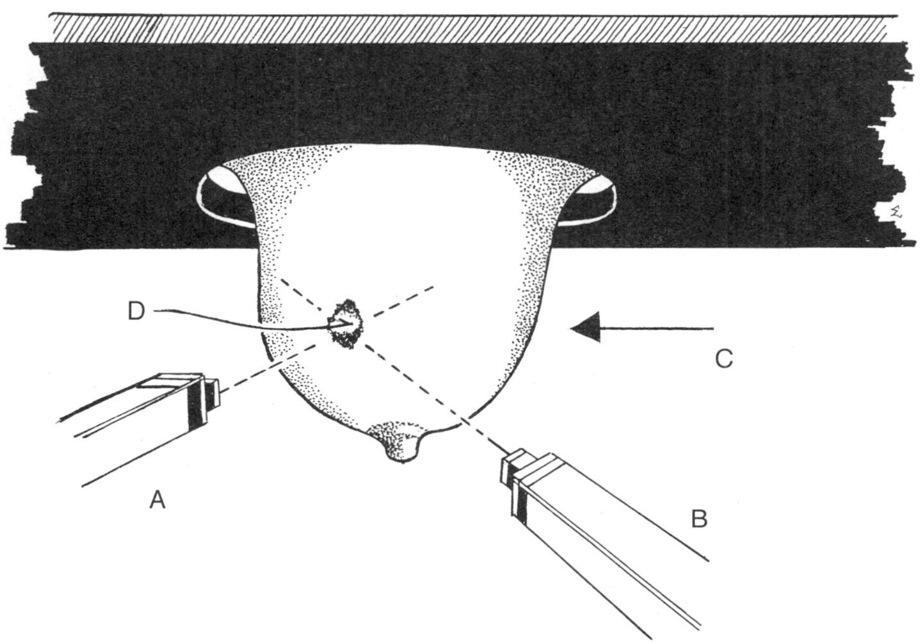

Figure 1.

PROCEDURE

- You'll be asked to lie face down on a special table with an opening in it. You will be positioned so that your breast falls through the opening (Fig. 1). In this position, gravity will pull the breast away from the chest so that more of it can be x-rayed.
- Your breast will be held in place gently by two plates. The front plate has a 2-inch by 2-inch window in it. The position of the breast will be adjusted so that the abnormal area will be in the center of the window.
- The x-ray machine will take pictures, each from a different angle (A and B). A computer will help determine the exact location of the lump (along the line of arrow C).
- A spot on the breast that is over the lump will be painted with an antiseptic solution.
- A very thin, short needle will be used to inject the skin in the painted area with an anesthetic to make it completely numb.
- Using the measurement developed by the computer that is part of the machine, a special needle will then be placed through the numbed area and down to the lump.
- Several pieces of tissue about the size of the lead in a wood pencil will be taken from different areas of the lump for examination in the pathology laboratory. You will hear clicking sounds during the biopsy but should not feel any pain.

Sometimes plans are made to do an open biopsy if the stereotactic needle biopsy shows cancer. This stereotactic technique is used to help the surgeon locate the lump in the breast because it cannot be felt. In such instances, the following takes place:

- When the lump is exactly localized as described above, a special wire (the size of a thin guitar string) is advanced through the needle down to the lump.
- The position of the wire is double-checked, and if it is in the right position, one drop of blue dye is injected into the lump through the needle. The needle is removed, leaving the wire through the skin with its tip in the lump (D). You then are taken to the outpatient operating room for an open biopsy.

THE BIOPSY

- The breast will be painted with an antiseptic solution and draped.
- A very thin needle will be used to inject anesthetic around the point at which the wire enters the breast as well as in the surrounding and deep tissue so that all of it will be numb. You may also be given medicine to make you feel drowsy.
- A cosmetic incision will be made right next to where the wire enters the breast. The wire will be followed down to its tip (and the drop of blue dye) where the lump is located.
- The breast tissue containing the lump will be removed.
- During the operation, you may feel some tugging but not pain.
- A special type of x-ray will be taken of the removed breast tissue with the wire in it to be certain that all that was suspicious on the mammogram actually was removed.
- After the above, the breast tissue (the open biopsy) is sent to the laboratory for examination.
- The incision will be closed in a cosmetic fashion.

POSTOPERATIVE CARE

- You will be taken to a recovery room. When your blood pressure, pulse, and breathing are stable and you are completely alert, you should be able to go home that same day with a responsible adult.
- Arrangements will be made for your medicine, follow-up office visit, stitch removal, and discussion of the laboratory findings.
- As with any operation, complications are always possible. Although they are uncommon with this type of operation, they can include bleeding and infection, and possibly others.

✚ HOME CARE

- Resume your usual activities.
- Unless instructed otherwise, you may shower as you wish and with any dressings on or off.
  - There may be narrow strips of tape across the incision. It's all right if they get wet; they will be removed in the doctor's office.
  - After you dry yourself, replace any dressings with clean, dry ones.
- Take medicine as prescribed for your pain.
- Wearing a loose bra at bedtime—mostly to keep your breasts from moving around too much as you shift during sleep—will make you more comfortable.
- You may drive your car as long as you are not taking medicines that reduce your alertness.
- You may return to work when you feel up to it.

✆ CALL OUR OFFICE IF

- The incision becomes red or swollen, or there is drainage from it.
- You develop a temperature higher than 100°F.
- You have any questions.

△ GENERAL INFORMATION

Annual breast checkup with mammography in healthy women can reveal small breast lumps that cannot be felt. Some of them turn out to be cancerous.

DIAGNOSIS

The majority (75%) of these breast lumps are not cancerous. In a woman whose mammogram indicates a risk of cancer of less than 2%, it is usually reasonable that she be observed carefully by her physician and have another mammogram in 4 months. Generally, if the risk of cancer is thought to be greater than 2%, removing some of the suspicious tissue for testing (a *biopsy*) is recommended. The biopsy can be done in one of several ways as follows:

Fine-Needle Aspiration Biopsy: The skin of the breast over the suspicious area is swabbed with an antiseptic solution. A fine needle is used to inject an anesthetic into the skin to make the area numb. Using x-ray or ultrasound as a guide, a fine needle is placed through the numbed skin and down into the suspicious mass, and some cells are removed.

Needle Core Biopsy: Sometimes, a larger needle is used so that several *cores* (that are about as thick as the lead in a pencil) of the suspicious area are removed.

In both instances, the specimens are sent to the pathology laboratory for examination.

Open Biopsy: Generally, if the risk of the mass being a cancer is substantially higher than 2%, removal of the entire lump by an operation is advised.

○ TREATMENT

You have an area on mammography that is sufficiently suspicious of being a cancer that the recommendation is to remove it by an operation.

So that the surgeon will know where to find the abnormality that cannot be felt, it will first have to be localized for the surgeon by x-ray. After careful consideration of all factors, the recommendation is that you have a breast biopsy done in this manner.

PREPARATION FOR THE PROCEDURE

- Do not eat or drink anything for 8 hours before the operation.
- Shower or bathe as usual on the morning of the operation.

PROCEDURE

- A mammogram will be taken, but this time a plastic plate with one or more openings (windows) in it will be used to compress the breast.
- The mammogram that is taken will now show the breast, the abnormality in it, and the openings of the compression plate.
- With your breast (and the plastic plate over it) still compressed on the mammogram machine, the skin over the abnormality in the breast will be matched with calibrations on the opening and this point on the skin marked with a small dot.
- A short, very fine needle may be used to inject an anesthetic in the area of the dot to make it numb. Then, a special needle with a wire in it about the size of a thin guitar string and a hooked tip will be placed through the numbed skin and down into the lump. Another x-ray is taken to make certain the needle tip is inside the abnormality.
- Next, the needle is removed, but the wire with the hooked tip is left in place. The hooked wire then will be taped securely to the skin.
- You will now be taken to the outpatient operating room for the open biopsy.

THE BIOPSY

- The breast will be swabbed with an antiseptic solution and surrounded with sterile sheets.
- An anesthetic will be injected around the point at which the wire enters the breast, as well as into the deep tissue so that all of this area will be numb. You may also be given medicine that will make you feel drowsy.
- A cosmetic incision will be made close to where the wire enters the breast. The wire will be followed down to its hooked tip that is in the abnormal tissue (Fig. 1).

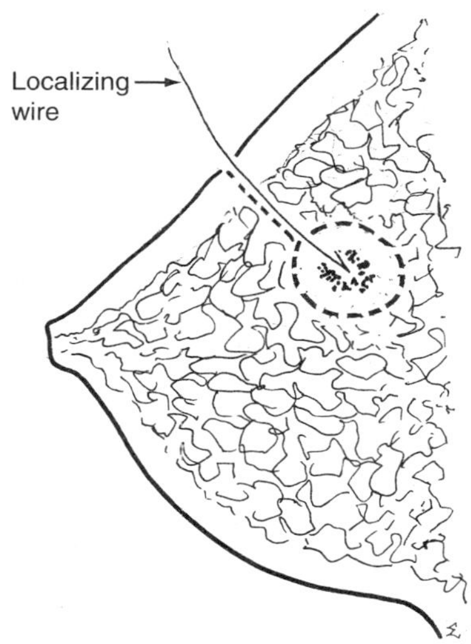

Figure 1.

- During the operation, you may feel some tugging but not pain.
- The entire suspicious tissue will be removed.
- A special type of x-ray will be taken of the removed breast tissue and the wire in it to be certain that the abnormality seen on the mammogram actually was removed.
- After the above, all of the removed tissue will be sent to the pathology laboratory for examination to

determine what it is and whether it was removed with clean borders.

- The incision will be closed in a cosmetic fashion.
- The operation usually takes about 1 hour.

POSTOPERATIVE CARE

- You will be taken to a recovery room. When your blood pressure, pulse, and breathing are stable and you are completely alert, you should be able to go home that same day with a responsible adult.
- As with any operation, complications are always possible. With this type of operation, they can include bleeding, infection, and possibly others.
- Arrangements will be made for any medicine, follow-up office visit, stitch removal, and discussion of the laboratory findings.

✚ HOME CARE

- Resume your usual activities.
- Unless instructed otherwise, you may shower if you wish and with any dressings on or off.
  - There may be narrow strips of tape across the incision. It's all right if they get wet; they will be removed in the doctor's office.
  - After you dry yourself, replace any dressings with clean, dry ones.
- Take medicine as prescribed for your pain.
- Wearing a loose bra at bedtime—mostly to keep your breasts from moving around too much as you shift during sleep—will make you more comfortable.
- Do not drive a car if you are taking medicines that reduce your alertness.

✆ CALL OUR OFFICE IF

- You develop any unusual signs or symptoms.
- The incision becomes red or swollen, or there is drainage from it.
- You develop a temperature higher than 100°F.
- You have any questions.

BREAST BIOPSY: Ultrasound-Guided

△ GENERAL INFORMATION

Thousands of women have breast masses that may cause some concern. These masses can be smaller than a pea or as large as an orange. There may be one mass or many masses. They can be solid or filled with fluid *(cysts)*. Some masses can be felt, whereas some are seen only on mammography. Most are benign, but some are malignant. Because not all masses are the same or have the same risk of being cancerous, they all do not need to have a sample (a *biopsy*) taken of them in the same way. The biopsy can be done in one of several ways.

DIAGNOSIS

The majority (75%) of these breast lumps are not cancerous. In a woman whose mammogram indicates a risk of cancer of less than 2%, it is usually reasonable that she be observed carefully by her physician and have another mammogram in 4 months. Generally, if the risk of cancer is thought to be greater than 2%, removing some of the suspicious tissue for testing (*a biopsy*) is recommended. The biopsy can be done in one of several ways as follows:

Fine-Needle Aspiration Biopsy: The skin of the breast over the suspicious area is swabbed with an antiseptic solution. A fine needle is used to inject an anesthetic into the skin to make the area numb. Using x-ray or ultrasound as a guide, a fine needle is placed through the numbed skin and down into the suspicious mass, and some cells are removed.

Needle Core Biopsy: Sometimes, a larger needle is used so that several *cores* (that are about as thick as the lead in a pencil) of the suspicious area are removed.

In both instances, the specimens are sent to the pathology laboratory for examination.

Open Biopsy: Generally, if the risk of the mass being a cancer is substantially higher than 2%, removal of the entire lump by an operation is advised.

○ TREATMENT

The advantages of using ultrasound to help guide the needle during biopsy of certain masses that can be seen but not felt are as follows:

- No incision is necessary.
- There is no elaborate preparation or unnecessary delay.
- It is accurate.
- It is not painful.
- It can be performed in the doctor's office.

After careful consideration of all factors, it is recommended that you have a breast biopsy using this technique (Fig. 1).

PREPARATION FOR THE CLOSED BIOPSY

- No special preparation is necessary.
- Inform the doctor or nurse if you are taking blood-thinning medicine (anticoagulants).

THE PROCEDURE

- You will lie on a comfortable table in the surgeon's office.
- Some lubricating solution will be placed over your breast.
- A gadget the size of a small deck of cards and connected to the ultrasound machine will be moved back and forth over the breast. This gadget aims harmless sound waves at the breast. The sound waves that bounce back (the echoes) are seen on the ultrasound screen. You will be able to see all this yourself as it is taking place.
- The entire breast will be examined and the position of the suspicious mass carefully noted.
- The skin over this area of the breast will be swabbed with an antiseptic solution and surrounded with sterile towels.
- A thin, short needle will be used to inject an anesthetic in the skin over the mass to make it numb.
- As everything is watched on the ultrasound screen, a special needle is placed through the numbed skin and into the mass. A short piece of the lump, as big around as the lead in a pencil (a *core biopsy*), is taken and the needle removed.
- The biopsy tissue is sent to the laboratory for examination.
- After a small tape bandage is placed over the needle puncture site, the procedure is over and you are free to leave.
- Arrangements will be made for you to learn of the results as soon as they are available.

✚ HOME CARE

- Resume your usual activities.

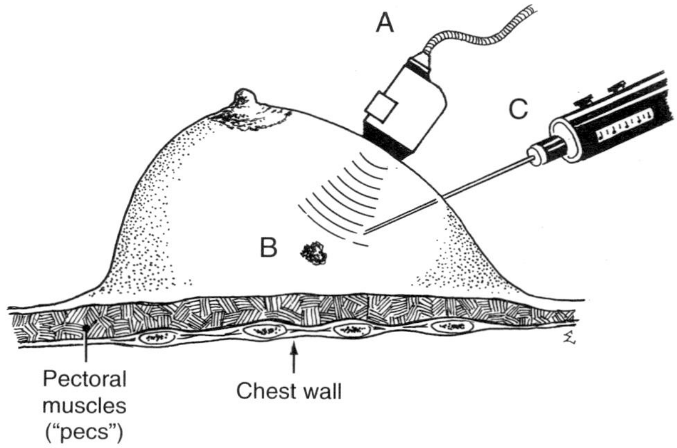

Figure 1. Ultrasound (A) is used to locate the breast lumps (B) that can be seen on a mammogram but cannot be felt. While observing the tumor with the ultrasound, the needle (C) is directed to the lump so that a piece of it can be taken for examination in the laboratory.

✆ CALL OUR OFFICE IF

- The breast swells, becomes extremely painful, or develops a blue area.
- You have any questions.

△ GENERAL INFORMATION

Cancer of the breast in men is rare, and its cause is not known. It occurs most often in an older man who just doesn't think of cancer when a breast lump appears. So he puts off a visit to the doctor.

COMMON SIGNS AND SYMPTOMS

There is a mass in the breast that has the following characteristics:

- Is irregular.
- Is firm to hard.
- Is fixed to the skin and possibly to the muscle underneath it.
- Does not hurt.

DIAGNOSIS

- Usually the diagnosis can be made by taking a detailed history, doing a thorough physical examination, and carefully considering the laboratory reports.
- Although gynecomastia, a harmless enlargement of the breasts (*both* breasts—something rarely seen with cancer) is always a possibility, the doctor must establish what the mass is.
- A mammogram sometimes can be helpful except that it is not easy to do it well on a breast that doesn't stick out like a woman's breast.
- One method is to insert a needle into the mass to obtain a tiny piece of it (called *needle aspiration biopsy*) for examination in the laboratory.
- Another method is to anesthetize the skin over the mass to make it completely numb. A small piece of the mass is taken (an *open biopsy*) for examination under the microscope.

○ TREATMENT

- The best chance for cure is to remove the cancer and the lymph nodes under the armpit.
- There is little tissue in and around a man's breast (compared with a woman's breast). Because of this, a cancer in a man's breast gets stuck to the muscle underneath it and to the skin over it very early.
- For the above reasons, the muscle under the breasts also has to be removed to get around the cancer properly. The operation to do this is called a *radical mastectomy*.

After careful consideration of all factors, the recommendation is that you have a radical mastectomy.

PREOPERATIVE CARE

- You will have a routine examination of your blood, urine, heart (EKG), and lungs (chest x-ray).
- A bone scan might be done to be certain the bones are not involved.
- Do not drink or eat anything for 8 hours before the operation.
- Shower as usual on the morning of the operation.
- You may be given medicine that will make you feel drowsy before you are brought to the operating room.

□ OPERATION

- You will be asleep for this operation.
- The skin over the cancer has to be removed with a wide margin to be certain no cancer is left behind. Because there is often little extra skin to begin with, the incision sometimes cannot be closed. In such an instance, a small piece of skin will be taken from your abdominal wall or thigh and placed over the open area on the chest wall (a *skin graft*). The area over the abdomen or thigh will make new skin.
- The operation usually takes about 2 hours.
- You will not need a blood transfusion.

POSTOPERATIVE CARE

- You will be taken to a recovery room and observed. When your blood pressure, pulse, and breathing are stable, you will be taken to a regular hospital room.
- There may be a thin plastic tube coming from the wound that will drain any fluid into a small plastic bag.
- There is moderate pain that will be controlled with medicine.
- That evening you will be helped to sit up in bed and the next day to get out of bed.
- You should be able to go home in several days.
- Your condition can be cured. Assessment of this can be made only after all the test results are back.
- As with any operation, complications are always possible. They can include bleeding, infection, and loss of the skin graft, among others.
- Arrangements will be made for your medicines, follow-up office visit, stitch or clip removal, discussion of the laboratory findings, instructions on wound care, an arm exercise program, and possible additional treatment.

✥ HOME CARE

- Continue with the program started in the hospital.
- You may walk about as you wish, even climb stairs.
- You may eat as you wish.
- Unless instructed otherwise, you may shower if you wish and with any dressings on or off.
  - There may be narrow strips of tape across the incision. It's all right if they get wet; they will be removed in the doctor's office.
  - After you dry yourself, replace any dressings with clean, dry ones.
- Arrangements can be made for a home visiting nurse if one is needed.

✆ CALL OUR OFFICE IF

- You develop any unusual signs or symptoms.
- The incision becomes red or swollen, or there is drainage from it.
- You develop a temperature higher than 100°F.
- You have any questions.

△ GENERAL INFORMATION

Modified radical mastectomy means the removal of the entire breast and the lymph nodes in the *axilla* (armpit). No muscles are removed (Fig. 1). (The operation in which muscle tissue is removed is called a *radical mastectomy.*) This operation of modified radical mastectomy is done to remove cancer that cannot be removed safely by a smaller operation, such as a *lumpectomy* (also known as *wide local excision*).

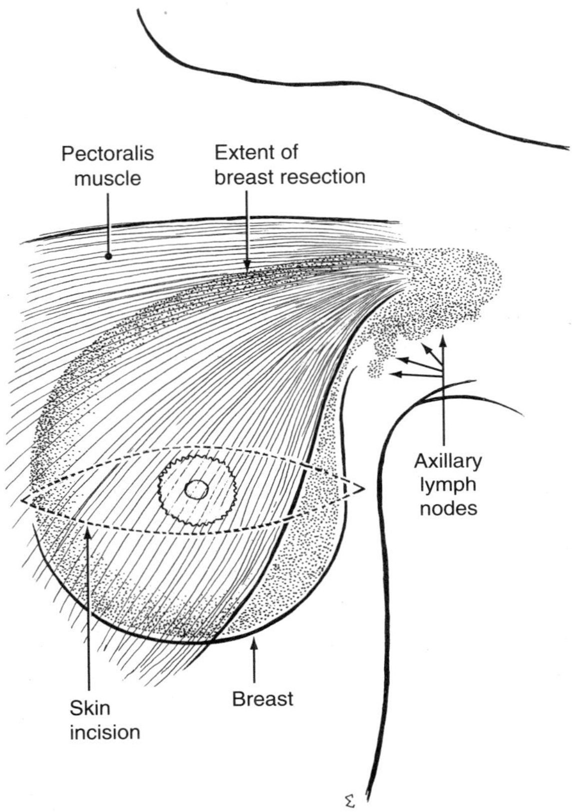

Figure 1. In a modified radical mastectomy, all the breast tissue and the lymph nodes in the axilla (armpit) are removed. The pectoral muscles (the "pecs") deep to the breast are not disturbed. A common type of skin incision is shown.

COMMON SIGNS AND SYMPTOMS

- A lump is felt by the person just by chance while dressing or taking a shower or by the doctor doing a routine examination.
- There is a vague aching over the area.
- There is dimpling of the skin, or the breast is slightly flattened over the area.

DIAGNOSIS

A biopsy will have been done by removing a small piece of breast tissue with a fine needle or possibly an open incision. Or, it may be agreed that the biopsy will be done while you are asleep under anesthesia. If the diagnosis is cancer, then the operation can be done at the same time.

○ TREATMENT

- The best chance to cure a cancer of the breast such as you have is by an operation, often followed by additional medical treatment.

There are several operations for breast cancer. Findings that indicate a modified radical mastectomy is appropriate include the following:

- There may be very little to feel, but the mammogram shows areas suspicious for cancer throughout the breast.
- A generous open biopsy is done, but under the microscope it can be seen that the tumor extends across all the margins of the biopsy specimen.
- The breast is small, and doing a lumpectomy to remove a fair-sized cancer to include normal tissue around the tumor doesn't leave much behind. Also, the tissue remaining has to receive x-ray treatments for 5 to 6 weeks.

After careful consideration of all factors, the recommendation is that you have a modified radical mastectomy.

PREOPERATIVE PREPARATION

- An examination of your blood, urine, heart (EKG), and lungs (chest x-ray) will be done.
- A bone scan may be done to be certain there is nothing abnormal.
- Do not eat or drink anything for 8 hours before the operation.
- Shower as usual the morning of the operation.
- You may be given medicine that will make you feel drowsy before you are brought to the operating room.

□ OPERATION

- You will be asleep for the operation.
- The operation usually takes about 2 hours.
- You will not receive a blood transfusion.
- The removed breast and lymph nodes will be sent to the laboratory to be examined by a pathologist.

POSTOPERATIVE CARE

- You will wake up in a recovery room. When your blood pressure, pulse, and breathing become stable, you will be taken to a regular hospital room.
- There will be a thin plastic tube coming from the wound that will drain any fluid into a small plastic bag.
- There is only moderate pain, and it will be controlled with medicine.
- The evening of the operation you will be helped to sit up and on the next day to get out of bed.
- You will be shown how to manage the thin plastic tube and its container; it's not difficult.

- You should be able to go home in several days.
- Your cancer can be cured. The chances of this can be estimated only after all the laboratory tests are back.
- Arrangements will be made for your follow-up office visit, pain medicine, stitch and tube removal, instructions on arm exercises, and discussion of the laboratory findings.
- As with any operation, complications are always possible. With this type of operation, they can include bleeding, infection, loss of some skin, arm swelling, and possibly others.

✣ HOME CARE

- You may walk about as you wish, even climb stairs.
- You may eat as you did before the operation.
- You will be given instructions on how to take care of the drainage bag; it's not difficult.
- Sponge bathe as you wish. After the first change of dressings, you may shower as you wish and with any dressings on or off.
  - When taking a shower, the small plastic bag for the draining fluid can be strapped around your waist or hung around your neck with a string.
  - There may be narrow strips of tape across the incision. It's all right if they get wet; they will be removed in the doctor's office.
  - After you dry yourself, replace any dressings with clean, dry ones.
- Arrangements can be made for a home visiting nurse if one is needed.
- Even though many of the lymph nodes were removed, enough of them remain in other parts of the axilla and above the collar bone to drain the arm under normal circumstances. Just the same, those that remain should not be abused if they are to do their job properly. They can be hurt by the following:
  - Infection: You should avoid injury to that arm, such as dirty scratches, splinters, and even needle sticks to draw blood.
  - X-rays to the axilla. You will not receive any x-ray treatments to your axilla.
  - Repeated hard work with that arm for long periods of time (examples: using that arm to pull weeds for an hour or two, to vacuum your entire house, or to wash all the windows in one session).
- Occasionally there will be some swelling of the hand or forearm. There are treatments for this.
- Driving a car with an automatic shift may not seem too demanding. However, you may have to slam on brakes or twist to turn the steering wheel and may strain your sutures or tear something. During your follow-up visit, let's discuss when you can resume driving.
- You may resume sexual activity whenever you choose.
- You may return to work when you feel up to it, but let's talk about it first during your follow-up office visit.

✆ CALL OUR OFFICE IF

- Your incision area becomes red or swollen, or there is drainage from it.
- The area in the axilla becomes swollen.
- Your hand or arm becomes swollen.
- You develop a temperature higher than 100°F.
- You have any questions.

△ GENERAL INFORMATION

This operation is the wide local excision of only the cancerous breast lump (a *lumpectomy*) instead of all of the breast *(modified radical mastectomy)*. The lymph nodes in the *axilla* (armpit) may be removed at the same time, usually through a separate cosmetic incision (Fig. 1).

When done under the right circumstances, this operation, including the x-ray treatments that follow, has the same cure rate as when the entire breast is removed, yet it is more pleasing cosmetically than removal of the breast.

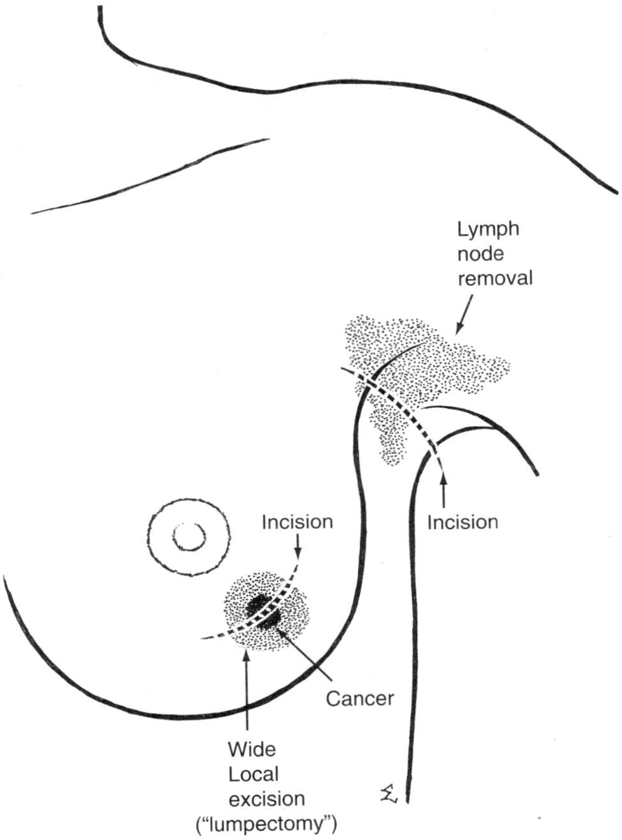

Figure 1. In this operation the cancer is excised widely enough that the borders of the removed tissue are free of cancer. The lymph nodes in the axilla (armpit) usually are removed through a separate incision. If the cancer is close to the axilla, the cancer and the lymph nodes can be removed through a single incision.

COMMON SIGNS AND SYMPTOMS

- There are few symptoms with early lesions. There may be a mild ache over the tumor.
- A breast lump may be felt by the person by chance while taking a shower, dressing, or doing a breast self-examination. Or it may be discovered by the doctor during a routine examination.
- There may be very little or nothing to feel, but the mammogram shows a suspicious abnormality.

DIAGNOSIS

A diagnosis can be made by several methods:

- The skin over the lump is made numb with an anesthetic, and a fine needle is used to obtain a tiny piece of it (a *fine-needle aspiration biopsy*) for examination in the laboratory.
- The skin is made numb, an incision is made over the lump, and a piece of it is removed (an *open biopsy*) for examination in the laboratory.
- The entire operation can be done in one step while you are asleep under anesthesia. The biopsy is performed, and while you are kept asleep a quick examination is made of the tissue in the laboratory. If the diagnosis is cancer, the remainder of the operation is completed.

PREOPERATIVE PREPARATION

- You will have an examination of your blood, urine, heart (EKG), and lungs (chest x-ray).
- If you have any bone symptoms or if the breast lump is sizable, a bone scan may be done to be certain there is no tumor in the bones.
- Do not eat or drink anything during the 8 hours before your operation.
- You may take a shower on the morning of the operation.
- You may be given medicine that will make you feel drowsy before you are brought to the operating room.

□ OPERATION

- You will be asleep for the operation.
- There will be one incision over the breast and a second one along a crease in the axilla. Sometimes the lump in the breast and the lymph nodes in the axilla are removed through one incision.
- The incisions will be made in a cosmetic fashion so that they will be the least visible.
- The removed breast tissue and lymph nodes will be sent to the laboratory to be examined by a pathologist.
- The entire operation usually takes about 2 hours.
- You will not receive any blood transfusion.

POSTOPERATIVE CARE

- You will wake up in a recovery room. When your blood pressure, pulse, and breathing are stable you will be taken to a regular hospital room.
- There is only moderate pain, and it will be controlled with medicine.
- There may be a small plastic tube from your axilla draining any fluid into a small plastic bag. You will be shown how to take care of this; it's not difficult.
- Do not start any arm exercises until you are shown how to do them by the surgeon.
- The need for any hormones or chemotherapy will be determined after all the laboratory tests on the removed tissue are completed.

- As with any operation, complications are always possible. Although they are uncommon with your type of operation, they can include bleeding, infection, and possibly others.
- Your condition can be cured. An estimate of your chances can be made only after all the test results are back.
- Arrangements will be made for your medicine, follow-up office visit, and stitch removal.

✚ HOME CARE

- You may walk about as you wish, even climb stairs.
- Unless instructed otherwise, you may shower as you wish and with any dressings on or off.
  - There may be narrow strips of tape across the incision. It's all right if they get wet; they will be removed in the doctor's office.
  - After you dry yourself, replace any dressings with clean, dry ones.
- Even though many of the lymph nodes were removed, enough of them remain in other parts of the axilla and above the collar bone to drain the arm. Just the same, those that are left behind should not be abused if they are to do their job properly. They can be hurt by the following:
  - Infection: You should avoid injury to that arm, such as dirty scratches, splinters, and even needle sticks to draw blood.
  - X-ray to the axilla: You will not receive any x-ray treatments to your axilla.
  - Repeated hard work with that arm for long periods of time (examples: using that arm to pull weeds for 2 to 3 hours, to vacuum your entire house, or to wash all the windows in one session).
- Occasionally there will be some swelling of the hand or forearm. There are treatments for this.
- Take medicine as prescribed for your pain.
- Wearing a loose bra at bedtime—mostly to keep your breasts from moving around too much as you shift during sleep—will make you more comfortable.
- Driving a car with an automatic shift may not seem too demanding. However, you may have to slam on brakes or twist to turn the steering wheel and may strain your sutures or tear something. During your follow-up visit let's discuss when you can resume driving.
- You may resume sexual activity whenever you choose.
- You may return to work when you feel up to it, but let's talk about it first during your follow-up office visit.

✆ CALL OUR OFFICE IF

- The incision on the breast or axilla becomes swollen or red, or there is drainage from it.
- You develop a temperature higher than 100°F.
- You have any questions.

AFTER CARE

- Arrangements will be made for the routine x-ray treatments to your breast starting 4 to 6 weeks after the operation, after everything has healed satisfactorily.
- The x-ray treatments will be given to you daily on an outpatient basis (five times per week) for 5 to 6 weeks. The details will be explained to you.

△ GENERAL INFORMATION

Fibroadenoma is a common noncancerous tumor of the breast seen most often in young women. There may be a relationship between fibroadenoma and some hormonal event. Fibroadenoma of the breast has nothing to do with fibroids of the uterus.

COMMON SIGNS AND SYMPTOMS

- The tumor feels like a smooth, rubbery mass that is freely movable. It feels like a "slippery olive."
- It usually does not hurt.
- It rarely changes in size with the menstrual cycles. It is different from fibrocystic changes of the breast. The latter are areas of nodularity or thickening that cause the breast to feel tender or painful and that change with the menstrual cycle.
- There may be more than one lump in a single breast or in both breasts.

DIAGNOSIS

A detailed history and physical examination by an experienced doctor can make the diagnosis accurately about 85% of the time. Methods that can help establish the diagnosis inlcude the following:

- Ultrasound: Harmless sound waves are aimed at the breast. The sound waves bouncing back (the echoes) from structures inside the breast are seen as pictures on a screen. This is a convenient, painless, and harmless way to look at certain kinds of lumps inside the breast.
- A mammogram may be ordered. It can show not only the nature of the tumor but also possibly another abnormality that cannot be felt (in either breast).

  If there's any question about the diagnosis, further evaluation may be necessary. Sometimes it is necessary to confirm the clinical diagnosis of a mass by examining a small amount of it (a *biopsy*) under the microscope. This can be done in one of several ways:
- *Fine-Needle Aspiration Biopsy*: This method is most suitable for women younger than 20 years of age. The breast is painted with an antiseptic solution, and then the skin over the mass is made numb with an anesthetic. A fine needle will be inserted through the numbed skin and into the mass. A few cells will be drawn off and sent to the laboratory for examination. A fine-needle aspiration biopsy is 85 to 95% accurate.
- *Core Needle Biopsy*: A slightly more accurate type of needle biopsy involves preparing the breast in the same manner but using a somewhat larger needle to core out a piece of tissue for the diagnosis. The ultrasound may be used to help aim the needle and to confirm that the tissue being sampled is really from the tumor.

○ TREATMENT

- Removing the mass (even if proved by biopsy to be fibroadenoma) is often advisable. At other times it may be reasonable to observe it for a while or even not to treat it at all.

Reasons for an Early Operation

- If a woman is trying to become pregnant. Breast examination and follow-up during pregnancy and breast-feeding is more difficult with a fibroadenoma present. Also, removal of an enlarging mass from a pregnant breast is much more difficult, and the wound heals less well.
- If it appears to be growing rapidly. A small percentage of fibroadenomas grow to a large size.
- If this tumor can be felt, it may be a continuous source of concern for a patient.

Reasons to Wait

- If on physical examination, ultrasound, or mammography, the mass appears to be a fibroadenoma and fine-needle aspiration supports this diagnosis, it is reasonable to observe this mass at regular intervals.
- The mass has been present for a period of time and has not grown at all.
- The person is young. The possibility that this is a fibroadenoma is high, and the risk of cancer is low.
- Incisions in locations other than the areola on a young, still-growing breast can be prone to form thick, wide scars.

After taking all of the above factors into consideration, the recommendation is that your tumor be removed.

PREOPERATIVE CARE

If you are younger than 35 years and are not going to have this operation under general anesthesia, only physical examination and blood count will be necessary. Otherwise, you will have a routine examination of your blood, urine, and lungs (chest x-ray).

- You may be given medicines that will make you feel drowsy before you are brought to the operating room.

□ OPERATION

- Depending on how deep the tumor is in the breast, the operation can be done under local anesthesia, along with medicine to make you feel drowsy, or under general anesthesia. Usually, the incisions for deep lesions can be a little shorter if the patient is asleep, or they can be placed more easily on the edge of the areola (which causes less scarring). The choice of the anesthetic will be discussed with you.
- The place of incision will be selected carefully and made so that it will show as little as possible.

- The entire specimen will be sent to the pathology laboratory for examination.
- There will be a cosmetic closure. You will have a scar. The size of the scar depends on how your skin heals. The operation generally takes 45 minutes.

POSTOPERATIVE CARE

- You will be taken to a recovery room. When your blood pressure, pulse, and breathing are stable and you are completely alert, you should be able to go home that same day accompanied by a responsible adult.
- As with any operation, complications are always possible. Although they are uncommon with your type of operation, they can include bleeding, infection, and possibly others.
- Arrangements will be made for your pain medicine, follow-up office visit, and stitch removal.

✚ HOME CARE

- Resume your usual activities.
- You may shower if you wish after 24 hours and with any dressings on or off.
  - There may be narrow strips of tape across the incision. It's all right if they get wet; they will be removed in the doctor's office.
  - After you dry yourself, replace any dressings with clean, dry ones.
- Wearing a loose bra at bedtime—mostly to keep your breasts from moving around too much as you shift during sleep—will make you more comfortable.

✆ CALL OUR OFFICE IF

- The incision becomes red or swollen, or there is drainage from it.
- You develop a temperature higher than 101°F.
- You have any questions.

BREAST PROSTHESIS REMOVAL

△ GENERAL INFORMATION

A breast prosthesis usually is put in place to make a small breast larger or to replace cancerous breast tissue that was removed during a *mastectomy*.

Most prostheses are made of a plastic bag in the shape of a breast that is filled with silicone fluid or with saline (a salt solution).

- Sometimes the plastic bag develops a leak or shows evidence of weakness.
- Sometimes too much scar tissue develops around a breast implant.

COMMON SIGNS AND SYMPTOMS

- Often there are no symptoms. The leak (or weakness) in the plastic bag is picked up on routine mammograms or on physical examination.
- Sometimes the breast has a vague pain that won't go away.
- A change in breast consistency (either firmer or softer) can be a sign of leakage of a gel-filled implant.
- If a saline-filled implant develops a leak, the breast will become smaller over 2 or 3 days.

DIAGNOSIS

- The diagnosis is made by taking a detailed history and doing a careful physical examination.
- Mammogram: This is one way to examine the breast for any fluid that has leaked from the prosthesis. Also, if the prosthesis was put in just to make a small breast larger, it is the way to examine the breast for a possible cancer.
- MRI (magnetic resonance imaging): No x-rays are used with this technique. Instead, magnetic fields and radio waves are used. A computer develops the pictures to show the breast from several angles. It is the best way to pick up a weakness or rupture in the wall of the prosthesis.

○ TREATMENT

- If the prosthesis is filled with silicone liquid and the silicone has leaked, then the plastic bag and all the silicone outside it must be removed.
- If the prosthesis is filled with saline and it leaks, the breast will collapse and the leaked saline will be absorbed by the body. It is advisable that the collapsed prosthesis be removed.
- Sometimes there is no leakage, but a weakness develops in the wall of the prosthesis. This prosthesis should be removed.
- Each patient, with the help of the surgeon, should decide whether to simply remove the implant or to replace the implant with a new one.

PREOPERATIVE PREPARATION

- You will have a routine examination of your blood and urine, and possibly other tests will be done, depending on your age and medical condition.
- Do not drink or eat anything for 8 hours before the operation.
- Shower as usual the morning of the operation.
- You may be given medicine that will make you feel drowsy before you are brought to the operating room.

□ OPERATION

- You will be asleep for the operation.
- Most of the time, the incision will be through the original one used to put in the prosthesis. It may be necessary to enlarge the incision (Fig. 1).
- The incision will be closed in a plastic fashion.
- The operation generally takes 2 to 4 hours.

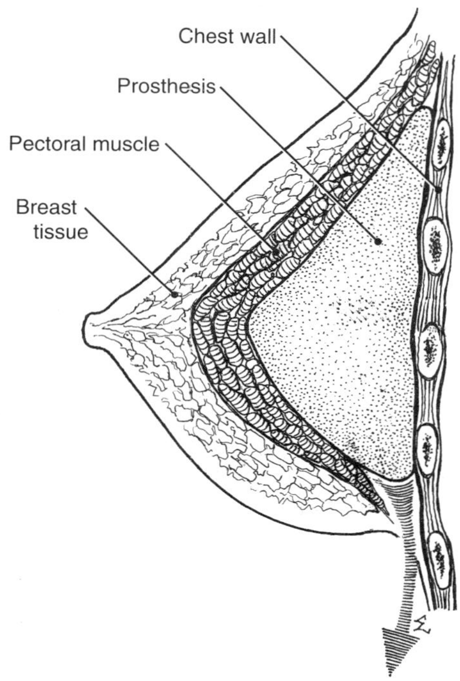

Figure 1. A breast prosthesis is most commonly placed under the pectoral muscles (the "pecs"). Removal of the prosthesis is usually done through the same skin incision used to insert it *(arrow)*. The empty space following removal can be left that way permanently or filled right away or later with another prosthesis depending on the reason it was removed, the local conditions present, and the desires of the patient.

POSTOPERATIVE CARE

- You will be taken to a recovery room and observed. When your blood pressure, pulse, and breathing are stable and you are completely alert, you should be able to go home that same day with a responsible adult.
- There may be a small plastic tube coming from the wound that is connected to a small plastic bag and drains any fluid that needs to come out from the

wound. You will be shown how to take care of it; it's not difficult.
- Antibiotics will be prescribed if the implant is replaced.
- Pain can be controlled with medicine.

HOME CARE

- You may walk about as you wish, even climb stairs, but don't overdo things.
- Take medicine as prescribed for your pain.
- Eat as you wish.
- Do not get the dressings wet.
- The dressings will be changed and any drains removed during your first postoperative office visit.
- Unless instructed otherwise, you may shower if you wish and with any dressings on or off.
  - There may be narrow strips of tape across the incision. It's all right if they get wet; they will be removed in the doctor's office
  - After you dry yourself, replace any dressings with clean, dry ones.
- Avoid vigorous exercises or heavy lifting for 1 month.
- Depending on the extent of the operation and the nature of your job, you may return to work as early as 1 week.

CALL OUR OFFICE IF

- The incision becomes red or swollen, or there is drainage from it.
- You develop a temperature higher than 100°F.
- You have any questions.

△ GENERAL INFORMATION

Some women who are scheduled to have their breasts removed because of cancer wish to have a breast reconstruction at the same time.

DIAGNOSIS

The diagnosis of cancer will have been made by a biopsy done before the scheduled mastectomy (Fig. 1). A biopsy of the suspicious tissue and examination of it under the microscope are always done before the breast is removed. Sometimes the diagnosis is made and the treatment is given during the same operation.

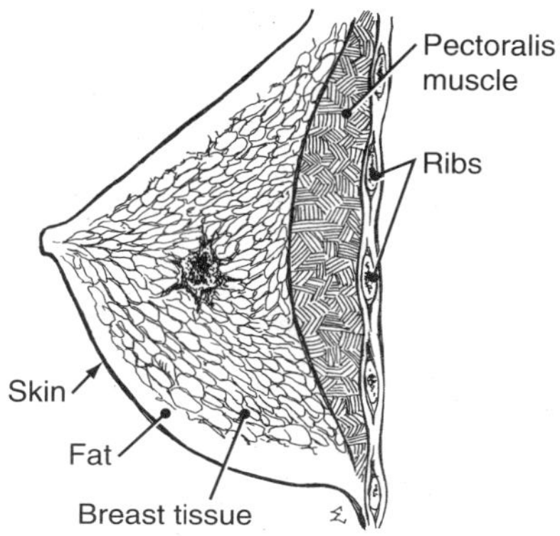

Figure 1. A breast with a cancer in its center. Notice the breast tissue is on top of the pectoral muscles. The pectoral muscles lie on the ribs.

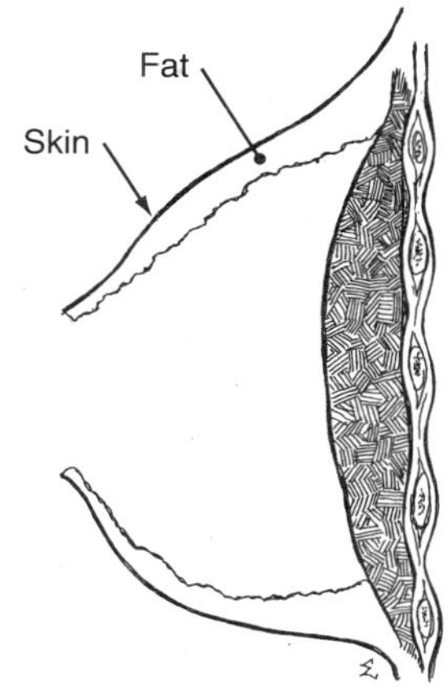

Figure 2. In a modified radical mastectomy, some skin, all of the breast tissue, and the lymph nodes in the axilla (armpit) are removed. The pectoral muscles are not removed.

○ TREATMENT

It has been determined that you are not a candidate for breast conservation. The reasons for this have been explained to you.

Characteristics of your cancer indicate that your best option for surgical treatment is to have your breast and the lymph nodes in your armpit removed (a *modified radical mastectomy*) (Figs. 2 and 3).

Several factors determine what can or will be done in performing your reconstruction. They cannot be known for sure before the operation.

- Occasionally, an implant may be put in position immediately, once the breast is removed.
- Sometimes the amount of skin the cancer surgeon needs to remove does not leave enough room for an implant to fit safely. The skin is tight and stretched and becomes pale to blue. There is a risk that if it is left this way, the skin may die and the wound may weaken, exposing the implant and requiring its removal. In such an instance, the prosthesis is not placed in position. Instead, a tissue expander (this is a flattened balloon) will be placed under the muscle and skin. Over a period of several months, the muscle and skin over the tissue expander will be stretched by the surgeon injecting saline (salt water solution) into the tissue expander. When the skin has ballooned up to match that of the opposite breast, the tissue expander will be removed and replaced with a permanent implant in a minor operation (often done on an outpatient basis).
- Occasionally, after the breast is removed, the skin is stunned and the tiny vessels in it (the *capillaries*) clamp down. Because of this, the skin might die if it is stretched too tightly over an implant. If this happens to you, a tissue expander will be inserted, as in the above situation.
- If there are no plans to place an implant or a tissue expander, the excess skin is trimmed and thrown away when removing the breast so that when the wound edges are sewn together the surface will be flat and smooth.
- It will be explained to you how a nipple and areola can be made and the best time to do this.

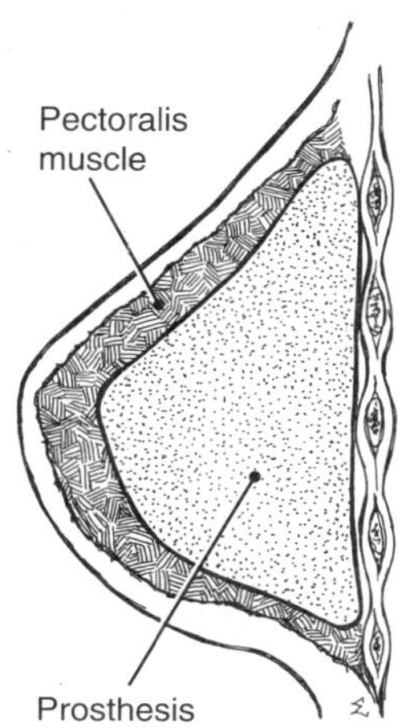

Figure 3. In the reconstruction, the prosthesis is placed under the pectoral muscles and over the ribs. This position gives the skin a better chance to establish a good blood supply from the muscle. Also, the new "breast" feels soft and more natural to the touch.

PREOPERATIVE PREPARATION

- You will have an examination of your blood, urine, heart (EKG), and lungs (chest x-ray).
- If you smoke, stop *now*. Nicotine can make the capillaries in the skin clamp down. This increases the risk that the skin over the prosthesis will die.
- Do not eat or drink anything for 8 hours before the operation.
- Shower as usual on the morning of the operation.
- You may be given medicine that will make you feel drowsy before you are brought to the operating room.

□ OPERATION

- When the cancer surgeon is through with removal of the breast, the plastic surgeon takes over.
- The plastic reconstruction generally takes about 2 hours.
- You will not receive a blood transfusion unless it is absolutely necessary.

POSTOPERATIVE CARE

- You will wake up in a recovery room. When your blood pressure, pulse, and breathing are stable, you will be taken to a regular hospital room.
- There may be a snug bandage around your entire chest.
- Pain will be controlled with medicine.
- There may be a small plastic tube coming to the outside from right next to the incision. It drains any fluid that may need to come out.
- That evening you will be helped to sit up in bed and on the next day to get out of bed.
- You should be able to go home in 1 to 2 days.
- As with any operation, complications are always possible, some of them serious. With this type of operation, they can include bleeding, loss of skin as well as the prosthesis, infection, and possibly others.
- Your cancer can be cured. An estimate of your chances can be made only after all the test results are back.
- Arrangements will be made for your medicines, follow-up office visits, stitch removal, discussion of any laboratory reports, and instructions on an arm exercise program.

✣ HOME CARE

- Continue with the program started while you were in the hospital.
- You may walk about as you wish, even climb stairs.
- After the first change of dressings in the surgeon's office, you will be told when you may begin taking showers and how to change your dressings. In the meantime, sponge bathe as you wish.
- You will be helped to select a bra that is suitable for wearing during the day as well as when you sleep.
- Driving a car with an automatic shift is not too demanding. But if you suddenly have to slam on the brakes or twist to turn the steering wheel, you may strain the sutures or tear something. During your follow-up visit let's discuss when you can resume driving.
- You may resume sexual activity whenever you choose.
- You may return to work when you feel up to it, but let's talk about it first during a follow-up office visit.

✆ CALL OUR OFFICE IF

- The incision becomes red or swollen, or there is drainage from it.
- You develop a temperature higher than 101°F.
- You have any questions.

BREAST RECONSTRUCTION: Latissimus Dorsi Muscle Flap

△ GENERAL INFORMATION

Some women who have had their breast removed because of cancer wish to have a breast reconstruction on that side. This may be done immediately following removal of the breast or at a later date. There are a number of ways to reconstruct the breast by using synthetic material (an implant) or the patient's own tissue.

CONSIDERATIONS

- A woman who has had a mastectomy (breast removal), possibly with some muscle also removed, who now has a flat chest and a moderately large opposite breast.
- Previous x-ray treatments to the breast or chest.
- A mastectomy (breast removal) is recommended, and immediate reconstruction is being considered.

○ TREATMENT

There are several requirements for breast reconstruction with the patient's own tissue:

- Muscle, fat, and some skin (that will make up the new breast) must be swung from a nearby area.
- This tissue needs to have a good blood supply coming to it as it is moved to its new location.

There are several reasons for using the patient's own tissue:

- The patient does not want any synthetic material in her body.
- The opposite breast is too large for even the largest implant, so they cannot be matched.
- The patient does not wish to have a larger opposite breast made smaller so that it can match the smaller size of the breast reconstructed with an implant.

The main choices for reconstruction are to swing tissue from the upper back *(latissimus dorsi flap)* or from the abdomen (transrectus abdominis muscle flap—TRAM flap).

- An individual may have had abdominal surgery in the past, so the TRAM flap cannot be used.
- An individual may be so thin that there is not enough fat to use in the TRAM flap.

After careful consideration of all factors, the recommendation is that you have your reconstruction using a latissimus dorsi flap. The reasons for this recommendation have been explained to you.

PREOPERATIVE PREPARATION

- You will have an examination of your blood, urine, heart (EKG), and lungs (chest x-ray).
- Do not eat or drink anything for 8 hours before the operation.
- Shower as usual on the morning of the operation.
- You may be given medicine that will make you feel drowsy before you are brought to the operating room.
- You will have an incision on both the back and the front of your chest (Figs. 1 and 2).
- It will be explained to you how a nipple and areola will be positioned at a later time.
- You will not receive a blood transfusion unless it is absolutely necessary.
- The operation usually takes about 3 to 4 hours.

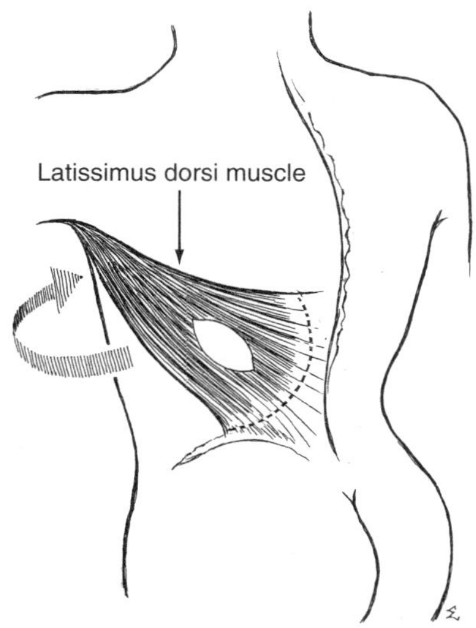

Figure 1. The latissimus dorsi muscle with an attached ellipse of skin is mobilized and swung toward the front of the chest. The muscle continues to get its nourishment from its original blood supply.

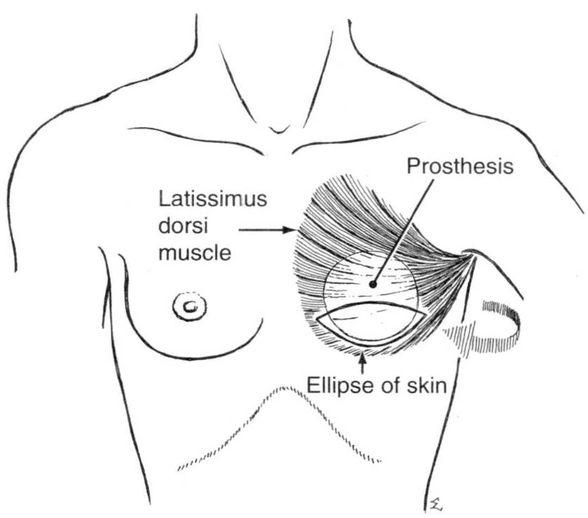

Figure 2. The muscle flap with the attached ellipse of skin and the skin already present are swung toward the front *(arrow)* and aligned with the opposite breast. In addition, a saline-filled prosthesis is placed under the muscle flap to help build a breast mound.

POSTOPERATIVE CARE

- You will wake up in a recovery room. When your blood pressure, pulse, and breathing are stable, you will be taken to a regular hospital room.
- That evening you will be helped to sit up in bed and on the next day to get out of bed.
- Pain can be controlled with medicine.
- There may be a small plastic tube coming out next to the incision to drain any fluids that need to come out. The tube will be removed in a few days.
- You should be able to go home in 2 to 3 days.
- With any operation, complications are always possible. With your type of operation, they can include loss of portion of the flap, infection, bleeding, and possibly others.
- Arrangements will be made for your pain medicine, follow-up office visit, stitch removal, and instructions on arm exercises.

✚ HOME CARE

- Continue with the program started while you were in the hospital.
- You may walk about as you wish, even climb stairs.
- Take medicine as prescribed for your pain.
- Before leaving the hospital, you will be told when you may begin taking showers.
- Include plenty of roughage and liquids in your diet to help prevent constipation.
- Driving a car with an automatic shift is not too demanding. But if you suddenly have to slam on the brakes or twist to turn the steering wheel, you may strain the sutures or tear something. During your follow-up visit let's discuss when you can resume driving.
- You may return to work when you feel up to it, but let's first talk about it during a follow-up office visit.

✆ CALL OUR OFFICE IF

- The incision becomes red or swollen, or there is drainage from it.
- You develop a temperature higher than 100°F.
- You have any questions.

BREAST RECONSTRUCTION: Transrectus Abdominis Muscle Flap (TRAM Flap)

△ GENERAL INFORMATION

Some women who have their breast removed because of cancer wish to have a breast reconstruction on that side. This may be done immediately following removal of the breast or at a later date. There are a number of ways to reconstruct the breast by using synthetic material (a *prosthesis*), the patient's own tissue, or a combination of both. One technique that uses only the patient's tissue is a TRAM flap.

CONSIDERATIONS

- A woman who has had a mastectomy (breast removal), possibly with some muscle also removed, and now has a flat chest and a moderately large opposite breast.
- A women who is scheduled to have a mastectomy and wishes to have an immediate reconstruction.

○ TREATMENT

There are several requirements for breast reconstruction with the patient's own tissue:

- Muscle, fat, and some skin (that will make up the new breast) must be swung from a nearby area.
- This tissue needs to have a good blood supply coming to it after it is moved to its new location.

Situations suitable for use of a patient's own tissue:

- The woman does not want any synthetic implant material in her body.
- Previous radiation treatment to the breast and chest wall has produced enough damage that the tissue used to create the new "breast" must be healthy as well as bring along its own blood supply.

The choices are to swing around tissue from your upper back (the *latissimus dorsi flap*) or upward from the abdominal wall (the *TRAM flap*).

After careful consideration of all factors, the recommendation is that your reconstruction should be done with a TRAM flap. One important reason for this choice is that you have enough extra tissue in your lower abdomen that can be used to make the new breast (at the same time, this will give you a "tummy tuck").

PREOPERATIVE PREPARATION

- You will have a routine examination of your blood, urine, heart (EKG), and lungs (chest x-ray).
- Stop smoking for 48 hours or longer before the operation. Nicotine can make small skin blood vessels clamp down and interfere with proper healing.
- Do not eat or drink anything for 8 hours before the operation.

□ OPERATION

- You will be asleep for the operation.
- You will have incisions on your chest wall and in your lower abdomen.
- Skin, fat, and muscle (along with their blood supply) from the abdomen will be swung up to your chest wall. This tissue will be fashioned into the shape of a breast and stitched in place (Figs. 1, 2, and 3).

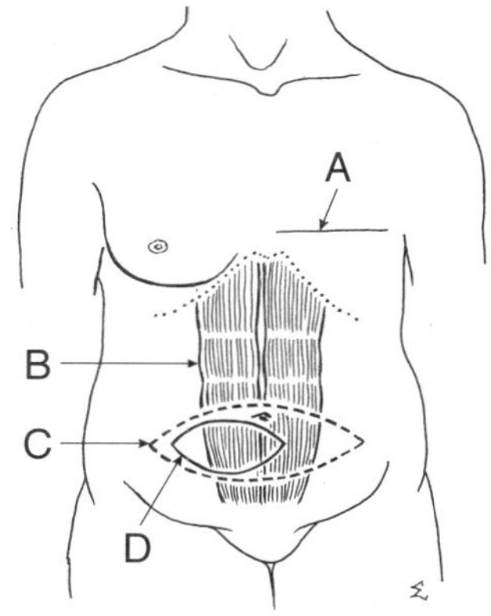

Figure 1. Normal anatomy. Notice excess abdominal skin and fat. A, Scar following left mastectomy. B, Skin, fat, and muscle flap to be transferred to left chest wall. C, Portion of skin around B that will be removed as part of the tummy tuck. D, Rectus abdominis muscle *(right)*.

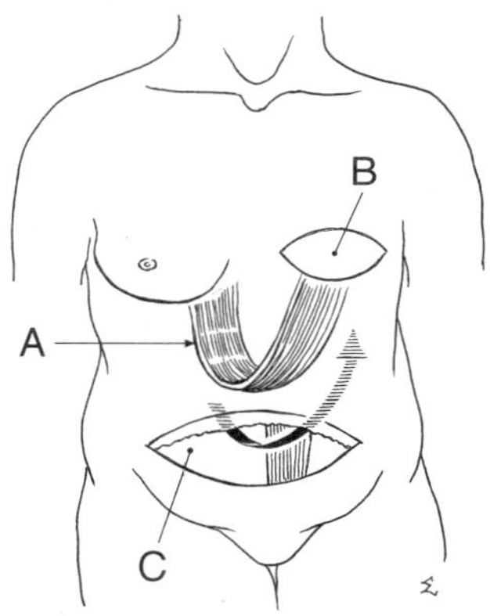

Figure 2. Lower portion of right rectus abdominis muscle (A) along with skin and fat (B) has been tunneled under abdominal skin and brought to the surface of the left chest wall. Incision (C) will be closed as part of the tummy tuck.

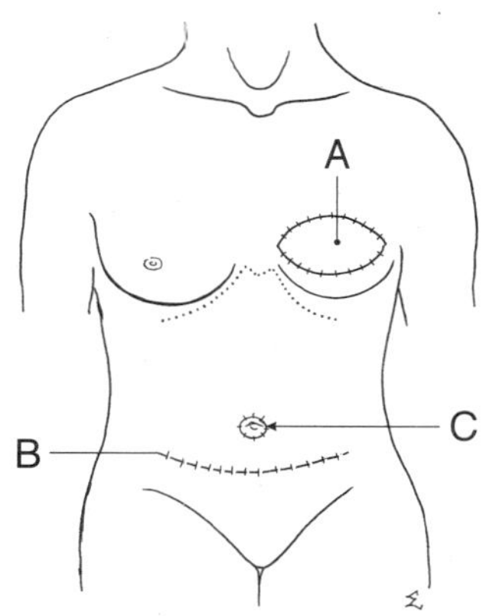

Figure 3. A, TRAM flap in position. B, Incision following tummy tuck. C, Umbilicus in new position. Notice abdomen is now more slim.

- An areola and nipple are usually "created" at a later time.
- The operation generally takes approximately 4 hours.

POSTOPERATIVE CARE

- You will be taken to a recovery room and observed. When your blood pressure, pulse, and breathing are stable, you will be taken to a regular hospital room.
- That evening you will be helped to sit up in bed and the next day to get out of bed.
- Pain will be controlled with medicine.
- There will be a small plastic tube coming from the abdominal incision draining extra fluid from the area.
- You should be able to go home in 5 to 7 days.
- Arrangements will be made for your medicine, follow-up office visit, stitch removal, and discussion of some abdominal exercises.
- As with any operation, complications are always possible. With your type of operation they can include bleeding, infection, wound separation, loss of a portion of the flap, and possibly others.

✚ HOME CARE

- You may walk about as you wish, even climb stairs.
- Before you leave the hospital you will be told when you can begin taking showers.
- Exercises will be prescribed for you to help make your abdomen become as strong as possible. However, it is not likely that you will have the same strength as before the operation.
- Include plenty of roughage and liquids in your diet to help prevent constipation.
- You may resume sexual activity whenever you choose.
- You may return to work when you feel up to it.

✆ CALL OUR OFFICE IF

- Your incisions become red or swollen or there is drainage from them.
- You develop a temperature higher than 101°F.
- You have any questions.

BREAST REDUCTION

△ GENERAL INFORMATION

Women with very large breasts (*macromastia*) can suffer in a number of ways, both physically and emotionally. This condition is seen in young girls to middle-aged women. The condition probably is caused by hormonal factors but is also associated with obesity. Often there is a family pattern of large breasts.

COMMON SIGNS AND SYMPTOMS

- Physical activity is limited. Exercise may be difficult or impossible.
- Often, the back and shoulders hurt because of the heavy weight they have to hold up.
- A stooped-over position may result because of the heavy breasts.
- The shoulder areas may be deeply grooved and even cut from the brassiere straps digging in.
- The skin under the breasts can be chronically irritated or even infected.
- Some persons may develop shyness or other personality changes because of their appearance and the effects of excessively large breasts.

DIAGNOSIS

- A diagnosis can be made by examining the breasts carefully and relating the findings to the patient's history.

○ TREATMENT

- Most women think about treatment for quite a while before seeking surgical help.
- Most women have tried to deal with the problem of very large breasts for a long time.
  - They are often either teased by their schoolmates or treated as sex objects.
  - Many have tried various awkward ways to minimize their breasts.
  - The physical handicap becomes an increasing problem with age.
  - Young as well as older women find it difficult to buy or wear tasteful clothing.
- The first choice is an operation to reduce the size of the breasts.
- The aims of the operation are the following:
  - To remove enough breast tissue to be able to construct a normal-appearing breast mound.
  - To reposition the nipple-areola in a suitable position in the "new" breast.

There are many operations to reduce large breasts. A common technique is shown (Figs. 1–3).

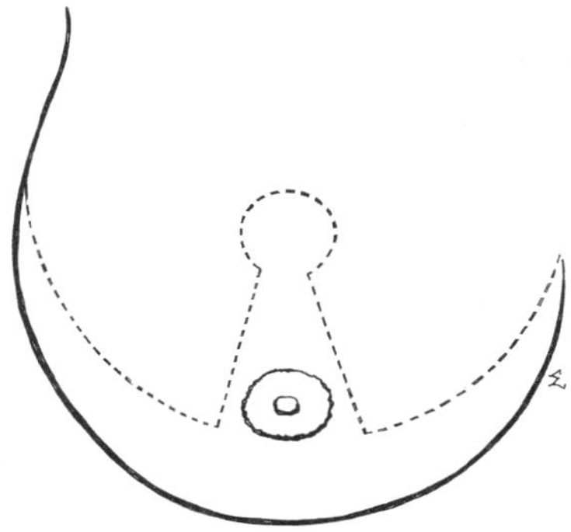

Figure 1. The skin and breast to be removed are shown within the dashed lines and the crease along the bottom of the breast. The nipple and areola (the dark skin around the nipple) will be left intact.

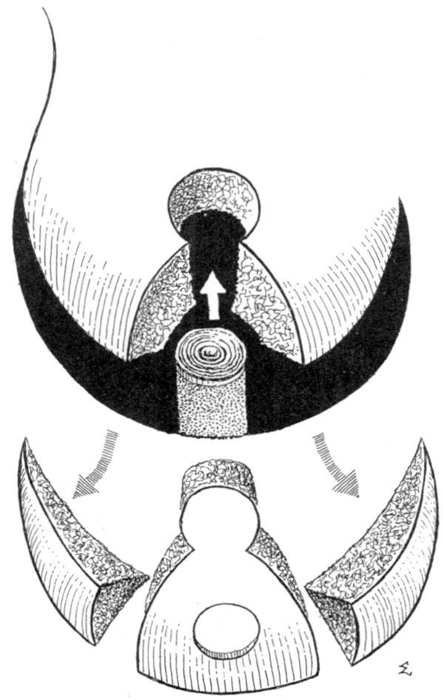

Figure 2. The removed breast tissue will be discarded. The nipple and areola will be moved upward to their new location *(white arrow)*.

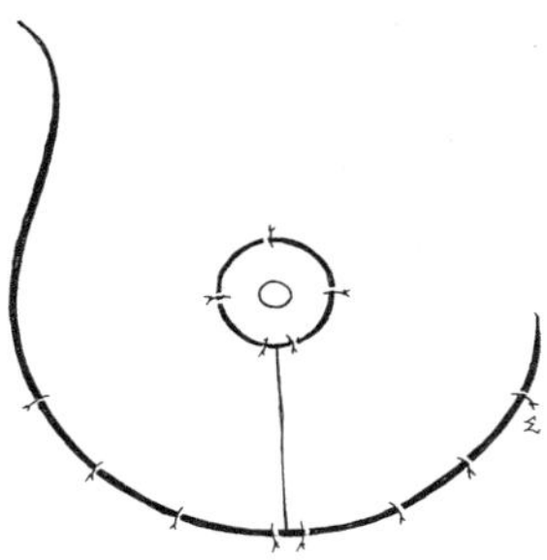

Figure 3. The reconstructed (smaller) breast.

PREOPERATIVE PREPARATION

- You will have an examination of your blood and urine. Other tests, for example, heart (EKG) and lungs (chest x-ray), will be required if you are older than 40 years of age or have medical problems.
- A careful examination of the breasts and a bilateral mammogram will be done for women older than 30 years of age.
- You will need to correct any problems of excess

weight as much as possible: otherwise, the purpose of the operation will be compromised. If you lose the weight *after* the operation, the new breast might sag somewhat.

- Smoking makes the small vessels of the skin clamp down. This can hurt the healing process. You should avoid smoking completely for at least 1 month before the operation.
- You should know that the following are common after this operation:
  - The sensation in your nipple probably will be decreased.
  - You likely will not be able to nurse an infant.
  - Reading your mammogram may become more difficult because of the scarring inside the breast.
  - The scars from the operation may be prominent.
- On the day of the operation, the places where the incisions will be made on your breasts and the new position of the nipple-areola will be marked with dissolving ink while you are in a sitting position.
- You may be given medicine that will make you feel drowsy before you are brought to the operating room.

☐ OPERATION

- You will be asleep for this operation.
- The operation generally takes 3 to 4 hours.

POSTOPERATIVE CARE

- You will be taken to a recovery room and observed. When your blood pressure, pulse, and breathing are stable, you will be taken to a regular hospital room.
- You will have a surgical dressing. Small plastic tubes will be coming from the breast incisions and will be connected to small plastic bulbs. They drain any extra fluid that needs to come out.
- That evening you will be helped to sit up in bed and on the next day to get out of bed.
- Your diet will first be liquids and then will be increased as tolerated.
- As with any operation, complications are always possible. With this type of operation, they can include bleeding, necrosis of skin or breast tissue, infection, and possibly others.
- You should be able to go home the day after the operation.
- Arrangements will be made for your medicine, follow-up office visit, and stitch removal.

✜ HOME CARE

- You may walk about as you wish, even climb stairs, but don't overdo things.
- Avoid heavy exercise, heavy lifting, or stress on the upper body for 1 month.
- Do not get the dressings wet; sponge bathe.
- The dressings will be changed and any drains removed during your first postoperative office visit.
- After the first change of dressings in the surgeon's office, you will be instructed on when you may shower and how to care for your dressings.
- You will wear a support bra for 4 to 6 weeks after surgery. Bring the bra with you during your first follow-up office visit.
- Most patients can return to nonphysical work within a week or two following breast reduction surgery.

✆ CALL OUR OFFICE IF

- The incisions become red or swollen, or there is drainage from them.
- You develop a temperature higher than 100°F.
- You have any questions.

△ GENERAL INFORMATION

After an operation in which your breast is removed (a *mastectomy*) and the lymph nodes in the (armpit) *axilla* are removed (an *axillary dissection*), the entire area aches for awhile and you won't feel like moving your shoulder joint; much of this is natural. Not moving the shoulder for too long, however, can make the area stiff, and then it's much more difficult to bring it back to normal again. This is especially true in an older person.

Although too little limbering up is not good, stretching the shoulder and arm a lot at one time and doing it too soon can cause tearing of some fine fibers and produce a sore shoulder. For the following few days you'll be more stiff than before.

Remember, too much motion too soon is not good, but not starting early enough to limber up also is not good. It's a matter of balancing things and developing a program to get your arm back to normal.

THE EXERCISES

The aim is to help you limber up your *shoulder,* not just to move your elbow and hand; the elbow rarely gets stiff. Also, with this exercise it is not just how high your hand reaches but how much your shoulder joint moves to let your arm and hand get up there.

Many exercises are recommended, and practically all of them are effective. One or more may be recommended for you. The following exercise is easy to do, takes little time, is logical, and works (Fig. 1). Start the exercise gradually, be consistent, and progress a little each day. Unless instructed otherwise, start the exercises a week after the operation.

- Stand facing a wall with your toes actually touching the wall (A). This way your arm can only travel straight up to reach its goal.
- Do not perform the exercise incorrectly (B). Notice the woman is not moving her stiff shoulder. She is bending at the waist to get the shoulder and the arm high; the shoulder joint itself is not really moving very much.
- Raise the arm on the nonoperated side straight up and press the palm against the wall (C). This keeps you from bending at the waist ("cheating") to help your hand reach up, in other words, your hand reaching high without your shoulder joint actually moving.
- On the first day, raise the arm on the operated side as high as is comfortable for you and mark this spot on the wall. Don't guess the spot; mark it.
- On the next day repeat this exercise three times in the morning and three times before bedtime.
- At the end of each day reach just one-half inch higher. Don't try to set a record; just one-half inch higher.
- Do this every day.
- You will be able to reach about 3 inches higher at the end of each week. Before long both arms will reach the same height.

Otherwise gradually perform normal activities. At least for the first 6 months, avoid performing hard activity in a repetitive manner with the affected arm (examples: weed pulling, pushing the vacuum cleaner for long periods, cleaning the whole house nonstop).

✆ CALL OUR OFFICE IF

- The hand (the back part) or the lower arm becomes swollen.
- There is redness of the arm.
- You develop a temperature higher than 100°F.

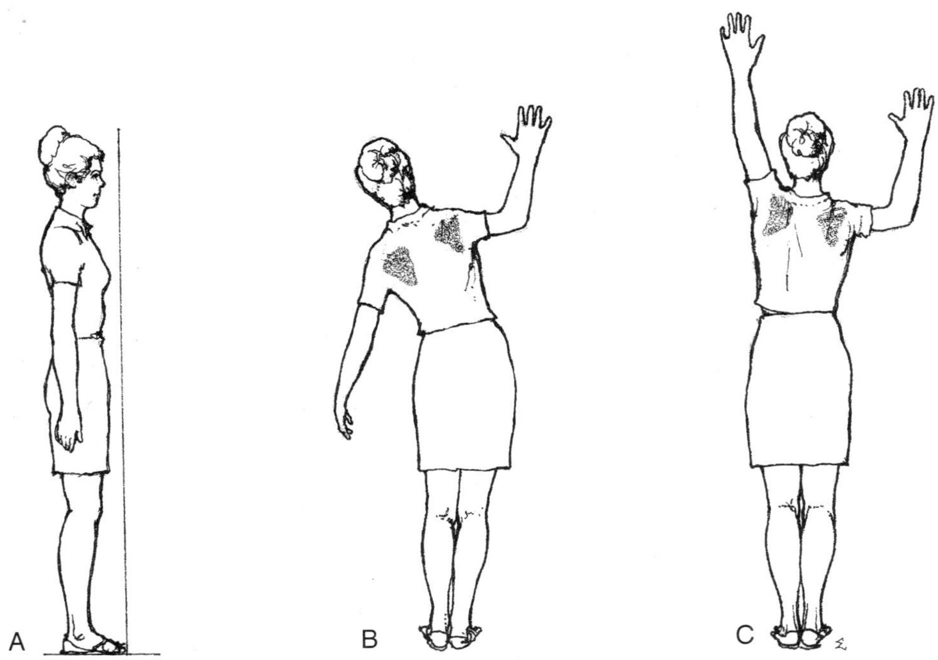

Figure 1.

△ GENERAL INFORMATION

Bronchoscopy is looking down the *trachea* (windpipe) and its branches. The reason for looking is to make a diagnosis of an abnormal shadow on an x-ray or because of symptoms that point to the lungs as the cause.

COMMON SIGNS AND SYMPTOMS

The symptoms or the signs could be anything related to the lungs. Examples include the following:

- A new and unexplained persistent cough.
- A significant change in a chronic cough.
- Something new seen on routine chest x-ray.
- A change in an old lung shadow.
- Constant pain over a spot on the chest wall.
- Coughing up of blood.
- Unexpected wheezing that is not caused by asthma or allergy.
- Possible aspiration of a foreign object.
- Foul sputum.

DIAGNOSIS

A diagnosis will be made after a number of procedures or tests are performed. Bronchoscopy is often one of those procedures.

It has been determined that you need a bronchoscopy to get some answers about your lung problem. In this way, a better decision can be made regarding the necessary treatment.

PREPARATION

- Do not eat or drink anything for 8 hours before the procedure.
- You will be given medicine that will make you feel drowsy and your mouth very dry before you are brought into the endoscopy room.

THE BRONCHOSCOPE

The bronchoscope is an optical instrument that is smooth, soft, and flexible with a light at its tip and is as thick as a lead pencil.

THE BRONCHOSCOPY

- In the endoscopy room your mouth and throat will be sprayed with an anesthetic solution that will make them numb. Also you will be given medicine that will make you feel very drowsy.
- The bronchoscope will be inserted into your mouth and down into the trachea and its branches.
- If anything suspicious is seen, a small portion of it will be taken (a *biopsy*) with the bronchoscope for examination in the pathology laboratory.
- Mucus also will be taken so that it can be examined for bacteria that might be the cause of your problem.
- Because everything has been made numb, you won't feel any pain with this procedure and you are not likely to gag.
- Generally, the bronchoscopy takes 15 to 20 minutes.
- After the bronchoscopy, you will wake up quickly. Most patients don't remember much of the procedure itself.

POSTPROCEDURE CARE

- You will remain in the endoscopy unit until your blood pressure, pulse, and breathing are stable and you are completely awake and alert. You then should be able to leave for home that same day accompanied by a responsible adult.

✚ HOME CARE

- Do not eat or drink anything until the numbness in your mouth and throat is completely gone. Usually this takes 1 to 2 hours. Otherwise, you won't feel the food or fluid in your throat, and it may go down your windpipe and cause you to choke.
- Do not drive or otherwise engage in activity that requires sharp judgment and reflexes for 24 hours.
- Resume your normal activities the following day.
- Arrangements will be made for you to get the results of any laboratory tests.

✆ CALL OUR OFFICE IF

- You cough up any blood other than blood-tinged mucus.
- You have severe difficulty breathing.
- You develop any unusual signs or symptoms.
- You develop a temperature higher than 101°F.
- You have any questions.

△ GENERAL INFORMATION

A bunion is a condition in which the great toe points towards the smaller toes (Figs. 1 and 2). The cause of bunions is not known, but bunions run in some families.

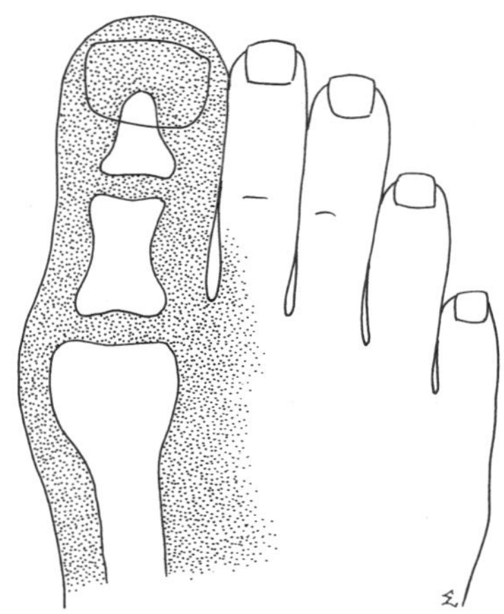

Figure 1. Normal great toe.

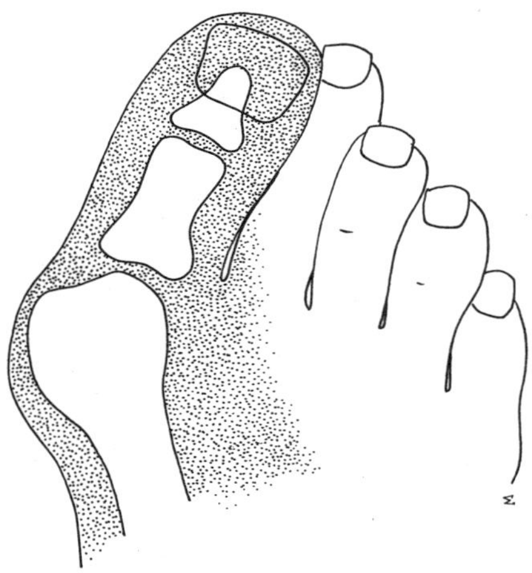

Figure 2. Bunion.

COMMON SIGNS AND SYMPTOMS

- The classic appearance of a bunion is the angulation of the great toe toward the second, third, fourth, and fifth toes.
- The large joint of the great toe sticks out toward the inner part of the foot.
- The pain is usually generalized pain of the great toe or pain associated with the wearing of shoes.

DIAGNOSIS

- Usually the diagnosis can be made by direct observation of the foot.
- An x-ray is required to determine the true nature of the bunion and to provide the necessary information on what operation would be necessary if the decision is to correct the problem.

○ TREATMENT

The treatment depends largely on the following:

- How much discomfort the bunion is producing.
- Whether it interferes with daily activities.
- Its appearance.

There are many different operations to correct bunions. In general, an operation involves reconstruction of the ligaments and other soft tissues around the great toe. In addition, most of the time one of the two bones on either side of the major joint of the great toe needs to be cut across and reset in the correct position. For these reasons, the operation is best done by a surgeon who has specific interest in the problem of bunions, has had focused training in these operations, and has had experience and demonstrated skill in performing these operations.

After careful consideration of all factors and a discussion with you, the plan is to proceed with an operation. The specific type of operation proposed will be discussed with you beforehand.

PREOPERATIVE PREPARATION

- You will have an examination of your blood and urine and possibly of your heart (EKG) and lungs (chest x-ray).
- Do not eat or drink anything for 8 hours before the operation.
- Shower or bathe as usual on the morning of the operation.
- You may be given medicine that will make you feel drowsy before you are brought to the operating room.

□ OPERATION

- The type of anesthesia used will be discussed with you beforehand.
- The operation usually lasts about 1 hour.

POSTOPERATIVE CARE

- You will be taken to a recovery room and observed. When your blood pressure, pulse, and breathing are stable and you are completely alert, you should be able to go home that same day with a responsible adult.
- Arrangements will be made for your medicine, follow-up office visit, and stitch removal.
- As with any operation, complications are always possible. With this type of operation, they can include a recurrence of the bunion, a leaning of the great toe in the opposite direction, stiffness, numbness, swelling, delayed healing, infection, and possibly others.

✚ HOME CARE

- Take it easy, and don't overdo things.
- Keep the foot elevated on one or two pillows as much as possible. This helps with the pain as well as in keeping the swelling down.

- Limit the amount of walking you do. This will be discussed with you after the operation.
- Do not get the dressing wet. You will need to sponge bathe for a while unless you can manage to bathe with your leg hanging outside of the tub.
- Take medicine as prescribed for your pain.
- Include plenty of roughage and liquids in your diet to help prevent constipation.
- Do not drive a car if you had the operation on your right foot or you have taken medicines that reduce your alertness.
- You may return to work when you feel up to it, but let's talk about it first during a follow-up office visit.

✆ CALL OUR OFFICE IF

- The incision becomes red or swollen, or there is drainage from it.
- You develop a temperature higher than 100°F.
- You have any questions.

△ GENERAL INFORMATION

Carcinoid tumor of the intestine is not common, but it is important because its behavior is unlike almost all other tumors of the intestine. It is found most often in the appendix, the nearby small intestine, or the rectum. A carcinoid tumor of the intestine can be as small as a cranberry or as large as a walnut.

COMMON SIGNS AND SYMPTOMS

There are different sets of symptoms depending on the size of the tumor, its location, whether it is benign or malignant, whether it has spread to other areas, and whether it produces a substance called *serotonin.*

- If the tumor affects the appendix, the symptoms can be those of appendicitis with pain in the right side of the abdomen.
- If it affects the nearby small intestine and blocks it, then it causes cramps, followed by severe pain, ballooning of the abdomen, and possibly peritonitis.
- If it is cancerous, it can spread—mostly to the liver. Here, the symptoms are pain in the right side of the abdomen and loss of appetite and weight, among others.
- If it is cancerous and makes serotonin, it can produce very dramatic and frightening symptoms because serotonin acts on the blood vessels. These symptoms include the following:
  - Sudden, sharp rises in the blood pressure.
  - Diarrhea along with cramping abdominal pain, usually after meals.
  - Severe flushing of the face.
  - Heart disease because of the damage to the heart vessels by serotonin.
  - Asthma because serotonin causes the bronchi (the small tubes that let air in and out of the lungs) to clamp down.

The grouping of the above symptoms is called the *carcinoid syndrome.*

DIAGNOSIS

- Anyone who has the above history or symptoms should be concerned about carcinoid syndrome.
- The diagnosis can be made by examining the urine and finding the chemical associated with serotonin. If the tumor does not produce serotonin, the test result will be negative, but that does not mean that carcinoid is not present.
- Most carcinoids are found at the time of an operation performed for abdominal pain for which the cause is not known.

○ TREATMENT

The treatment for carcinoid is to remove the tumor for the following reasons:

- It may be causing pain just like appendicitis.
- It may be blocking the intestine, so the blockage needs to be removed and the cut ends of the bowel reconnected.
- Perhaps the blocked bowel can be fixed, but the tumor has also spread to other organs that cannot be removed. The benefit here is the relief from the blockage.
- The carcinoid may be in the liver, and all of it cannot be removed. Even so, the bulk of the tumor should be removed if it can be done safely because the more tumor that is removed, the more of the very disabling symptoms can be reduced. Malignant carcinoid often is slow growing so that if the tumor can be kept to a minimum, a person can live more comfortably and longer.

Most of the things that can and possibly will be done during the operation will be discussed with you further and in greater detail.

PREOPERATIVE PREPARATION

- You will have an examination of your blood, urine, heart (EKG), and lungs (chest x-ray).
- CT scan (computed tomography scan): These special x-rays are taken by a machine that is shaped like a huge doughnut. You will lie on a table inside the hole in the "doughnut." The x-rays are taken as very thin slices through the abdomen. This makes it possible to see the fine details in the liver and other organs in the body.
- MRI (magnetic resonance imaging): No x-rays are used with this technique. Instead it is done with harmless magnetic fields and radio waves. A computer develops the pictures to show organs from several angles. It is valuable for examining the liver, blood vessels, and nerve tissue, as well as bone.
- Do not eat or drink anything for 8 hours before the operation.
- Shower as usual on the morning of the operation.
- You may be given medicine that will make you feel drowsy before you are brought to the operating room.

□ OPERATION

- It is not possible to know beforehand exactly what the operation will involve because a lot depends on what is found. The possibilities will be discussed with you before the operation.
- You will be asleep for the operation.
- During the operation, your heart, blood pressure, and the oxygen levels in your blood will be watched closely.
- You will not receive a blood transfusion unless it is absolutely necessary.

POSTOPERATIVE CARE

- You will be taken to a recovery room and observed. When your blood pressure, pulse, and breathing are stable, you will be taken to a regular hospital room.
- You will have a thin plastic tube in your nose. It goes down to your stomach to suck up the air you swallow. It will be removed when your bowels start working.

- Pain can be controlled with medicine. The nurse will give it to you, or you can give yourself a preset amount of pain medicine when you feel you need it. This is done with a device called patient-controlled analgesia (PCA) that is connected to the tubing giving you intravenous fluids.
- That evening you will be helped to sit up in bed and on the next day to get out of bed.
- When your bowels start working, the tube in your nose will be removed and you will be started on a liquid diet that will be increased as you tolerate it.
- As with any operation, complications are always possible. With this type of operation, they can include only limited improvement of symptoms, wound infection, pneumonia, heart and lung problems, and possibly others.
- Arrangements will be made for your medicine, follow-up office visit, and stitch or clip removal.

✚ HOME CARE

- Continue with the program started while you were in the hospital.
- You may walk about as you wish, even climb stairs, but don't overdo things.
- You may eat as you did before the operation.
- You may shower as you wish and with any dressings on or off.
  - There may be narrow strips of tape across the incision. It's all right if they get wet; they will be removed in the doctor's office.
  - After you dry yourself, replace any dressings with clean, dry ones.
- Your incision and the muscles of the abdomen may ache, especially at the end of the day and after you have been standing for a long period. You can support your abdomen by wearing a girdle that is snug (but not too tight). Wearing the girdle over a cotton undergarment is easier on your incision and the stitches.
- Include plenty of roughage and liquids in your diet to help prevent constipation.
- You may return to work when you feel up to it, but first let's talk about it during your follow-up office visit.
- Driving a car with an automatic shift may not seem too demanding. However, you may have to slam on the brakes or twist to turn the steering wheel and may strain your sutures or tear something. During your follow-up visit, let's discuss when you can resume driving.
- You may resume sexual activity whenever you choose.
- You may return to work when you feel up to it.

✆ CALL OUR OFFICE IF

- You develop any unusual signs or symptoms.
- The incision becomes red or swollen, or there is drainage from it.
- You develop a temperature of over 100°F.
- You have any questions.

△ GENERAL INFORMATION

Blood travels from the heart to the brain through four arteries: the left and right *common carotid arteries* and the two smaller *vertebral arteries*. The common carotid arteries divide into the important *internal carotid arteries* and the less important *external carotid arteries*. Carotid endarterectomy is an operation in which a seriously narrowed carotid artery is opened up to allow better flow of blood to the brain.

The usual cause of this narrowing is a cholesterol deposit (*atheroma*) at the beginning of the internal carotid artery (*white arrow*). This condition is most often seen in older men.

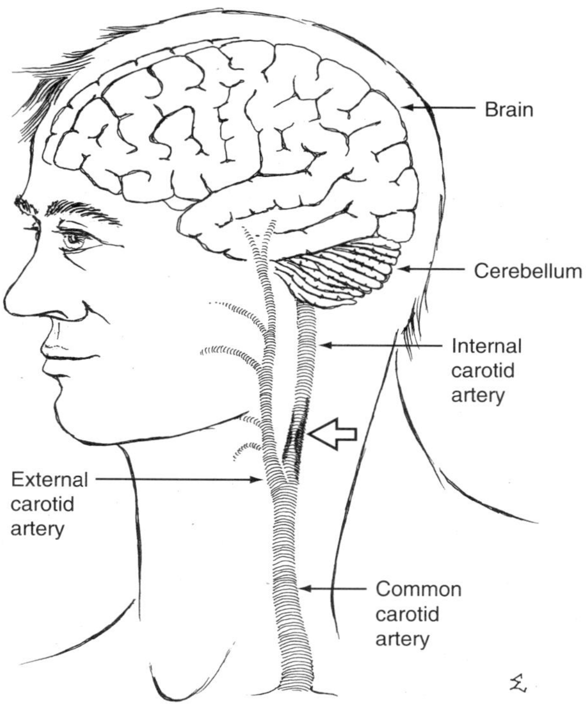

Figure 1.

COMMON SIGNS AND SYMPTOMS

- Sometimes the artery may be partially narrowed, and there may be no symptoms at all.
- If there is enough narrowing, it may produce symptoms. These symptoms last less than 24 hours—usually from a few minutes to a few hours—often with complete recovery. They may include the following:
  - Weakness or paralysis of the muscles of the face, arm, or leg on one side.
  - Slurred speech.
  - Occasionally a shade-like blindness of one eye.

Because these symptoms of insufficient blood to a body part (*ischemia*) don't last too long, this condition is called transient ischemic attack (TIA).

DIAGNOSIS

- Usually, the diagnosis is made by taking a detailed history and doing a thorough physical examination.
- The surest way to make the diagnosis is to perform an arteriogram. This is the injection of a special dye into the neck arteries. X-ray pictures are taken of the dye as it travels through the carotid arteries to the brain. In this way, one can see which arteries are involved, the extent of the narrowing, and the status of the arteries in the brain.

○ TREATMENT

- Transient ischemic attacks are a *warning* of impending stroke.
- The most important thing is to correct the narrowing *before* a stroke happens, because correcting the carotid narrowing after the stroke happens won't make the stroke go away. It will not improve an already paralyzed arm or a blind eye.
- After careful consideration of all factors, the recommendation is that you have an operation to open up the narrowed carotid artery.

PREOPERATIVE PREPARATION

- There will be a careful examination of your blood, urine, heart (EKG), and lungs (chest x-ray) to see that you don't have anything seriously wrong in these areas.
- Particular attention will be given to the heart and its own blood vessels (the coronary arteries) to be certain they are not involved in any important way.
- The arteries to your legs will be examined for any narrowing, as they are often affected.
- Do not eat or drink anything for 8 hours before the operation.
- Shower (and shave) as usual before the operation.
- You may be given medicine that will make you feel drowsy before you are brought to the operating room.

□ OPERATION

- The incision will be on the side of your neck. The carotid artery will be exposed. A detour will be put in the carotid artery in the area of blockage so that blood flows to your brain without interruption while the narrowed artery is being cleared out. When everything is fixed, the detour will be removed and the incision closed.
- The operation generally takes 2 hours.

POSTOPERATIVE CARE

- You will be taken to the Surgical Care Unit, where the doctors and nurses are experienced in taking care of patients like yourself. As soon as you are coming along well enough, you will be transferred to a regular hospital room.
- Pain can be controlled with medicine.

- In the evening you will be helped out of bed, and on the next day you will be walking and discharge plans will begin.
- Your diet will be increased as tolerated.
- As with any operation, complications are always possible, some of them serious. With your type of operation, they can include stroke, pneumonia, heart problems, wound infection, bleeding into the neck wound, and possibly others.
- You should be able to go home possibly the next morning or in a few days, depending on your progress.
- Arrangements will be made for your medicine, follow-up office visit, and stitch removal.

✚ HOME CARE

- Resume your usual activities.
- You may walk about as you wish, even climb stairs.
- You may shower as you wish and with any dressings on or off.
  - There may be narrow strips of tape across the incision. It's all right if they get wet; they will be removed in the doctor's office.
  - After you dry yourself, replace any dressings with clean, dry ones.
- You can safely shave close to the incision and the stitches (an electric shaver may be best). Then you can replace the dressings with clean dry ones.
- You can shave over the incision any time after the stitches and the strips of tape are removed.
- Driving your car may be important to you, but when you can do this safely depends on the medicines you are taking and your condition in general. During the follow-up visit let's discuss when you can resume driving.
- You may resume sexual activity whenever you choose.
- The side of your neck will be numb from the surgical incision. This shouldn't be a cause for concern, as it usually disappears in a few months.

✆ CALL OUR OFFICE IF

- You have any symptoms similar to the old ones or any new or unusual symptoms.
- The incision becomes red or swollen, or there is drainage from it.
- You develop a temperature higher than 100°F.
- You have any questions.

△ GENERAL INFORMATION

Carpal tunnel syndrome is caused by compression (squeezing) of the *median nerve* as it passes through a canal or tunnel through the wrist and palm along with nine tendons (Fig. 1). The median nerve is one of the main nerves providing sensation to the hand. When the nerve is even slightly compressed (such as from swelling of the tendons) symptoms such as tingling or numbness result.

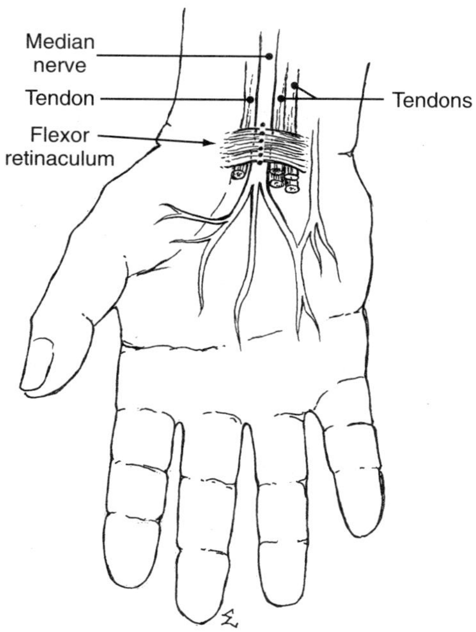

Figure 1. The median nerve, along with a number of tendons, passes through the crowded carpel tunnel. Under the tunnel are bones and over it is a band of tough tissue (the flexor retinaculum). In this operation, the flexor retinaculum is divided *(dotted line)* to relieve the squeeze on the median nerve.

COMMON SIGNS AND SYMPTOMS

- There is numbness or a "pins-and-needles" feeling in the thumb, index, and middle fingers, especially at night or early in the morning. This is sometimes relieved by shaking or moving the hand.
- There can be a feeling of weakness or fatigue with use, and possibly clumsiness of the hand.

DIAGNOSIS

- Usually, the diagnosis can be made by taking a detailed history and doing a thorough physical examination.
- A pins-and-needles sensation is usually noted in the fingers when the nerve is tapped or pressed at the wrist.
- Special electrical studies (nerve and conduction tests or *electromyogram*) of the median nerve and the muscles in the hand can be used to confirm the diagnosis.

○ TREATMENT

- Decrease activities that can aggravate the condition (such as prolonged typing).
- Wear a wrist splint, especially during sleep. This keeps the wrist from bending downward through the night, which can further pinch the nerve.
- Take a nonsteroidal medicine or receive a cortisone injection into the wrist to reduce any swelling of the tendons.
- An operation can be used to release the ligament on top of the nerve to give it more room to "breathe." This is required if
  - The previously suggested treatments help for short periods of time only.
  - The muscles of the hand at the base of the thumb show any shriveling (*atrophy*) from severe compression of the nerve.

PREOPERATIVE PREPARATION

- Do not eat or drink anything for 8 hours before the operation.
- Shower as usual before the operation.
- You may be given medicine that will make you feel drowsy before you are brought to the operating room.

□ OPERATION

- The operation generally is preceded by injection of an anesthetic that will make only the arm or hand numb. You can request medicine to make you feel drowsy during the operation.
- The nerve can be freed from the snug tunnel in several ways:
  - The surgeon can make an incision over the nerve in the wrist and palm. This lets the surgeon see the nerve clearly. The scar can range from 1 to 2½ inches.
  - The surgeon can insert a special optical instrument with a light at its tip through a smaller incision. This also allows sectioning of the ligament on top of the nerve so that the compression can be relieved.
- The recommended operation and the reason for it will be explained to you in the office.
- The operation generally takes less than 1 hour.

POSTOPERATIVE CARE

- You will be taken to a recovery room. When your blood pressure, pulse, and breathing are stable and you are completely alert, you will be able to go home that same day with a responsible adult.
- Pain can be controlled with medicine.
- Arrangements will be made for your follow-up office visit and stitch removal.
- As with any operation, complications are always possible. Although they are uncommon with your type of operation, they can include damage to the nerves in this area, bleeding, separation of the incision, and infection. Also, it is always possible that

some or all of your symptoms might not be completely relieved.

✣ HOME CARE

- Keep the hand elevated as much as possible for the first 1 to 2 days. When sitting or sleeping, place the arm and hand on one or two pillows.
- Try to keep your fingers moving if they are left out of the dressing. This keeps the tendons gliding past the nerve in the canal and helps reduce stiffness of the fingers.
- You may sponge bathe as you wish. If you would like to take a shower, the hand and entire lower arm must be protected so they do not get wet. This precaution is necessary only until the first dressing change. After that you may shower with the dressings on or off.
- Driving your car may be important to you, but driving with your operated, bandaged hand is not advisable and using only one hand can be dangerous. During your follow-up visit let's discuss when you can resume driving.

✆ CALL OUR OFFICE IF

- The incision becomes red or swollen, or there is drainage from it.
- You develop a temperature higher than 100°F.
- You have any questions.

CENTRAL VENOUS CATHETERIZATION

△ GENERAL INFORMATION

Placing an intravenous (commonly called an *IV*) catheter is common practice in a hospital and especially before an operation. This makes it possible to give the patient various types of fluids, medicines, and chemicals. Such an IV is most commonly placed in a vein in the arm. A vein in the arm (or leg) is called a *peripheral vein.*

Quite often, a larger catheter needs to be used and so must be placed in a larger vein. Such veins are called *central veins* and are available and easiest to reach in the neck or just under the *clavicle* (collarbone) (Fig. 1). A central catheter is long enough that, once it is placed in the vein, it can be advanced so the tip of it is close to the heart. In addition, a central venous catheter may have more than one tunnel in it so that different medicines can be given at the same time but through separate tunnels.

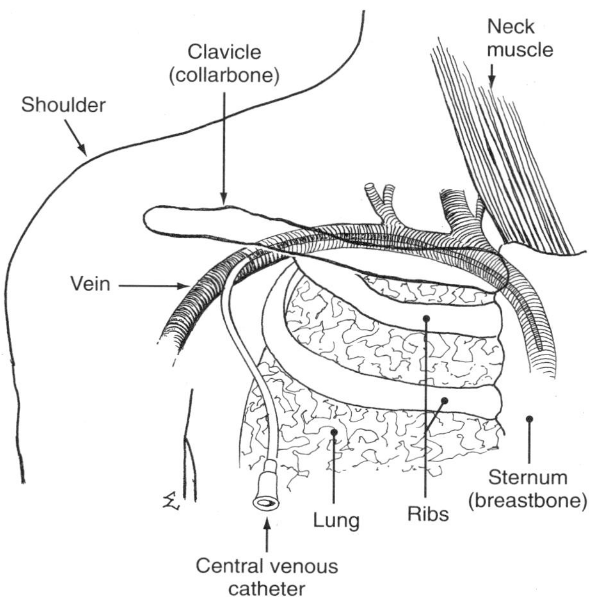

Figure 1. The central venous catheter typically is inserted into the vein (subclavian) at a point just under and at the outer side of the clavicle. It is then threaded to a point just outside the heart.

INDICATIONS FOR PLACING A CENTRAL VENOUS CATHETER

- **Inability to Place a Catheter in a Peripheral Vein:** Peripheral veins may not be found or may be difficult to cannulate. This does not occur often; it is more common in patients who have received chemotherapy or steroids or in patients who have had their peripheral veins used so many times in the past that all the good peripheral veins have clotted.
- **Need to Monitor the Pressure of Venous Blood:** In contrast to IV catheters in a peripheral vein, catheters in a central vein make it possible to measure the pressure in the veins leading into the heart; thus, it is called *central venous pressure.* Knowing the central venous pressure makes it possible for the doctor to estimate the volume of blood in the patient's blood stream and the amount of fluids to give. This type of monitoring is not necessary in most patients. Factors that determine whether central venous pressure monitoring is required during the operation include the following:
  - The extent of the problem requiring the operation.
  - The extent of the operation planned.
  - Associated medical problems.

  In healthy patients, measuring the heart rate, blood pressure, and urine output is enough to determine the amount of intravenous fluid to give a patient. However, patients with associated diseases, such as of the heart, or those with kidney failure may require a central venous catheter because the blood pressure and pulse are not accurate enough measurements of blood volume. In addition, if the operation is very extensive or lasts a long time, central venous pressure measurement is helpful in determining whether more intravenous fluid is required. In a patient with persistently low blood pressure, central venous pressure monitoring is helpful to the doctor in deciding whether decreased volume of blood is the cause of the low blood pressure.
- **Large Blood Loss Anticipated During the Operation:** Central venous catheters are available in many sizes. The larger ones are significantly larger than those commonly used in peripheral IV catheters. A large central venous catheter can be used to give blood or other fluids rapidly to replace such blood loss with intravenous fluid or blood products during the operation.
- **Need for Drug and Special Fluid Administration:** Sometimes it is necessary to administer certain medications and nutrition (intravenous nutritional feedings). Such medicines and nutritional fluids are irritating to the vein. Administering them into smaller peripheral veins often damages and clots these veins. For this reason, such fluids are given through a central venous catheter in which the blood flows more swiftly.
- **Air Embolism:** During an operation, air may enter the venous circulation. This relates primarily to neurosurgical procedures. A central venous catheter allows for withdrawal of such air as may enter the veins.
- **Facilitates Other Procedures:** When a central venous catheter is already in place, it is much easier, simpler, and faster to place things through the vein that are necessary to treat certain problems, for example, to insert a wire for a temporary heart pacemaker or a pulmonary artery catheter.

PROCEDURE

Placing a central venous catheter during an operation can be done with the patient awake (with medicine beforehand to cause drowsiness) or asleep. In addition, the patient may be given oxygen and have the heart monitored (with an EKG) while this is being done. In nonsurgical patients, the procedure is done in the patient's room. Medication is given to relax the patient.

The catheter may be placed in the *internal jugular vein* (in the neck), the *external jugular vein* (in the neck), the *subclavian vein* (under the clavicle), or the *femoral vein* (in the groin region). Because there's a right and a left side for each location, eight sites are available. The internal jugular and subclavian veins are the most common sites of insertion. The decision on which of the above locations to place the catheter is based on how long the catheter will have to stay in place, the possible complications associated with each location, how easy it is to insert the catheter in a specific circumstance, and physician preference.

A central venous catheter is placed under sterile conditions. The area where the catheter will be inserted is swabbed with an anesthetic solution and surrounded with sterile draping towels. The draping towels will likely cover your face; don't let this alarm you. You may be positioned so that your head is lower than your feet. This encourages the veins to swell and makes it easier to insert the catheter. When placing catheters in peripheral veins, the veins can be seen. Central venous veins, however, usually cannot be felt or seen; they are located by knowing where they are and using anatomic landmarks to get to the right spot. For this reason, inserting a central venous catheter requires greater knowledge and skill than placing a catheter in a peripheral vein.

A fine needle will be used to inject an anesthetic in an area to make it numb. A needle is placed into the central vein, and a long, thin wire (the size of a guitar string) is inserted through the needle and into the vessel. The needle is then removed, and the catheter is threaded over the wire into the vein. The wire is removed, and the central venous catheter is secured to the skin with sutures.

POSSIBLE COMPLICATIONS

As with any procedure, complications are always possible. With this procedure, they can include the following:

- **Puncture of the Artery:** Central veins are located next to the major arteries. The internal jugular vein is next to the *carotid* artery; the subclavian vein is next to the *subclavian* artery; and the femoral vein is next to the *femoral* artery. About 3 to 10% of the time there is an unintentional puncture of one of these arteries. Such a complication usually causes no problem if it is recognized promptly and the needle is withdrawn. If, however, a large central catheter needs to be inserted into the vein and such a catheter is unintentionally inserted into the artery, significant problems can result.
- **Pneumothorax:** The lung also is close to the central veins and can be punctured when attempting to insert a needle into the vein. Air can then escape from the lung to form a *pneumothorax*, which is a collection of air outside the lung but inside the chest cavity. A chest x-ray is taken after central venous catheter insertion to pick up a pneumothorax if it has occurred. A pneumothorax may resolve on its own or may require a tube inserted into the chest cavity to drain the air.
- **Arrhythmias:** Arrhythmias are changes in the normal beat of the heart. They occur when the catheter or the wire used to help insert the catheter passes into the heart and irritates it. Arrhythmias are usually temporary and stop when the wire or catheter is withdrawn slightly. An EKG will be used to monitor your heart for arrhythmia.
- **Nerve Injury:** Nerve injury is possible from direct trauma by the needle. This is a rare complication.
- **Infection:** Central venous catheters tend to be left in place for a longer time than peripheral venous catheters. For this reason, sterile technique is followed even more carefully when inserting these catheters. In addition, the catheter insertion site is inspected on a regular basis for signs of infection. Even so the site of central catheter insertion may become infected. Such a localized infection may spread into the blood stream and cause generalized infection.

Other complications can occur but are rare.

As you can now appreciate, central venous catheters can have a critical role in making some operations possible, safer, and more successful.

△ GENERAL INFORMATION

The cervix is at the bottom of the uterus and can be seen at the deepest part of the vagina.

Sometimes, suspicious abnormalities are seen in the cells scraped off the cervix during a Papanicolaou (Pap) smear. These abnormalities may range from minor ones to finding precancerous cells. Sometimes, however, even though cells scraped off during the Pap smear are abnormal, no certain abnormality can be seen with the naked eye.

In such circumstances, a colposcopy may be performed with a special instrument called a *colposcope.* The colposcope has lenses in it that magnify things six to 40 times, making it possible for the doctors to see tissue much more clearly. A biopsy (removal of a tiny piece of tissue) can be performed on any abnormal area for examination under the microscope.

In your case, based on the results of all the tests done, the recommendation is that the most appropriate treatment of your problem is an office procedure called *cryotherapy* of the cervix. This involves freezing (to death) tissue with a special instrument designed for this purpose.

This procedure is typically performed for mild abnormalities of the cervix after the gynecologist has made certain that no severe disorders are present. It may also be used when the cervix shows changes related to a virus that commonly infects the cervix, called human papillomavirus or HPV. This virus can create abnormal Pap smear results. Cryotherapy treats the abnormal areas by freezing the cells that are causing the problem.

PREOPERATIVE PREPARATION

- Do not douche or otherwise place anything into your vagina for 24 hours before the procedure.
- Shower as usual on the day of the procedure.

THE CRYOTHERAPY

- You will be positioned on the examining table just as for a pelvic examination.
- A speculum will be placed to expose the cervix completely.
- Your doctor may visualize the cervix again with the colposcope before performing the cryotherapy or the colposcopy may be done for the first time, depending upon your prior Pap smear results.
- The doctor will then pick the appropriate-sized cryotherapy probe to treat the abnormal area on the cervix based on the lesion size and location (Fig. 1).

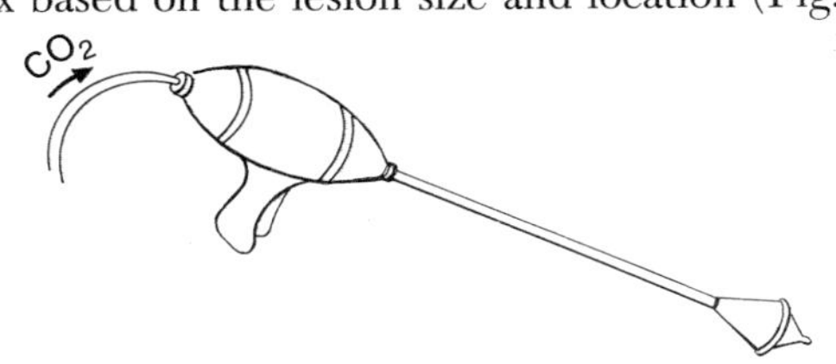

Figure 1. One of several models of the cryoprobe.

- The doctor will place the probe on the surface of the cervix and hold it there for several minutes while a very cold solution passes through the probe to freeze the surface of the cervix. This will not be painful to you, but you will feel a cold sensation in the vagina. This freezing is typically done two times to ensure that the entire abnormal area has been treated (Figs. 2 and 3).

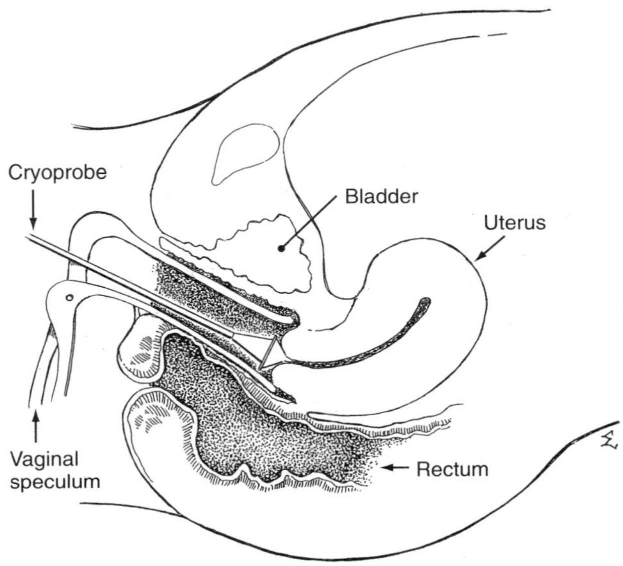

Figure 2. The speculum in the vagina keeps the vaginal walls apart. The tip of the cryoprobe is applied against the cervix.

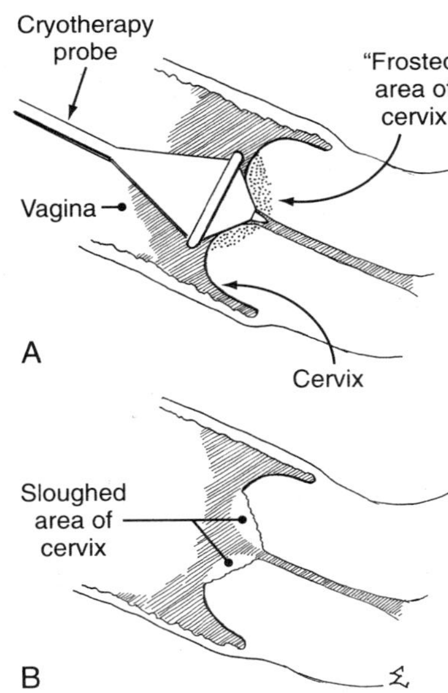

Figure 3. *A,* The cryoprobe is causing the portion of the cervix it is touching to become "frosted" and destroyed. *B,* The "frosted," destroyed portion of the cervix sloughs, and the resulting raw areas usually heal in several weeks.

AFTER THE CRYOTHERAPY

- You will be allowed to dress and return to your usual activities as soon as the freezing therapy is completed.
- Arrangements will be made for your follow-up office visit.

✣ HOME CARE

- Resume your usual activities.
- Do not douche or place anything into the vagina until your doctor instructs you that it is safe to do so. In the meantime, a sanitary pad should be sufficient for the expected discharge.
- You should not expect to see bleeding following a cryotherapy, but you will experience a significant amount of discharge in the weeks following the therapy. This is due to shedding of the cells that are destroyed with the treatment.
- During the office visit, let's discuss when it will be safe to resume sexual intercourse.
- You may return to work when you feel up to it.

✆ CALL OUR OFFICE IF

- There is any bleeding from your vagina beyond spotting.
- You develop a temperature higher than 100°F.
- You have any questions.

△ GENERAL INFORMATION

Sometimes suspicious abnormalities are seen in the cells scraped off the cervix during a Papanicolaou (Pap) test. On examination with the eye, no certain area of abnormality can be seen, so a more detailed investigation with a special microscope, called a *colposcope,* is required. Otherwise, there is a serious risk that a cancer may be missed. You may have already had this colposcopy, complete with biopsies of the cervix.

Based on the colposcopic examination and the result of any biopsies taken, it has been determined that the most appropriate treatment of your problem is a procedure called laser ablation of the cervix.

○ TREATMENT

This procedure is typically performed for mild to moderate abnormalities of the cervix after it has been determined that you do not have any severe disorders. It may also be used when the cervix shows changes related to a virus that commonly infects the cervix, called human papillomavirus or HPV. This virus can create abnormal Pap smear results. If it also infects the vaginal skin or the skin immediately outside of the vagina or anus, it may cause the growth of genital warts. The laser method of treatment of the cervix may be chosen if you have one or more of these wart growths that can be treated with the laser at the same time.

The intent of this type of treatment of the abnormal areas of the cervix is to laser off the top layer of cells where the abnormality is located.

PREOPERATIVE PREPARATION

- Do not douche or otherwise introduce anything into your vagina on the day before the procedure.
- Do not eat or drink anything for 8 hours before the procedure.
- Shower as usual on the day of the procedure.
- Medicine may be given to you that will make you feel drowsy before you are brought to the operating room.

THE LASER ABLATION PROCEDURE

- If the cervix alone is being treated, the procedure may be performed in the doctor's office. However, laser ablation will be done as an outpatient procedure in a surgical area if warty areas on the vagina or the skin outside the vagina are being treated at the same time.
- You will be given either general anesthesia and be totally asleep or a spinal block. The choice will be discussed with you beforehand.
- You will be positioned on the examining table the same as for a pelvic examination.
- A speculum will be placed in your vagina to visualize the cervix completely. Because it is important that the laser beam not touch the walls of the vagina, you will notice that the speculum is opened a bit more for this procedure than it is for a routine pelvic examination.
- The cervix will be examined again with the colposcope to identify the abnormal areas on the cervix.
- If the procedure is performed in the office, the cervix will be made numb by injecting anesthetic medicine around it.
- You will be warned before these injections, but typically they do not hurt as much as would a shot in your arm. Many patients do not feel them at all, and others note only a cramping type of discomfort.
- Two pieces of equipment will be turned on; they are noisy. One sucks away the smoke that is produced by the laser, and the other is the laser machine itself.

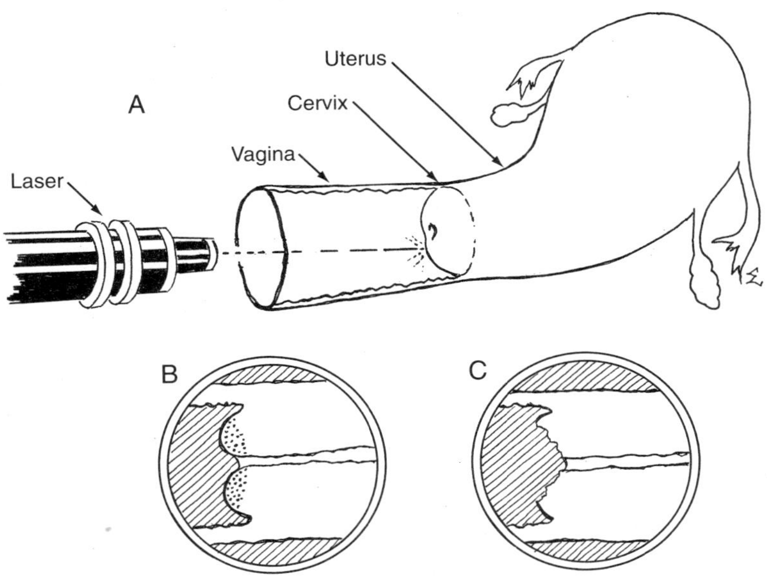

Figure 1. *A,* The vaginal speculum (not shown) will be placed with care so that the cervix is completely exposed. The affected area of the cervix will be vaporized by the pinpoint laser beam. *B,* Side view of the cervix before the laser treatment. The diseased area is stippled. *C,* The defect that results after the diseased area is vaporized, and the vaporized tissue sloughs off.

- The laser beam will be used to burn off the abnormal top layer of cells from the cervix (Fig. 1).
- If warty growths are also present, these will be lasered off at this time.
- If there is any bleeding from the laser site on the cervix, a dark brown solution may be applied to the cervix to control it. A white pasty cream (Silvadene cream) will be applied to any areas from which warty growths were lasered off of the skin, and a dressing will be placed over these areas.

AFTER THE LASER PROCEDURE

- You will be taken to a recovery room and observed. When your blood pressure, pulse, and breathing are stable and you are completely alert, you should be able to go home with a responsible adult. If the procedure is done in the office, you may drive yourself home if you choose.

✣ HOME CARE

- Resume your usual activities.
- Do not place anything in your vagina. Do not douche, use a tampon, or engage in sexual intercourse until you have been seen during your follow-up office visit to determine how well the cervix is healing.
- Sanitary napkins are satisfactory for the normal small amount of bleeding or discharge that is seen after laser ablation. The discharge may be brown in appearance, especially if the solution to control bleeding is used.
- You may shower if you wish, but do not start taking baths until we first talk about it.
- If you have also had warty growths treated with the laser, you will be instructed on changing the dressings over these areas and on the application of the Silvadene cream. Those areas will be tender.
- Take pain medicine that is prescribed for you.

✆ CALL OUR OFFICE IF

- There is any bleeding from your vagina beyond "spotting."
- You develop a temperature higher than 100°F.
- You develop any foul-smelling vaginal discharge.
- You have any questions.

CERVIX: Loop Electrocautery Excision Procedure (LEEP)

△ GENERAL INFORMATION

Sometimes suspicious abnormalities are seen in the cells scraped off the cervix during a Papanicolaou (Pap) smear. Your primary doctor has determined that the most appropriate treatment of these abnormalities is an office or outpatient procedure called a loop electrocautery excision procedure, or LEEP. Your doctor may already have investigated these abnormalities on the cervix and taken small pieces of them (called *biopsies*) with the use of a special microscope called a *colposcope*. Or, depending on the extent of abnormality noted on the Pap smear, the colposcopy may be planned as part of your LEEP.

○ TREATMENT

This procedure is performed when biopsies taken during your initial examination confirm abnormal areas on the cervix. Also, sometimes the findings from the cells scraped off during the Pap smear and the cells seen on biopsy are not in agreement. In this circumstance, it is important for your physician to know which test is actually more correct. At other times, LEEP may be performed if the colposcopic examination was not satisfactory to your physician because it was not possible to visualize an area of abnormality on the cervix entirely.

The LEEP involves removing the entire area of abnormal tissue from the cervix with a very fine wire so that it may be sent to the pathologist for more complete evaluation under the microscope. Some other treatments for abnormalities of the cervix actually destroy the problem tissue so that it is not available for microscopic examination. Therefore, a LEEP is used anytime the physician wants to ensure removal of the entire area that is affected or when microscopic examination of tissue is necessary to determine the true extent of abnormality.

PREOPERATIVE PREPARATION

- Do not douche, use a tampon, or otherwise place anything into the vagina for 24 hours before the procedure.
- Do not eat or drink anything on the morning of the operation.

THE LEEP

- You will be positioned on the examining table the same as for a pelvic examination.
- A speculum will be placed to visualize the cervix completely. Because it is important that the wire used for the LEEP does not touch the walls of the vagina—it is hot—you will notice that the speculum is opened a bit more for this procedure than for a routine pelvic examination (Fig. 1).
- A special solution will be placed on the cervix, which helps bring out the abnormal areas.

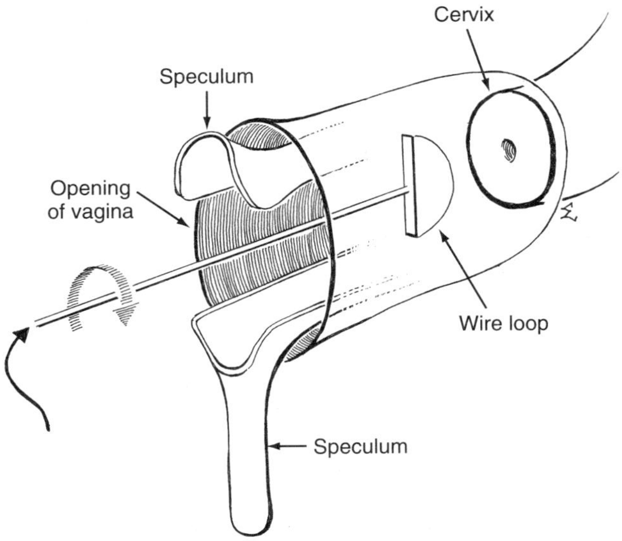

Figure 1. The vaginal speculum is positioned with special care to separate the walls of the vagina from the hot wire loop. The loops are of various sizes and shapes, and the one chosen depends on how much cervical tissue the surgeon intends to remove.

- The cervix will be visualized again with the colposcope, either to verify the abnormal area if colposcopy has been performed previously, or to evaluate the cervix completely if colposcopy is performed as a part of your LEEP.
- The appropriate size and shape of the wire to be used for the LEEP will be selected and will depend on the size and location of the abnormal area on your cervix.
- Your cervix will then be made numb with an anesthetic injected on each side of the cervix. You will be told just before these two injections are made, but typically they do not hurt as much as a shot in your arm would. Some patients do not feel them at all, and others note only a cramping type of sensation.
- Two pieces of equipment will be turned on. One makes a noise like a vacuum; it pulls out any smoke from the tissue cutting. The other is the laser, which makes a buzzing or humming sound during the actual procedure. These noises should not concern you.
- The wire loop is then used to remove the abnormal tissue from the cervix very much like a warm wire cutting through hard butter (Fig. 2). Mild cramping may be noticed. Each of the one or two passes through the cervix takes only about 5 seconds and should not hurt you at all. It is important, however, that you remain still while the wire loop is in the

vagina so that it does not touch the walls of the vagina or shift off course as it is passing through the cervix.

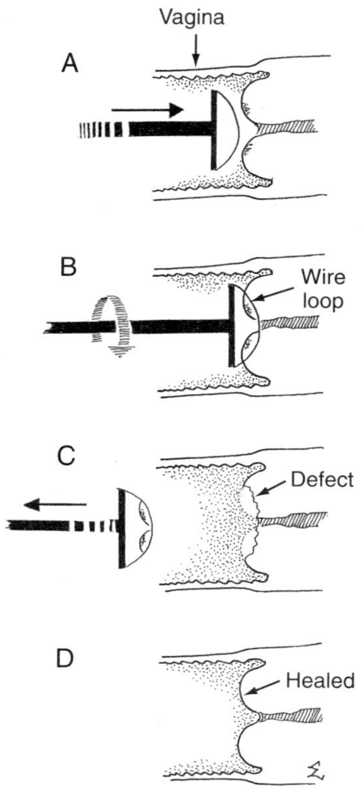

Figure 2. The sequence of events in the performance of the biopsy. *A*, The wire is advanced in the cervix. *B*, The wire loop cuts a predetermined amount of tissue. *C*, The wire loop is withdrawn, bringing the specimen with it. The defect in the cervix is shown. *D*, The cervix usually heals in several weeks.

- If there is any bleeding from the LEEP site, a different type of probe may be placed on the cervix to stop it, or a special solution that stops bleeding may be placed on the cervix. This solution is dark brown in color and may cause a dark brown discharge from the cervix for several days following the procedure.

AFTER THE LEEP

- You will be able to dress and return home or to work as soon as the procedure is completed.

HOME CARE

- Resume most of your usual activities.
- Do not douche, use a tampon, or engage in sexual intercourse until you have been seen during your follow-up office visit to determine how well the cervix is healing. This will likely be several weeks while the cervix heals.
- Sanitary pads are satisfactory for the normal small amount of bleeding or discharge that is seen after LEEP. The discharge may be brown in appearance, especially if the solution to control bleeding is used.
- You may shower if you wish, but do not start bathing until we discuss it during your follow-up visit.

CALL OUR OFFICE IF

- There is any bleeding from your vagina beyond spotting or a very light flow.
- You develop a temperature higher than 100°F.
- You notice a foul-smelling discharge.
- You have any questions.

△ GENERAL INFORMATION

Cancer of the cervix is a common type of cancer in women occurring most often between the ages of 35 to 55 years.

COMMON SIGNS AND SYMPTOMS

- In the early stage, there may be no symptoms at all.
- Later, there may be vaginal spotting between menstrual periods or after intercourse.
- There may be a persistent vaginal discharge.

DIAGNOSIS

- The diagnosis usually can be suspected from the history and physical examination.
- The diagnosis is most often made with a Papanicolaou (Pap) smear during a routine office examination. The surface of the cervix is scraped, and cells from this area are examined by specialists in the laboratory.

You may have some or all of the following tests:

- **Colposcopy:** This is a special instrument that magnifies the cervix six to 40 times, making it possible to have a closer and more complete look at the surface and inside the opening of the cervix.
- **Biopsy:** If there is a suspicious area, a small piece is removed for examination in the laboratory.
- **Conization:** Sometimes it is necessary to remove the entire surface of the cervix for microscopic examination of this tissue to be sure nothing is missed. The surface of the cervix will heal over gradually.

○ TREATMENT

- Either an operation to remove the cancer or the destruction of it with x-ray is effective if performed properly. The choice of treatment is influenced by the location of the cancer on the cervix, how deeply it has penetrated, its appearance under the microscope, the presence of tumor elsewhere in the body, and your general condition.

After careful consideration of all factors, the recommendation is that you have an operation in which your uterus, ovaries, and surrounding lymph nodes are removed. This will give you the best chance for cure.

PREOPERATIVE PREPARATION

- There will be an examination of your blood, heart (EKG), and lungs (chest x-ray).
- CT scan (computed tomography scan): These special x-rays are taken by a machine that is shaped like a huge doughnut. You will lie on a table inside the hole in the doughnut. The x-rays are taken as very thin slices through the area of the abdomen and pelvis. This makes it possible to see the fine details in these areas.
- Cystoscopy: This procedure looks inside your bladder with an instrument called a *cystoscope* that is hollow, is about as big around as a pencil, and has lenses in it and a light at its tip.
- Proctoscopy: This is an examination of your rectum with a hollow instrument somewhat similar to the cystoscope for any extension of tumor from the cervix that is just in front of the rectum.
- You will be instructed on how to clean out your bowels.
- Do not douche or use a tampon on the day of the operation.
- You may be given some medicine that will make you feel drowsy before you are brought to the operating room.

□ OPERATION

- You will be asleep for the operation.
- The incision will be in your lower abdomen.
- Your uterus, tubes, ovaries, and a very short length of your upper vagina will be removed (Fig. 1).
- The operation usually takes about 3 hours.

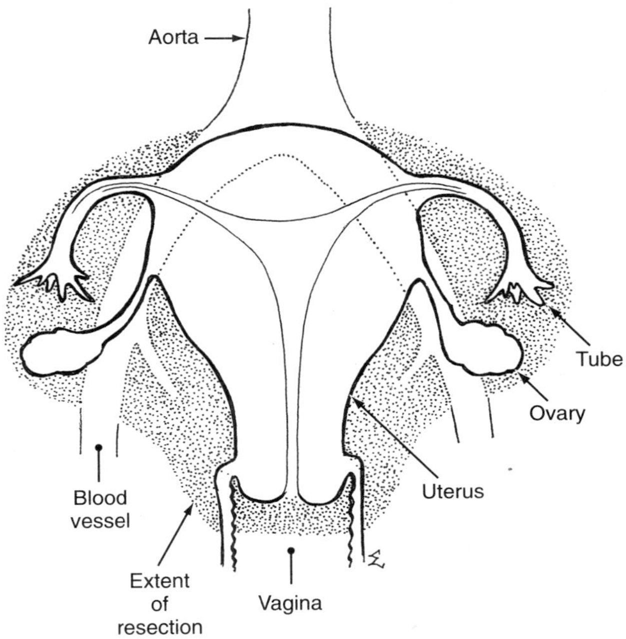

Figure 1. The tissue removed during an operation for cancer of the cervix is indicated by the stippled area. It includes the uterus, tubes, ovaries, a portion of the upper part of the vagina, and the tissue and lymph nodes along the surrounding blood vessels.

POSTOPERATIVE CARE

- You will be taken to a recovery room and observed. When your blood pressure, pulse, and breathing are stable, you will be taken to a regular hospital room.
- You may have a thin plastic tube in your nose until your bowels start working.

- That evening you will be helped to sit up in bed and the next day to get out of bed.
- There will be a catheter in your bladder to drain the urine.
- Pain will be controlled with medicine.
- Your diet will be liquid first and then will be increased as you tolerate it.
- As with any operation, complications are always possible, some of them serious. With this type of operation, they can include bleeding, leakage of urine because of breakdown of tissue, bowel obstruction, blood clots, peritonitis, heart problems, and possibly others.
- You should be able to go home in about 1 week.
- Arrangements will be made for your pain medicines, follow-up office visit, and stitch removal.
- Your condition can be cured. An estimate of your chances can be made only after all the test results are back.

✣ HOME CARE

- You may walk about as you wish, even climb stairs, but don't overdo things.
- Take medicine as prescribed for your pain.
- You may eat as you wish, but include plenty of roughage and liquids in your diet to help prevent constipation.
- You may shower if you wish and with any dressings on or off.
  - There may be narrow strips of tape across the incision. It's all right if they get wet; they will be removed in the doctor's office.
  - After you dry yourself, replace any dressings with clean, dry ones.
- Do not start bathing before we discuss it during your follow-up office visit.
- Do not lift anything heavier than 5 pounds. Ask someone to do it for you.
- Do not douche, use tampons, or engage in sexual intercourse until you have been seen during your follow-up office visit to determine how well the tissue is healing.
- Your incision and the muscles of the abdomen may ache, especially at the end of the day and after you have been standing for a long period. You can support your abdomen by wearing a girdle that is snug (but not too tight). Wearing the girdle over a cotton undergarment is easier on your incision and the stitches.
- Do not be surprised if it takes time for your bladder to start working normally. You may have to go home with a catheter for several weeks.

✆ CALL OUR OFFICE IF

- You develop any unusual signs or symptoms.
- The incision becomes red or swollen, or there is drainage from it.
- You develop a temperature higher than 100°F.
- You have any questions.

△ GENERAL INFORMATION

This is a condition in which there is an infection in the bile ducts, the tubes that carry bile (it has the consistency of olive oil) from the liver to the gallbladder and then into the intestine. The main section of the bile duct is about the size of a pencil. Sometimes the bile duct becomes blocked by gallstones, scar tissue, or cancer. This can cause the bile that cannot get by the blockage to become infected (called *suppurative cholangitis*) and is a serious problem.

COMMON SIGNS AND SYMPTOMS

- High fever that goes up and down.
- Pain over the liver, mostly in the right side of the upper abdomen.
- Jaundice (yellow eyes and skin).
- Shaking chills.
- Shock, confusion, and even unconsciousness if the condition becomes advanced.
- Some patients with cholangitis have only a few of these symptoms.

DIAGNOSIS

- It is possible to make the diagnosis by taking a detailed history, doing a thorough physical examination, and evaluating the test results carefully.

You will have some or all of the following tests:

- **Ultrasound:** Harmless sound waves are aimed at the area of your liver. The sound waves bouncing back (the echoes) from this area are seen as a picture on a screen. This is a convenient and painless way to examine the area in which the bile ducts are blocked and to look for gallstones.
- **Percutaneous Cholangiogram:** You will be given medicine to make you feel very drowsy. A spot on the skin over the liver is made numb with an anesthetic. Then a special fine needle is inserted through the numbed skin and into the liver until a bile duct is reached. Dye is injected into the bile duct as x-ray pictures are taken to show the area of blockage. At the same time, some bile is removed to see the type of bacteria growing in it. Often, a small tube is left with one end in the bile duct and the other end to the outside of the skin to allow the infected bile to drain.
- **ERCP (endoscopic retrograde cholangiopancreatography):** This is done using a special optical instrument with a light at its tip called a *gastroscope*. It is smooth, flexible, and as big around as the tip of your little finger. Your mouth and throat will be made numb with an anesthetic spray. Also, you will be given medicine to make you feel drowsy. The gastroscope is advanced gently down your throat and into your stomach and then out of the stomach into the duodenum to the spot where the bile duct enters the intestine. From the tip of the gastroscope an even thinner tube is made to come out. It is pushed up into the bile ducts, a dye is injected, and x-ray pictures are taken of the dye as it flows in the ducts to see where they are blocked.
- **CT scan (computed tomography scan):** These special x-rays are taken by a machine that is shaped like a huge doughnut. You will lie on the table inside the hole in the "doughnut." The x-rays are taken as very thin slices through the liver area. This makes it possible to see the fine details in the gallbladder and ducts. Also, the liver tissue itself can be examined to see if abscess cavities are present.

○ TREATMENT

- There are two aims in the treatment:
  - To control the infection that is present.
  - To correct the condition that caused the infection in the first place.
- Often, an operation is necessary to do the above.
- If a person is only mildly sick then there is time to do a number of these tests. If the person is very sick, however, then everything must be done more quickly. Such a patient can die if the infection is not cleared promptly.

After careful consideration of all factors, it is recommended that you have an operation to correct the problem.

PREOPERATIVE PREPARATION

- You will have an examination of your blood, heart (EKG), and lungs (chest x-ray) in addition to the other tests mentioned before.
- Do not eat or drink anything for 8 hours before the operation.

□ OPERATION

- You will be asleep for the operation.
- The exact operation that will be done depends on what is found. This will be explained to you further.

POSTOPERATIVE CARE

- You will be taken to the Surgical Care Unit, where the doctors and nurses are very experienced in taking care of patients like yourself. As soon as you are coming along well enough, you will be transferred to a regular hospital room.
- You will have a thin plastic tube in your nose until your bowels start working.
- There may be a small rubber tube coming out just next to the incision. This is *temporary* and drains your bile into a small bag on your side.
- Pain will be controlled with medicine.
- That evening you will be helped to sit up in bed and on the next day to get out of bed.
- You will be given an incentive spirometer. Breathing into this as you are instructed will help you expand your lungs and reduce the risk of developing pneumonia.

- You will go home as soon as it is safe to do so. Usually, this is in a week or so.
- Arrangements will be made for your medicine, follow-up office visit, and stitch or clip removal.

✚ HOME CARE

- You may walk about as you wish, even climb stairs, but don't overdo things.
- You will be shown how to take care of the little tube draining the bile; it's not difficult.
- You may eat as you did before the operation but include plenty of roughage in your diet to help prevent constipation.
- Unless instructed otherwise, you may shower as you wish and with any dressings on or off. After you dry yourself, replace any dressings with clean, dry ones.
- Take medicine as prescribed for your pain.
- Don't drive a car until we first discuss it during your office visit.
- You may return to work when you feel up to it.

✆ CALL OUR OFFICE IF

- You develop any unusual signs or symptoms.
- The incision becomes red or swollen, or there is drainage from it.
- You develop a temperature higher than 101°F.

CHOLECYSTECTOMY: Laparoscopic

△ GENERAL INFORMATION

Cholecystectomy is removal of the gallbladder that is located under your liver on the right side of your upper abdomen. The reason for removing the gallbladder is that it contains stones that cause inflammation and even infection.

COMMON SIGNS AND SYMPTOMS

- There is pain over the gallbladder on the right side of the upper abdomen.
- Often the pain comes on after a heavy meal. It may come and go or be there all the time.
- The pain may shoot to the back and to the tip of the right shoulder blade.
- There is loss of appetite or nausea. Sometimes there is vomiting, which may have a bitter taste.
- There may be fever and chills.
- There is tenderness over the gallbladder. This may be mild, or it may be very severe.
- A fullness may be felt over the gallbladder area.

DIAGNOSIS

- Usually the diagnosis can be made by taking a detailed history, doing a thorough physical examination, and considering the laboratory reports carefully.

  The tests will include some of the following:
- *Blood*: The blood will be analyzed for evidence of infection (elevation of the white blood cell count), anemia, or abnormalities of the liver. *Urine*: A urinalysis is done to look for red blood cells or white blood cells. *Heart* (EKG): A heart attack sometimes behaves just like a gallbladder attack. *Lungs* (chest x-ray): Occasionally, pneumonia or pleurisy can produce some of these symptoms.
- *X-ray of the abdomen*: Kidney stones and, at times, gallstones can be seen.
- *Ultrasound*: Harmless sound waves are aimed at the gallbladder area. The sound waves bouncing back (the echoes) from this area are seen as a picture on a screen. This is a convenient and painless way to examine organs and tissues inside most areas of the body. Gallstones can be seen using this technique.

○ TREATMENT

- The best treatment is to remove the gallbladder.
- Until a few years ago, most gallbladders were removed through an approximately 6-inch incision on the abdomen. With newer techniques, it now is possible to do the operation *laparoscopically*. This is done by using a hollow optical instrument with a light at its tip that is about as big around as the tip of your little finger. Three, possibly four, of these instruments are placed in the upper part of the abdomen through tiny incisions. There is much less pain and a faster recovery when the gallbladder is removed this way.

  After careful consideration, it is recommended that you have your gallbladder removed with a laparoscope. It has been explained to you why this operation is best suited for you.
- You should realize, however, that when the surgeon places the instruments in the abdomen, what is seen in the gallbladder area may be more complicated than what was expected. If this happens, it would not be safe to try to remove the gallbladder by laparoscopy. The abdomen will need to be opened so that the gallbladder and everything around it can be dissected safely.

PREOPERATIVE PREPARATION

- Do not take aspirin for 7 days before the operation. Take medications as directed by your physician.
- Do not eat or drink anything for 8 hours before the operation.
- Shower or bathe as usual on the morning of the operation.
- You may be given medicine that will make you feel drowsy before you are brought to the operating room.
- You will be given an antibiotic.

□ OPERATION

- You will be asleep for the operation.
- There will be three, possibly four, incisions, each about ¼ inch long through which the instruments will be introduced. The incisions will be placed in the navel and over the gallbladder (Fig. 1).
- You will not receive a blood transfusion unless it is absolutely necessary.
- The operation usually takes about 1½ hours.

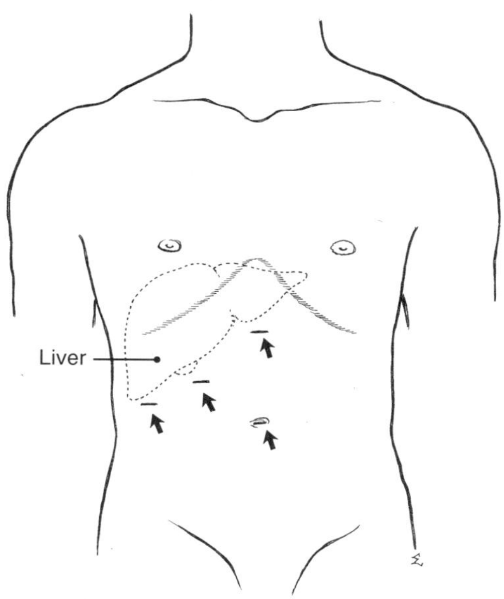

Figure 1. The location and the relative size of the incisions used to introduce the laparoscopes are shown.

POSTOPERATIVE CARE

- You will wake up in a recovery room. When your blood pressure, pulse, and breathing are stable, you will be taken to a regular hospital room. Occasionally, a patient feels well enough to go home the same day. Otherwise, you should be able to go home in 1 to 2 days.
- You may have a thin plastic tube in your nose for a day.
- You may have a thin plastic tube (drain) coming out of your side.
- That evening you will be helped to sit up in bed and on the next day to get out of bed.
- Pain can be controlled with medicine. The nurse will give it to you, or you can give yourself a preset amount of pain medicine when you feel you need it. This is done with a device called patient-controlled analgesia (PCA) that is connected to the tubing giving you intravenous fluids.
- You may have some discomfort in your right shoulder.
- Arrangements will be made for your medicine, follow-up office visit, and stitch or clip removal.
- As with any operation, complications are always possible. Although they are uncommon with this type of operation, they can include bleeding, peritonitis, injury to the bile ducts, and possibly others.

✚ HOME CARE

- You may walk about as you wish, even climb stairs.
- Take medicine as prescribed for your pain.
- You may eat as you did before the operation, but avoid fatty foods for a month or so.
- You may shower as you wish and with any dressings on or off.
  - There may be narrow strips of tape across the incision. It's all right if they get wet; they will be removed in the doctor's office.
  - After you dry yourself, replace any dressings with clean, dry ones.
- Do not drive your car for 1 week and then only if you have no pain and can move freely.
- You may resume sexual activity whenever you choose.
- You may return to work when you feel up to it.

✆ CALL OUR OFFICE IF

- You develop any unusual signs or symptoms, fainting, dizziness, or severe pain in the chest or abdomen.
- The incision becomes red or swollen, or there is drainage from it.
- You develop a temperature higher than 100°F.
- You have any questions.

△ GENERAL INFORMATION

Cholecystectomy is removal of the gallbladder that is located under your liver on the right side of your upper abdomen. The most common reason for removing the gallbladder is that it contains stones that cause it to become infected.

COMMON SIGNS AND SYMPTOMS

- There is pain over the gallbladder on the right side of the upper abdomen.
- Often the pain comes on after a heavy meal. It may come and go or be there all the time.
- The pain may shoot around to the back and to the tip of the right shoulder blade.
- There is loss of appetite or nausea. Sometimes there is vomiting, which may have a bitter taste.
- There may be fever and chills.
- There is tenderness over the gallbladder. This may be mild, or it may be very severe.
- A fullness may be felt over the gallbladder area.

DIAGNOSIS

- Usually the diagnosis can be made by taking a detailed history, doing a thorough physical examination, and considering the laboratory reports carefully.

The tests will include some and maybe all of the following:

- You will have an examination of your blood, urine, heart (EKG), and lungs (chest x-ray).
- *X-ray of the abdomen*: Kidney stones and at times gallstones can be seen.
- *Ultrasound*: Harmless sound waves are aimed at the gallbladder area. The sound waves bouncing back (the echoes) from this area are seen as a picture on a screen. This is a convenient and painless way to examine organs and tissues in this area.
- *Radionuclide scan*: A special dye is injected into your vein. The photographs taken of this dye as it travels to the liver, bile ducts, and gallbladder can show the condition of the bile ducts and gallbladder.

○ TREATMENT

- If you are seen soon after the gallbladder attack, the best treatment is to remove the gallbladder. Just waiting and watching has some disadvantages:
  - Your condition may become worse.
  - It may take quite a few days for the infection to quiet down.
  - You will need the operation eventually.

There are several ways to remove the gallbladder.

- **Laparoscopic:** This is done with instruments that are about as thick as your little finger and have lenses and a light in them. Three or four of them are introduced into the abdomen through tiny incisions over the gallbladder, and the gallbladder is removed in this manner. The *advantages* of this method are that there is less pain after the operation, the recovery is faster, and the scars are tiny. The *disadvantages* are that it is not safe if there is a lot of scar tissue in the area from inflammation of the gallbladder or from a previous operation.
- **Open:** This is done through an incision over the gallbladder. The *advantage* of this technique is that the tissue (even heavy scar tissue) around the gallbladder area can be seen and dissected more safely. The *disadvantages* are that there is more discomfort after the operation, the recovery time is longer, and there is a visible scar.

After taking all factors into consideration, it is recommended that you have a cholecystectomy performed through an open incision.

PREOPERATIVE PREPARATION

- Do not eat or drink anything for 8 hours before the operation.
- You may be given medicine that will make you feel drowsy before you are brought to the operating room.

□ OPERATION

- You will be asleep for the operation.
- The incision will be crosswise over your gallbladder or up and down between the breast bone and the navel.
- The operation usually takes about 1½ hours (Fig. 1).

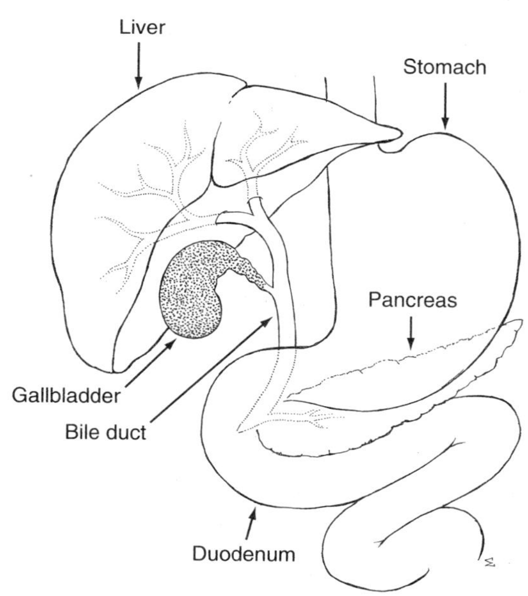

Figure 1. The gallbladder *(stippled area)* is removed during this operation.

POSTOPERATIVE CARE

- You will be taken to a recovery room and observed. When your blood pressure, pulse, and breathing are stable, you will be taken to a regular hospital room.

- You may have a thin plastic tube in your nose for a day or so.
- You may have a thin plastic tube coming out from the side of your abdomen temporarily.
- That evening you will be helped to sit up in bed and on the next day to get out of bed.
- Pain will be controlled with medicine.
- When you start to eat, your diet will be as you tolerate it.
- You should be able to go home in about 2 to 4 days.
- Arrangements will be made for your medicine, follow-up office visit, and stitch or clip removal.
- As with any operation, complications are possible. With this type of operation, they can include infection, pneumonia, heart problems, blood clots, and possibly others.

✣ HOME CARE

- You may walk about as you wish, even climb stairs.
- You might go home with the drain in your abdomen still in place and with dressings over it. You will be shown how to take care of it; it's not difficult.
- Take medicine as prescribed for your pain.
- Unless instructed otherwise, you may shower as you wish and with any dressings on or off. There may be narrow strips of tape across the incision. It's all right if they get wet. They will be removed in the doctor's office. After you dry yourself, replace any dressings with clean, dry ones.
- Include plenty of roughage and liquids in your diet to help avoid constipation.
- Do not drive unless you can move freely and without pain and you are not taking medicines that decrease your alertness.

✆ CALL OUR OFFICE IF

- The incision becomes red or swollen, or there is drainage from it.
- You have severe pain in your abdomen or behind your breast bone.
- You develop a temperature higher than 100°F.
- You have any questions.

△ GENERAL INFORMATION

Circumcision is removal of the foreskin of the penis. There can be several reasons for a circumcision:

- The foreskin is too long and tight, and it is very difficult to pull it back completely to clean the "head" *(glans)* of the penis that is under the foreskin.
- Irritation under the foreskin because of the moisture and the material that collects there (called *smegma*).
- A lesion on the foreskin.
- Appearance.
- Painful urination.
- Concern about the greater risk of cancer of the penis when the foreskin is present.
- Itching under the foreskin.
- The foreskin pulls back and becomes swollen, seriously choking the glans or the penis.
- An undesirable odor in the constantly moist foreskin.

DIAGNOSIS

- The diagnosis usually can be made from the history and physical examination.
- The penis is inspected before the circumcision because a circumcision might make an existing problem worse. Or another problem (and *not* the foreskin) may be the cause of some of your symptoms.

○ TREATMENT

If the reasons already mentioned apply to you, the treatment to correct the problem is a circumcision.

PREOPERATIVE PREPARATION

- Do not eat or drink anything for 8 hours before the operation.
- You will have an examination of your blood to be certain that it clots normally.
- You will be given medicine that will make you feel drowsy before you are brought to the operating room.

□ OPERATION

- The operation usually is done under local anesthesia. A very thin needle is used to inject an anesthetic in the tissue to make this entire area numb. Also, you will be given medicine that will make you feel very drowsy.
- During the operation you may feel some tugging but not pain.
- Absorbable stitches will be used.
- The operation is straightforward and usually takes about 1 hour.

POSTOPERATIVE CARE

- You will be taken to a recovery room. When your blood pressure, pulse, and breathing are stable and you are completely alert, you should be able to go home that same day with a responsible adult.
- Arrangements will be made for your medicine and follow-up office visit.

✙ HOME CARE

- For the first 24 hours, lie down as often as possible. It may help reduce any swelling.
- Take medicine as prescribed for your pain.
- It is important that you not have an erection of your penis. This can be painful and can put strain on the stitches. Avoid conditions that may arouse you sexually.
- You may be given some medicines to "relax" you and to decrease the chance you will be sexually aroused.
- You may shower as you wish. Pat yourself dry gently.
- Wear the type of shorts (boxer or jockey) that keep you most comfortable.
- Driving a car with an automatic shift is not too demanding. But if you suddenly have to slam on the brakes or twist to turn a wheel, you may strain the sutures or tear something. Remind me during the follow-up visit to discuss with you when you can resume driving.
- You should not engage in sexual intercourse until you are healed completely.
- You may return to work as soon as you feel up to it.

✆ CALL OUR OFFICE IF

- There is any bleeding from the incision.
- You cannot urinate.
- The penis swells and continues to remain swollen.
- You develop a temperature higher than 100°F.
- You have any questions.

△ GENERAL INFORMATION

Circumcision is removal of the foreskin of the penis. There can be several reasons for wanting a circumcision:

- Religious practice, as, for example, with Muslims and Jews.
- The parents feel that
  - It is difficult or cumbersome to pull back the foreskin regularly to clean the area.
  - It will protect the infant from urinary tract infections.
  - It will prevent infection and irritation under the foreskin.

PREOPERATIVE PREPARATION

- There may be testing of the blood to see that it clots normally.
- A general physical examination may be performed. The procedure should not be done in premature infants or in those with any other illness unless the most careful consideration has been given by the pediatrician and the parents.
- The penis and scrotum should be examined carefully to be certain no abnormalities are present. A circumcision can worsen some conditions or make it much more difficult to correct them later.

□ OPERATION

Infant

- It can be done with or without local anesthesia, depending on the custom of the surgeon or the desires of the parents.
- The procedure takes about 5 minutes.
- A petroleum jelly–covered dressing is applied loosely around the tip of the penis.
- The infant can be taken home directly after the procedure.

Child

- Do not let the child eat or drink anything for 6 hours before the operation.
- The operation is done under general anesthesia.
- The operation usually takes 30 minutes.
- A light petroleum jelly dressing will be applied around the circumcision.
- The child will be taken to a recovery room. As soon as the child's blood pressure, pulse, and breathing are stable and he is fully alert, he may be taken home.

✙ HOME CARE

- Resume the usual activities.
- Make every attempt to change the diapers as soon as possible when they are soiled.
- The child may be bathed, but do not let him soak any more than is necessary to complete the bathing.

✆ CALL OUR OFFICE IF

- There is bleeding from the circumcision.
- The child cannot urinate.
- The penis becomes red and appears infected.
- The infant or child develops a temperature higher than 101°F.
- You have any questions.

CLAVICLE (COLLARBONE) FRACTURE: Adult

△ GENERAL INFORMATION

Most commonly, fracture of the *clavicle* (the collarbone) is the result of a direct injury to the middle of the clavicle or a fall on an outstretched hand.

COMMON SIGNS AND SYMPTOMS

- There is a deformity over the clavicle.
- It is difficult to move the shoulder.
- Sometimes the fracture may cause nerve problems of the shoulder and arm.

DIAGNOSIS

- The diagnosis is suspected from the history and the physical examination.
- X-rays of the clavicle will confirm the diagnosis (Fig. 1).

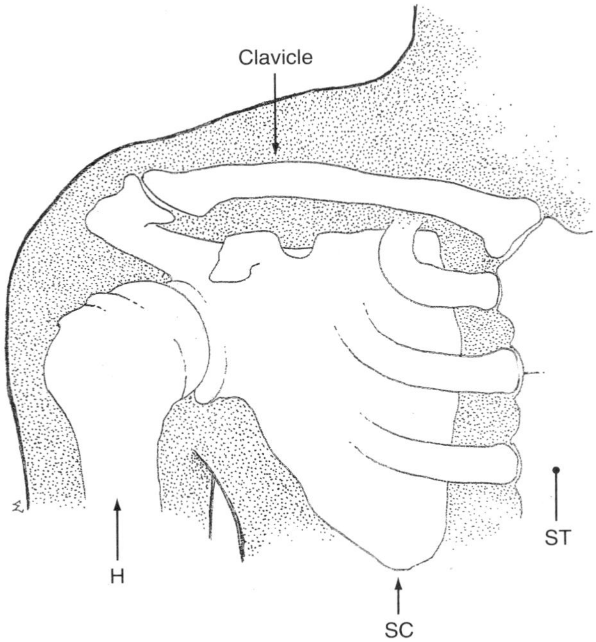

Figure 1. The clavicle can fracture in a variety of ways. The treatment of each depends on the individual clinical and technical circumstances. H, Humerus (upper arm bone); SC, scapula (shoulder blade); ST, sternum (breastbone).

- Often an operation is not required for a clavicle fracture except in the following circumstances:
  - When the end of the fractured clavicle has punctured the skin.
  - When there is involvement of nearby nerves or blood vessels.
  - When the fractured ends of the clavicle are too much out of line.
  - X-rays of the chest, neck, and spine may have determined that there is injury to these areas.

After careful consideration of all factors, the recommendation is that you have an operation for your fractured clavicle.

SURGICAL TREATMENT

- The most effective surgical treatment is to realign the two ends of the fractured fragments to their normal position and then hold them in place with a plate and screws. If the fracture has multiple pieces, then adding a bone graft to the repair may improve the chances of healing. Clavicle fractures generally heal within 8 weeks.

PREOPERATIVE PREPARATION

- You will have an examination of your blood, urine, heart (EKG), and lungs (chest x-ray).
- Do not eat or drink anything for 8 hours before the operation.
- You may be given medicine that will make you feel drowsy before you are brought to the operating room.

□ OPERATION

- You will be asleep for the operation.
- An incision will be made that can be closed in a cosmetically pleasing manner.
- The two ends of the fracture will be brought together and stabilized in an appropriate manner.
- The operation usually takes about 2 hours.
- A dressing will be applied at the incision site, and the arm will be placed in a sling.

POSTOPERATIVE CARE

- You will be taken to a recovery room and observed. When your blood pressure, pulse, and breathing are stable, you will be taken to a regular hospital room for an overnight stay. Occasionally, it is possible to go home the same day as the operation. Otherwise you will remain in the hospital a day or so.
- That evening you will be helped to get out of bed and sit in a chair.
- Your pain will be controlled with medicine.
- Arrangements will be made for your medicine, follow-up office visit, and stitch removal.
- As with any operation, complications are always possible. Although they are uncommon with this type of operation, they can include failure of the fracture to heal, injury to the nerves in this area, and possibly others.

✚ HOME CARE

- You may walk about as you wish, even climb stairs, but don't overdo things.
- Your arm should remain in a sling until it is determined by the surgeon that you can begin to move the shoulder. You may move your hand and wrist as tolerated.
- Take medicine as prescribed for your pain.
- Eat as you wish but include plenty of roughage and liquids in your diet to help prevent constipation.

- You may bathe with help. The area of the operation should be kept as dry as possible until the sutures have been removed. Replace any dressings that get wet with clean, dry ones.
- Do not drive until we first talk about it during your follow-up office visit.
- You may return to work when you feel up to it. However, strenuous work is not possible until as late as 3 months and heavy work until as late as 6 months.

✆ CALL OUR OFFICE IF

- The incision becomes red or swollen, or there is drainage from it.
- You develop a temperature higher than 100.5°F.
- You develop numbness and tingling in the arm or neck.
- You develop shortness of breath.
- You have any questions.

CLAVICLE (COLLARBONE) FRACTURE: Infant, Child, or Adolescent

△ GENERAL INFORMATION

The *clavicle* (collarbone) is the bone that connects the arm with the trunk. The clavicle is one of the most frequently broken bones in children (Fig. 1).

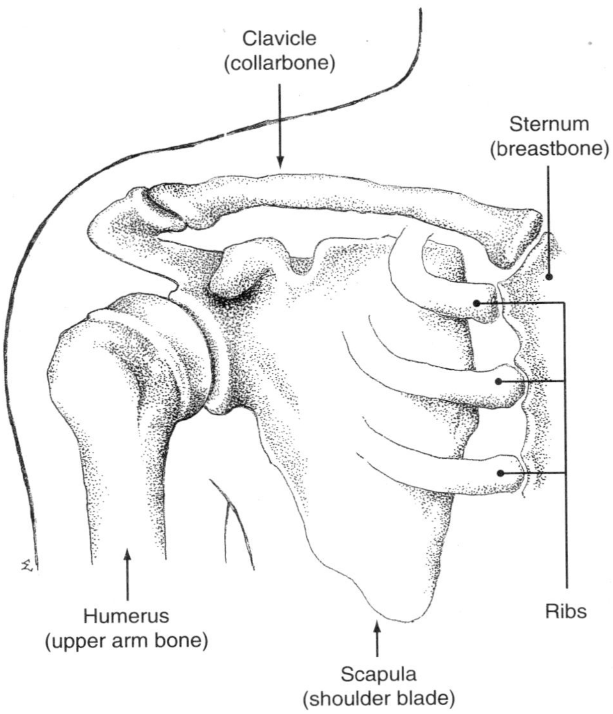

Figure 1. Normal bone anatomy of the shoulder area.

COMMON SIGNS AND SYMPTOMS

Infants

- The clavicle may be deformed.
- Usually there is swelling over the fracture.
- The infant doesn't want to move the arm because of the pain. This is sometimes called "pseudoparalysis," but very rarely is anything wrong with the nerves.

Children or Adolescents

- There is pain and swelling over the fracture.
- The clavicle usually shows some deformity.
- There is painful motion at the shoulder joint.

DIAGNOSIS

History

Infant

- Commonly, there is a history of a difficult birth.

Child or Adolescent

- Most commonly, there is a history of a fall on an outstretched arm or a direct injury to the middle of the clavicle.

Physical Examination

Infant

- Sometimes when examining the infant gently, the broken bone can be felt crackling under the skin.
- The infant won't move the arm.

Child or Adolescent

- Often the broken bone can be felt under the skin.
- The clavicle may be crooked.
- When the shoulder is moved, there is pain over the fracture.
- X-rays of the clavicle show the fracture, which can be as follows (Fig. 2):
  - It can be fractured, but not through and through (this usually is referred to as a *greenstick fracture*) (*A*).
  - It can be a through and through fracture but can have one of the following appearances:
    - It is not out of place (*B*).
    - The clavicle is bent at the fracture (*C*).
    - The broken ends of the clavicle have slid over each other but are still touching (*D*).
    - The broken ends are widely separated from each other (*E*).

The above variations are important because they determine the type of therapy that is necessary.

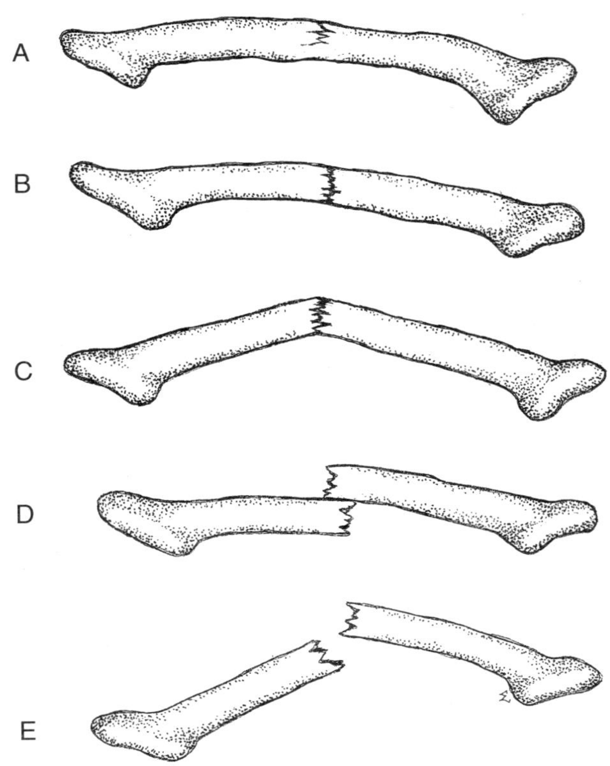

Figure 2. The most common types of fractures in an infant or a child.

○ TREATMENT: *No Operation*

Infant

- If there are no symptoms, no specific orthopedic treatment is necessary. The infant should be handled gently, however.
- If there is pain on touching the fracture site or there is pseudoparalysis, the arm is immobilized by pinning the shirtsleeve on the injured arm to the body of baby's shirt with a safety pin for 1 or 2 weeks until the tenderness disappears.

Note: The arm will be examined carefully and repeatedly for any neurologic problems, especially in those infants who do not move the arm.

Child or Adolescent

- A bandage (called a *figure of eight*) is applied. The purpose of this bandage is to pull the shoulders back. It helps prevent the clavicle from moving too much.
- The above therapy does not require an anesthetic; it is done on an outpatient basis.
- Usually the figure-of-eight bandage is kept on for 2 weeks. If pain is still present after 2 weeks, the bandage is kept on for another week or so longer.
- Usually physical therapy is not required.
- Full range of motion can be expected once the pain from the fracture disappears.
- Any deformity of the clavicle usually corrects itself with time.

✚ HOME CARE

- Pain medicine is required only occasionally.
- The figure-of-eight bandage needs to be checked every day to see that it is snug. The buckles in the back need to be adjusted as necessary.
- Check the elbow, wrist, and hand to see that they move as well as those in the unaffected arm.
- Check the fingers twice a day to make certain there is no change in color.
- The figure-of-eight bandage presses against the moist skin in the armpit, which can irritate the area. Use some gauze with ordinary rubbing alcohol on it to keep the area clean.

○ TREATMENT: *Operation*

- An operation is rarely required and only in the following instances:
  - When a nerve is caught in the fracture area.
  - When the fracture does not heal, usually because the broken ends were too far apart.
  - When the fracture is an outer end (distal) fracture through the growth plate with significant displacement and deformity.
  - The operation is done under general anesthesia.
  - An incision is made that can be closed in a cosmetically pleasing fashion.

POSTOPERATIVE CARE

- At the completion of the operation, your child will be taken to a recovery room and observed. After the blood pressure, pulse, and breathing are normal, the child usually can be taken home that same day. Occasionally, a 1- or 2-day hospital stay is necessary.
- Arrangements will be made for medicine, instructions on care, and the postoperative office visit.

✚ HOME CARE

- Pain medicine is required only occasionally.
- Sponge bathe. Let's discuss when tub baths or showers are appropriate.
- Keep the dressings dry. If they get wet, replace them with clearn, dry ones.

✆ CALL OUR OFFICE IF

- There is a change in color of the fingers, or the fingers or wrist cannot be moved as well as those on the unaffected arm.
- Any unusual signs or symptoms develop.

△ GENERAL INFORMATION

The small intestine travels through the lower part of the abdomen. In the right lower part of your abdomen, it enters the colon. At the point it enters the colon, the small intestine has a fairly reliable one-way valve: digested food can go from the small intestine into the colon, but it cannot go back from the colon into the small intestine (Fig. 1).

Sometimes the colon becomes blocked by a cancer or by a benign condition. The stool cannot go forward past the blockage in the colon, yet digested food keeps on coming into the colon from the small intestine. The colon keeps on growing larger; because of the valve, the stool cannot back up into the small intestine. This is called a *closed loop syndrome*—a very dangerous situation (see Fig. 1).

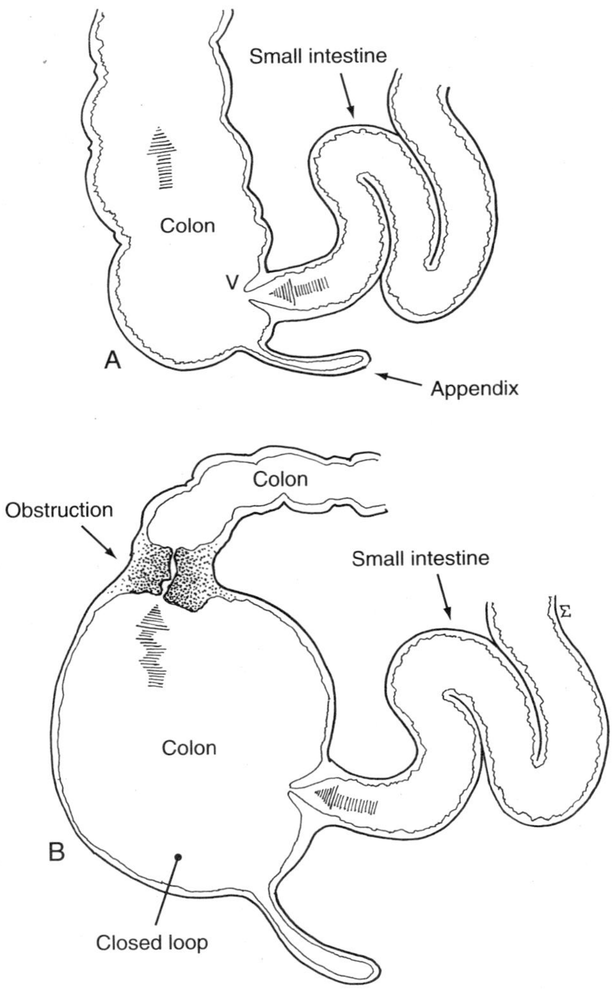

Figure 1. *A*, Normally, the contents of the small intestine pass through a one-way valve (V) into the colon, from which they eventually exit as stool. *B*, If the colon is blocked by a growth or scarring, the contents cannot pass, but neither can they back up into the small intestine. As a result, the colon becomes distended and is at risk of bursting.

COMMON SIGNS AND SYMPTOMS

- Because liquid stool and air keep entering the blocked colon, there are severe cramps as the colon tries to push ahead the stool and air inside it.
- The colon can become very distended.
- There is tenderness over the distended colon on the right side.

DIAGNOSIS

- Usually the diagnosis can be made by taking a detailed history, doing a thorough physical examination, and considering the laboratory reports carefully.
- An x-ray of the abdomen will show the hugely distended colon. If the colon begins to get larger than about 5 inches, it may burst.
- The white blood cell count may be elevated, and there may be some fever.
- The right side of the abdomen is tender when pressure is applied over it.

○ TREATMENT

The treatment is an operation—which should be done as soon as possible—to relieve the distention. If an operation is not done, the colon may balloon up enough to burst. If this happens, the risk of dying is very high.

PREOPERATIVE PREPARATION

- You will have an examination of your blood, urine, heart (EKG), and lungs (chest x-ray).
- You may be given medicine that will make you feel drowsy before you are brought to the operating room.

□ OPERATION

- You will be asleep for the operation.
- It is not possible to know beforehand the exact operation that will be performed. Generally, however, the blocked bowel, along with the growth causing the blockage, is removed and the intestines reconnected. *Sometimes* it is necessary to perform a temporary colostomy. Such a temporary colostomy will be closed at a later date.
- You will not receive a blood transfusion unless it is absolutely necessary.
- The operation usually takes about 2 to 3 hours.

POSTOPERATIVE CARE

- You will be taken to a recovery room and observed. When your blood pressure, pulse, and breathing are stable, you will be taken to a regular hospital room.
- You will have a thin plastic tube in your nose. It goes down to your stomach to suck up the air you swallow. It will be removed when your bowels start working.
- That evening you will be helped to sit up in bed and on the next day to get out of bed.
- Pain can be controlled with medicine. The nurse will

give it to you, or you can give yourself a preset amount of pain medicine when you feel you need it. This is done with a device called patient-controlled analgesia (PCA) that is connected to the tubing giving you intravenous fluids.
- When your bowels start working, the tube in your nose will be removed and you will be started on a liquid diet that will be increased as you tolerate it.
- You should be able to go home in about 1 week.
- Arrangements will be made for your medicine, follow-up office visit, and stitch or clip removal.
- As with any operation, complications are always possible. With this type of operation, they can include infection, blood clots, bleeding, pneumonia, bowel obstruction, and possibly others.

✣ HOME CARE

- Continue with the program started while you were in the hospital.
- You may walk about as you wish, even climb stairs, but don't overdo things.
- You may eat as you did before the operation but be certain to include plenty of roughage and fluids in your diet to help prevent constipation.
- You may shower as you wish and with any dressings on or off.
  - There may be narrow strips of tape across the incision. It's all right if they get wet; they will be removed in the doctor's office.
  - After you dry yourself, replace any dressings with clean, dry ones.
- Take medicine as prescribed for your pain.
- Your incision and the muscles of the abdomen may ache, especially at the end of the day and after you have been standing for a long period. You can support your abdomen by wearing a girdle or similar garment that is snug (but not too tight).
- Driving a car with an automatic shift might not seem to be too demanding. However, you may have to slam on the brakes or twist to turn the steering wheel and may strain your sutures or tear something. During your follow-up visit, let's discuss when you can resume driving.
- You may resume sexual activity whenever you choose.
- You may return to work when you feel up to it.

✆ CALL OUR OFFICE IF

- You develop any unusual signs or symptoms.
- The incision becomes red or swollen, or there is drainage from it.
- You develop a temperature higher than 100°F.
- You have any questions.

△ GENERAL INFORMATION

This is a condition of the *aorta*, the large vessel that is about as large around as a broom handle that comes off the heart and goes down the chest and into the abdomen and legs (Fig. 1). Very infrequently, a person is born with a very short area of narrowing of the aorta in the chest; this narrowing can be as small around as angel hair spaghetti and is called *coarctation of the aorta.* Blood has a difficult time passing through such a narrow channel, so blood pressure builds up behind the narrowing. Also, detour vessels begin to develop around the narrowed aorta to get the blood where it's supposed to go.

COMMON SIGNS AND SYMPTOMS

Most people do not have any symptoms even though their blood pressure is high because of the blocked blood flow. Often, the diagnosis is made during a routine physical examination.

- Symptoms are more common in adults. These symptoms may include headache, shortness of breath, a pounding or throbbing sensation in the head, dizziness, chest pain, and eye problems, among others.

DIAGNOSIS

- There is high blood pressure in the arms and a low or an absent pulse in the legs.
- The vessels in the neck and shoulder may be enlarged; one can see the pulses in them.
- A murmur can be heard in the left side of the chest; this is the blood squirting through the narrow channel.
- A chest x-ray may show changes that are telltale signs of a coarctation.
- The electrocardiogram (EKG) will show that the heart is strained.

Some or all of the following tests may need to be done:

- Cardiac catheterization: A very fine plastic tube is inserted into a blood vessel in the arm or neck and advanced to the heart. Measurements of pressure in the various chambers of the heart help make the diagnosis.
- Injecting a special liquid into the aorta and taking x-ray pictures of it as it flows through the aorta will show the narrowed area.
- Echocardiogram: Harmless sound waves are aimed at the heart. The sound waves bouncing back (the echoes) from this area are seen as a picture on a screen. This is a convenient and painless way to examine the blood vessels coming from the heart.

○ TREATMENT

- The treatment is an operation to remove the narrowed area.
- The operation is best done between the ages of 3 and 4 years, but if the clinical condition is bad, the operation is done at any age.
- Sometimes the diagnosis is not apparent or does not produce symptoms until the person becomes an adult. In such an instance, an operation is necessary.
- The most common causes of death in patients who do not have an operation are rupture of the aorta, failure of the heart, infection of the heart, and rupture of a weak vessel (aneurysm) in the brain, causing a stroke.

PREOPERATIVE PREPARATION

- The necessary medical preparation for the operation will have been done while making the diagnosis.
- Do not eat or drink anything for 8 hours before the operation.
- You may shower or bathe on the morning of the operation.
- You may be given medicine to make you feel drowsy before you are brought to the operating room.

□ OPERATION

- You will be asleep for the operation.
- The incision will be in the left chest.

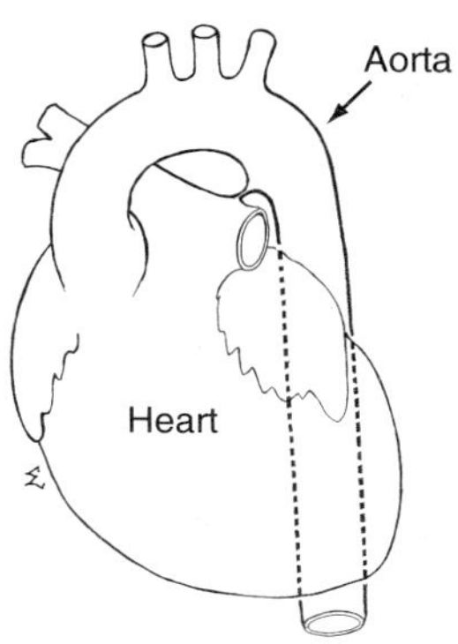

Figure 1.

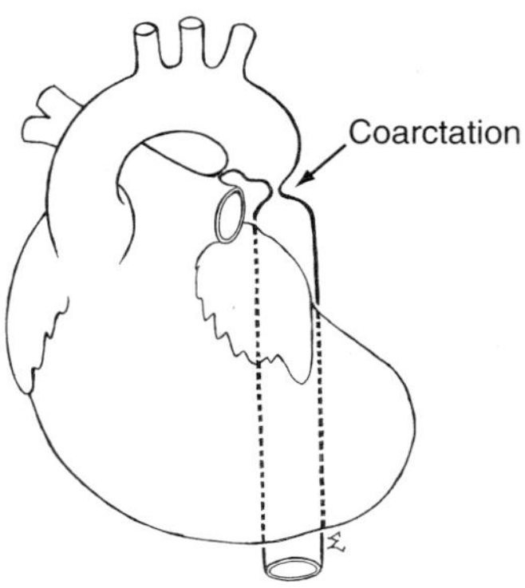

Figure 2.

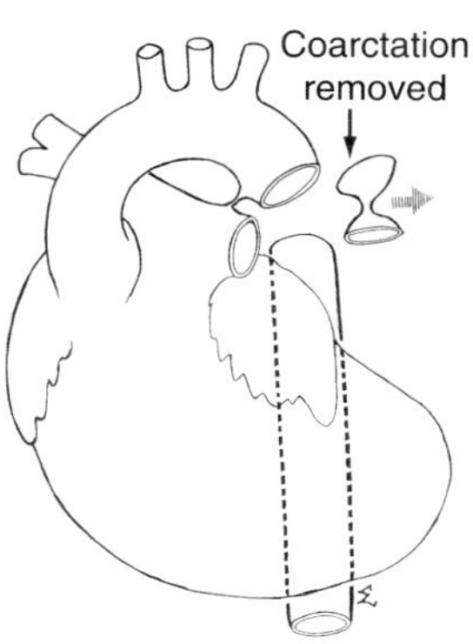

Figure 3.

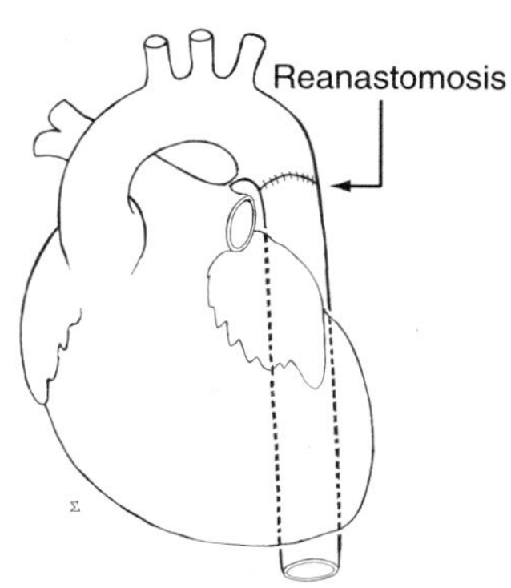

Figure 4.

- The usual operation consists of removing the narrowed area and reconnecting the normal ends of the aorta (Figs. 2–4).
- The operation usually takes about 2 hours.

POSTOPERATIVE CARE

- You will be taken to a recovery room and observed. When your blood pressure, pulse, and breathing are stable, you will be taken to a regular hospital room.
- A small plastic tube will be coming out through your chest for a day or two. It was placed there to drain any excess fluid.
- You may have a catheter in your bladder for a day or so.
- That evening you will be helped to sit up in bed and on the next day to get out of bed.
- You will be given an incentive spirometer. Breathing into this as you are instructed will help you expand your lungs and reduce the risk of developing pneumonia.
- Your diet will first be liquids and then will be advanced to solid foods as you tolerate them.
- You should be able to go home in about 1 week.
- As with any operation, complications are always possible. With this type of operation, they can include bleeding in the chest, infection, heart problems, hoarseness, continued fluid accumulation in the chest, paralysis from the waist down (rarely), and possibly others.
- Arrangements will be made for your medicine, follow-up office visit, and stitch removal.

✚ HOME CARE

- Continue with the program started while you were in the hospital.
- You may walk about as you wish, even climb stairs, but don't overdo things.
- You may eat as you wish but include plenty of roughage and liquids in your diet to help prevent constipation.
- Take the medicines prescribed for you.
- Unless advised otherwise, you may shower as you wish and with any dressings on or off. After you dry yourself, replace any dressings with clean, dry ones.
- Engaging in sexual intercourse too soon can be harmful to your recovery. If you wish, let's talk about this during your follow-up visit.
- Sometimes the blood pressure takes quite a while to come down to normal levels. Rarely, it never comes down to normal.
- Don't plan to return to work until we have talked about it during one of your follow-up visits.

✆ CALL OUR OFFICE IF

- The incision becomes red or swollen, or there is drainage from it.
- You develop a temperature higher than 100°F.
- You have any questions.

△ GENERAL INFORMATION

This is a condition of the *aorta*, the vessel that is as large as your middle finger and comes off the heart and goes down the chest and into the abdomen and legs (Fig. 1). Very infrequently, a child is born with a very short area of narrowing of the aorta in the chest; this narrowing can be as small around as angel hair spaghetti and is called *coarctation of the aorta*. Blood has a difficult time passing through such a narrow channel, so blood pressure builds up behind the narrowing. Also, detour vessels begin to develop around the narrowed aorta to get the blood where it's supposed to go.

COMMON SIGNS AND SYMPTOMS

Most children do not have any symptoms even though their blood pressure is high because of the blocked blood flow. Often, the diagnosis is made during a routine school health examination.

- If the narrowing is severe, the heart is so strained that the infant may die unless an operation is done quickly.
- Symptoms are more common in adults. These symptoms may include headache, shortness of breath, a pounding or throbbing sensation in the head, dizziness, chest pain, and eye problems, among others.

DIAGNOSIS

- There is high blood pressure in the arms and a low or an absent pulse in the legs.
- The vessels in the neck and shoulder may be enlarged; one can see the pulses in them.
- A murmur can be heard in the left side of the chest; this is the blood squirting through the narrow channel.
- The electrocardiogram (EKG) will show that the heart is strained.

Some or all of the following tests may need to be done:

- Cardiac catheterization: A very fine plastic tube is inserted into a blood vessel in the arm or neck and advanced to the heart. Measurements of pressure in the various chambers of the heart help make the diagnosis.
- Injecting a special liquid into the aorta and taking x-ray pictures of it as it flows through the aorta will show the narrowed area.
- Echocardiogram: Harmless sound waves are aimed at the heart. The sound waves bouncing back (the echoes) from this area are seen as a picture on a screen. This is a convenient and painless way to examine the blood vessels coming from the heart.

○ TREATMENT

- The treatment is an operation to remove the narrowed area.
- The operation is best done between the ages of 3 and 4 years. If the clinical condition is serious, however, the operation needs to be done whatever the age.
- The most common causes of death in patients who do not have an operation are rupture of the aorta, failure of the heart, and infection of the heart.

After careful consideration of all factors, the recommendation is that your child have an operation to correct the coarctation of the aorta.

PREOPERATIVE PREPARATION

Most of the necessary preparation for the operation will have been done while making the diagnosis.

- Do not allow your child to eat or drink anything for 8 hours before the operation.

□ OPERATION

- The operation will be done under general anesthesia.
- The incision will be in the left chest.
- The usual operation consists of removing the narrowed area and reconnecting the normal ends of the aorta (Figs. 2–4).
- The operation usually takes about 2 hours.

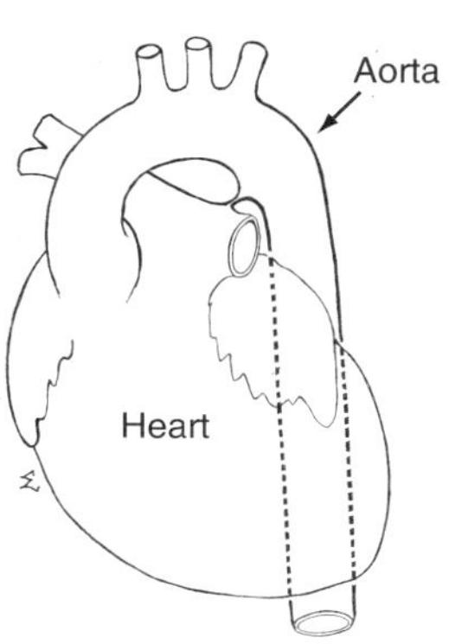

Figure 1.

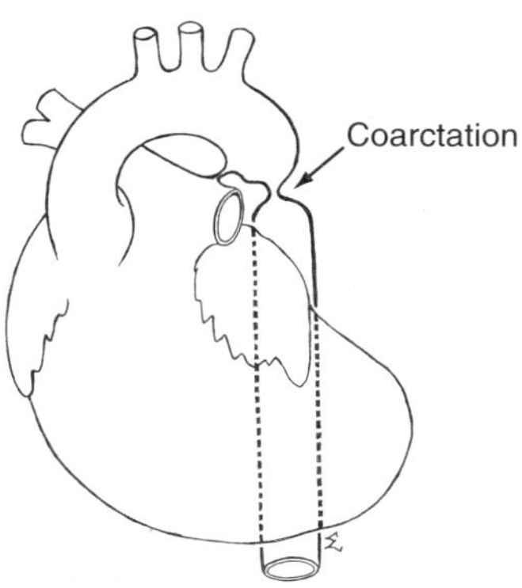

Figure 2.

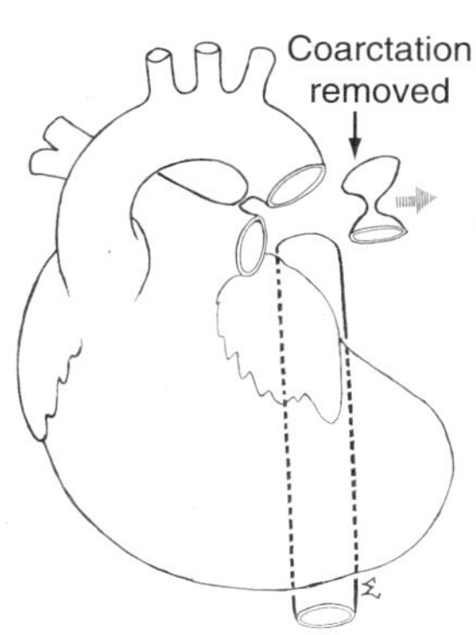

Figure 3.

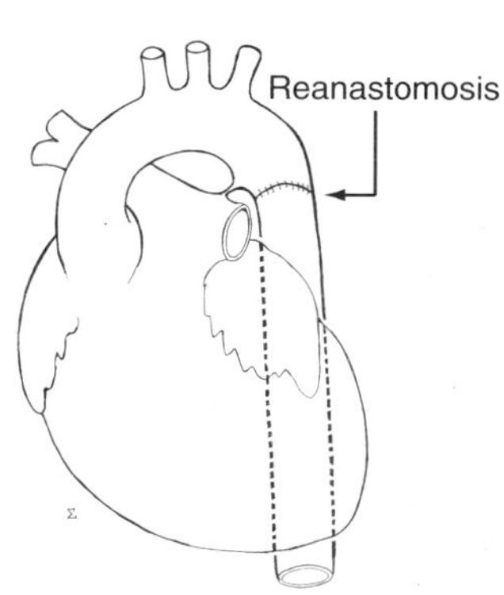

Figure 4.

POSTOPERATIVE CARE

- Your child will be taken to a surgical care unit, where the doctors and nurses are very experienced in taking care of such patients, and later will be transferred to a regular room.
- Your child will be encouraged to move as soon as he or she wishes.
- Pain will be controlled with medicine.
- A small plastic tube coming from the chest will be removed in a day or so.
- There may be a catheter in the urinary bladder for a day or so.
- Your child will be encouraged to move as much as possible, yet be comfortable.
- The diet will first be liquids and then solid foods as they are tolerated.
- Your child should be able to go home in about 1 week.
- As with any operation, complications are always possible. With this type of operation, they can include bleeding in the chest, infection, heart problems, hoarseness, fluid accumulation in the chest, paralysis below the waist (rarely), and possibly others.
- Arrangements will be made for medicine and the follow-up office visit.

✚ HOME CARE

- Continue with the program started in the hospital.
- Unless instructed otherwise, sponge bathe the child as necessary, but do not get any dressings wet.
- The diet can be as tolerated.

✆ CALL OUR OFFICE IF

- The incision becomes red or swollen, or there is drainage from it.
- The child develops a temperature higher than 101°F.
- You have any questions.

△ GENERAL INFORMATION

Colles' fracture is a fracture of the wrist usually caused by a fall on the palm of an outstretched arm (Fig. 1). It is most common in persons older than 50 years of age.

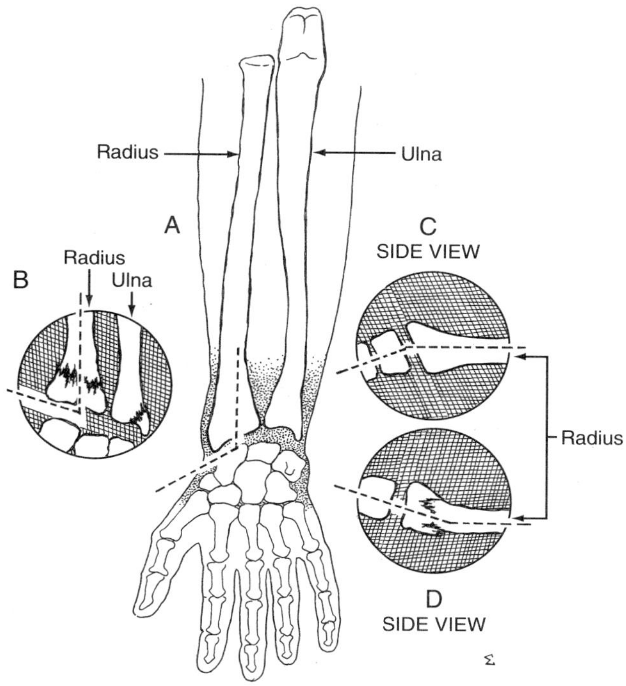

Figure 1. *A*, Normal relationship of the bones of the wrist, back to front view. Notice the radius is longer than the ulna. With a Colles' fracture, significant changes occur in the position of the radius. *B*, The radius is fractured and pushed back so that it now is shorter than the ulna, causing the wrist to angle more toward the thumb. *C*, Side-to-side view of a normal radius, showing the downward slant of the joint. *D*, Side-to-side view showing the radius fractured, pushed back, and the joint now having an upward slant.

COMMON SIGNS AND SYMPTOMS

The symptoms vary, depending on the extent of the fracture, how widely the fracture segments are separated, and the time since the injury.

With minimal injury, there is very little deformity, minimal tenderness over the fracture, and slight swelling over the point of fracture. With modest injury, the arm just above the wrist is bent upward (it looks like a fork facing down), there is acute tenderness over the fracture, and there is moderate swelling over this area. The hand cannot be turned palm up. With severe injury, all the above signs and symptoms are more marked. In addition, there may be symptoms caused by pressure on the nerve from swelling or from a fragment of bone.

DIAGNOSIS

- The diagnosis usually can be made by taking a detailed history of how the injury occurred and doing a thorough physical examination. The surest way to make the diagnosis is by taking appropriate x-rays of the wrist.

Note: Very infrequently, it is not a Colles' fracture that is producing the symptoms but a fracture of one of the small bones of the wrist. Such a fracture may need entirely different management. This is the reason that your x-rays will be looked at with great care to be certain that such a fracture is not missed.

- Symptoms of pressure on the nerve require prompt attention to remove this pressure to avoid possible permanent damage.

○ TREATMENT

The aim of treatment is to restore the function of the arm to as normal a condition as possible and with the least deformity. The treatment of Colles' fracture is heavily influenced by the age, sex, and occupation of the person; other associated injuries or diseases that may complicate matters; and, most important, how badly the bone is broken and how severely the wrist is deformed.

Minimal Deformity

For an older patient, a priority is to restore normal function as soon as possible.

- Often, there is no attempt to have a perfect alignment.
- A simple splint is applied from the elbow to the crease in the palm.
- After 3 to 4 weeks, the splint is removed and progressive motion is begun.

For a younger patient, the priority is to prevent displacement. A forearm cast is applied from the crease in the palm to below or above the elbow.

- A repeat x-ray is taken 2 days later to be certain the bones have not changed their alignment.
- The cast is removed in 6 weeks and graduated motion is started.

Marked Displacement

- In such cases, the displaced bones should be realigned and then firmly immobilized in that position until they heal.
- A repeat x-ray is taken in 2 days to be certain the bones have not changed their alignment.
- The cast is removed in 6 weeks and graduated motion is started.

After reviewing your case, the recommendation is that you have a resetting of the fractured bones to a more normal position.

PREMANIPULATION

- Except for older persons or those with associated injuries or illnesses, laboratory tests are not always necessary.

- Do not eat or drink anything for 8 hours before the procedure.
- You may be given medicine beforehand that will make you feel drowsy.

REDUCTION OF FRACTURE

An *open* operation is rarely necessary for a Colles' fracture. If you need an open operation, the entire procedure will be discussed with you before anything is planned or done.

- The anesthesia for a *closed* reduction of a Colles' fracture can be given in several ways, depending on the individual clinical and technical circumstances. *Local anesthesia:* A local anesthetic is injected into the fracture itself with a fine needle. *Regional block:* The nerves that supply sensation to the arm are temporarily anesthetized by injecting a local anesthesia around them. *General anesthesia*: You are completely asleep during reduction of the fracture. The choice of anesthetic will be discussed with you beforehand.
- The fractured bones will be realigned by pulling and bending the wrist and then applying a cast to hold them in this corrected position.
- The cast usually extends from the crease in the palm to below or above the elbow.
- The hand will purposely be angled away from the thumb and toward the palm. This is necessary to retain the proper position of the broken bones while they are healing.
- You will be taken to a recovery room and observed. When your blood pressure, pulse, and breathing are stable, you should be able to go home that same day with a responsible adult. On occasion, however, it may be necessary for you to stay in the hospital overnight.
- Arrangements will be made for your pain medicine, follow-up x-rays, and office visit.

✚ HOME CARE

- You will be fitted with a sling that fits around your neck and under the cast to hold your arm more comfortably.
- For the first several days lie down as much as possible and keep the arm elevated on two or three pillows. This elevation will help keep down the swelling of the tissue, which now is inside the rigid cast.
- Move your fingers at every opportunity.
- Take medicine as prescribed for your pain.
- Eat as you wish.
- You may bathe or shower as you wish, but don't get the plaster cast wet. A small plastic trash bag fitted over the entire arm and sealed at the top with tape usually is satisfactory.
- During a follow-up visit, you will have x-rays to check the position of the bones. Following this, you may have your cast changed to one that goes to just below the elbow.
- Usually, the cast is removed in 6 weeks and a program of graduated exercises of the wrist begun.
- Satisfactory return of motion varies quite a bit, depending again on how severely the bones were broken, how far they were separated, and your age and general condition.
- As with any operation, complications are always possible. With this type of operation, they can include stiffness of the wrist joint, inability to turn the forearm freely, pressure on the nerve to part of the hand, and shoulder stiffness (especially if exercises are neglected). Infrequently, there is a severely disabling complication of marked pain, tenderness, and swelling of the hand, with severe stiffness of the fingers and shoulder.

Important: Notify the doctor *promptly* if you cannot move your fingers, if they become bluish, if you feel a pins-and-needles sensation in them, or if you feel increasing pain in the fracture under the cast. If you cannot reach the doctor, go to the local hospital emergency room promptly.

✆ CALL OUR OFFICE IF

- You have any questions.

COLON CANCER: Laparoscopic-Assisted Resection

△ GENERAL INFORMATION

Colon cancer is an uncontrolled growth in an area of the colon (large bowel). It is very common and occurs mostly in older men and women. The cause of the type of cancer you have is not known.

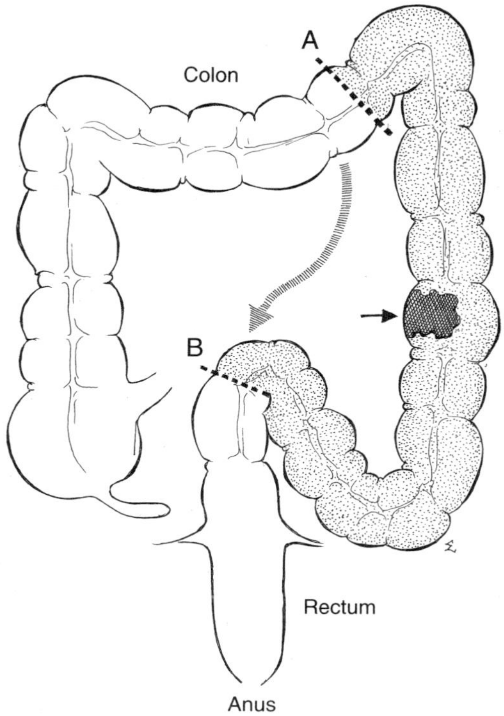

Figure 1. A cancer of the left colon is shown. The part of the colon to be removed is stippled.

COMMON SIGNS AND SYMPTOMS

- In the early stage, there are usually no symptoms. If the stool is tested, it may show the presence of blood.
- The blood in the stool may vary in color from bright red to maroon, or even black. Later, there may be red blood in the stool, or the stools may be almost black from old blood in them.
- If the cancer begins to block the colon, there may be a sense of fullness, cramping, constipation, or narrowing of the stool.
- As the colon finally pushes the firm stool and liquid above it through the narrowing passage, what comes out is often a mixed solid and liquid diarrhea.
- There may be anemia because of slow bleeding from the tumor.

DIAGNOSIS

- Usually, the diagnosis begins by taking a detailed history and doing a thorough physical examination.
- You will have an examination of your blood, urine, heart (EKG), and lungs (chest x-ray).
- *Barium enema:* This is done by placing liquid barium (it has the color and consistency of buttermilk) into the rectum and colon (just like a regular enema) and taking x-ray pictures as it flows throughout the large bowel. The results help to determine the cause of the symptoms.
- *Colonoscopy:* This is done with an optical instrument that is smooth, flexible, and as big around as your little finger and with a light at its tip. During the procedure you will be given medicine that will make you feel drowsy. The tip of the instrument will be lubricated and then gently inserted into your anus and advanced throughout the colon, which will be inspected carefully. If any suspicious tissue is seen, a small piece of it can be taken (a *biopsy*) for laboratory examination.
- *CT scan* (computed tomography scan): These special x-rays are taken by a machine that is shaped like a huge doughnut. You will lie on a table inside the hole in the "doughnut." The x-rays are taken as very thin slices through the area of the entire abdomen. This makes it possible to see details inside the abdominal cavity.

○ TREATMENT

- The treatment is an operation to remove the part of the colon with the cancer in it and then to reconnect the cut ends (Figs. 1 and 2).

After careful consideration of all factors, the recommendation is that you have this operation with laparoscopic assistance.

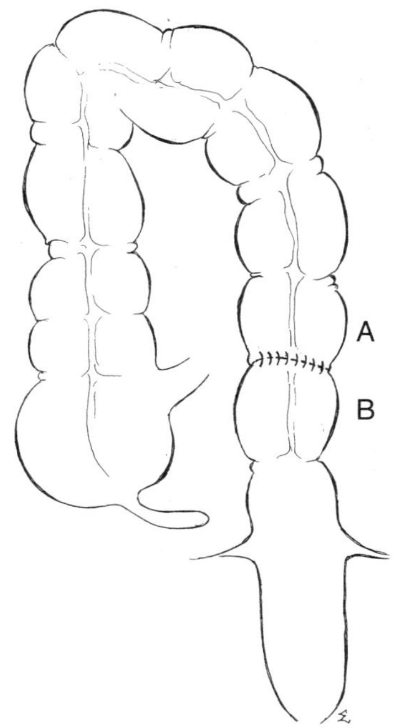

Figure 2. Following removal of the cancer, A has been connected to B so that the contents of the colon can travel in a normal manner.

PREOPERATIVE PREPARATION

- You will have an examination of your blood, urine, heart (EKG), and lungs (chest x-ray).
- You will be instructed on how to clean out your bowel.
- Do not eat or drink anything for 8 hours before your operation.
- Shower (and shave) as usual on the morning of the operation.
- You may be given medicine that will make you feel drowsy before you are brought to the operating room.

☐ OPERATION

- You will be asleep for the operation.
- Your abdomen will be scrubbed with an antiseptic solution and surrounded with sterile drapes.
- The instrument used (a *laparoscope*) is smooth, has lenses in it, is as big around as your little finger, and has a light at the tip. Three or four laparoscopes will be placed in your abdomen through tiny incisions. The affected colon will be dissected inside the abdomen with the laparoscopes until it is free. A short incision will be made in your abdomen over the colon containing the cancer, and only the part of the colon with the cancer in it will be brought to the outside. **Note:** Sometimes, after the laparoscopes have been introduced in the abdomen, it is determined that this technique is not a suitable or safe way to remove the colon with the cancer in it. If that is the case with you, then an open incision will be made. The part of the colon with the cancer will be removed, the open ends reconnected, and the colon replaced in the abdomen.
- You will not receive a blood transfusion unless it is absolutely necessary.
- The operation usually takes about 3 hours.

POSTOPERATIVE CARE

- You will be taken to a recovery room and observed. When your blood pressure, pulse, and breathing are stable, you will be taken to a regular hospital room.
- You may have a thin plastic tube in your nose. It goes down to your stomach to suck up the air you swallow. It will be removed when your bowels start working.
- That evening you will be helped to sit up in bed and on the next day to get out of bed.
- Pain will be controlled with medicine. The nurse will give it to you, or you can give yourself a preset amount of pain medicine when you feel you need it. This is done with a device called patient-controlled analgesia (PCA) that is connected to the tubing giving you intravenous fluids.
- You will be given an incentive spirometer. Breathing into this as you are instructed will help you expand your lungs and reduce the risk of developing pneumonia.
- After the tube in your nose is removed, you will be started on a liquid diet that will be advanced to solid food as you tolerate it.
- As with any operation, complications are always possible. With this type of operation, they can include peritonitis, bleeding, bowel obstruction, pneumonia, and possibly others.
- You should be able to go home in about 4 days.
- Arrangements will be made for your medicine, follow-up office visit, and stitch removal.

✚ HOME CARE

- Continue with the program started while you were in the hospital.
- You may walk about as you wish, even climb stairs, but don't overdo things.
- Take medicine as prescribed for your pain.
- You may eat as you did before the operation, but include plenty of roughage and liquids in your diet to help prevent constipation.
- Unless instructed otherwise, you may shower if you wish and with any dressings on or off.
    - There may be narrow strips of tape across the incision. It's all right if they get wet; they will be removed in the doctor's office.
    - After you dry yourself, replace any dressings with clean, dry ones.
- Driving a car with an automatic shift may not seem too demanding. However, you may have to slam on brakes or twist to turn the steering wheel and may then strain your sutures or tear something. So during your follow-up visit, let's discuss when you can resume driving.
- You may resume sexual activity whenever you choose.
- You may return to work when you feel up to it.

✆ CALL OUR OFFICE IF

- You develop any unusual signs or symptoms.
- You develop cramps or become bloated.
- You do not have a bowel movement for 2 to 3 days.
- You develop a temperature higher than 100°F.
- The incisions become red or swollen, or there is drainage from them.
- You have any questions.

COLON CANCER: Open Resection

△ GENERAL INFORMATION

Colon cancer is a new uncontrolled growth in the area of the colon (large bowel) (Fig. 1). It is very common and occurs mostly in older men and women. The cause of the type of cancer you have is not known.

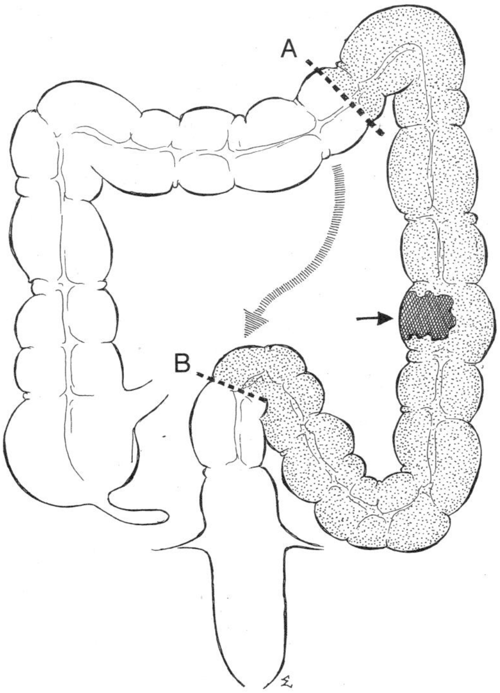

Figure 1. A cancer of the left colon is shown. The part of the colon to be removed is stippled.

COMMON SIGNS AND SYMPTOMS

- In the early stage, there are usually no symptoms. If the stool is tested, it may show the presence of blood.
- The blood in the stool may vary in color from bright red to maroon, or even black.
- If the cancer begins to block the colon, there may be a sense of fullness, cramping, constipation, or narrowing of the stool.
- As the colon pushes stool through the narrowing passage, all the stool and the liquid above it come out as a mixed solid and liquid diarrhea.
- There may be anemia because of slow bleeding from the tumor.

DIAGNOSIS

- Usually, the diagnosis begins by taking a detailed history and doing a thorough physical examination.
- You will have an examination of your blood, urine, heart (EKG), and lungs (chest x-ray).
- *Barium enema:* This is done by placing liquid barium into the rectum and colon (just like a regular enema) and taking x-ray pictures. The results help to determine the cause of the symptoms.
- *Colonoscopy:* This is done with an optical instrument with a light at its tip. It is smooth, flexible, and as big around as your little finger. During the procedure you will be given medicine that will make you feel drowsy. The tip of the instrument will be lubricated and then gently inserted into your anus. It can be used to inspect your entire colon. If suspicious tissue is seen, a small piece of it can be taken (a *biopsy*) for laboratory examination.
- *CT scan* (computed tomography scan): These special x-rays are taken by a machine that is shaped like a huge doughnut. You will lie on a table inside the hole in the "doughnut." The x-rays are taken as very thin slices through the area of the abdomen. This makes it possible to see the fine details in the abdomen.

○ TREATMENT

- The treatment is an operation to remove the part of the colon with the cancer and then to reconnect the colon (Fig. 2). After careful consideration of all factors, it is recommended that you have an open operation to accomplish this.

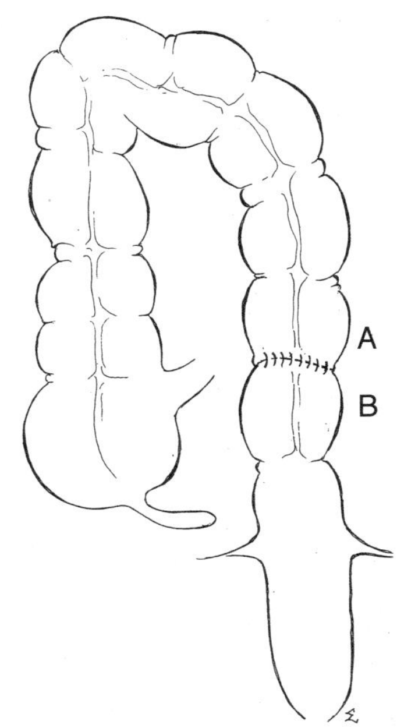

Figure 2. Following removal of the cancer, A has been connected to B so that the contents of the colon can travel in a normal manner.

PREOPERATIVE PREPARATION

- During the day before the operation, drink only liquids. At 2:00 P.M. drink a 10-ounce bottle of cold citrate of magnesia.
- Have only a clear liquid (e.g., jello, broth) for supper.

- Do not eat or drink anything for 8 hours before your operation.
- Shower (and shave) as usual on the morning of the operation.
- You may be given medicine that will make you feel drowsy before you are brought to the operating room.

☐ OPERATION

- You will be asleep for the operation.
- Very infrequently, a *temporary* colostomy (bowel opening on the side of your body) has to be done for safety reasons. If you have a colostomy, it will be closed a few weeks later.
- You will not receive a blood transfusion unless it is absolutely necessary.
- The operation usually takes 2 hours.

POSTOPERATIVE CARE

- You will wake up in a recovery room. When your blood pressure, pulse, and breathing are stable, you will be taken to a regular hospital room.
- You may have a thin plastic tube in your nose. It goes down to your stomach to suck up the air you swallow. It will be removed when your bowels start working.
- That evening you will be helped to sit up in bed and on the next day to get out of bed.
- Pain can be controlled with medicine.
- After the tube in your nose is removed you will be started on a liquid diet; this will be advanced to solid food as you tolerate it.
- As with any operation, complications are always possible. With your type of operation, they can include peritonitis, bleeding, bowel obstruction, and pneumonia, among others.
- You should be able to go home in about 1 week.
- Arrangements will be made for your medicine, follow-up office visit, and stitch removal.

✣ HOME CARE

- Continue with the program started while you were in the hospital.
- You may walk about as you wish, even climb stairs.
- You may eat as you did before the operation but include plenty of roughage and liquids in your diet to help prevent constipation.
- Unless instructed otherwise, you may shower if you wish and with any dressings on or off.
  - There may be narrow strips of tape across the incision. It's all right if they get wet; they will be removed in the doctor's office.
  - After you dry yourself, replace any dressings with clean, dry ones.
- Don't lift anything heavier than 5 pounds. Have someone do it for you.
- Driving a car with an automatic shift is not too demanding. But if you suddenly have to slam on the brakes or twist to turn a wheel, you may strain the sutures or tear something. So, during your follow-up visit let's discuss when you can resume driving.
- You may resume sexual activity whenever you choose.
- You may return to work when you feel up to it, but let's first talk about it during your follow-up visit.

✆ CALL OUR OFFICE IF

- You develop any unusual signs or symptoms.
- You develop cramps or become bloated.
- You do not have a bowel movement for 2 to 3 days.
- You develop a temperature higher than 100°F.
- The incision becomes red or swollen, or there is drainage from it.
- You have any questions.

△ GENERAL INFORMATION

A colon polyp is a growth on the lining (the *mucosa*) of the colon. It may form a bulge (a *sessile polyp*), or it may be at the end of a stalk *(pedunculated polyp)*.

Polyps can be as small as a split pea or as large as a walnut—even larger. Most polyps are benign, but some can be cancerous. The larger the polyp, the greater the risk that it is cancerous.

The cause of most polyps is unknown.

COMMON SIGNS AND SYMPTOMS

Most polyps do not produce any signs or symptoms. They are found by chance during a routine examination of the lower or large bowel.

- Some polyps bleed because they have been scratched by stool rubbing against them, or because they have cancer in them that has become ulcerated.
- Rarely, they are large enough to cause some blockage and produce cramps.

DIAGNOSIS

- *Barium enema:* Barium (it has the color and consistency of buttermilk) is placed into the large bowel like a regular enema, and x-ray pictures are taken. If a polyp is seen with this examination and a *biopsy* (removal of a small piece of it for examination in the laboratory) or removal of the entire polyp is thought to be necessary, then another procedure needs to be done.
- *Flexible sigmoidoscopy:* Most polyps are seen through a flexible sigmoidoscope. This is a flexible, rather short instrument as thick as your little finger with a light at its tip. It is inserted through the anus and into the rectum and lower part of the colon. About half of the polyps occur this low and can be seen with this examination. Because of its short length, however, only the bottom one-third of the colon can be examined in this manner.
- *Colonoscopy:* If a polyp is found during flexible sigmoidoscopy, then the entire large bowel must be examined with a colonoscope to be certain there is nothing else higher up. A colonoscopy also is necessary if the results of the flexible sigmoidoscopy examination are negative yet symptoms suggestive of a polyp are present. Colonoscopy is done with a long, optical instrument that is smooth, flexible, as big around as your little finger, and with a light at its tip.

PREPARATION FOR COLONOSCOPY

- It is important that the bowel be as clean as possible for this examination; otherwise it will be difficult to see things clearly and to perform a biopsy accurately. There are a number of ways to cleanse your colon for the examination. You'll be given instructions on how to do this.

THE COLONOSCOPY

- A small needle will be placed in your vein so that relaxing medicines can be given to make you feel very drowsy during the procedure.
- You will be lying on your side.
- The lubricated colonoscope will be introduced through the anus and gently advanced up into the rectum and colon.
- You may feel mild cramping while this is done.
- Your entire large bowel will be examined thoroughly.
- If a polyp is seen, a decision will be made on whether to remove all of it at that time, perform a biopsy of it, or make plans for an operation.
- If only an examination is performed, the colonoscopy lasts about 30 minutes or so. You will become alert quickly and probably remember very little of the procedure.

POSTCOLONOSCOPY CARE

- You will be kept in the endoscopy unit until your blood pressure, pulse, and breathing are stable and you are alert. You should then be able to leave the unit with a responsible adult.
- Arrangements will be made for your follow-up office visit to discuss the results of the colonoscopy, any biopsy results, and any recommendation for further treatment.

✙ HOME CARE

- Resume your usual activities.
- Avoid foods with a lot of roughage in them for the first day.
- Your first bowel movement may be mostly red or maroon blood clots. If the blood is bright red and liquid or comes out in this fashion more than once, notify the doctor promptly.

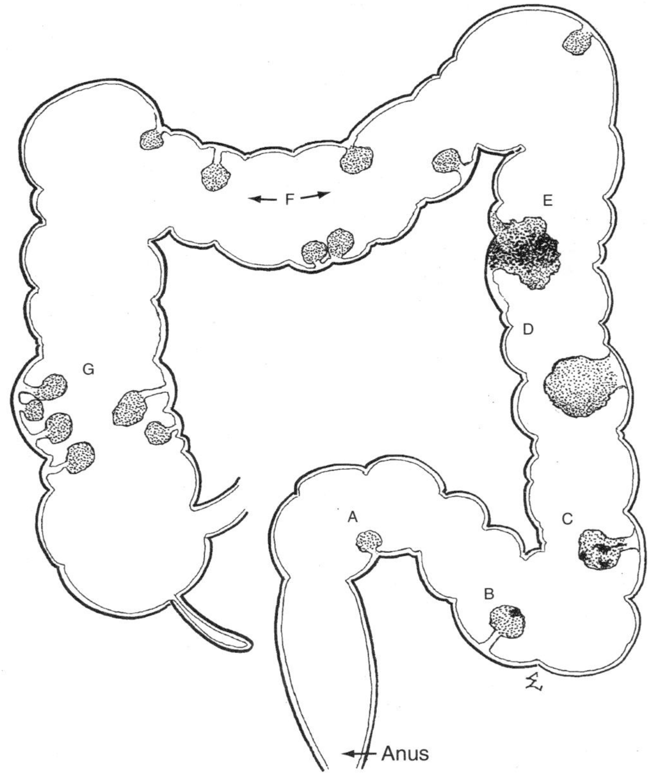

Figure 1.

○ TREATMENT

The usual options in the treatment of colon polyps depend on a number of factors. They include the following (Fig. 1):

- A single polyp can be removed entirely through the colonoscope, and when examined under the microscope it is shown to be entirely benign (A). In such circumstances, usually no further treatment is necessary at that time.
- An excised single polyp has cancer but only at its tip (B). In such circumstances and if the stalk of the polyp is entirely negative, than usually no further treatment is necessary at that time.
- The excised polyp is cancerous in several areas (C).
- The polyp cannot be removed as one piece through the colonoscope. Or, the biopsy results of one area are benign, but the diagnosis of other areas of the polyp is not known (D).
- The polyp is cancerous and does not have a stalk (E).

In the above three situations (C, D, and E), the treatment is usually an operation.

- There are multiple polyps present. They may each be in a different location (F), or they may be grouped in the same area (G). In such instances, commonly some portion of the colon needs to be removed. How much is removed depends on a number of factors specific to a particular patient.

As you see, the possible treatments can range from observation only to resection of a portion or even most of the colon.

Any recommendations will be discussed with you in detail before anything is planned or done.

△ GENERAL INFORMATION

Colonoscopy is a procedure in which the inside of the entire colon can be looked at with an instrument called a *colonoscope*. Also, if something abnormal is seen, a small piece of it (a *biopsy*) can be taken for examination in the pathology laboratory.

The inside of the bowel can also be examined by filling the bowel with barium and taking x-ray pictures of it (a *lower GI series*). For some diseases, it is the best way to make a diagnosis. An important drawback to a barium enema is that the bowel lining cannot be looked at directly. Also, a biopsy cannot be done at that time if something abnormal is seen. The person needs to return for a colonoscopy.

THE COLONOSCOPE

- The colonoscope is a smooth, flexible, optical instrument about as thick as the tip of your little finger. It has lenses in it as well as a light at its tip that lets the operator see what is ahead.
- The colonoscope has several small tunnels in it.
  - One tunnel is used to suck out any mucus that might be in the way.
  - Another tunnel is used to pass a very thin wire with a biting tip as small as a sesame seed at its end that can be used to take a biopsy.

The colonoscope is 3 feet long so that it can be passed up to the very beginning of the large bowel. The end held by the operator has a knob and several buttons that are used to steer the tip of the colonoscope as it is passed up the colon. The buttons are used to control the suction and other functions.

PREPARATION FOR THE COLONOSCOPY

- The bowel must be cleansed of all stool so that the lining can be seen clearly. You will be instructed on how to clean your bowel.
- Do not eat or drink anything for 8 hours before the procedure.

THE COLONOSCOPY PROCEDURE

- A thin needle will be used to start some fluids in your vein.
- The procedure will begin with you lying on your side.
- Medicine will be injected through the needle in your vein, and you will feel very drowsy.
- The colonoscope will be lubricated thoroughly and inserted gently through the anus and into the colon. You will be vaguely aware of what is happening, or you may simply doze off. The instrument will be advanced through the entire colon for a thorough examination (Fig. 1).
- You will be able to hear and cooperate with the doctor as you are asked to change your position, but you will not be too aware of what is happening.
- When the procedure is completed, the relaxing medicine is stopped, and within a few minutes you will be fully awake.
- The procedure takes 15 to 30 minutes. Many patients remember so little of the procedure they think it took just several minutes, or they may not remember anything at all about it.
- Your blood pressure, pulse, and breathing will be watched until they are stable. When you are completely alert, you should be able to go home with a responsible adult.

Colonoscopy has become an important way to examine the inside of the entire colon directly.

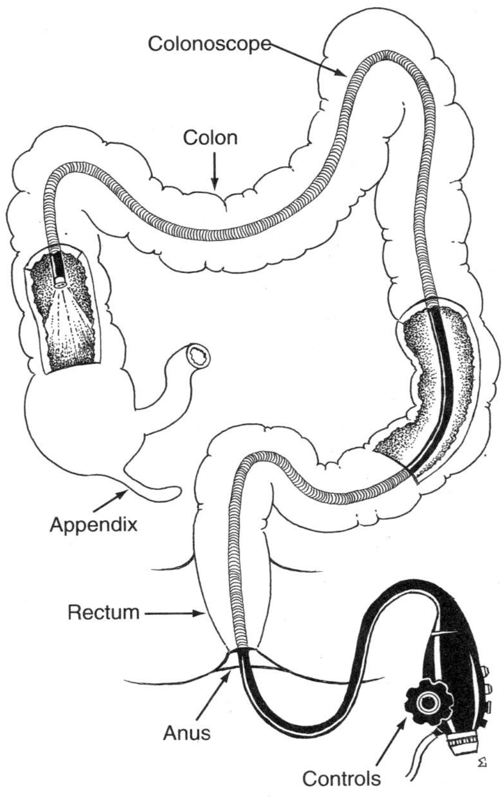

Figure 1. The lubricated colonoscope is inserted in the anus and then advanced through the entire colon. On occasion it can even be advanced up the small intestine (the ileum) for a short distance. The controls are used to steer the direction of the tip of the colonoscope as well as to regulate suction and other functions.

△ GENERAL INFORMATION

A *colostomy* is the making of an opening in the colon and bringing it out through the skin so that its contents (stool) can pass directly to the outside.

SOME REASONS FOR A COLOSTOMY

- The bowel is blocked enough that no stool, or very little stool, can get past the blockage to reach the outside in the normal manner. The most common causes of such blockage can be a cancer or scarring from a chronic infection. Soon the bowel balloons up because of the blockage. A colostomy needs to be done promptly; otherwise the ballooned bowel may burst.
- Part of the colon and rectum has been removed and the cut ends reconnected, but there is too great a risk that the new connection might leak. For safety reasons, a *temporary* colostomy is done so that the stool does not pass across the new connection. When after a few weeks the new connection is well healed, the temporary colostomy is closed.
- There is a hole in the bowel from injury or infection, and there is general infection inside the abdomen (called *peritonitis*). The part of the bowel with the hole in it is removed, but it is too risky to connect the ends because so much infection is present already. The ends are brought to the outside. When after a few weeks the infection heals, the ends of the bowel are reconnected.
- The colostomy is performed because the anus and rectum are removed, usually to cure a cancer.

DIAGNOSIS

The diagnosis of a blockage that needs to be relieved by a colostomy is made in different ways for different conditions. Some of the methods of making the diagnosis include the following:

- A history of changing bowel habits and constipation, with or without a history of infection.
- Examination of the blood, urine, heart (EKG), and lungs (chest x-ray).
- Swelling of the abdomen.
- An x-ray of the swollen abdomen that shows a large amount of air in the colon up to the point of blockage.
- Barium enema: Barium (it has the color and consistency of buttermilk) is placed in the colon (very much like a regular enema) as you lie on the x-ray table. The barium is observed as it flows throughout the colon. This will show the blocked colon and often what is causing the blockage.
- Flexible sigmoidoscopy: This is done with an optical instrument with a light at its tip that is smooth, flexible, and as big around as your little finger. It can be used to inspect the inside of the lower one-fourth of your large bowel.
- Colonoscopy: This is done with an optical instrument with a light at its tip that is smooth, flexible, and as big around as your little finger. During the procedure, you will be given medicine that will make you feel drowsy. The tip of the instrument will be inserted into your anus gently and then advanced until your entire large bowel is examined. If suspicious tissue is seen, a small piece of it can be taken (a *biopsy*) for laboratory examination.
- Performing an operation and unexpectedly finding the blockage and determining at that moment that a temporary colostomy is necessary.

PREOPERATIVE PREPARATION

There are several types of colostomy, each serving a specific need. The choice for you will be discussed with you beforehand. Any abnormalities in addition to the colon problem will be corrected as much as possible, depending on how much time is available.

For an Emergency Colostomy

- Fluid will be started in your vein.
- A thin plastic tube may need to be passed into the stomach to suck up air that is trapped there.

For an Elective Colostomy

- You will be given instructions on how to prepare your bowel.

□ OPERATION

- You may be given medicine that will make you feel drowsy before you are brought to the operating room.
- You will be asleep for the operation.
- The skin of your abdomen will be scrubbed with an antiseptic solution and surrounded with sterile drapes.
- The location of the incision will depend on the type of colostomy performed and the reason for it.
- You will not receive a blood transfusion unless it is absolutely necessary.
- The colostomy bag will be fitted while you still are in the operating room.

POSTOPERATIVE CARE

- You will wake up in a recovery room. When your blood pressure, pulse, and breathing are stable, you will be taken to a regular hospital room.
- That evening you will be helped to sit up in bed and on the next day to get out of bed.
- Pain can be controlled with medicine. The nurse will give it to you, or you can give yourself a preset amount of pain medicine when you feel you need it. This is done with a device called patient-controlled analgesia (PCA) that is connected to the tubing giving you intravenous fluids.
- As soon as possible and while you are in the hospital, the surgical team of doctors, nurses, and technicians will help you learn how to take care of your colostomy. It is not difficult.
- You'll be given information on your diet and how it may influence the working of your colostomy.

- You should be able to go home in 3 to 10 days, depending on the reason for the colostomy.
- Arrangements will be made for your medicine, follow-up office visit, and stitch or clip removal.
- As with any operation, complications are always possible. With your type of operation, they can include infection, bleeding, bowel obstruction, heart or lung problems, and possibly others.

✚ HOME CARE

- You may walk about as you wish, even climb stairs, but don't overdo things.
- Take medicine as prescribed for your pain.
- You will be given a suggested diet; however, you will soon find out for yourself if you need to adjust your diet so that your colostomy will work in the best manner.
- Almost all patients develop their own way and routine for colostomy care so that it doesn't interfere too much with their daily schedule. You'll find the best way to take care of yours.
  - Many patients take an enema each morning or every other morning to empty the colon of stool and then wear a small plastic bag over the opening for safety's sake. Only occasionally will stool come out into the bag.
  - Other patients do not use an enema but simply leave the bag in place, discarding it when stool empties into it and then replacing it with a new one.
- Arrangements can be made for a home visiting nurse if one is needed.

Many thousands of patients have a colostomy; you may already know some. There probably are persons at work or other acquaintances who have a colostomy, and you don't know about it because you have not been told and you cannot tell. Remember, it is possible to lead a life that is pretty close to what you were used to. It will take a little time to learn the new routines, but before you know it you'll have them under control.

✆ CALL OUR OFFICE IF

- You develop any unusual signs or symptoms.
- Your colostomy does not work for 36 hours.
- The incision becomes red or swollen, or there is drainage from it.
- You develop a temperature higher than 100°F.
- You have any questions.

△ GENERAL INFORMATION

Sometimes, suspicious abnormalities are seen in the cells scraped off the cervix during a Papanicolaou (Pap) smear. These abnormalities may range from minor ones that persist on repeated Pap smears, and, therefore, require more detailed evaluation, to cells that may be precancerous. On examination with the naked eye, no certain areas of abnormality can be seen, even though abnormal cells were obtained from the cervix. For this reason, investigation with a special microscope called a *colposcope* is necessary. This instrument has lenses in it that magnify what is being examined from 6 to 40 times. If this examination is not done and the problem not treated, there is the potential risk of progression of this abnormal area to a more serious and even potentially cancerous lesion.

PREOPERATIVE PREPARATION

- The procedure may be done if you are menstruating lightly, but it is preferable to schedule it for a time when you are not bleeding.
- A colposcopy is approached differently if you are pregnant, so be certain to tell the gynecologist if you know or think you are pregnant.
- You may have a light breakfast that morning.
- Shower or bathe on the morning of the examination.
- Do not douche or otherwise introduce anything into your vagina for at least 24 hours before the examination.
- Empty your bladder before you enter the gynecologist's office; it will make your examination more comfortable.

THE COLPOSCOPIC EXAMINATION

Colposcopy is not painful. To you, this examination may seem like a particularly long speculum or pelvic examination.

- You will be positioned on the examining table as you would for any other pelvic examination. A speculum will be introduced into your vagina.
- A dilute vinegar solution will be applied to the cervix. This solution helps highlight any abnormal cells on the cervix.
- The doctor will then spend several minutes looking at your cervix carefully through the colposcope. A cotton-tipped applicator may be used to move your cervix slightly during the examination to be certain the entire surface of the cervix can be seen.
- The vaginal tissue also will be examined. If the doctor is concerned about abnormal areas here, the vagina also will be brushed with a dilute vinegar solution and examined through the colposcope.
- The doctor may identify one or more areas of abnormality on the cervix on which biopsies should be performed. This is done by removing a tiny bit of tissue (the size of a grain or two of rice) with a special instrument. Most patients don't feel anything during the biopsy, although occasionally a "pinch" may be felt.
- Any bleeding from the vaginal site is stopped with a special solution that is applied with a cotton-tipped applicator.

AFTER THE COLPOSCOPY

- You can get dressed directly after the examination and be ready to go home.
- The doctor will review with you the general findings from the examination.
- Any tissue taken during the biopsy will be sent to the pathology laboratory for a thorough, careful examination. The results will not be known for several days.
- If a biopsy has been performed, you should not douche or place anything in the vagina for the period of time you are told. This precaution is necessary to allow the biopsy site to heal properly.
- You may see some "spotting" following the examination. This is common and expected.
- You should also expect to see some brown discharge from the vagina for several days. This is because the solution that was used to stop the bleeding from the biopsy site is brown.
- Sanitary pads should be sufficient for any such discharge that may occur.

ANY FURTHER TREATMENT

After the results of the biopsies have been returned, there will be a discussion with you about possible further treatment. Further treatment may include the following:

- A simple follow-up Pap smear at a later time.
- Cryosurgery: This is the destruction of local tissue by freezing it with a special instrument.
- Laser therapy: This is pinpoint destruction of the abnormal tissue with a special (laser) light beam.
- Removing a larger portion of the cervix, either in the office or in the operating room.
- Hysterectomy.

As you see, treatment for any one individual depends on the biopsy findings and the needs and expectations of the patient.

✆ CALL OUR OFFICE IF

- There is true bleeding beyond simple "spotting" from the vagina.
- You develop a temperature higher than 100°F.
- You have any questions.

COLPOSCOPY OF THE CERVIX WITH BIOPSY

△ GENERAL INFORMATION

The cervix is at the bottom of the uterus and can be seen at the deepest part of the vagina. *Colposcopy* is a direct examination of the surface of the cervix with an instrument (a colposcope) that has lenses in it and can magnify things from 6 to 40 times. This magnification gives the gynecologist the advantage of being able to see with ease small changes on the surface of the cervix that are difficult or impossible to see with the naked eye. Also, this instrument makes it possible for the gynecologist to see the magnified view in two dimensions *(stereoscopic)*.

Colposcopy is most useful when a routine Papanicolaou (Pap) smear shows some abnormalities. These abnormalities may range from minor ones that persist to cells that may be precancerous. These changes must be investigated further; otherwise there is the risk that this abnormal area may progress to become a more serious and even potentially cancerous lesion.

PREOPERATIVE PREPARATION

- Do not douche or otherwise place anything in your vagina for 24 hours before the procedure.
- Shower as usual on the morning of the examination.
- Colposcopy is approached differently if you are pregnant, so be certain to tell the gynecologist if you know that you are or if you think you might be pregnant.
- Empty your bladder just before you enter the gynecologist's office to make your examination more comfortable.

THE COLPOSCOPIC EXAMINATION

- Colposcopy is not painful. It essentially is like a long speculum examination.
- You will be positioned on the examining table the same as for a regular pelvic examination.
- The regular vaginal speculum will be inserted.
- A dilute vinegar solution will be applied to the cervix. This solution helps highlight any abnormal cells on the cervix.
- The doctor will spend several minutes looking at your cervix through the colposcope. A cotton-tipped applicator may be used to move your cervix slightly during the examination to be certain the entire surface of the cervix can be seen.
- The vaginal tissue will be examined also. If the doctor is concerned about abnormal areas, the vagina also will be brushed with a dilute vinegar solution and examined through the colposcope.
- The doctor may identify one or more areas on the cervix that are sufficiently abnormal that samples need to be taken for a biopsy. This is done by removing a tiny bit of tissue (the size of a grain or two of rice) from the cervix with a special instrument. Most patients don't feel anything during the biopsy, although occasionally a "pinch" may be noted.
- There also may be sampling of the tissue in the canal of the cervix, which is the part that leads up to the uterus (Fig. 1 stippled area, indicated by arrow). This is called an *endocervical canal* sampling (ECC). It is done with a special instrument that scrapes the canal rather than taking a bite of the tissue. This sampling typically causes a cramping sensation; the actual scraping, however, lasts for only about 10 seconds.
- Any bleeding from the biopsy area is stopped with a special solution that is applied with a cotton-tipped applicator.

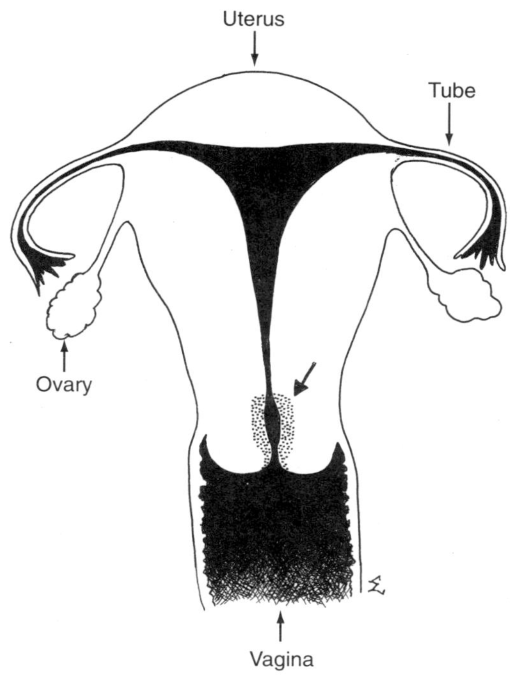

Figure 1.

AFTER THE COLPOSCOPY

- You may get dressed directly after the examination.
- The doctor will review with you the general findings from your examination.
- If a biopsy has been performed, you should not douche or place anything in your vagina for several days. Your doctor will let you know the exact length of time. This precaution will allow the biopsy site to heal properly.
- You may see some "spotting" following the examination. This is common and expected.
- You should expect to see some brown discharge from the vagina for several days. This is because the solution that was used to stop the bleeding from the biopsy site is brown. A sanitary napkin should be sufficient to collect such discharge.

ANY FURTHER TREATMENT

After the results of the biopsies have been returned, there will be discussion with you about possible further treatment. Further treatment may include the following:

- A simple follow-up Pap smear at an appropriate time.
- Cryosurgery: This is destruction of the tissue by freezing it with a special instrument.
- Laser therapy: This is pinpoint destruction of the abnormal tissue with a special (laser) light beam.
- Removing a larger portion of the cervix, either in the office or in the operating room.
- Hysterectomy.

As you can see, treatment for any individual depends on the biopsy results and the needs and expectations of the patient.

✆ CALL OUR OFFICE IF

- There is true bleeding beyond simple "spotting" from the vagina.
- You develop a temperature higher than 100°F.
- You have any questions.

△ GENERAL INFORMATION

The heart pumps blood and the oxygen in it to all parts of the body through arteries of various sizes. The heart gets its own blood supply and oxygen from the arteries that can be seen on the surface of the heart and are called *coronary arteries*. Sometimes these arteries become partially narrowed by cholesterol deposits (called *atherosclerosis*) in their walls. These narrowings can prevent enough blood and its oxygen from passing through the artery and to the heart muscle. Not enough oxygen to the heart muscle causes discomfort in the chest, called *angina*. In addition, if the pumping ability of the heart decreases, irregular heartbeats can occur. If the coronary artery is blocked completely, the heart muscle supplied by this artery dies. This is a *myocardial infarct*. The aim, of course, is to keep this from happening in a person who has significant narrowing of the coronary arteries.

○ TREATMENT

Certain types of narrowing can be approached in ways that do not involve opening the chest and grafting new vessels to the heart. Two of these ways would be *medical management* and *coronary angioplasty*.

Medical Management

- Certain medicines are now available that can control blood pressure, heart rate, and irregular heartbeats. These can decrease the episodes of chest pain while at the same time helping the patient tolerate more activity.
- A proper diet is necessary to try to prevent the atherosclerosis from progressing.
- Activities that put unnecessary or too much strain on the heart should be avoided.
- Excess weight should be taken off.
- If you smoke, you should stop.

Often such measures work well and for long periods of time. Unfortunately, in some patients the atherosclerotic process continues and the symptoms of chest pain are not controllable. In such instances, a procedure called *coronary angioplasty* can be performed.

Coronary Angioplasty

- There will be an examination of your blood, urine, heart (EKG), and lungs (chest x-ray).
- Do not eat or drink anything for 12 hours before the procedure.
- On the day of the procedure, you will be taken to the cardiac catheterization laboratory.
- Fine wires taped to your skin will be connected to recording machines to watch the performance of your heart during the procedure.
- You will be given medicine that will make you feel drowsy and relaxed.
- The groin area will be painted with an antiseptic solution and draped with sterile towels. The skin in the groin area over the femoral artery will be made numb with a local anesthetic.

Balloon Technique

A flexible catheter no larger than angel hair spaghetti will be placed through the numbed skin and into the femoral vessels. At the tip of the catheter is a balloon that can be inflated up to the size of a small pea. The catheter with the balloon deflated is advanced up and into the coronary artery, exactly in the narrow area of the artery. The balloon then is inflated to dilate that artery. This allows more blood to flow through the coronary artery and into the heart muscle (Figs. 1–3).

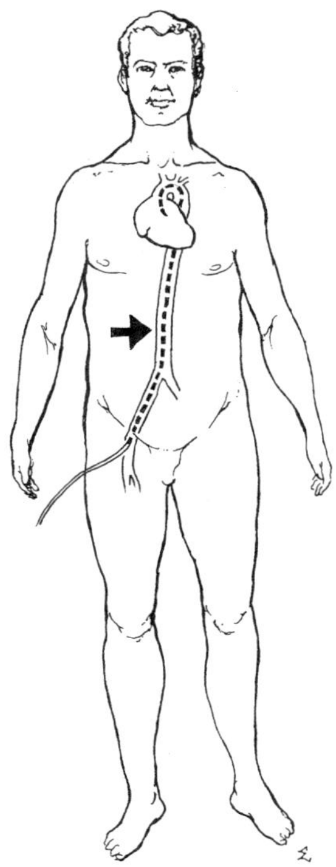

Figure 1. The balloon catheter is inserted into the groin artery and advanced upward inside the aorta toward the heart.

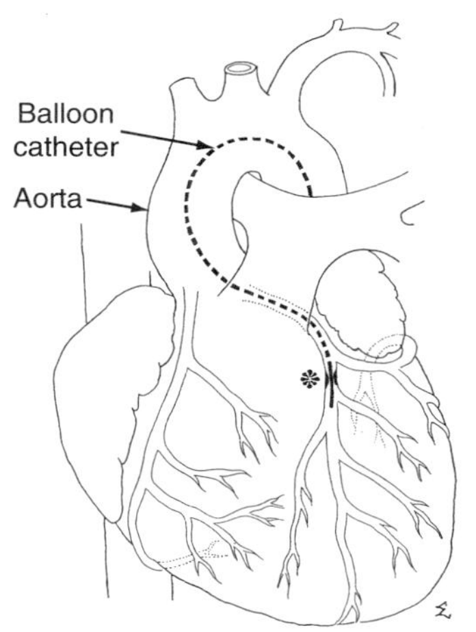

Figure 2. The balloon catheter has been advanced from the aorta into the affected artery. The balloon is positioned across the seriously narrowed area of the coronary artery *(asterisk)*.

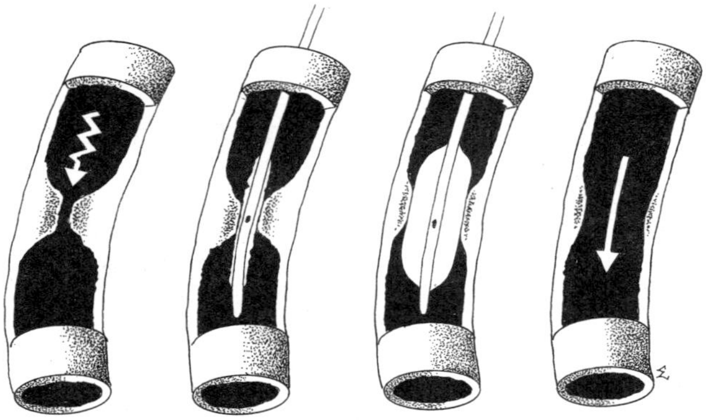

Figure 3. Segment of narrowed coronary artery. Sequence of angioplasty: *A,* Severe narrowing of the coronary artery prevents adequate flow of blood to the heart muscle; *B,* Deflated balloon catheter is positioned across narrow area in artery. *C,* Balloon is inflated, compressing atheroma against wall of coronary artery. *D,* Balloon is deflated and removed. Flow through artery is improved significantly.

Rotorooter Method

In this method, a tiny, precisely designed, swiftly rotating blade is at the tip of the angioplasty catheter. This blade can shave off tiny amounts of tissue with which it comes in contact. The rotating blade is slowly advanced to cross the area that is made narrow by the atherosclerosis. The blade cuts away the atheroma to make the passage larger. This opens the vessel to let more blood flow into the heart muscle.

The procedure takes approximately 2 to 3 hours, depending on how many vessels need to be dilated. During this time, you will be awake but drowsy. Very minimal amounts of pain are experienced. At the completion of the procedure, the catheter will be removed but a very thin wire will be left in place overnight.

AFTER THE ANGIOPLASTY

- A snug bandage will be placed over the groin, and you will be taken to a hospital room.
- You will be expected to lie flat for as long as the thin wire is in place and for 6 hours after the wire has been removed.
- Your heart, groin, and pulse will be monitored very carefully during this time.
- Most patients are able to go home in 2 to 3 days.
- As with any procedure, complications are possible. With this type of procedure, they can include bleeding from the catheter site or injury to the femoral artery. There can be complete blockage of the coronary artery, with a high risk of a heart attack unless something is done promptly to remove the blockage. Coronary artery blockage requires an immediate open-heart operation by a cardiac surgeon to prevent the heart muscle from dying. This is why a cardiac surgeon is available during the angioplasty in the unlikely event that such a blockage develops.

CALL THE CARDIOLOGIST IF

- There is any swelling, tenderness, or discharge in the area where the catheters were inserted.
- There is any pain in the leg, around the knee, or in the calf area.
- You develop a temperature higher than 100°F.
- You develop any unusual signs or symptoms.
- You have any questions.

CORONARY ARTERY BYPASS

△ GENERAL INFORMATION

The heart has its own arteries *(coronary arteries)*, which are the first branches of the big artery from the heart (the *aorta*). They carry blood to the heart muscle itself. If the coronary arteries don't work well, the heart doesn't work well. The coronary arteries are spread strategically over the surface of the heart and give off several large branches that in turn give off many smaller branches. These smaller branches go into the heart muscle itself and nourish it. Sometimes one or more of these arteries becomes partially blocked by cholesterol deposits (called *atherosclerosis*).

COMMON SIGNS AND SYMPTOMS

- There may be pain in the chest, shoulder, or arm and in a number of other places *(angina)*.
- This pain may start while working, but it can start while at rest.
- An individual may tire easily.
- There may be few or no symptoms, but the electrocardiogram shows serious changes.
- There may be a change in the rhythm of the heart.

○ TREATMENT

- Often, taking medicines and changing one's lifestyle can help slow down or even totally prevent the blockage from getting worse.
- At other times, placing special tiny tubes inside the narrowed coronary artery to stretch and keep it open or reaming out the blocked area will solve the problem.
- Unfortunately, in some persons the narrowing continues to get worse, or the blockage is too advanced to correct it; a new artery is necessary.

After careful consideration of all factors, it is recommended that the blocked areas in your coronary artery be bridged with a segment of new artery so that more blood can reach your heart muscle.

PREOPERATIVE PREPARATION

- Your lungs (chest x-ray), kidneys, and blood vessels to your brain and legs will be examined with special care.
- Don't eat or drink anything for 8 hours before the operation.
- You may be given medicine that will make you feel drowsy before you are brought to the operating room.

□ OPERATION

- You will be asleep for the operation.
- The incision will be in an up-and-down direction over the center of your breastbone.
- The artery under the breastbone *(internal mammary artery)* may be dissected free so that it is available for later use.
- Some plastic tubes will be placed in your major blood vessels. These will be used to connect you to the heart-lung machine (the "pump").
- After the heart is exposed and all is ready, the heart-lung machine takes over, supplying your body with blood and oxygen.
- The heart itself is then stopped, and the blocked arteries are exposed.
- At the same time, some members of the surgical team will remove a length of vein from your leg to be used as new coronary arteries.
- The vein or the internal mammary artery, or both, will be connected to the coronary arteries on the far side of the blocked areas (Fig. 1).
- The heart is then restarted. The heart-lung machine is stopped and disconnected.
- The entire operation usually takes 3 to 5 hours.

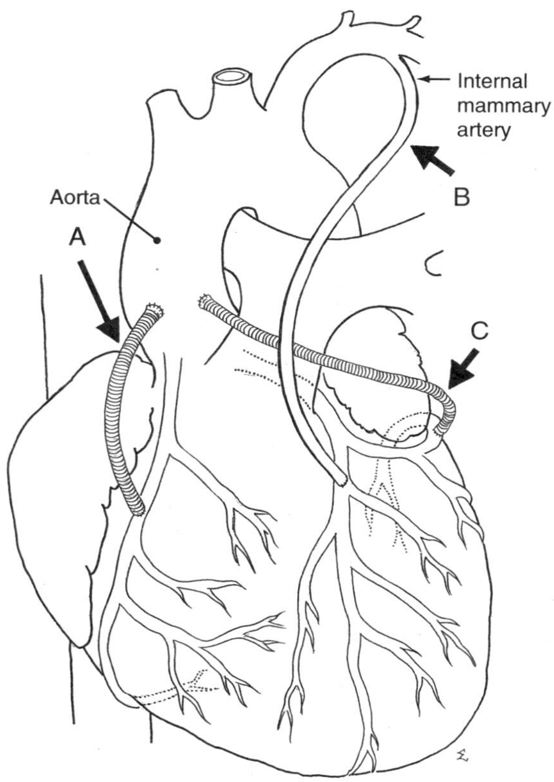

Figure 1. Blocked coronary arteries can be bypassed in several ways. Some examples are as follows: A, Vein graft from aorta to right coronary artery; B, internal mammary artery to left anterior descending coronary artery; C, vein graft from aorta to circumflex coronary artery.

POSTOPERATIVE CARE

- You will be taken to the Surgical Care Unit for a day or so, where the doctors and nurses are very experienced in taking care of patients like yourself.
- There may be a tube down your windpipe *(trachea)* for a day so that the surgical team can be certain you are getting the correct amount of oxygen. You will not be able to speak during this time, but the nurses will be at your bedside.

- Pain will be controlled with medicine.
- At first your diet will be liquids, and then it will be increased to solid food as you tolerate it.
- You will be given an incentive spirometer. Breathing into this as you are instructed will help you expand your lungs and reduce the risk of developing pneumonia.
- Arrangements will be made for your medicine and follow-up office visit.
- As with any operation, complications are always possible, some of them serious. With your type of operation, they can include heart problems, clotting of the new artery, infection, and possibly others.

✚ HOME CARE

- You may walk about as you wish, but don't overdo things. Take a short nap—maybe half an hour—twice a day, or as necessary.
- Take medicine as prescribed for your pain.
- You may eat as you wish. Include plenty of roughage and liquids in your diet to help prevent constipation.
- Unless instructed otherwise, you may shower if you wish and with any dressing on or off. There may be narrow strips of tape across the incision. It's all right if they get wet; they will be removed in the doctor's office. After you dry yourself, replace any dressings with clean, dry ones.
- Do not drive until we first talk about it during your follow-up office visit.
- Hold off on resuming sexual activity until we talk about it first.
- Let's discuss when it is advisable for you to return to work.

✆ CALL OUR OFFICE IF

- You develop any of the symptoms you had before the operation.
- Any incision becomes red or swollen, or there is drainage from it.
- You develop a temperature higher than 100°F.
- You have any questions.

△ GENERAL INFORMATION

Dramatic improvements have been made in modern surgery so that it is now possible to perform operations that were thought to be impossible not many years ago. Despite all this progress, it is still difficult to keep the lungs clear after an operation. In fact, the lungs are the most common cause of problems in the surgical patient.

The windpipe *(trachea)* is about as big around as a dust mop handle. As the trachea goes down into the lungs, it divides into smaller and smaller branches—eventually smaller than the lead in a pencil—until these branches reach the air sacs (the *alveoli*). The alveoli are lined by a thin membrane: on one side of this membrane is air and on the other side is the blood flowing in the capillaries. Through this remarkable membrane (a *semipermeable membrane*, because air but not blood can pass across it) fresh air that you breathe in can get to the blood and bad air (CO_2) in the blood can be removed as you exhale. This happens with every breath.

There are two properties of the alveoli (and so of the lung) that are interesting:

- The lung is elastic like a balloon. It likes to collapse, but inside the chest it cannot do that. There actually is a vacuum between the lung and the chest wall. As the chest expands, the lungs must follow the chest wall and all the alveoli open up. However, if the chest does not expand enough, some of the alveoli stay collapsed. Remember this point.
- The air tubes of the lungs are lined by microscopic hairs (called *cilia*) that are always waving in one direction—toward the outside. Although they are only microscopic, all of them together help move mucus (which is normal) from inside the lungs to the outside. This helps keep the lungs clean of dust and other particles we breathe in. Otherwise, the mucus would plug up these tiny tubes. If the tubes become blocked, the lung tissue (being elastic) collapses. This condition is called *atelectasis*. The collapsed lung tissue is spongy to soggy and has bacteria in it that got there from the air we breathe. It is the perfect place and condition for the start of an infection that can lead to pneumonia.

Even though they should, patients don't want to move or breathe deeply after an operation because it hurts. They surely don't like to cough because that hurts even more. One important reason for giving you pain medicine is to lessen the pain with coughing.

You will be given an incentive spirometer. Breathing into this as you are instructed will help you expand your lungs and reduce the risk of developing pneumonia.

ABOUT SMOKING

Smoking does several things to the lungs:

- It stimulates them to make much more mucus. Any steady smoker knows this.
- Also, it stuns (and sometimes cripples or even destroys) the tiny hairs. This prevents them from pushing out the mucus. In addition, the irritation from the anesthetic causes more mucus to form.

Not smoking for 1 week can make a big difference.

- It lets the stunned cilia recover and work better.
- It means that less mucus is likely to be present to plug up your lungs.

So, *stop smoking* at least 1 week before your operation. This will help reduce the risk of developing a serious lung infection following your operation.

△ GENERAL INFORMATION

Crohn's disease is a chronic inflammation of the small and large intestines and often of other areas in the abdomen. It can even affect organs outside the abdomen. Mostly the disease begins at the age of 10 to 15 years and can affect anyone.

Sometimes the condition gets better by itself or with a little treatment only to come back some years later in the same area or in a different area, and even in a different manner. At other times Crohn's disease may be slowed down a bit with treatment but always keeps progressing.

Although there are many theories on what causes Crohn's disease, none has been proven.

COMMON SIGNS AND SYMPTOMS

- There is colicky pain, especially after eating.
- Diarrhea is common because the bowel is inflamed or working forcefully to overcome a partial blockage, or because the food in it is improperly digested.
- The scarred small bowel can develop enough blockage that there is severe cramping pain or swelling of the abdomen.
- There may be poor nutrition or not enough nutrition because food is not being absorbed properly. Or the person avoids eating so as not to develop the cramping pain.
- There is weight loss because of the above.
- Anemia from bleeding or poor nutrition is common.
- There is a general ill feeling because of inflammation and infection of all the tissue.

DIAGNOSIS

An absolutely certain diagnosis can't be made in one specific way or even in several ways. Rather, the diagnosis is made by putting together the information from the history, the symptoms, the physical examination and laboratory tests, and the way the disease has behaved.

- Blood and urine tests can show the degree of anemia or infection in the body.
- Careful examination of the area around the anus may show infection there.
- Colonoscopy: This is done with an optical instrument with a light at its tip that is smooth, flexible, and as big around as your little finger. During the procedure you will be given medicine that will make you feel drowsy. The tip of the instrument will be lubricated, gently introduced through the anus, and advanced along the large bowel. It can be used to inspect your entire large bowel and even a short distance into the small intestine. If suspicious tissue is seen, a small piece of it can be taken (a *biopsy*) for laboratory examination.
- Barium enema: Barium (it has the color and consistency of buttermilk) is placed in the colon like a regular enema, and x-rays are taken from various angles. These x-rays can show the area of the colon that is affected.
- Ultrasound: Harmless sound waves are aimed at the area of your abdomen. The sound waves bouncing back (the echoes) from this area are seen as a picture on a screen. Ultrasound is a convenient and painless way to examine organs and tissues inside this area of your body.
- Small bowel x-rays: You will be given barium to swallow. X-rays will be taken of the barium as it travels through your small bowel to try to pick up areas of involvement.

○ TREATMENT

Medical

Generally, the treatment is medical with several aims:

- To provide nutrition that is easy for the body to utilize because the diseased intestine may not be able to do this with a regular diet.
- To use medication to prevent or treat infection.
- To attempt to boost the person's immune system.

Surgical

Surgery is reserved for specific problems. Eventually, however, most patients need an operation of one type or another. Mostly the operation is to relieve symptoms rather than to cure the disease. An operation may be necessary for the following:

- An abscess that needs to be drained.
- A connection (a *fistula*) between one portion of the bowel and another segment. Or there may be a connection from the bowel through the skin to the outside.
- Uncontrolled bleeding from the inflamed bowel.
- Blockage, mostly of the small bowel. This is because the small intestine is so inflamed and swollen that little can pass through it. At other times the intestine is not actually blocked but so swollen that it cannot squeeze down to move food along.
- Complications affecting the bladder from inflamed intestine resting on the bladder. Sometimes the inflamed intestine breaks through and makes a connection into the bladder.
- Cancer in the diseased colon.

After the most careful consideration of all factors, the recommendation is that you have an operation for your present problem. The exact nature of the operation can vary depending on what is found during the operation and what is needed to correct it. However, every effort is made *not* to remove intestine because this leaves you with less intestine to digest your food. The emphasis is to fix things so that food can pass through your intestine.

Trust and confidence in the surgeon are necessary, and a discussion before the operation is the best way for you to better understand the course of action. For this reason, there will be a discussion with you at length about your problem and the solutions to it. You are encouraged to ask all the questions you wish.

PREOPERATIVE PREPARATION

- You should be in the best possible condition to reduce the risks of an operation. This may consist of at least some of the following:
  - Giving you extra fluid by vein.
  - Starting antibiotics.
  - Giving you blood transfusions to correct any anemia.
  - Improving your nutrition.
- Do not eat or drink anything for 8 hours before the operation.
- You will have an examination of your blood, urine, heart (EKG), and lungs (chest x-ray).

□ OPERATION

- You will be asleep for the operation.
- The length of the operation depends on what is found and what needs to be done.

POSTOPERATIVE CARE

- As with any operation, complications are always possible, some of them serious. With this type of operation, they can include peritonitis, pneumonia, heart attack, blood clots and fistula, and possibly others.
- Arrangements will be made for your medicines, follow-up office visit, and stitch or clip removal.
- Some specific instructions will depend very much on the specific nature of your problem, the treatment you receive, and how much and how swiftly you recover. For this reason, some specific instructions will not be given to you until shortly before you leave the hospital.

✚ HOME CARE

- Follow the instructions given to you while you were in the hospital.
- You may walk about as you wish, even climb stairs, but don't overdo things.
- Be certain to take the medicines as prescribed for you.
- A diet will be suggested to you if this is necessary.
- Arrangements will be made for a home visiting nurse if one is needed.
- Unless instructed otherwise, you may shower as you wish and with any dressings on or off. After you dry yourself, replace any dressings with clean, dry ones.
- You may return to work when you feel up to it.
- Do not drive a car unless you can move freely and without pain and you are not on medicines that decrease your alertness.

✆ CALL OUR OFFICE IF

- Any of your previous symptoms return, or if you develop unusual signs and symptoms.
- The incision becomes red or swollen, or there is drainage from it.
- You develop a temperature higher than 100°F.
- You have any questions.

△ GENERAL INFORMATION

A CT scan (computed tomography scan) is a special way of taking x-rays of any part of your body. A computer in the x-ray machine can show pictures as though they were very thin slices across the area being examined.

Imagine that you have a loaf of raisin bread and you want to know how many raisins are inside it and exactly where they are located. You might also want to know if there are things other than raisins inside.

By cutting the loaf into very thin slices and examining each slice carefully, you could find all the raisins. Also, you would know in which part of the slice (top, bottom, side) each raisin is located. In addition, by knowing which slice of bread you were looking at, you could tell in which section of the loaf any raisin was located. As a bonus, you might also find things in each slice that you didn't suspect—or that shouldn't be there.

So the CT scan lets you "look in" at each slice of the body without having to cut anything open to find out what is inside.

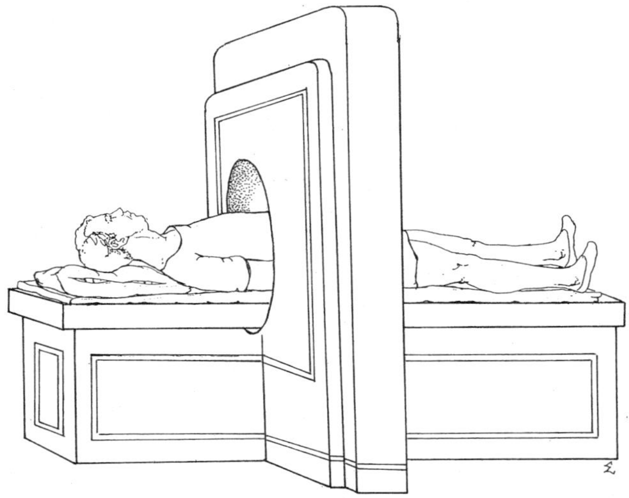

Figure 1.

PREPARATION

- Wear comfortable clothing because you will have to lie on the x-ray table for a while.
- You may be asked to drink a small amount of a special fluid. This will help make the details in the different organs and tissues sharper.

THE PROCEDURE

- You will need to remove any pieces of metal that might get in the way of the x-rays and cover something important (examples: belt buckles, necklaces, broaches).
- You will lie on a padded table and be made comfortable.
- The CT scan machine is shaped like a huge doughnut. The table on which you are lying is made to slide in the hole of this "doughnut" (Fig. 1).
- The machine will be turned on. You won't feel a thing as the machine moves one-fourth inch every minute as it passes across the part of your body being examined.
- You will need to lie still while this is going on.
- The procedure will take anywhere from 15 minutes to an hour or so, depending on how much of your body is being examined. After this, you are free to leave. There are no aftereffects.
- All these x-ray slices, with their many shadows in each slice, will be assembled and examined carefully by specialists in this field. They will look at everything—normal or abnormal. In addition, they will know from your doctor what the problem is and any things they should look for specifically.

The findings will be reported to your doctor, who will discuss them with you.

△ GENERAL INFORMATION

The ulnar nerve is one of the nerves that supplies sensation and motion to the arm below the elbow. It travels behind the inside of the elbow. It is often sensitive if struck or leaned on (the "funny bone").

The ulnar nerve can be compressed or can even become "stuck" behind the elbow. This can be associated with activities that require repetitive bending and extending the elbow (Fig. 1).

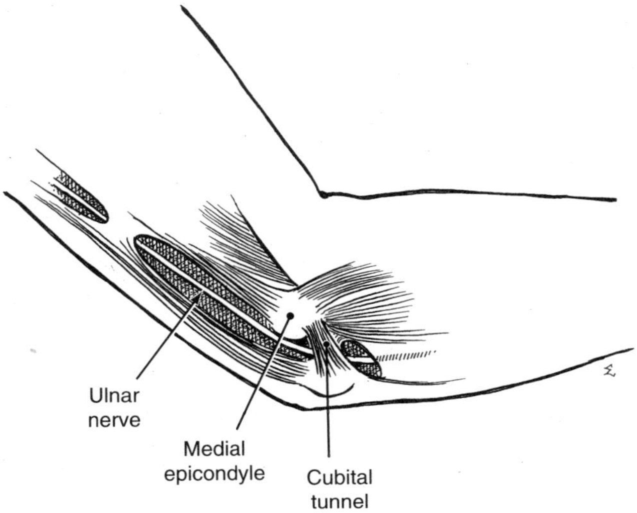

Figure 1. Inner aspect of left elbow. The ulnar nerve is squeezed as it passes under the cubital tunnel. The purpose of the operation is to release the fibers that squeeze the nerve.

COMMON SIGNS AND SYMPTOMS

- The symptoms of ulnar nerve compression include tingling or numbness down the inside of the forearm, which can radiate into the ring and small fingers.
- A vague aching or soreness about the medial elbow can also be present.
- If this condition is allowed to progress to the late stages, the hand may develop a deformity in which the ring and small fingers stay bent ("claw" deformity). This makes it difficult to perform fine movements with the fingers.

DIAGNOSIS

- The diagnosis is made by the history of symptoms, the physical examination, and often the results of special electrical studies.
- Commonly, symptoms can be reproduced by tapping on the ulnar nerve at the elbow or by maintaining the elbow in a bent position.
- Studies of how well the nerve carries the impulse and electromyography (EMG) studies may be performed by a neurologist. These studies can confirm the diagnosis of ulnar nerve compression at the elbow.

○ TREATMENT

- Conservative treatment should be tried first. It begins with an elbow pad, which provides protection for the nerve from direct trauma, such as leaning on the nerve during work or while driving.
- Patients with this condition often sleep with their elbows bent, which tents the nerve. A long arm elbow splint worn at night to keep the arm straight during sleep is often helpful in relieving symptoms.
- If the symptoms are not relieved with these conservative measures or if loss of sensation or function is present, an operation may be required.

After careful consideration of all factors, the recommendation is that you have an operation to try to help with your problem.

PREOPERATIVE PREPARATION

- You will have an examination of your blood and possibly your heart (EKG) in preparation for the operation.
- Do not eat or drink anything for 8 hours before the operation.
- Shower or bathe as usual on the morning of the operation.
- You may be given medicine that will make you feel drowsy before you are brought to the operating room.

□ OPERATION

- The operation will be performed either under general anesthesia, with you totally asleep, or under regional anesthesia. Regional anesthesia involves the use of a fine needle to inject an anesthetic into the arm nerve to make only the arm numb. Also, you may be given medicine to make you stay drowsy.
- The incision will be over the inside of your elbow. The ulnar nerve will be freed from any areas of compression.
- Typically, the ulnar nerve will then be moved to a more forward location on the elbow to take tension off the nerve. This will allow it to become lax when the elbow is bent.
- During the operation, you may feel some tugging but not pain.
- The operation usually takes 1 to 2 hours.

POSTOPERATIVE CARE

- You will be taken to a recovery room and observed. When your blood pressure, pulse, and breathing are stable and you are completely alert, you should be able to go home that same day with a responsible adult.
- There will be a bandage on your arm and possibly a splint, which will not allow you to move your elbow.
- As with any operation, complications are always possible. With this type of operation, they can include bleeding, temporary worsening of numbness or tingling (due to nerve manipulation during the operation), infection, and possibly others.
- Arrangements will be made for your medicine, follow-up office visit, and stitch removal.

✣ HOME CARE

- You may walk about as you wish, even climb stairs, but don't overdo things.
- Take medicine as prescribed for your pain.
- Most of your discomfort will resolve within several days after the operation.
- You may eat as you did before the operation.
- You may bathe or shower, but you will have to keep your dressings dry. One way of doing this is to place your entire arm in a plastic trash bag and seal the opening with tape.
- Soon after the operation, your dressings will be removed and you will begin to move your elbow so it does not become stiff. Therapy may be prescribed to help you regain your elbow motion and function.

✆ CALL OUR OFFICE IF

- You develop any unusual signs or symptoms.
- The incision becomes red or swollen, or there is drainage from it.
- You develop a temperature higher than 100°F.
- You have any questions.

△ GENERAL INFORMATION

In the normal female anatomy, the vagina is immediately in front of the rectum and behind the bladder (Fig. 1). The rectum is separated from the vagina by a thick sheet of muscle and tissue that can stretch remarkably. During childbirth, the vaginal tissue is stretched, and afterward it recovers its strength but is not quite the same as before childbirth. This happens with each childbirth. Later, with older age, the tissue relaxes even more. The result is that this weak tissue bulges into the vagina. If the bulge is in the front of the vagina, it is called a *cystocele* (Fig. 2).

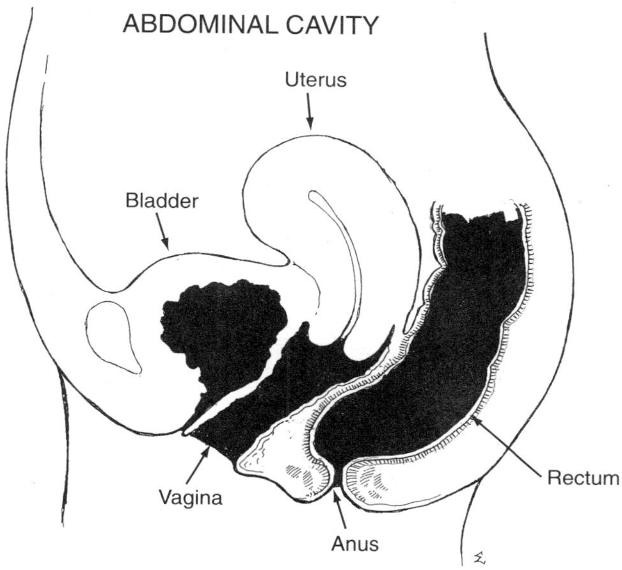

Figure 1. Side view of pelvis: normal anatomy.

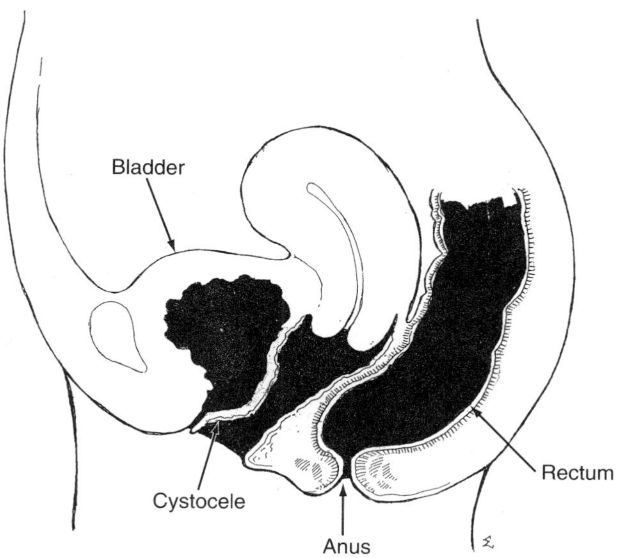

Figure 2. The cystocele shown is typical. It can, however, vary in size and shape. This influences somewhat the technique of therapy.

COMMON SIGNS AND SYMPTOMS

- A bulge in the front wall of the vagina.
- The bulge in the front wall of the vagina probably involves the tissue that is part of the *urethra*—the short tube through which the urine in the bladder comes to the outside. This relaxed, weak tissue does not squeeze down as tightly as it used to. When there is stress such as coughing, lifting something heavy, or similar activity, there can be a little leakage of the urine.

DIAGNOSIS

- Usually the diagnosis can be made by taking a detailed history and doing a thorough physical examination of this area of your body.
- The bulge in the front part of the vagina becomes more obvious when "pushing down" as though having a bowel movement. Sometimes some urine may be seen to leak out during this part of the examination.
- Ultrasound: A probe (something like an enema tip) is placed inside your vagina. From the tip of this probe, harmless, painless sound waves are aimed at the area of the cystocele. The sound waves bouncing back (the echoes) from this area are seen as pictures on a television screen. They show tissues in the vagina and where areas are weak. This information helps the surgeon determine how they will be repaired.
- Cystoscopy: This is looking into your bladder with an instrument that is smooth, as big as the tip of your little finger, and with lenses in it and a light at its tip.
- Manometry: This test is done with a tiny tube placed in your urethra. It measures how well the muscles around the urethra work.

○ TREATMENT

It has been determined that the front part of your vagina is weakened (you have a cystocele) and that it needs to be repaired.

PREOPERATIVE PREPARATION

- You will have an examination of your blood, urine, heart (EKG), and lungs (chest x-ray).
- Do not eat or drink anything for 8 hours before the operation.
- Do not douche or place anything in your vagina on the day of the operation.
- You may be given medicine that will make you feel drowsy before you are brought to the operating room.

□ OPERATION

- You will be asleep for the operation or be offered a spinal type of anesthesia.
- The incision will be at the front part of your vagina.
- You will not need a blood transfusion.
- The operation usually takes about 2 hours.

POSTOPERATIVE CARE

- You will be taken to a recovery room and observed. When your blood pressure, pulse, and breathing are stable, you will be taken to a regular hospital room.
- There will be a catheter in your bladder. This will make it easier for the urine to drain from the bladder and will keep urine away from the healing tissue.
- Pain will be controlled with medicine.
- That evening you will be helped to sit up in bed and on the next day to get out of bed.
- Your diet will be as you tolerate it.
- You should be able to go home in about 3 days.
- As with any operation, complications are always possible. With your type of operation, they can include bleeding, infection, separation of the incision, difficulty passing urine, and possibly others.
- Arrangements will be made for your medicine and follow-up office visit. The stitches will be absorbed by your body.

✚ HOME CARE

- You may walk about as you wish, even climb stairs, but don't overdo things.
- Do not douche or place anything in your vagina until you discuss this with the surgeon. A sanitary pad can be used for any light drainage that may occur.
- Don't lift anything heavier than 5 pounds. Ask someone to do it for you.
- Be careful that you do not become constipated.
  - Include enough roughage and plenty of liquids in your diet.
  - You may need some help with a mild laxative (example: milk of magnesia).
- You may shower as you wish for the first week. After that, you may include tub bathing if this is your preference.
- Take medicine as prescribed for your pain.
- Engaging in sexual intercourse too soon can be harmful to your recovery. If you wish, let's talk about this during your follow-up visit.
- You may return to work when you feel up to it.

✆ CALL OUR OFFICE IF

- There is drainage from the incision.
- You develop a temperature higher than 100°F.

D&C (DILATION AND CURETTAGE)

△ GENERAL INFORMATION

D&C stands for *dilation* (stretching) of the cervix and *curettage* (scraping) of the lining of the uterus.

The uterus has a lining (the *endometrium*) that serves many functions and also can be the location of a number of problems. Starting at puberty and ending at menopause, the endometrium is renewed each month. The discarded endometrium is menstruation fluid.

COMMON SIGNS AND SYMPTOMS

Some conditions that may require the endometrium to be scraped include the following:

- An incomplete, spontaneous abortion in the first few months of pregnancy. The scraping is done to reduce the loss of blood or the risk of infection.
- Excessive bleeding not associated with menstruation in the following situations:
  - Looking for an abnormal growth.
  - A thick endometrium that builds up because it did not come out completely during the previous menstrual periods.
- Bleeding ("spotting") after the menopause, because such bleeding means the endometrium has to be examined to be sure that there is no cancer present.

DIAGNOSIS

The reason for the D&C is to establish or confirm a diagnosis.

PREOPERATIVE PREPARATION

- You will have an examination of your blood, urine, heart (EKG), and lungs (chest x-ray).
- Do not douche the day of the procedure.
- Do not eat or drink anything for 8 hours before the procedure.
- Shower (not bathe) as usual the morning of the procedure.
- You may be given medicine that will make you feel drowsy before you are brought to the operating room.

□ OPERATION

- The operation will be done under quick-acting general anesthesia.
- The opening of the cervix, which is smaller than a straw, is gradually stretched with special instruments until it is opened to about the size of a pen.
- This permits the special scraping instruments of various sizes to be used inside the uterus.
- The scraping procedure is done in a very methodical and thorough fashion to make certain no area is missed (Fig. 1).
- The procedure usually takes about 30 minutes.

POSTOPERATIVE CARE

- You will wake up in the recovery room, and when your blood pressure, pulse, and breathing are stable and you are completely alert, you should be able to go home that same day with a responsible adult. Occasionally, it is necessary for you to remain in the hospital overnight.
- As with any operation, complications are always possible. Although they are uncommon with this type of operation, they can include injury to the uterus during the D&C, bleeding, infection, and possibly others.

✚ HOME CARE

- Resume your usual activities.
- Shower (not bathe) as you wish.
- Do not douche or use a tampon until you speak with the doctor during your follow-up visit.
- Sexual intercourse may be resumed once the bleeding has stopped completely—usually about 5 to 7 days after the procedure.

✆ CALL OUR OFFICE IF

- You have persistent abdominal pain.
- You have abnormal vaginal bleeding.
- You develop a temperature higher than 100°F.
- You have any questions.

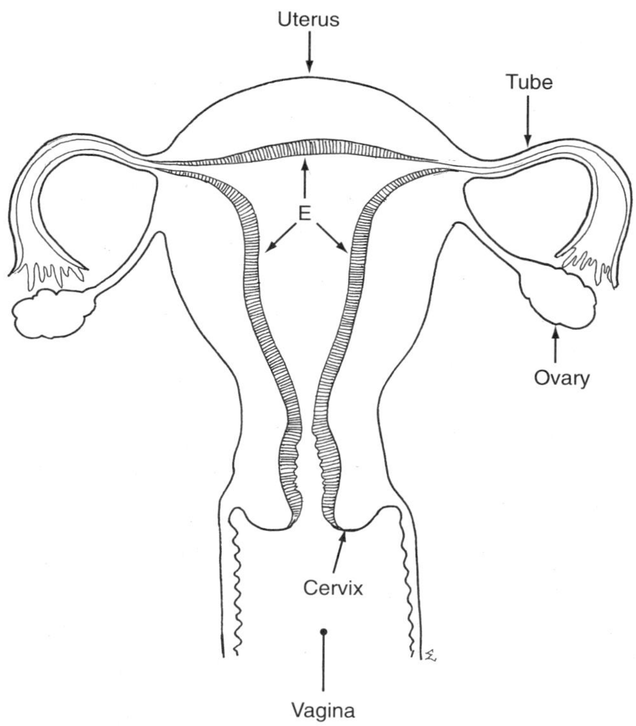

Figure 1. The tissue removed during a dilation of the opening in the cervix and curettage of the lining of the uterus is indicated by the cross-hatched lines (E).

△ GENERAL INFORMATION

The tendons that extend (straighten) your thumb pass across the wrist through a canal over the wrist bone just beneath the base of your thumb (Fig. 1). These tendons can become swollen or inflamed (called *tendinitis*), which will lead to pain when the tendons are pulled through this tight canal. The disease is named after the doctor who first described it.

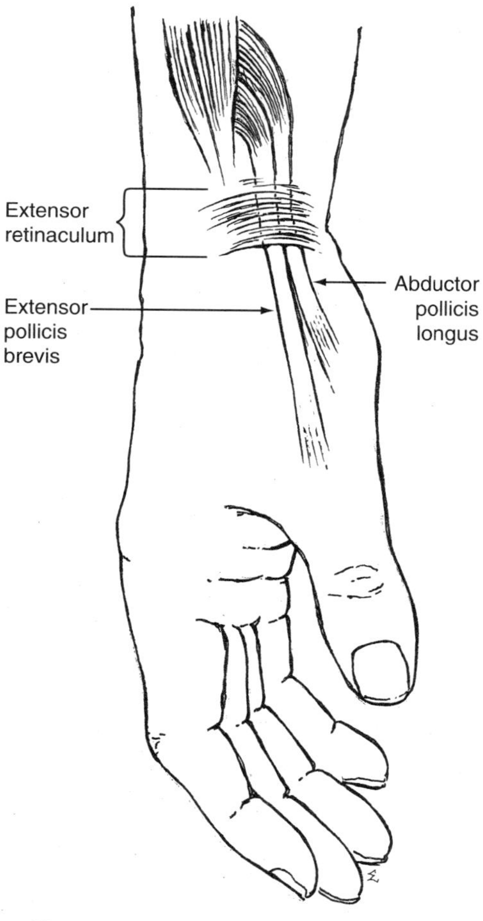

Figure 1. The tendon that opens the thumb is squeezed and inflamed by a ligament lying over it. The operation to correct this involves cutting the ligament so that the thumb tendon is free to move.

COMMON SIGNS AND SYMPTOMS

- Symptoms begin with pain along the thumb side of the wrist. This can be a very sharp, severe pain that makes it difficult to use the hand.
- Activities such as pinching or gripping that require the tendon to be pulled through its canal can aggravate the condition and increase the pain.
- Most of the time there is only low-grade discomfort when the wrist or thumb is moved in an exaggerated way. More severe involvement can lead to pain that can prevent a good night's sleep.
- Tingling or numbness is not part of this condition. It is not a nerve condition but a tendon problem.
- De Quervain's disorder is often associated with the repetitive use of the hands or with overactivity that can lead to inflammation of the tendons, which then causes the symptoms.

DIAGNOSIS

- The diagnosis is usually made by taking a detailed history of the symptoms and performing a thorough physical examination. More sophisticated studies are generally not needed.
- X-rays may be taken to be certain there are not other conditions that are causing the pain at the base of the thumb.
- Specific thumb and wrist motions tend to reproduce the symptoms and will help make the correct diagnosis.
- Sometimes a clicking or grinding sensation can be felt over the region in the wrist where the inflamed and swollen tendons are being pulled through the tight canal.

○ TREATMENT

Treatment usually begins with conservative measures; they are successful in a large percentage of cases.

- Injections of cortisone around the tendon can diminish the inflammation and lessen the symptoms. Often, more than one injection is necessary.
- You may need to wear a splint to try and rest the inflamed tendons. Also, activities that tend to aggravate the condition will need to be modified.

If you continue to have symptoms that inhibit your activities despite the above treatments, an operation may be necessary. This consists of releasing the tight canal that the tendons pass through. It will heal back at a larger size, which will not tend to catch on the tendons and cause recurrence of the inflammation.

PREOPERATIVE PREPARATION

- You will have an examination of your blood and possibly of your heart (EKG) before the operation.
- Do not eat or drink anything for 8 hours before the operation.
- Shower or bathe as usual on the morning of the operation.
- You may be given medicine that will make you feel drowsy before you are brought to the operating room.

□ OPERATION

- The operation will be done under one of two types of anesthesia. *Local anesthesia:* A fine needle is used to inject the tissue over the canal to make the area numb. *Regional anesthesia:* The nerve supplying the arm will be injected with anesthesia.
- During the operation, you may feel some tugging but not pain.
- The operation generally takes less than 1 hour.

POSTOPERATIVE CARE

- You will be taken to a recovery room. When your blood pressure, pulse, and breathing are stable and you are completely alert, you should be able to go home that same day with a responsible adult.
- As with any operation, complications are always possible. With this type of operation, they can include injury to the small nerves that supply sensation and that lie over the inflamed compartment at the base of the thumb and wrist. Even careful retraction of these nerves can lead to loss of sensation (temporary or permanent) on the finger side of the incision at the base of the thumb. Scar sensitivity is another common complication. Fortunately, this usually resolves with time.
- Arrangements will be made for your medicine, follow-up office visit, and stitch removal.

HOME CARE

- Resume your usual activities when possible.
- Take medicine as prescribed for your pain.
- Arrangements may be made for you to see a therapist who will help you regain motion and function of your thumb and wrist.

CALL OUR OFFICE IF

- You develop any unusual signs or symptoms.
- The incision becomes red or swollen, or there is drainage from it.
- You develop a temperature higher than 100°F.
- You have any questions.

△ GENERAL INFORMATION

Persons who suffer from progressive kidney failure will gradually have an accumulation of waste products in their body. Since the kidneys are the organs that remove these waste products, they can no longer perform this function when they are diseased. These waste products are poisons, and if they accumulate to a high enough level, death is inevitable.

Fortunately, there are many ways to treat kidney failure, and all these depend on finding other ways to remove the poisonous waste products from the body. *Dialysis* is a term used to describe the mechanical removal of waste products from the body. Dialysis can be done either by cleaning the blood *(hemodialysis)* or by using other organs of the body to function as an artificial kidney. The organ most commonly used is the abdominal cavity, or *peritoneum*, so dialysis within the abdominal cavity is called *peritoneal dialysis*.

HOW PERITONEAL DIALYSIS WORKS

Peritoneal dialysis uses the ability of the peritoneum to act as a kidney. When a dilute salt solution is placed in the abdominal cavity, the waste products from the patient's own tissues will diffuse slowly across the peritoneum into the salt solution. The peritoneum has microscopic openings that let molecules of the waste products pass into the salt solution in the abdominal cavity, where the concentration of molecules is lower. After 4 to 6 hours, the concentration of waste products in the solid body tissue will be the same as that of the fluid in the abdomen and no further diffusion will occur. In peritoneal dialysis, therefore, the used fluid needs to be removed regularly and fresh fluid placed in the abdominal cavity to have additional continuous removal of the waste products. It is necessary to have some tubing device by which the salt solution can be administered to pass both into and out of the abdominal cavity on a regular basis. Such catheters are referred to as peritoneal dialysis catheters, and the most common such catheter is frequently referred to as a Tenckhoff catheter (Fig. 1).

Peritoneal dialysis requires considerable participation by the patient. It cannot be performed if patients are not interested and cooperative and meticulously clean in their hygiene. These concerns will be discussed with you by your nephrologist (kidney doctor), and it is the nephrologist who will decide if peritoneal dialysis is appropriate for you. If peritoneal dialysis is recommended, then patients are referred to a surgeon for the placement of the peritoneal dialysis catheter.

After careful consideration of all factors, the recommendation is that you have an operation to make it possible for you to have peritoneal dialysis.

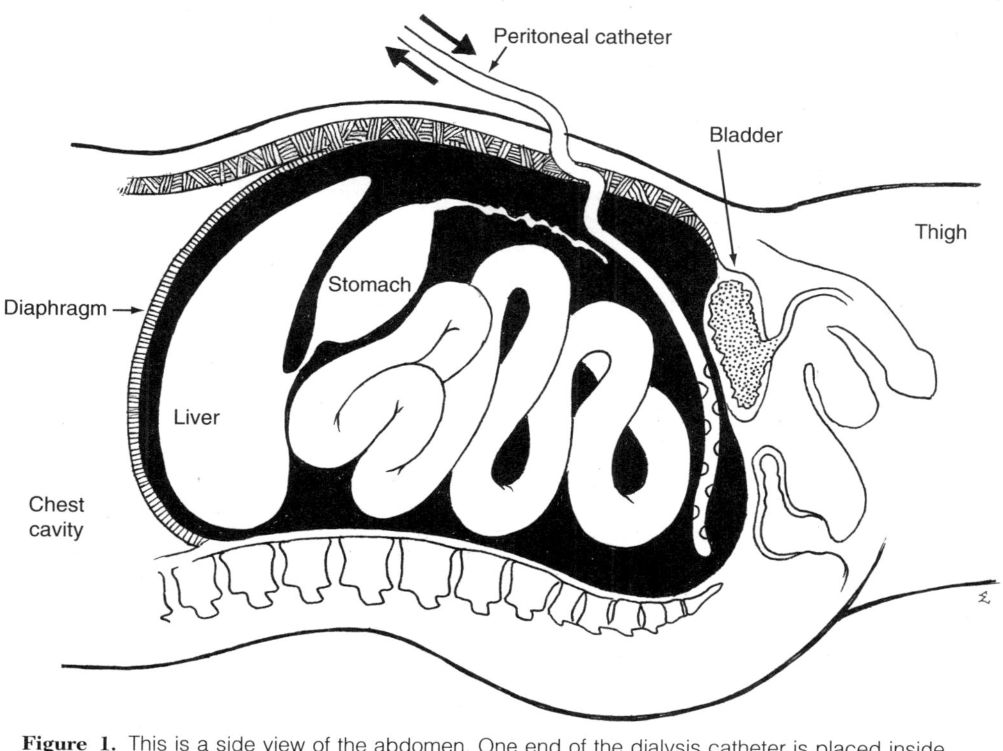

Figure 1. This is a side view of the abdomen. One end of the dialysis catheter is placed inside the abdominal cavity through a short incision. The tip of the catheter is directed so that it lies in the pelvic (or lowest) part of the abdominal cavity. In this position it can most effectively suck out the dialysis fluid that is introduced as part of the treatment. Fluid is instilled into the abdominal cavity *(arrow pointing inward)* and after a determined period is removed *(arrow pointing outward)*.

PREOPERATIVE PREPARATION

- A physical examination is done to be as certain as possible that there is no active infection elsewhere in the body and to determine the best place for the abdominal incision.
- You will be told of any special preparations necessary on your part.
- You will be instructed on how to clean out your bowel.
- Shower or bathe on the morning of the operation.

☐ OPERATION

- The insertion of a Tenckhoff catheter is almost always done on an outpatient basis.
- Your abdomen will be scrubbed with an antiseptic solution and then surrounded with sterile drapes.
- A fine needle will be used to inject anesthetic in the skin to make the area numb. In addition, you will be given medicine to keep you drowsy during the operation. The usual incision is 2 to 3 inches long and runs up and down the side of the umbilicus. One end of the dialysis catheter is placed in the abdomen. The other end is tunneled under the skin and brought out in a separate spot. Usually, this is just under the ribs. This location is not cosmetically acceptable to some patients who wear bikini bathing suits. If so, arrangements can be made so that the catheter comes out through the skin in a less visible part of the body. This will be discussed with you beforehand.
- After the catheter is inserted into the abdominal cavity and brought to the outside, fluid is administered through the catheter and then allowed to drain out. This is done to make certain the catheter is working properly.
- The operation usually takes about 1½ hours.

POSTOPERATIVE CARE

- You will be taken to a recovery room and observed. When your blood pressure, pulse, and breathing are stable and you are completely alert, you should be able to go home that same day with a responsible adult.
- Arrangements will be made for your medicine, follow-up office visit, and stitch or clip removal.
- As with any operation, complications are always possible. Although they are uncommon with this type of operation, they can include infection, catheter malfunction, and possibly others.

✚ HOME CARE

- Resume your usual activities.
- Most patients who have peritoneal dialysis catheters placed do not begin this treatment for several weeks. This is to allow the tissue around the catheter ample time to heal and so reduce the likelihood of infection.
- When you return to the surgeon's office, the incision will be examined and the decision made on when the nephrologist can begin the treatments of peritoneal dialysis.
- When dialysis fluid is placed into the abdominal cavity, it occasionally gives rise to a sense of fullness in the lower abdomen. Also, there may be a sensation of the need to urinate or to move your bowels. The sensation will pass quickly as the fluid is drained. These sensations do not recur once dialysis is done on a regular basis.

✆ CALL OUR OFFICE IF

- You develop any unusual signs or symptoms.
- The incision becomes red or swollen, or there is drainage from it.
- You develop a temperature higher than 100°F.
- You have any questions.

DIALYSIS SHUNT (ARTERIOVENOUS SHUNT)

△ GENERAL INFORMATION

Dialysis is the mechanical removal of waste products from the body. *Hemodialysis* is a type of dialysis to clean the blood. It is a medical procedure by which a very thin tube is placed in a blood vessel and used to take blood and pass it through a machine that cleans it of waste products usually removed by normal kidneys. The clean blood is then returned to the bloodstream.

WHY DIALYSIS IS DONE

Dialysis is done for persons whose kidneys are not well enough to remove waste products from their bodies. If dialysis is not performed, these people go into kidney failure and eventually die from the buildup of poisonous waste products. Alternative therapy may include placing a catheter into the abdominal cavity and using it to instill a special cleansing fluid into the abdominal cavity. After a short while, the fluid is removed and it brings some of the waste products with it. This form of dialysis is called *peritoneal dialysis*.

HOW DIALYSIS WORKS

To do a hemodialysis, it is necessary to take blood from a vessel that has a lot of blood flowing through it. The artery in the wrist is such a vessel. Unfortunately, it is very difficult to safely stick the artery with a needle too many times. The vein is such a vessel that a technician can easily see and stick with a needle. Unfortunately, the blood does not flow through it fast enough to perform the dialysis procedure. Besides, if the vein is stuck too often, the blood in it will clot.

The solution is to connect the artery directly to the vein so that the vein now has a lot of blood flowing through it (Fig. 1). This is called a *shunt;* the medical term is *arteriovenous shunt*, or *arteriovenous fistula.*

TYPES OF SHUNTS

There are two types of shunt: A shunt can be made by connecting the artery to the vein directly. This is a *natural* shunt. If for some reason the artery and vein cannot be connected directly, a small plastic tube is used to make the connection. This is a *graft* shunt.

When a shunt needs to be used (whichever type you have), a special needle is placed into the vein or plastic connection so that blood can be taken swiftly and sent to the cleaning *(dialysis)* machine. After the blood has been cleansed, it is returned to the same vein by another needle (Fig. 2). A surgical operation is necessary to make a shunt.

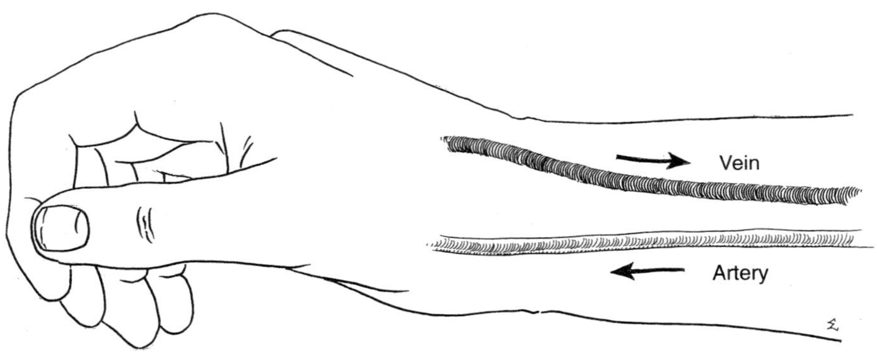

Figure 1. Shunts for use in dialysis can be placed in a number of areas of the body. The most common is just above the wrist between the artery *(radial)* and the vein *(cephalic)*.

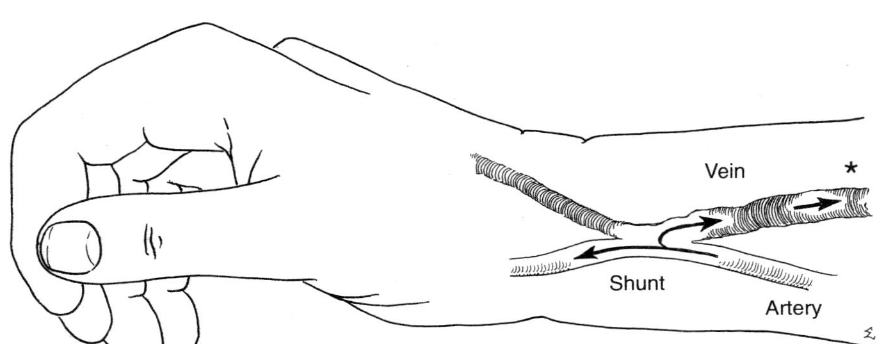

Figure 2. After the anastomosis is made, the flow of blood in the vein is greatly increased. The needle for use during the dialysis is placed in the vein anywhere along the area marked with an asterisk.

PREOPERATIVE PREPARATION

- Do not eat or drink anything for 8 hours before the operation.
- Shower as usual on the morning of the operation.
- You may be given medicine that will make you feel drowsy before you are brought to the operating room.
- The doctor will tell you if you have to make any changes in your medicines before the operation.

☐ OPERATION

- On the morning of the operation, some blood may be taken to be examined for the level of chemicals in it.
- A fine needle will be used to place an anesthetic in the skin of the wrist area to make it numb. Also, you may be given medicine that will make you feel drowsy during the operation.
- You may feel some tugging during the operation but not pain.
- The operation usually takes about 2 hours.

POSTOPERATIVE CARE

- You will be taken to a recovery room. When your blood pressure, pulse, and breathing are stable and you are completely alert, you should be able to go home that same day with a responsible adult.
- Arrangements will be made for your medicine, follow-up office visit, and stitch removal.

✣ HOME CARE

- Keep the dressings dry until the stitches are removed. If the dressings get wet, replace them with sterile dry ones.
- Do not use dressings that place pressure on the shunt or completely encircle the arm or wrist.
- Exercise your natural shunt by squeezing a rubber ball 10 times, four times a day. This is not necessary if you have a graft shunt.

HOW TO PROTECT YOUR SHUNT

All of the following are to help prevent cutting off the flow in your shunt because that would cause the shunt to clot and stop the flow permanently.

- Do not sleep on your shunt.
- Do not wear jewelry or tight sleeves on the arm that has the shunt.
- Do not carry anything hanging over the arm with the shunt.
- Do not let anyone take your blood pressure or take blood from the arm with the shunt.
- Check the shunt for any problems every morning and evening:
  - Loss of the "thrill" over the shunt.
  - Loss of pulsation over the shunt.
  - Pain or hardness in the area of the shunt.
  - A red or swollen incision, or one that is draining.
- If any of the above are present, *do not* pick at your shunt. Use the telephone number given to you to contact the doctor or nurse promptly. If this is not possible, go to a hospital emergency room.
- If there is bleeding from the needle puncture site, keep continuous gentle pressure on the puncture site for 30 minutes with a piece of sterile gauze. If it still bleeds when you remove the pressure, reapply the pressure and call the doctor or go to a hospital emergency room.

The shunt you have is very important to your health. If it is properly taken care of, it can last you quite a long while.

To reduce irritation or stimulation of the digestive tract that occurs with an ulcer, it is recommended that you adopt a bland diet (diet for chronic peptic ulcer disease). Although you likely will be prescribed a medication to help treat your ulcer, some foods are known to be irritating to the stomach or intestines. Everyone has different tolerances; therefore, there is no need to eliminate any food from your diet unless it bothers you on a regular basis.

HELPFUL HINTS

- Eat meals at scheduled times, and add smaller, more frequent meals if food gives you relief.
- Avoid foods that cause you discomfort.
- Avoid lying down after eating, and limit late-night snacking to prevent acid buildup during sleeping.
- Continue to eat a well-balanced diet, selecting a variety of foods from all the food groups.
- Known gastric irritants include caffeine, alcohol, chocolate, pepper, and chili powder.

FOODS TO AVOID

- Coffee, tea, chocolate, cocoa, alcohol, and carbonated beverages.
- Spicy salad dressings or other spicy condiments.
- Any foods made with black pepper, chili powder, chili peppers, or red or white pepper.
- Spicy products such as Mexican foods, hot and spicy Chinese foods, chili, spicy meats, pepper, or spicy cheeses.
- Chocolate or coffee-flavored desserts.

SAMPLE MENU

Breakfast
Apple juice
Scrambled eggs
Whole wheat toast with margarine and jelly
Banana
Milk

Snack
Graham crackers
Milk

Lunch
Garden vegetable soup
Turkey sandwich with lettuce and mayonnaise
Pear halves
Iced tea

Snack
Apple
Cheese and crackers

Dinner
Tossed salad with vinegar and oil dressing
Dinner roll with margarine
Baked fish
Fluffy rice
Steamed carrots
Peanut butter cookies
Milk

DIET AND NUTRITION: Diet Following Ostomy Placement

You have recently had surgery for placement of an ostomy tube. It is recommended that for 6 to 8 weeks you follow the dietary guidelines listed below to help eliminate problems with clogging of your ostomy tube, gas (bloating), and unpleasant odors. After 6 to 8 weeks, you can start introducing new foods, one at a time, to be certain that they do not cause discomfort and that you can tolerate them. Carbon filters and deodorants also help eliminate problems with gas and odors.

HELPFUL HINTS

- Moderation is the key—most foods do not have to be eliminated completely.
- Experiment and keep track of irritating foods.
- Soluble fiber can help prevent loose stools, so be sure to include rice, oatmeal, bananas, and applesauce in your diet.
- Soft, cooked, or pureed vegetables should be used initially.
- Remove skin and seeds from fruits and vegetables.
- Water (fluid) is necessary to keep you from becoming dehydrated. It is recommended that you drink at least 8 to 10 glasses of liquid a day. You need to discuss the need for increases in fluid with your doctor if you experience symptoms of dehydration, including dry mouth, rapid decline in weight, constipation, dizziness, or a combination of these.
- Chew slowly with mouth closed to keep extra air from entering the intestines. Avoid chewing gum or drinking through a straw to prevent gas production.
- Chew all food well, and choose a variety of foods.
- Smaller, more frequent meals may make adjusting to foods easier, and skipping meals may cause watery stools and increase gas.
- Broil, roast, grill, or boil meats instead of frying.

Foods that may control odors: Tomato, cranberry, and orange juice; parsley; spinach; buttermilk; yogurt.
Foods that may control diarrhea: Applesauce, boiled rice, boiled milk, tapioca, marshmallows, peanut butter, bananas.
Foods that may eliminate constipation: Increase in fluids, cooked fruits and vegetables, coffee, and fresh fruit.
Foods that may help to form bulk: Bran, corn, lettuce, noodles, raw vegetables and fruit, whole wheat bread

FOODS TO AVOID

Stoma-Obstructing Foods
Nuts and seeds
Popcorn
Lobster
Crab
Fibrous foods
Corn
Mushrooms
Shrimp
Coconut

Color-Changing Foods
Strawberries
Iron pills
Red Jell-O
Beets
Licorice
Red food coloring

Colon-Irritating Foods
Raw vegetables and fruit
Green leafy vegetables
Prunes
Milk
Alcoholic beverages
Raisins
Whole grain wheat
Spices
Bran cereals

Gas-Producing Foods
Cabbage
Beans
Beer
Milk
Gum
Onions
Cucumbers
Broccoli
Cauliflower
Alcohol
Nuts
Radishes
Turnips
Carbonated drinks

Odor-Producing Foods
Fish
Peanut butter
Asparagus
Garlic
Strong cheese
Onions
Cod liver oil
Baked beans
Eggs

After 6 to 8 weeks, gradually add new foods, one at a time, to make sure they do not cause problems. Slowly add milk products, and if side effects occur, retry at a later time.

SAMPLE MENU

Breakfast
Apple juice
Cream of wheat
Milk (if tolerated)
Plain bagel with jelly and margarine
Coffee or tea

Snack
Banana
Low-fat yogurt

Lunch
Chicken rice soup (with clear broth)
Egg salad sandwich on white bread made with low-fat mayonnaise
Canned sliced peaches
Cranberry juice

Snack
Pretzels
Iced tea

Dinner
Dinner roll with low-fat margarine
6 ounces pot roast with carrots and potatoes
Low-fat yogurt
Angel food cake
Coffee or tea

Some dietary changes may help diminish problems with heartburn or gastroesophageal reflux. It is recommended, therefore, that you follow this special diet to help decrease reflux.

HELPFUL HINTS

- Beverages to avoid include those containing alcohol or caffeine, coffee (regular and decaffeinated), and carbonated beverages.
- Relax, eat slowly, and eat at scheduled times.
- Avoid eating for about 3 hours before bedtime.
- Avoid larger meals; eat smaller amounts at more frequent times.
- Avoid foods that irritate you; eat a variety of foods.
- Eat less citrus-type fruit, and include more melon.
- Avoid fatty foods, which can take longer to digest than less fatty foods.
- Add flavor to foods with the use of herbs or broths.
- Replace heavy sauces with low-fat cheese, low-fat margarine, or seasonings, such as garlic or onion powder.

FOODS TO AVOID THAT MAY CAUSE DISCOMFORT

- High-fat starches including regular snack crackers, croissants, biscuits, cookies, and rice or pasta with heavy sauces, spices, or cream.
- Citrus-type fruits: lemons, oranges, pineapples, tangerines, and their juices.
- Fried vegetables and those in heavy sauces or with added butter.
- Gas-forming vegetables, such as cabbage, should be used only as tolerated.
- Tomatoes or tomato products.
- Spiced meats or processed lunch meats.
- Higher-fat meats (large degree of marbling), poultry (with skin), or fish (fatty types).
- All fried meats, poultry, and fish.
- Nuts and peanut butter.
- Whole milk products, heavy cream, and regular cheeses.
- High-fat snacks: potato chips, tortilla chips, high-fat or spicy dips, cakes, pies, pastries, chocolate, creamed candies, regular ice creams, and coconut.
- Regular salad dressings with spices and high-fat condiments such as mayonnaise.
- Creamed soups, gravies, butter, and margarine.

SAMPLE MENU

Breakfast
Grape juice
Oatmeal
Skim milk
Low-fat blueberry muffin with low-fat margarine

Snack
Low-fat yogurt
Strawberries
Iced tea (as tolerated)

Lunch
Salad greens with low-fat dressing
Tuna fish (packed in water) with low-fat mayonnaise and chopped celery on whole wheat toast
Low-fat cottage cheese with peaches
Apple juice

Dinner
Vegetable soup (with clear broth)
Grilled skinless chicken breast with preferred seasonings
Green beans with margarine
Baked potato with low-fat sour cream
Iced tea
Angel food cake

Snack
Cantaloupe wedge
Graham crackers

To prevent or treat constipation, it is recommended that you follow a high-fiber diet. A high-fiber diet contains at least *20 to 35* grams of fiber per day. Fiber grams of foods are typically listed on all packaged foods. The amounts listed are for individual servings.

HELPFUL HINTS

- Add fiber to your diet gradually. Increasing fiber too quickly can cause gas, cramping, diarrhea, or bloating.
- Fiber absorbs large amounts of water. Drink plenty of fluids with increased fiber intake—at least 8 cups per day to prevent constipation.
- Look at food labels for those foods containing whole grain or whole wheat first in the ingredient list. Wheat flour usually means white flour, which is low in fiber.
- Highest fiber-containing foods (with 6 grams or more per serving) include kidney, baked, and navy beans and "all bran"–type cereals.
- Most fiber-containing foods have between 1 and 4 grams of fiber per serving.

WAYS TO INCREASE DAILY FIBER INTAKE

Fruits and Vegetables

- Eat raw fruits and vegetables, as they typically contain more fiber than cooked or canned products or juice.
- Eat dried fruit.
- Remember that the skin of fruits and vegetables contains fiber.

Bread, Cereals, Rice, and Pasta

- Whole grain, whole wheat, cracked wheat, stone ground, whole oat, or rye breads and crackers.
- Whole wheat pastas.
- Barley, bulgur, millet, and wild and brown rice.
- Cereals made with wheat, corn, oat, or rice bran, whole grains, or wheat germ.

Meats, Fish, Poultry, Dried Beans, Eggs, and Nuts

- Excellent fiber sources include baked beans and kidney, pinto, lima, garbanzo, and navy beans; lentils; yellow or black-eyed peas; split green peas; nuts; and seeds.

Milk, Yogurt, and Cheese

- There is little fiber in these types of products, but fiber can be added to them (by adding fruit or nuts to yogurt).

Sweets and Snacks

- Popcorn, desserts with raw fruit, cakes and cookies made with oatmeal, whole wheat pretzels.

SAMPLE MENU

Breakfast

"All bran"–type cereal
Whole wheat toast with margarine
Apple
Coffee

Snack

Graham crackers
Water or milk

Lunch

Split pea soup
Turkey sandwich on whole wheat bread with mayonnaise, lettuce, and tomato
Orange
Fruit milkshake
Water or iced tea

Snack

Whole wheat blueberry muffin with margarine
Iced tea

Dinner

Cucumber and shaved carrot salad with vinegar and oil–type dressing
Baked fish
Brown rice with peas
Rye bread with margarine
Water
Oatmeal raisin cookies

Snack

Banana
Chunky peanut butter on whole grain toast
Water

Patients with diverticulosis can follow a high-fiber diet to prevent inflammation of the intestines, constipations, and hemorrhoids. Certain fiber-containing foods cannot be eaten by patients with diverticulosis, as they may settle in pockets in the colon and cause irritation. The foods to avoid include nuts, seeds, kernels, and foods that contain them, such as berries, popcorn, corn, chunky peanut butter, figs, jams, preserves, and foods with poppy, sesame, or caraway seeds.

DIET AND NUTRITION: High-Protein, High-Calorie Diet

To help maintain your weight, gain weight, improve your body's protein (stores), or a combination of these, it is recommended that you try to incorporate the following dietary recommendations into your daily eating plan.

HELPFUL HINTS

- Add whole or 2% milk to prepare hot cereals, soups, hot chocolate, and puddings.
- Have high-calorie snacks to munch on, such as dried fruit, nuts, cheeses, peanut butter, and crackers.
- Eat high-calorie desserts, such as ice cream, regular yogurt, milkshakes, puddings, and candies.
- Add cheeses to salads, vegetables, omelets, soups, noodles, sauces, and casseroles.
- Add extra butter and regular margarines to vegetables, soups, rice, pasta, cooked cereals, and potatoes.
- Use regular mayonnaise, salad dressings, and sour cream.
- Use more syrups, sugar, jellies, jams, and honey.
- Choose canned fruit with heavy syrup.
- Choose frozen vegetables and entrees with sauces, creams, and gravies.
- Add hard-boiled eggs to soups, salads, and sandwiches.
- Make double-strength milk by adding 1 cup of dry milk powder to 1 quart of whole or 2% milk to use in recipes and for drinking.
- Add peanut butter to plain crackers, breads, celery, and fruit slices.
- Add milkshakes and instant breakfast mixes to daily meals. Discuss possibility of commercially available nutritional beverages.
- Add nuts, seeds, and wheat germ to cereals, salads, fruit, yogurt, and ice cream.
- Add chopped-up or ground meat to soups and casseroles.
- Smaller, more frequent meals may help meet calorie needs when large portions or multiple varieties of foods cannot be eaten at one time.
- Plan daily meals in advance to help ensure availability of foods at hand.
- Keep track of daily intake, and include time and amount consumed.

SAMPLE MENU

Breakfast
Cooked cereal with fortified milk
Grape juice
Blueberry muffin with margarine
Coffee or tea with milk and sugar or honey

Snack
Yogurt with added dry fruit and granola cereal
Instant breakfast drink

Lunch
Deviled eggs
Turkey sandwich with mayonnaise, lettuce, tomatoes, and cheese
Apple
Milkshake

Snack
Pound cake with strawberries
Coffee or tea with sugar or honey and milk

Dinner
Bread sticks
Pizza with meat and vegetables
Chocolate milk

Snack
Cheese and crackers
Milkshake or liquid yogurt

DIET AND NUTRITION: Low-Residue, Low-Fiber Diet

It is recommended that you follow a low-residue, low-fiber diet for one or more of the following reasons: rest for your stomach and intestines before or after surgery, acute problems with Crohn's disease, diverticulitis, or diarrhea and stomach cramping.

HELPFUL HINTS

- This diet is to be used on a short-term basis, until you can return to a regular diet.
- Avoid foods that you know cause discomfort.
- Know the ingredients used to prepare the foods you eat.
- The principal foods to avoid are milk products (residue producing) and those with high fiber.
- Introduce foods gradually back into your daily diet once problems have subsided.
- Remove skin from vegetables and fruits before cooking.
- Refined wheat pastas, cereals, and breads and white rice are typically low in fiber and should be used.
- Strain all vegetable and fruit juices.

FOODS TO AVOID

- Foods with whole grains, seeds, nuts, dried fruit, bran, oatmeal, graham crackers, or coconut.
- Foods with greater than 1 gram of fiber listed in the nutrition facts section of the food package.
- Prune juice (or prunes), raw fruit, and all berries.
- Tough meats with gristle, lunch meats with seeds or casings, peanut butter, highly seasoned or fried meat, fish, or chicken.
- Dry beans, peas, or lentils.
- Raw vegetables, sauerkraut, winter squash, peas, and vegetables with seeds.
- Brown or wild rice, potatoes with skin on them, and whole grain pasta products.
- Limit milk products to 2 cups per day.
- Popcorn, raisins, fresh herbs, sesame, caraway and poppy seeds, olives, pickles, and relish.

SAMPLE MENU

Breakfast
Apple juice
Plain bagel with butter and jelly
Farina with slices of canned peaches
Milk (1 cup)
Coffee or tea

Snack
Half portion of cottage cheese
Fruit cocktail

Lunch
Chicken noodle soup
Saltine crackers
Tuna fish (packed in water) sandwich on toast with light mayonnaise on white toast
Cooked carrots with margarine
Vanilla wafers
One-half cup milk
Iced tea

Snack
Ripe banana
Pretzels
Iced tea or water

Dinner
Plain roll with margarine
Baked, skinless chicken breast with white rice and gravy
Green beans
Angel food cake
Coffee, tea, or iced tea

DIET AND NUTRITION: Mechanical Soft Diet

It is recommended that you follow a mechanical soft diet because you are having problems with chewing or swallowing your food. The mechanical soft diet contains foods that are chopped, liquefied in a blender, and ground. To make foods easier to eat, liquids are added to regular foods.

HELPFUL HINTS

- Pour syrups, honey, or juices over bread products such as pancakes, French toast, waffles, and muffins.
- Soften crackers and other breads in soups.
- Eat rice (except wild), noodles, and pastas.
- Use gravies, broth, and sauces on ground meats, poultry, or other dishes.
- Eat plain yogurts or yogurts without added fruit.
- Eggs (cooked), cooked dry beans and peas, and creamy peanut butter are good sources of protein that can be used.
- Choose cheeses that are soft, including cottage cheese, ricotta, and highly processed spreads without nuts.
- Well-cooked soft (or mashed) vegetables without skin, mashed potatoes, and vegetable juices are well tolerated.
- Choose cooked or canned fruit without seeds or skin or fruit juices, or mix regular fruits with yogurt or ice cream in a blender to make milkshakes.
- Chew all foods well, and eat slowly to make swallowing food easier.

FOODS TO AVOID

Raw fruits and vegetables
Coconut
Dried fruits
Nuts and seeds
Foods that do not fit into the guidelines listed above

SAMPLE MENU

Breakfast
Apple juice
Farina with butter
Scrambled eggs
Banana
Milk
Coffee or tea

Snack
Fruit milkshake

Lunch
Vegetarian vegetable soup
Grilled cheese sandwich
French fries
Canned pears
Vanilla pudding with whipped topping
Iced tea

Snack
Fruit cocktail
Iced tea

Dinner
Dinner roll with butter
Spaghetti with meatballs
Green beans (soft)
Sliced peaches
Angel food cake
Milk
Tea or coffee or iced tea

Snack
Chocolate chip cookies softened with milk

Because of your recent operation, it is advisable that you follow a soft diet until you can tolerate all foods in your regular diet. This diet helps you avoid foods that may be irritating to you following the operation.

HELPFUL HINTS

- Broil, roast, bake, or stew meats.
- Fruits and vegetables should be well cooked or canned.
- Caffeine-free drinks are allowed.
- Eat fat in moderation.

FOODS TO AVOID

Caffeinated beverages or desserts.
Any foods containing nuts, seeds, raisins, prunes, coconut, or dates.
Fried foods.
Highly spiced entrees or condiments.
Hot sauce, horseradish, pepper, and seeded mustards.
Chocolate.
Sharp or highly seasoned cheeses.
Heavy sauces or gravies.
Highly processed lunch meats, sausage, and hotdogs.
Bran or whole grain cereals and breads.
Wild rice.
Potato skins.
Corn, radishes, turnips, chili peppers, pinto beans, Brussels sprouts, onions, broccoli, cabbage, split peas, dried beans, parsnips.
Fruit with skin or seeds.
Chunky peanut butter.

SAMPLE MENU

Breakfast
Orange juice
Banana
Pancakes with margarine and syrup
Corn flakes
Milk
Decaffeinated coffee or tea

Snack
Fruit cocktail

Lunch
Shredded lettuce salad with dressing
Hamburger on bun with catsup
Cooked carrots
Canned pears
Red gelatin with whipped cream
Milk
Decaffeinated iced tea

Snack
Frozen yogurt
Vanilla wafers

Dinner
Cream of spinach soup
Vegetable beef stew with biscuit
Rice
Fruit cocktail
Tapioca pudding
Decaffeinated tea, coffee, or iced tea

Because you are unable to eat or cannot eat enough food to meet your daily nutritional needs, you will need to receive all or part of your nutrition through a tube feeding (enteral feeding). The tube feeding formula is available in liquid form, which goes into your feeding tube. The tube feeding formula is made of the same nutrients found in regular foods.

HELPFUL HINTS

- Keep track of supplies, and make sure all supplies are correct for your tube feeding regimen.
- Most enteral solutions do not require refrigeration. However, "leftovers" from preparation of your feeding formula should be refrigerated and used within 24 hours.
- To prevent contamination and reduce the risk of infection, solutions and supplies should be handled properly.
  - Wash your hands and equipment before beginning your feeding.
  - Do not use feeding formulas that are past their expiration date.
  - Use a clean area for feeding preparation.
- If medications need to be added through your feeding tube, make sure you have had proper instructions on how to put the medicine in the tube (not all medicines can be crushed or added directly to the food without causing problems).
- Gastric residuals (the amount of stomach juices and formula left in your stomach) may need to be checked regularly to make sure the tip of the feeding tube is still in the stomach and that the tube feeding is still being absorbed. Checking gastric residuals is done with a syringe before the start of the feeding.
- If gastric residuals are greater than 150 ml, the tube feeding should be stopped and the residual checked again 30 to 60 minutes later. If then it is within normal limits, tube feeding can be restarted with continued monitoring of gastric residuals. If gastric residual amounts continue to be high, contact the individual familiar with your tube feedings.
- Keep daily records of the following:
  - Amount of feeding formula used per day.
  - Other fluids given per day.
  - Other foods eaten (if you can eat).
  - Amount of urine and an estimate of the amount of stool you make.
  - Your body weight and temperature.
  - Medications taken through the tube.
  - Daily activities and problems.

METHODS OF TUBE FEEDING

Gravity Drip: The formula bag hangs from a pole with a stand, and the feeding drips into your feeding tube. You should sit at at least a 30-degree angle when receiving your feedings and remain upright for 60 minutes following feedings.

Equipment
Formula.
Gravity bag set.
Syringe for flushing (clearing the feeding tube) and adding additional water.

Bolus: This method allows you to put the feeding formula directly into your feeding tube with a syringe. These feedings should be given over at least a 15-minute time period. The bolus method allows you to get feedings at times you would normally eat meals. This method is not tolerated by all patients.

Equipment
Formula.
Syringe for adding feedings to feeding tube.
Additional syringe for flushing (clearing the feeding tube) and adding additional water.

Pump: An electric pump is hooked up to your feeding tube to be certain the correct amount of formula is given over a set period of time.

Equipment
Pump mounted on a pole.
Feeding bag and pump tubing.
Formula.
Syringe for flushing (clearing the feeding tube) and adding additional water.

PROBLEMS TO WATCH FOR

Diarrhea
Nausea
Vomiting
Constipation
Excessive weight gain
Clogged feeding tube

Any of the above problems should be reported to your doctor and the health care professional helping you monitor your tube feedings.

△ GENERAL INFORMATION

The wall of the colon can develop little sacs (called *diverticula*) that usually range in size from that of a pea to a grape. This condition is called *diverticulosis* and is very common, especially in the elderly. Most of the time, the diverticula produce no trouble whatsoever. However, if these sacs fill with stool and it gets trapped, it can irritate the sacs and they can become infected. This is called *diverticulitis*.

Diverticulosis occurs most commonly in the end of the colon *(sigmoid)*, but other areas of the colon can also be affected. The cause of diverticulosis is not truly known, but it is associated with chronic constipation.

COMMON SIGNS AND SYMPTOMS

- Pain, especially in the left part of the lower abdomen, from inflammation of the sacs.
- Constipation, because the bowel is in spasm or is swollen and narrowed and the solid stool cannot get by easily.
- Diarrhea, because stool is finally pushed through the narrowed area and rushes out as liquid bowel movement.
- Fever, from infection or an abscess in this area.

Other symptoms depend on how badly the area is infected and what other organ may be touching the colon (examples: bladder, small intestine, and others).

DIAGNOSIS

- Usually, the diagnosis can be made by taking a detailed history, doing a thorough physical examination, and considering the laboratory reports.
- Examination of the blood and urine may be done to look for evidence of infection.
- Flexible sigmoidoscopy: This is done with an optical instrument with a light at its tip that is smooth, flexible, and as big around as your little finger. It can be used to inspect the inside of the lower one fourth of your large bowel.
- Lower gastrointestinal (GI) series: A special liquid dye is placed into the colon very much like an enema. X-ray pictures are taken as this liquid flows throughout the colon. This procedure can give an accurate diagnosis most of the time.

○ TREATMENT

Most patients with diverticulosis have no symptoms, so they do not need treatment. They are encouraged to include enough roughage and liquid in their diet so they don't become constipated.

Medical Therapy: For most patients who do have symptoms, the treatment is medical and usually includes the following: medicine to reduce the spasm of the irritated colon, antibiotics to fight infection, and a diet to avoid constipation.

Surgical Therapy: An operation is appropriate when there are repeat attacks, or the attacks are becoming more severe and lasting longer. An operation in these circumstances can be done when it is convenient.

An operation needs to be done urgently in the following circumstances:

- An abscess develops.
- Obstruction does not let up.
- The colon has made a connection with another organ.

An emergency operation is necessary if the following occurs:

- An abscess has burst, and there is generalized peritonitis.
- There is hemorrhage from that area of the colon that won't stop.

After careful consideration of all factors, the recommendation is that you have the part of your colon with the diverticulitis resected.

PREOPERATIVE PREPARATION

- You will have an examination of your blood, urine, heart (EKG), and lungs (chest x-ray).
- You may have an x-ray examination of your colon to look for other possible lesions.
- Ultrasound: Harmless sound waves are aimed at the area of your abdomen. The sound waves bouncing back (the echoes) from this area are seen as a picture on a screen. Ultrasound is a convenient and painless way to examine organs and tissues inside this area of your body.
- The inside of your bladder may be looked at (a *cystoscopy*) to determine whether the bladder is affected by the inflamed colon, which is right next to it.
- A CT scan may be done. This special x-ray is taken by a machine that is shaped like a huge doughnut. You will lie on a table inside the hole in the "doughnut." The x-rays are taken as very thin slices through the area of the abdomen. This makes it possible to see the fine details in this area.
- You'll be given specific instructions how to clean out your bowel.
- Do not eat or drink anything for 8 hours before the operation.

□ OPERATION

- You will be asleep for the operation.
- The operation depends on what is found and can be one of the following (Fig. 1):
  - Remove the diseased colon and reconnect everything, all in the same operation.
  - Remove the diseased colon and do a *temporary* colostomy.
  - Remove the inflamed part of the colon and reconnect everything. However, for safety reasons, there may have to be a *temporary* colostomy so that the stool does not flow past the new connection for a few days.
  - Drain the abscessed area and do a *temporary* colostomy.

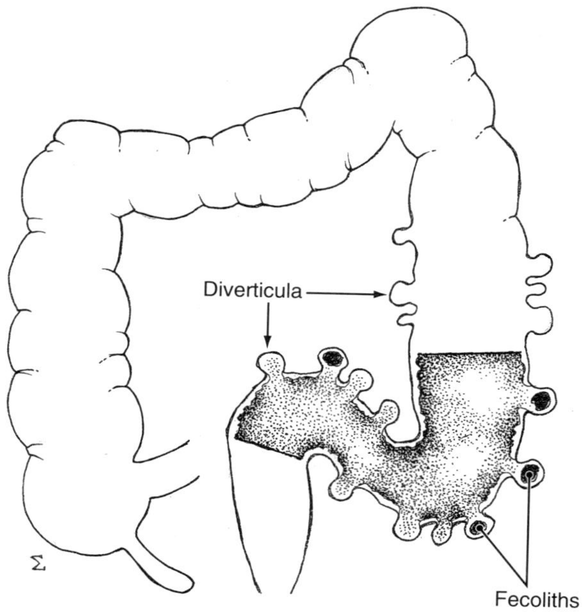

Figure 1. Diverticulitis can affect any part of the colon, although the stippled area shown (the sigmoid colon) is the most common. Of the several operations available to correct the problem, the one shown here (removal of the sigmoid and connection of the cut ends) is used most often.

POSTOPERATIVE CARE

- You will be taken to a recovery room and observed. When your blood pressure, pulse, and breathing are stable, you will be taken to a regular hospital room.
- There will be a small plastic tube in your bladder for a few days.
- That evening you will be helped to sit up in bed and on the next day to get out of bed.
- If you have a thin, plastic tube in your nose, it will be removed as soon as your bowels start working. You then will be started on a liquid to soft diet.
- Pain will be controlled with medicine.
- As with any operation, complications are always possible. With this type of operation, they can include bleeding, wound infection, leakage where the colon was reconnected, pneumonia, heart problems, and possibly others.
- You should be able to go home in about 5 days.
- Arrangements will be made for your medicine, follow-up office visit, and stitch or clip removal.

✣ HOME CARE

- You may walk about as you wish, even climb stairs, but don't overdo things.
- You will be given a suggested appropriate diet to follow during your convalescence.
- Take the medicines prescribed for you.
- Unless instructed otherwise, you may shower if you wish and with any dressings on or off. After you dry yourself, replace any dressings with clean, dry ones.
- You may return to work when you feel up to it.

✆ CALL OUR OFFICE IF

- You have any questions.
- The incision becomes red or swollen, or there is drainage from it.
- You develop a temperature higher than 100.5°F.

DUODENAL ULCER: Antrectomy and Vagotomy

△ GENERAL INFORMATION

This is an ulcer in the wall of the beginning of the *duodenum*, which is the part of the intestine just past the stomach (Fig. 1). It occurs mostly in younger and middle-aged adults and is almost never cancerous. Several causative factors for this ulcer are too much acid in the stomach, the right amount of acid but a weakened lining of the duodenum from taking certain medicines (example: aspirin), and a special type of infection. Often the reason for the ulcer is not apparent.

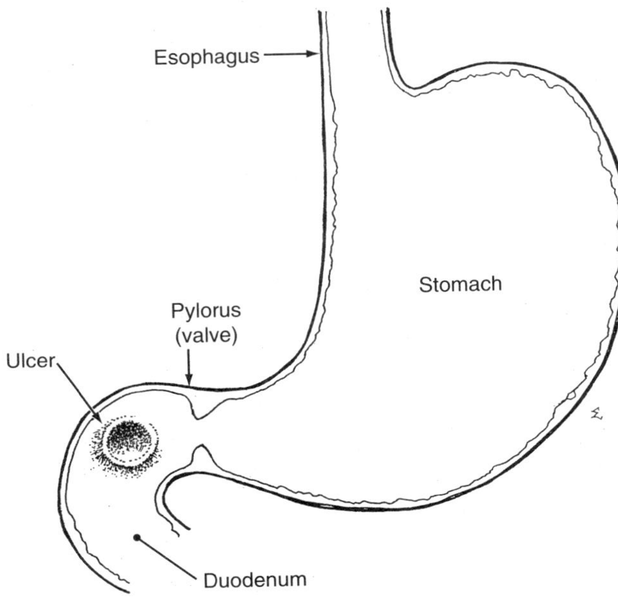

Figure 1.

COMMON SIGNS AND SYMPTOMS

- Severe boring pain in the pit of the stomach or just to the right of it. Typically, it begins 30 to 45 minutes after a meal or in the middle of the night.
- Often the pain is lessened by eating soothing or mild food or by taking medicine to block the stomach from making acid or reduce the amount of acid in the stomach. There may be nausea or vomiting, either from spasm of the stomach or from bleeding into it. With bleeding, the bowel movement becomes very dark.

DIAGNOSIS

- *Stomach x-rays (upper GI series):* Liquid barium is swallowed, and x-rays are taken of it as it goes down the esophagus into the stomach and out the duodenum. This is a way to see abnormalities such as an ulcer in this area.
- *Gastroduodenoscopy:* The surest way to make the diagnosis is by gastroduodenoscopy. This is done with a long, smooth, flexible optical instrument that has a light at its tip and is as thick as your little finger. Your mouth and throat will be sprayed with an anesthetic to make them feel numb. Also, you will be given medicine to make you feel drowsy during the procedure. The instrument will be passed gently through your mouth down to the stomach and then out to the duodenum. The entire area will be examined thoroughly.

○ TREATMENT

- Most ulcers are successfully treated medically. Some, however, may respond for only a short period or not at all to medicine and so require an operation for cure. These ulcers may hemorrhage or make a hole in the duodenum, so that an emergency operation is necessary; they may narrow or even close the outlet of the stomach, causing vomiting and weight loss. After careful consideration of all factors, it is recommended that you have an operation for your condition.
- There are several operations for this condition. The one most suitable for you is *antrectomy*. This involves removing the lower portion of the stomach and reconnecting the cut ends so that you can eat as before (Fig. 2). Also, the *vagus* nerves that stimulate the stomach to make acid are cut; this is termed *vagotomy*.

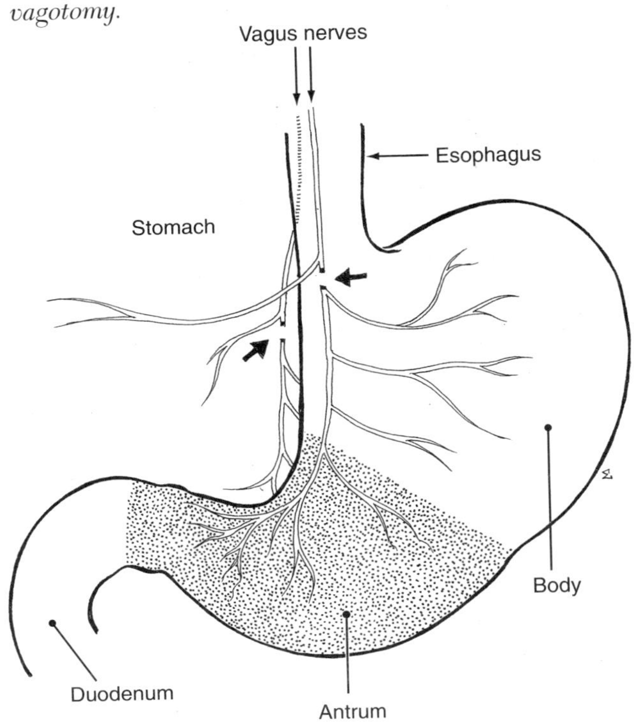

Figure 2. In this operation the distal part of the stomach (the antrum) is removed *(between the dashed lines)* and the cut ends are reconnected. The vagus nerves *(arrows)* are divided.

PREOPERATIVE PREPARATION

- You will have an examination of your blood, urine, heart (EKG), and lungs (chest x-ray).
- Do not take aspirin or anti-inflammatory agents for 1 week before the operation.
- Do not eat or drink anything for 8 hours before the operation.
- You may be given medicine that will make you feel drowsy before you are brought to the operating room.

☐ OPERATION

- You will be asleep for the operation.
- The operation usually takes about 2 hours.

POSTOPERATIVE CARE

- You will be taken to a recovery room and observed. When your blood pressure, pulse, and breathing are stable, you will be taken to a regular hospital room.
- You may have a thin plastic tube in your nose. It goes down to your stomach to suck up the air you swallow. It will be removed when your bowels start working.
- Pain will be controlled with medicine.
- That evening you will be helped to sit up in bed and on the next day to get out of bed.
- You will be given an incentive spirometer. Breathing into this as you are instructed will help you expand your lungs and reduce the risk of developing pneumonia.
- When the tube from your nose is removed, you will be started on a liquid diet and then switched to a soft diet as you tolerate it. Initially, you will need to eat small meals and to eat more often.
- You should be able to go home in about 3 to 5 days.
- Arrangements will be made for your medicine, follow-up office visit, and stitch removal.
- As with any operation, complications are always possible. With your type of operation they can include pneumonia, heart problems, poor emptying of the stomach, wound infection, and a sensation of flushing, fainting, or diarrhea after eating certain foods.

✚ HOME CARE

- Continue with the diet program started while you were in the hospital.
- You may walk about as you wish, even climb stairs, but don't overdo things.
- Take medicine as prescribed for your pain.
- Unless instructed otherwise, you may shower as you wish and with any dressings on or off. There may be narrow strips of tape across the incision. It's all right if they get wet; they will be removed in the doctor's office. After you dry yourself, replace any dressings with clean, dry ones.
- Do not drive a car unless you can move freely and without pain and are not on medicines that decrease your alertness.
- You may return to work when you feel up to it.

✆ CALL OUR OFFICE IF

- You develop any unusual signs or symptoms.
- You feel nauseated or vomit.
- The incision becomes red or swollen, or there is drainage from it.
- You develop a temperature higher than 101°F.

△ GENERAL INFORMATION

This is an ulcer in the wall of the beginning of the *duodenum*, which is the part of the intestine just past the stomach (Fig. 1). It occurs mostly in younger and middle-aged adults and is almost never cancerous. Several causative factors for this ulcer are too much acid in the stomach, the right amount of acid but a weakened lining of the duodenum from taking certain medicines (example: aspirin), and a special type of infection. Often the reason for the ulcer is not apparent.

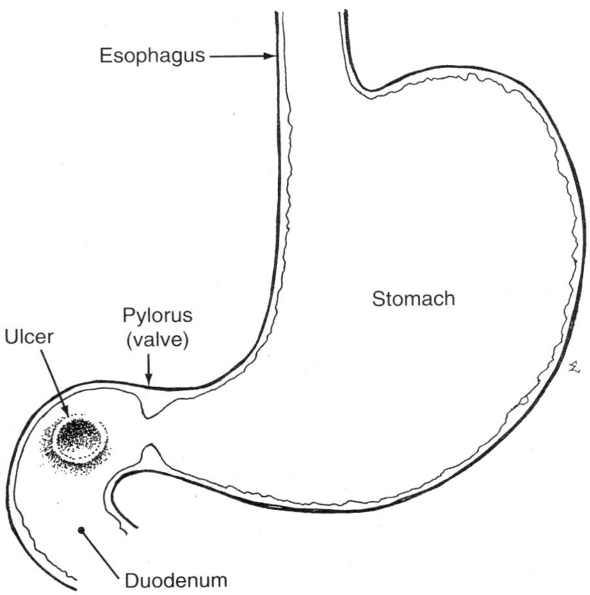

Figure 1.

COMMON SIGNS AND SYMPTOMS

- Severe boring pain in the pit of the stomach or just to the right of it. Typically, it begins 30 to 45 minutes after a meal or in the middle of the night.
- Often the pain is lessened by eating soothing or mild food or by taking medicine to block the stomach from making acid or reduce the amount of acid in the stomach. There may be nausea or vomiting, either from spasm of the stomach or from bleeding from it. With bleeding, the bowel movement becomes very dark.

DIAGNOSIS

- *Stomach x-rays (upper GI series):* Liquid barium is swallowed, and x-rays are taken of it as it goes down the esophagus into the stomach and out the duodenum. This is a way to see abnormalities such as an ulcer in this area.
- *Gastroduodenoscopy:* The surest way to make the diagnosis is by gastroduodenoscopy. This is done with a long, smooth, flexible optical instrument that has a light at its tip and is as thick as your little finger. Your mouth and throat will be sprayed with an anesthetic to make them feel numb. Also, you will be given medicine to make you feel drowsy during the procedure. The instrument will be passed gently through your mouth down to the stomach and then out to the duodenum. The entire area will be examined thoroughly.

○ TREATMENT

- Most ulcers are successfully treated medically. Some, however, may respond for only a short period or not at all to medicine and so require an operation for cure. These ulcers may hemorrhage or make a hole in the duodenum, so that an emergency operation is necessary; they may narrow or even close the outlet of the stomach, causing vomiting and weight loss. After careful consideration of all factors, it is recommended that you have an operation for your condition.
- There are several operations for this condition. The one most suitable for you is to leave the stomach and ulcer in place but to selectively cut the nerves that stimulate such high levels of acid production. This is called *highly selective vagotomy* (Fig. 2).

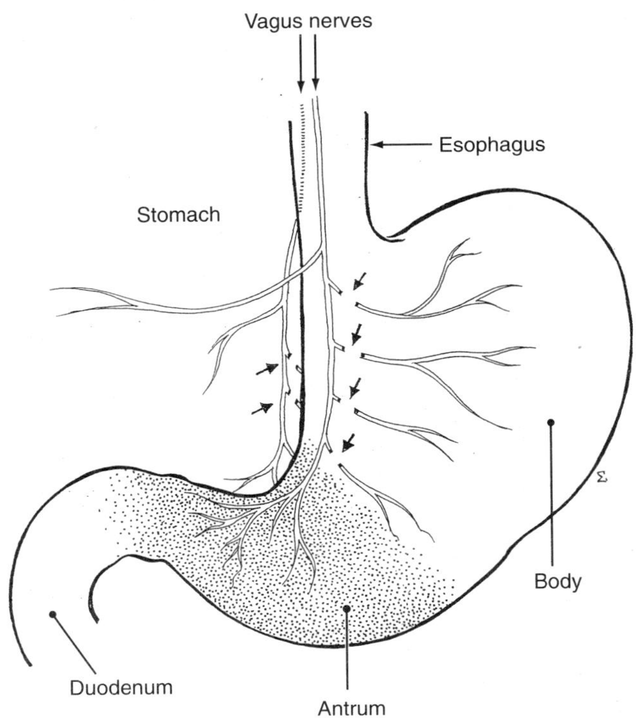

Figure 2. In this operation, no part of the stomach is removed. Instead, selected nerves that stimulate the stomach to make high levels of acid are cut *(arrows)*. The nerve supply of the distal part of the stomach *(stippled area)* is intact and can work normally.

PREOPERATIVE PREPARATION

- You will have an examination of your blood, urine, heart (EKG), and lungs (chest x-ray).
- Do not take aspirin or anti-inflammatory agents for 1 week before the operation.
- Do not eat or drink anything for 8 hours before the operation.
- You may be given medicine that will make you feel drowsy before you are brought to the operating room.

□ OPERATION

- You will be asleep for the operation.
- The operation usually takes about 2 hours.
- *Note:* Occasionally, on opening the abdomen, the conditions found are such that a highly selective vagotomy cannot be done. If that is the case with you, then removing the distal part of your stomach or widening the outlet of your stomach will be necessary.

POSTOPERATIVE CARE

- You will be taken to a recovery room and observed. When your blood pressure, pulse, and breathing are stable, you will be taken to a regular hospital room.
- You may have a thin plastic tube in your nose. It goes down to your stomach to suck up the air you swallow. It will be removed when your bowels start working.
- Pain will be controlled with medicine.
- That evening you will be helped to sit up in bed and on the next day to get out of bed.
- You will be given an incentive spirometer. Breathing into this as you are instructed will help you expand your lungs and reduce the risk of developing pneumonia.
- When the tube from your nose is removed, you will be started on a liquid diet and then switched to a soft diet as you tolerate it. Initially, you will need to eat small meals and to eat more often.
- You should be able to go home in about 3 to 5 days.
- Arrangements will be made for your medicine, follow-up office visit, and stitch removal.
- As with any operation, complications are always possible. With your type of operation they can include pneumonia, heart problems, poor emptying of the stomach, wound infection, and a sensation of flushing, fainting, or diarrhea after eating certain foods.

✚ HOME CARE

- Continue with the diet program started while you were in the hospital.
- You may walk about as you wish, even climb stairs, but don't overdo things.
- Take medicine as prescribed for your pain.
- Unless instructed otherwise, you may shower as you wish and with any dressings on or off. There may be narrow strips of tape across the incision. It's all right if they get wet; they will be removed in the doctor's office. After you dry yourself, replace any dressings with clean, dry ones.
- Do not drive a car unless you can move freely and without pain and are not on medicines that decrease your alertness.
- You may return to work when you feel up to it.

✆ CALL OUR OFFICE IF

- You develop any unusual signs or symptoms.
- You feel nauseated or vomit.
- The incision becomes red or swollen, or there is drainage from it.
- You develop a temperature higher than 101°F.

△ GENERAL INFORMATION

Dupuytren's contracture involves an abnormal thickening of the *fascia* (the tissue layer between the muscle and the skin) in the palm. Progression of this disease is unpredictable and varies from individual to individual.

Dupuytren's contracture tends to run in families, most commonly in northern Europeans. It is also associated with diabetes mellitus, medications taken for seizures, and alcohol use.

COMMON SIGNS AND SYMPTOMS

- Early in the condition, small, firm knots or nodules arise in the palm. Typically, these are not tender.
- Advanced disease results in longitudinal "cords" that run in the same direction as the fingers. They pull the fingers into the palm and do not allow them to straighten out completely (Fig. 1).
- The ring and little finger are most commonly affected.
- Tingling and numbness are not part of this condition.

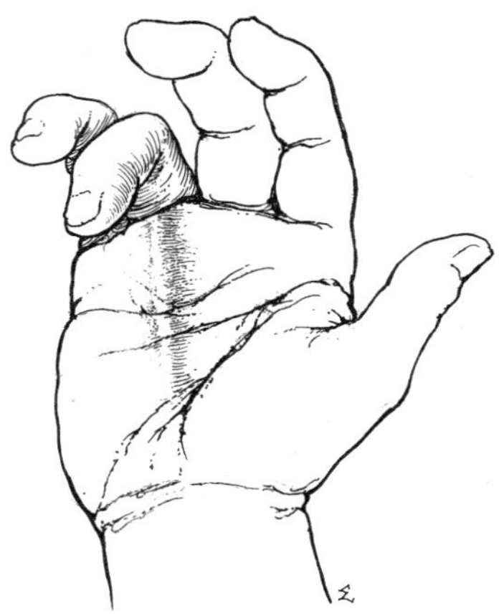

Figure 1. In this disease, scar tissue forms in the deeper tissue in the palm of the hand. As the disease progresses, the scar tissue pulls down the fingers (involvement of one finger is shown here). With even further progression, the fingers—typically the last two or three—can be pulled down severely, making it difficult to use the hand.

DIAGNOSIS

- The diagnosis is relatively straightforward. Dupuytren's contracture manifests with a characteristic history and results on physical examination.
- Special tests are not required to make the diagnosis of this condition.

○ TREATMENT

- Splinting or stretching the fingers does not change the natural history of the condition.
- Physical therapy also is not helpful in straightening out the fingers.
- When there are just nodules, they can typically be ignored. Removal of early nodules does not tend to halt progression of the disease; it can even stimulate a rapid progression of the disease.
- Cords also are typically watched until they cause the fingers to lose their ability to straighten out. Then an operation may be necessary if the bound-down fingers interfere with function of the hand.
- An operation is the only treatment available when progression of the contracture prevents acceptable function. The delicate operation consists of removal of the diseased tissue. The most difficult problem is protection of the nerves and blood vessels to the fingers as the diseased tissue is removed.

PREOPERATIVE PREPARATION

- You will have an examination of your blood and possibly your heart (EKG) before the operation.
- Do not eat or drink anything for 8 hours before the operation.
- Shower or bathe on the morning of the operation.
- You may be given medicine that will make you feel drowsy before you are brought to the operating room.

□ OPERATION

- The operation will be done either under regional anesthesia (only the arm will be made numb, and you will be given medicine to keep you drowsy) or under general anesthesia.
- During the operation, you may feel some tugging but not pain.
- The operation can be tedious and may take several hours depending on how many fingers are involved and the extent of the involvement.

POSTOPERATIVE CARE

- You will be taken to a recovery room. When your blood pressure, pulse, and breathing are stable and you are completely alert, you should be able to go home that same day with a responsible adult.
- Arrangements will be made for your medicine, follow-up office visit, and stitch removal.
- As with any operation, complications are always possible. With your type of operation, they can include damage to the nerves or blood vessels to the fingers, skin healing problems, or stiffness (loss of mobility following surgery). Also, some patients have a recurrence of the diseased tissue shortly after the operation even though the operation was done properly. Progression of the disease is again unpredictable, and excision of the tissue is not a "cure" in all patients.

✣ HOME CARE

- You may walk about as you wish, even climb stairs.
- You may shower if you wish, but you must not get the dressings wet. A method to prevent this is to fit a small plastic trash bag over your *entire* arm and seal it with tape around the open end.

- Soon after surgery you will probably be sent to a therapist. Rehabilitation is very important following most operations for Dupuytren's contracture, and you will have to work very hard to regain your finger motion and function.
- Swelling is common, and your physical therapist will work on ways to diminish this. If it increases within the first several weeks following the operation, please contact us.
- Often, the surgical wound is not closed completely. The skin can contract when the fingers are bent for a long period of time; when they then are straightened out by an operation, there may not be enough skin available for closure. Your therapist will teach you how to care for your wounds. These usually heal in a few weeks.
- Because the fingers were bent down for a long time, you will have a splint made by the therapist so that you can keep your fingers straight during the time between exercise sessions and during sleep. Often this splint is worn for many months during sleep following the operation to decrease the risk of the condition returning.

✆ CALL OUR OFFICE IF

- You develop any unusual signs or symptoms.
- The incision becomes red or swollen, or there is drainage from it.
- You develop a temperature higher than 100°F.
- You develop an increase in swelling, with stiffness and loss of motion of your fingers.
- You have any questions.

DYSPLASTIC NEVI

△ GENERAL INFORMATION

A *dysplastic nevus* is a lesion (commonly called a *mole*) that has a distinctive appearance to the naked eye and under the microscope. This appearance is not that of a malignant mole (scientifically called a *malignant melanoma*).

However, if

- A person has *many* such dysplastic nevi,
- A person with dysplastic nevi has had in the past a malignant melanoma,
- A person with dysplastic nevi has a family history of multiple dysplastic nevi or malignant melanoma,

then this person has *dysplastic nevus syndrome*. This means that the dysplastic nevi in such a person have a high risk (sometimes up to 100%) of becoming malignant over time.

The overwhelming majority of ordinary nevi are benign. Also, a person with just one dysplastic nevus and a negative family history for dysplastic nevi or malignant melanoma does not have the high risk mentioned above. However, dysplastic nevi seen under the circumstances mentioned earlier need very special attention.

COMMON SIGNS AND SYMPTOMS

- Dysplastic nevi usually do not appear in childhood but rather in puberty—age 11 or older—the same age as for ordinary moles. The exceptions are those that appear on the scalp.
- An increased number of ordinary moles beginning at age 5 to 8 years of age may be a clue that the person will develop the dysplastic nevus syndrome.

Characteristics of Dysplastic Nevi

- They are found in the same areas of the body as ordinary moles but are seen most commonly on the trunk, particularly on the back.
- Dysplastic nevi usually are larger than 5 mm (the size of the hole in a looseleaf page).
- Usually, most of the dysplastic nevus is flat with a slight bump in its center.
- The borders are fuzzy and irregular. They are described as having a "fried egg" appearance.
- They usually do not have a uniform color. The nevi may be tan to tan-brown, dark brown, or pink-brown. A pink base is especially characteristic of dysplastic nevi.
- Moles that are blue-black in color should arouse suspicion that they are malignant melanomas rather than dysplastic nevi.

DIAGNOSIS

- The diagnosis begins with a detailed, precise history of the person's skin problem, as well as a history of any problems in family members.
- There is a meticulous examination of the skin over the entire body done under fluorescent lighting.
- The exact diagnosis can be made only by examining tissue under the microscope.

○ TREATMENT

The treatment depends on what is seen, suspected, or known.

- Because dysplastic nevi are multiple (often in the many dozens), it is not reasonable or desirable to remove all of them.
- A person with multiple lesions and a positive family history should have any suspicious nevi removed. In addition, several nonsuspicious ones should be removed and examined under the microscope to document that this person has dysplastic nevus syndrome.
- If any excised dysplastic nevi have highly suspicious findings when they are examined under the microscope, they should be re-excised with wider margins around the border. The same treatment is recommended for nevi that were cut across while they were being removed.

A person with a dysplastic nevus syndrome should have the following:

- Detailed, colored, overview photographs of the entire body with close-up photographic views of individual moles. One set of photographs is kept in the medical record and the other set given to the patient. The patient and the partner or friend are taught to examine all of the lesions every month or so and to compare them with the photograph. Any changes should be promptly reported to the physician.
- Any changed lesions and all scalp lesions should be excised.

After careful consideration of all factors, the recommendation is that you have some of your lesions removed by an operation.

PREOPERATIVE PREPARATION

- Do not eat or drink anything for 4 hours before the operation.
- Shower or bathe as usual on the morning of the operation.

□ OPERATION

- The operation will be done under local anesthesia.
- The area of the nevus will be swabbed with an antiseptic solution and surrounded with sterile towels. A fine, short needle will be used to inject anesthetic to make the entire area numb. The lesion will be removed through a cosmetic incision and closed in a similar fashion. The entire specimen will be sent to the laboratory for microscopic examination.

POSTOPERATIVE CARE

- You will be taken to a recovery room and observed. When your blood pressure, pulse, and breathing are stable and you are completely alert, you should be able to go home that same day with a responsible adult.
- Arrangements will be made for your medicine, follow-up office visit, and stitch removal.

✚ HOME CARE

- Resume your usual activities.
- Take medicine as prescribed for your pain.
- You may shower if you wish and with any dressings on or off.
  - There may be narrow strips of tape across the incision. It's all right if they get wet; they will be removed in the doctor's office.
  - After you dry yourself, replace any dressings with clean, dry ones.
- Do not drive if you are taking any medicines that might reduce your alertness.
- You may return to work when you feel up to it.

✆ CALL OUR OFFICE IF

- There is bleeding from the incision.
- The incision becomes red or swollen, or there is drainage from it.
- You develop a temperature higher than 100°F.
- You have any questions.

LONG-TERM CARE

- You will need to be examined at regular intervals, even if you believe nothing further is wrong with your skin.
- Minimize exposure to the sun. Avoid sunburn. When out in the sun, use a strong sunscreen.
- Persons with the dysplastic nevus syndrome should have members of their family (parents, brothers and sisters, and children 10 years of age or older) examined.

△ GENERAL INFORMATION

Echocardiography comes from "echo" (bouncing back of sound waves), "cardio" (the heart), and "graphy" (a picture). It refers to a group of tests that use ultrasound to examine the heart and record the data (as a picture) that bounce back from the heart.

Echocardiography is an accurate and reliable method of examining the heart muscle, its valves, and its function without having to enter the person's body. It is called a *noninvasive* test.

HOW ECHOCARDIOGRAPHY WORKS

Echocardiography uses high-frequency sound waves called *ultrasound*. These are harmless sound waves that cannot be heard; they can be picked up only by special sensors. The sound waves vibrate many thousands of times per second (the *pitch*), and these vibrations can be adjusted as necessary. The sound waves bouncing back (the *echoes*) from the heart structures are converted into pictures on a small television screen.

THE ECHOES

The electronic and computer equipment that sends out the sound waves toward the heart also collects and analyzes the echoes. When the information is electronically processed it can determine the following:

- The overall size of the heart.
- The thickness of the heart walls and valves.
- The overall movement and function of the heart.

Doppler Scanning: The direction and speed of blood flow in the heart and through the valves are determined by color flow Doppler signals, generated by echoes bouncing back from moving red blood cells in the heart. Color Doppler scanning is a routine part of an echocardiogram. This makes it possible to determine the following:

- Whether there is any restriction to the normal flow of blood through the heart chambers or valves (as occurs with a heart valve *stenosis*).
- Whether there is any abnormal leaking through a heart valve (valve insufficiency).
- Whether there is any abnormal flow of blood between the heart chambers.

HOW THE TEST IS DONE

- No advance preparation is necessary.
- You will be asked to disrobe from the waist up and put on a gown that can be opened in the front.
- You will be positioned on a comfortable table on your left side or back.
- Lubricating jelly, which improves sound transmission, will be applied on the skin of your chest. The gadget (called a *probe*) that sends out the sound waves is as big as a pack of cigarettes. It is connected to the ultrasound machine.
- The probe is placed on the chest over the heart and moderately firm pressure is applied, but this is not painful. The ultrasound beam penetrates the skin and muscle over your heart. The probe is aimed at your heart, and the echoes that are received are transformed into pictures. The reason the probe is moved to various spots and you are asked to change position is to be able to get the sound waves to reach the heart and bounce back without bumping into any solid objects such as bones along the way. When they do bump into objects, the resulting picture is not clear. Air in your lungs keeps the sound waves from getting to the heart, so you may be asked to hold your breath at times or to slow down your breathing.
- The procedure is done on an outpatient basis. The findings will be analyzed by a specialist and the results reported to your doctor.

OTHER USES OF SOUND WAVES TO STUDY THE HEART AND VESSELS

Intraoperative: When a person has an open heart operation and is asleep under general anesthesia, the surgeon can place the ultrasound probe directly on the heart or near the heart (by way of the esophagus, your swallowing tube) to examine its insides before it is opened. At the end of the operation and while the person is still in the operating room, the heart can be checked again.

Heart Size and Condition: A thin tube the size of spaghetti with an ultrasound probe at its tip can be placed in a vein or artery and advanced into the heart. The sound waves and echoes can be used to measure the size of the heart chambers and the condition of its valves. This is *invasive* echocardiography because the probe enters the inside of the heart.

Vessel Measurement: A tube the size of spaghetti with a probe that sends sound waves in all directions can be positioned in a coronary artery during a heart catheterization (also an invasive use of ultrasound). The sound waves strike the inside of the artery and bounce back. With this technique, it is possible to determine the condition of the wall of an artery. This is called *intravascular ultrasound*.

As you can see, the use of sound waves to examine the heart and blood vessels is a way to get information never before possible and with minimal risk. Ultrasound makes it possible for the surgeon to perform an operation more safely and with greater likelihood of success.

△ GENERAL INFORMATION

Empyema is a collection of infected fluid in the chest cavity. It can follow a number of conditions and includes the following:

- Pneumonia that infects the chest cavity as well as the lungs.
- A lung abscess that has ruptured and spilled its pus into the entire chest cavity.
- Infection that came up through the diaphragm from an abscess below.
- Infection that was introduced by a needle puncture or some foreign body associated with trauma.

COMMON SIGNS AND SYMPTOMS

- Persistent fever, especially following a lung infection.
- Evidence of infection after a lung operation.
- Difficulty with breathing.

DIAGNOSIS

- A chest x-ray shows that fluid is present.
- Usually the diagnosis can be made by taking a detailed history, doing a thorough physical examination, and considering the laboratory reports carefully.
- Some fluid from the chest is withdrawn with a needle and syringe to see which bacteria are present and to which antibiotic they may respond (a *culture*).
- CT scan (computed tomography scan): These special x-rays are taken by a machine that is shaped like a huge doughnut. You will lie on the table inside the hole in the "doughnut." The x-rays are taken as half-inch slices through the chest and upper part of the abdomen. This makes it possible to see the fine details in the organs in and below the chest cavity.

○ TREATMENT

There are several ways to treat empyema. They depend on the cause of the empyema, how long it has been present, any previous therapy, response to this type of therapy, and the condition of the person with empyema.

Medical: The first treatment should be antibiotic therapy—if possible, with an antibiotic that is known to be effective against the bacteria found in the fluid.

Needle Aspiration: Removing all the fluid in the chest with a needle. This is easier if the infected fluid is thin. This technique is successful about 15% of the time.

Tube Drainage: The skin over the chest is painted with an antiseptic solution and surrounded by sterile towels. The skin then is made numb by injecting an anesthetic with a fine, short needle. A small flexible plastic tube is placed through the skin into the chest cavity. Suction is then applied to the tube to remove the infected fluid. Sometimes the chest cavity is also rinsed with an antibiotic solution.

Thoracotomy: In more involved cases, an operation may be necessary to open the chest to remove the infected substance, because it has clotted and wrapped itself around the lung, preventing it from expanding.

Your condition is such that you do need an operation. The reasons for this have been explained to you.

PREOPERATIVE PREPARATION

- You will have an examination of your blood, urine, heart (EKG), and lungs (chest x-ray).
- Do not eat or drink anything for 8 hours before the operation.
- Shower as usual on the morning of the operation.
- You may be given medicine that will make you feel drowsy before you are brought to the operating room.

□ OPERATION

- You will be asleep for the operation.
- You will not receive a blood transfusion unless it is absolutely necessary.
- The operation usually takes 3 hours.

POSTOPERATIVE CARE

- You will be taken to the Surgical Care Unit, where the doctors and nurses are very experienced in taking care of patients like yourself. As soon as you are coming along well enough, you will be transferred to a regular hospital room.
- There will be one or two clear plastic tubes coming from your chest for several days to drain any further fluid that may accumulate.
- That evening you will be helped to sit up in bed and on the next day to get out of bed.
- Pain can be controlled with medicine. The nurse will give it to you. Or you can give yourself a preset amount of pain medicine when you feel you need it. This is done with a device for patient-controlled analgesia (PCA) that is connected to the tubing giving you intravenous fluids.
- You will be given an incentive spirometer. Breathing into this as you are instructed will help you expand your lungs and reduce the risk of developing pneumonia.
- Your diet will be as you tolerate it.
- You will be able to go home when your chest condition is stable and continuing to improve.
- As with any operation, complications are always possible. With this type of operation, they can include continued drainage of pus, heart problems, leakage of air from the surface of the lung, and possibly others.
- Arrangements will be made for your medicine, follow-up office visit, and stitch removal.

✚ HOME CARE

- Continue with the program started while you were in the hospital.
- You may walk about as you wish, even climb stairs.
- You may eat as you did before the operation.

- Occasionally the tube coming from your chest is left in place to drain even more fluid that needs to come out. You will be shown how to change the dressings; it's not difficult.
- You may shower as you wish and with any dressings on or off.
  - There may be narrow strips of tape across the incision. It's all right if they get wet; they will be removed in the doctor's office.
  - After you dry yourself, replace any dressings with clean, dry ones.
- Don't lift anything heavier than 5 pounds. Ask someone to do it for you.
- You can help "loosen" your shoulder by using your arm on the side of the incision. Also, a good exercise is to stand next to a wall and "climb up" the wall with your hand.
- Walking and otherwise moving about—in moderation—is good for your circulation, your breathing, and your muscle tone. Remain active as long as it doesn't hurt you or tire you.
- Driving a car with an automatic shift is not too demanding. However, if you suddenly have to slam on the brakes or twist to turn the steering wheel, you may get into an accident. Or you may strain the sutures or tear something. During your follow-up visit, let's discuss when you can resume driving.
- You may resume sexual activity whenever you choose.
- You may return to work when you feel up to it, but let's first talk about it during your follow-up office visit.

✆ CALL OUR OFFICE IF

- You develop any unusual signs or symptoms.
- The incision becomes red or swollen, or there is drainage from it.
- You develop a temperature higher than 101°F.
- You have any questions.

△ GENERAL INFORMATION

This is a condition in which the tissue lining the inside of the uterus (the *endometrium*) is found in places *outside* the uterus, mostly in the pelvis (Fig. 1). Endometriosis is seen in younger women. The cause is not truly known.

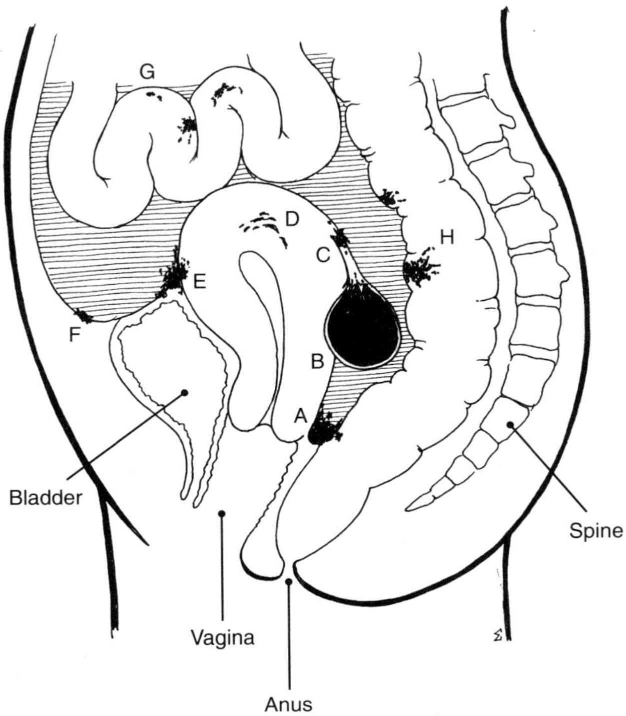

Figure 1. Tissue that normally lines the inside surface of the uterus (the *endometrium*) can, in some patients, be found outside the uterus. Most commonly, this tissue is found in the pelvis, although it can be anywhere in the abdominal cavity, and even, occasionally, outside the abdominal cavity. A, Behind the uterus (posterior cul-de-sac); B, old blood collected in the ovary forms a cyst; C, in the fallopian tube; D, in the wall of the uterus; E, between the uterus and the bladder; F, on the lining (peritoneum) of the abdominal wall; G, on the surface of the small intestine; H, surface of the colon.

COMMON SIGNS AND SYMPTOMS

- Mild (to severe) pain in the pelvis shortly before and usually during the first few days of the menstrual period.
- Low back pain.
- Pain during sexual intercourse.
- Abdominal cramps.

DIAGNOSIS

- In a young woman with a number of the above symptoms, the diagnosis can be suspected, but usually it is necessary to follow the patient for a while to be fairly certain.
- Some or all the following tests will need to be done:
  - *Laparoscopy*: It is done with a *laparoscope* that is an optical instrument about as big around as your little finger with a light at its tip. Under general anesthesia, a small incision is made at your navel, and the instrument is inserted into the abdomen. All the organs inside the pelvis can be looked at directly. If necessary, a small piece of tissue is taken (a *biopsy*) for examination in the laboratory.
  - *Ultrasound*: Harmless sound waves are aimed at the area of your pelvis. The sound waves bouncing back (the echoes) from this area are seen as a picture on a screen. Ultrasound is a convenient and painless way to examine organs and tissues in the pelvis.
  - *CT scan (computed tomography scan)*: These special x-rays are taken by a machine that is shaped like a huge doughnut. You will lie on a table inside the hole in the "doughnut." The x-rays are taken as half-inch slices through the area of your pelvis. This makes it possible to see fine details in the tissues in your pelvis.

○ TREATMENT

- Treatment depends on how much and where the endometriosis is located, your age, and whether you wish to have children (because in severe cases one of the treatments is to remove the uterus and ovaries).
- Generally, nonprescription pain medicines can help make the symptoms tolerable.

Hormone Therapy: A number of combinations of hormones can be effective. All of them have some side effect on most patients. The condition may come back when these hormones are stopped.

Surgical Therapy: Several operations are available for specific situations:

- Through the laparoscope, areas in the pelvis that cause the most trouble can be treated with laser.
- Sometimes the ovaries become ballooned *(cystic)* and painful from the old blood building up in them each month. Part, or all, of the ovaries can be removed by an operation.
- The uterus, tubes and ovaries can be removed.

After careful consideration, the recommendation is that you have an operation.

PREOPERATIVE PREPARATION

- You will have an examination of your blood, urine, heart (EKG), and lungs (chest x-ray).
- Do not eat or drink anything for 8 hours before the operation.
- Do not douche or use a tampon on the day of the operation.

□ OPERATION

- The planned operation was discussed with you in detail during your office visit.
- You will be asleep during the operation.

POSTOPERATIVE CARE

- You will be taken to a recovery room and observed. When your blood pressure, pulse, and breathing are stable, you will be taken to a regular hospital room.

- That evening you will be helped to sit up in bed and on the next day to get out of bed.
- Pain will be controlled with medicine.
- You should be able to go home in about 2 to 4 days.
- As with any operation, complications are always possible. Although they are uncommon with your type of operation, they can include wound infection, bleeding, and injury to the intestines, among others.
- Arrangements will be made for your medicine, follow-up office visit, and stitch removal.

✥ HOME CARE

- You may walk about as you wish, even climb stairs.
- Take medicine as prescribed for your pain.
- You may eat as you did before the operation.
- Unless instructed otherwise, you may shower as you wish and with any dressings on or off. There may be narrow strips of tape across the incision. It's all right if they get wet. They will be removed in the doctor's office. After you dry yourself, replace any dressings with clean, dry ones.
- Include plenty of roughage and liquids in your diet to help avoid constipation.
- Do not drive a car until you can move freely and without pain.
- You may return to work when you feel up to it.
- At your follow-up visit let's talk about when you can resume sexual intercourse.

✆ CALL OUR OFFICE IF

- You develop any unusual signs or symptoms.
- The incision becomes red or swollen, or there is drainage from it.
- You develop a temperature higher than 100°F.

△ GENERAL INFORMATION

Enteroclysis is the x-ray examination of the entire small intestine with barium. Some indications for enteroclysis include the following: to determine whether there is a partial small bowel obstruction; to confirm the presence of Crohn's disease and to determine its extent; to help diagnose and evaluate a malabsorption state; to try to discover the cause of obscure gastrointestinal bleeding; and to evaluate the status of the small intestine in patients, who should not be exposed to a long and tiring customary small bowel follow-through.

PREPARATION FOR THE EXAMINATION

The following is one way to adjust your diet in preparation for the examination.

On the Day before the Examination: (1) Have a light meatless breakfast. (2) For the rest of the day have only a *clear* liquid diet. Do not eat or drink any dairy products. (3) Drink one 8-ounce glass of water at 1:00, 2:00, 3:00, 4:00, 5:00, and 7:00 P.M. and at bedtime. (4) At 6:00 P.M. drink a cold, full (10-ounce) bottle of citrate of magnesia. (5) At 8:00 P.M. swallow whole four Dulcolax tablets with a glass of water.

On the Morning of the Examination: Do not eat, drink, smoke, or chew gum.

THE EXAMINATION

- You will be asked to remove your outer clothing and put on a gown.
- You will have a preliminary x-ray of your abdomen.
- Your throat and nose will be sprayed with an anesthetic solution to make them numb.
- A thin, flexible plastic tube will be lubricated and passed through your nose and down your esophagus into the stomach and then just past the stomach into the duodenum.
- You will be positioned on an x-ray table.
- Liquid barium (it has the color and consistency of buttermilk) will be inserted through the tube. The barium will proceed down the small intestine.
- You may develop a full feeling during this time. Taking deep breaths may help you relax.
- X-rays will be taken as the barium travels down the length of the small intestine.
- The table on which you will lie and the x-ray machine over it will move in several directions during the examination. Also, you will be asked to roll from side-to-side as well as to lie on your abdomen.
- During the examination, mild pressure will be applied to your abdomen with a compression device.
- The x-rays will be taken at intervals as determined by the radiologist and until all of the intestine has been examined. The examination generally takes about 30 to 45 minutes.

AFTER THE EXAMINATION

- After the examination you are free to go about your business as usual.
- Drink more than the average amount of fluid. This will help prevent you from becoming constipated.
- The next bowel movement or two will be white in color because of the barium.

All of the x-rays taken during the examination will be assembled and evaluated with care. The results will be discussed with you when they are available.

△ GENERAL INFORMATION

When a patient has pain after an operation, the medicine to relieve it usually is given as a shot in the arm or buttocks or as a pill by mouth. The pain medicine thus has an effect, but it is throughout the entire body even though the pain is in only one area of the body. Very commonly, when medicine is given this way the patient is not inclined to breathe deeply, feels sleepy, and feels unable or unwilling to do much except doze off. Such effects from pain medicine often prevent a patient from doing all the things necessary to bring about a speedy recovery. *Epidural analgesia* is a method of relieving the pain mostly where it exists and sparing the rest of the body from the effects of this medicine.

HOW EPIDURAL ANALGESIA WORKS

The *spinal column* goes from the skull to the waist. It is made up of bones *(vertebrae)* that are shaped somewhat like 1-inch slices of salami and that are stacked one on top of the other. In the back of the vertebrae is a tunnel that is as big as the tip of your little finger. Through this tunnel runs the *spinal cord*. The spinal cord is surrounded by a thin but tough sleeve of tissue (the *dura*). Inside the dura is the spinal fluid (as well as the spinal cord).

On its way downward, the spinal cord gives off nerve branches on both sides. These nerves go through the dura and then to the various parts of your body. They carry sensation (including the sensation of pain) back to the brain. In turn, the brain can signal down the spinal cord and out through these nerves to make the muscles move.

With epidural analgesia, the anesthetic medicine is placed around the particular nerves as they come out through the dura to carry sensations from the brain to your body and to carry sensations of pain from the body back to the brain.

OPERATIONS FOR WHICH EPIDURAL ANESTHESIA IS COMMONLY USED

- Hip, leg, knee, and foot operations.
- Abdominal operations.
- Lung surgery.
- Vascular operations inside the abdomen or the legs.

In general, postoperative epidural analgesia can be used for operations of the chest, abdomen, and lower body.

Some patients may especially benefit from epidural analgesia as opposed to pain medicine by vein or mouth.

- Patients with emphysema, difficulty breathing, or lung problems.
- Patients who have poor circulation to the legs.
- Patients who are having knee or hip surgery that requires physical therapy or a continuous motion machine after the operation.

THE PROCEDURE

- The anesthesiologist may have you sit upright or lie on your side.
- An antiseptic solution will be swabbed over your back and the area surrounded with sterile towels.
- A small amount of local anesthetic will be used to numb the skin.
- A special needle will be placed through the numbed skin and between the vertebrae to just outside the dura. A very fine plastic catheter (tube) will be passed through the needle so that the tip of the catheter lies just next to the nerves. The needle is now removed. The tip of the catheter is right next to the nerves, and the other end of the catheter is to the outside (Fig. 1).
- Occasionally a person feels a twinge of pain for a second or two when this is done.
- The catheter is taped securely in place. You can lie on your back without causing harm to yourself or damage to the tube.
- The catheter is now ready for use. Anesthetic medicine can be injected into it slowly as necessary. This medicine will bathe the nerves that surround it.

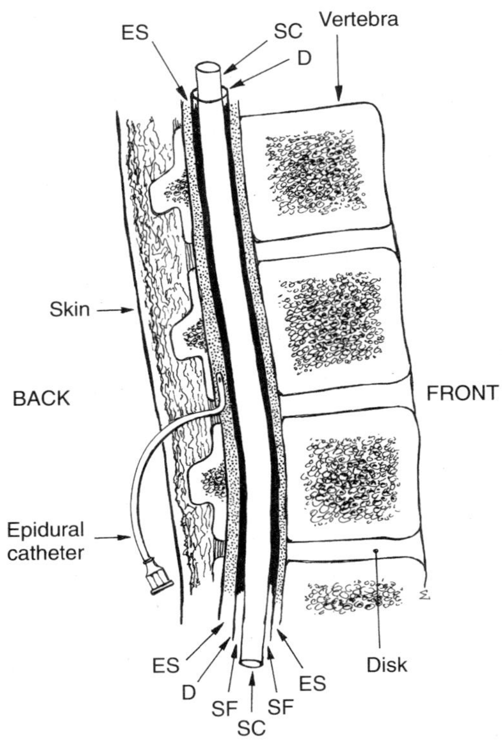

Figure 1. The epidural catheter is positioned as shown either in the operating room before the operation is started or after it is completed, or at any time in the postoperative period. ES, Epidural space; D, dura; SF, spinal fluid; SC, spinal cord.

CONDITIONS IN WHICH EPIDURAL ANALGESIA IS USUALLY NOT USED

- When patients are taking blood thinners such as heparin or warfarin (Coumadin).
- When patients have had previous extensive back surgery.

WHAT TO EXPECT AFTER YOUR OPERATION WHILE THE EPIDURAL CATHETER IS IN PLACE

- You will be comfortable but not totally numb.
- You will be more alert than if you had your pain medicine by needle or by mouth.
- If you feel discomfort, promptly tell the nurse. The infusion medicine may be increased; if you are experiencing numbness, the medicine may be decreased.
- You may need a catheter to drain your bladder because you may not feel the need to empty your bladder on your own.
- The epidural catheter may be removed in 1 to 3 days following the operation.
- Some patients experience a mild amount of itching. If this happens, you'll be given medicine to decrease it.
- Your leg muscles may not be working at their best. Please do not get out of bed without help.

COMPLICATIONS

As with any procedure, complications are always possible. Although they are most uncommon with this type of procedure, they may include headache, injury to a nerve, bleeding, and possibly others.

As you see, postoperative epidural analgesia is a safe and effective way to control your pain after an operation and at the same time make it possible for you to be more alert. This in turn gives you a better chance for an improved and safer recovery.

△ GENERAL INFORMATION

These are injections of steroids (cortisone medicines) into the space just outside the covering (the *dura*) of the spinal cord. Because the injection is outside *(epi)* the dura, it is called an *epidural* injection. This procedure has nothing to do with spinal anesthesia used for operations.

The spinal cord travels from the brain to the waist in a tunnel in the back part of the spine. About every inch along the way, the spinal cord gives off branches to the right and left. These branches carry sensations from the brain to various parts of the body to make things move. Also, these branches send back a variety of sensations (e.g., pain) through the cord and then to the brain (Fig. 1).

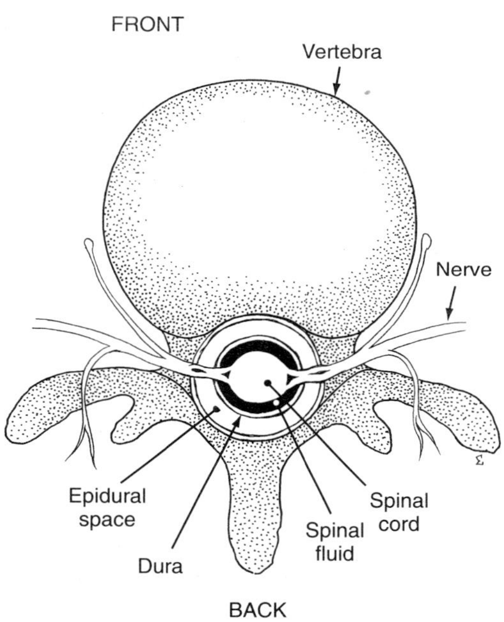

Figure 1.

These injections are performed when it is thought that inflammation is part of the process that causes the pain. A steroid medicine, which is a very potent anti-inflammatory drug, works best when it is injected into the area where the inflammation is occurring. Because the nerves of the spinal cord pass through the epidural space, the medicine comes in contact with them. The injections can be made anywhere along the spine: neck *(cervical)*, midback *(thoracic)*, lower back *(lumbar)*, and tailbone *(caudal)*.

PERSONS WHO MAY BENEFIT

Epidural injections are considered after the usual medicines have been tried and no longer are helpful. They are performed most commonly for people who suffer neck or back pain caused by herniated disk, degenerated disk, arthritis of the facet joints, or spinal stenosis.

PREPARATION FOR EPIDURAL INJECTION

- You will need to have a general evaluation by your primary doctor.
- Usually, an MRI or a CT scan of the affected area is done to be certain that there is not something unexpected or unusual causing the pain.
  - *MRI (magnetic resonance imaging)*: No x-rays are used with this technique. Instead, it is done with harmless magnetic fields and radio waves. A computer develops the pictures to show organs from several angles. It is especially valuable for examining your blood vessels, nerves, and bone tissue.
  - *CT scan (computed tomography scan)*: These special x-rays are taken as very thin slices through the area in question. A CT scan makes it possible to see the fine details in the nerves and bones in this area.
- Do not eat or drink anything for 8 hours before the procedure.
- Arrange for someone to drive you home afterward.

PROCEDURE

- You will be awake and not sedated during the procedure.
- You will probably be asked either to lie on your side or to sit up for this procedure.
- You will be asked to curl up so that the area of the spine is curved outward as much as possible.
- Your back will be prepared with an antiseptic solution, and the affected area will be surrounded with sterile towels.
- A short, thin needle will be used to inject an anesthetic into the skin to make it numb.
- The epidural needle will then be inserted through the numbed skin and advanced slowly. When the epidural space is reached, the injection will take a few seconds and the needle will be withdrawn.
- You will be asked to lie down on the side of your body that is most affected.

AFTER THE PROCEDURE

- Your blood pressure, pulse, and breathing will be checked frequently over the next 15 to 20 minutes. When they are stable, you should be able to go home directly with a responsible adult.
- If a local anesthetic was used along with the steroid, you may experience some *temporary* numbness and possibly weakness in the affected arm or leg.
- The effect of the steroid medicine may not begin for 24 to 72 hours.
- Occasionally, the steroid is irritating and may even temporarily worsen your pain. Your usual pain medicine should be sufficient to deal with this.
- Slowly resume your usual activities.

POSSIBLE COMPLICATIONS

As with any procedure, complications are always possible, some serious. With this procedure, they can include the following:

- A headache over the next day or two.
- During injections, some patients have a lowering of their blood pressure and pulse and may feel nauseated or faint. If this occurs, lying down and resting usually will allow things to correct themselves. Occasionally, however, fluids need to be started by vein and medication given.
- Diabetics will notice their blood sugar rising for several days after the injection and may require adjustment in their medications or diet.
- Rarely, *temporary* weakness and a drop in blood pressure occurs. Fluids may need to be started in your vein and possibly medicines given to minimize these symptoms.
- Very rarely, there may be bleeding into the epidural space. This is a very serious complication that may require an emergency operation to prevent paralysis from occurring.

FOLLOW-UP

Often, more than one epidural injection is required. However, a maximum of 3 to 6 months is the limit, usually at 2-week intervals.

ERCP (ENDOSCOPIC RETROGRADE CHOLANGIOPANCREATOGRAPHY)

△ GENERAL INFORMATION

ERCP stands for *endoscopic* (passing a tube into a cavity) *retrograde* (doing it against the main stream) *cholangio* (the bile ducts) *pancreato* (the pancreas duct) *graphy* (a picture). ERCP is a way to look at your bile ducts, pancreatic ducts, and pancreas. First, look at the illustration and you'll understand things better (Fig. 1).

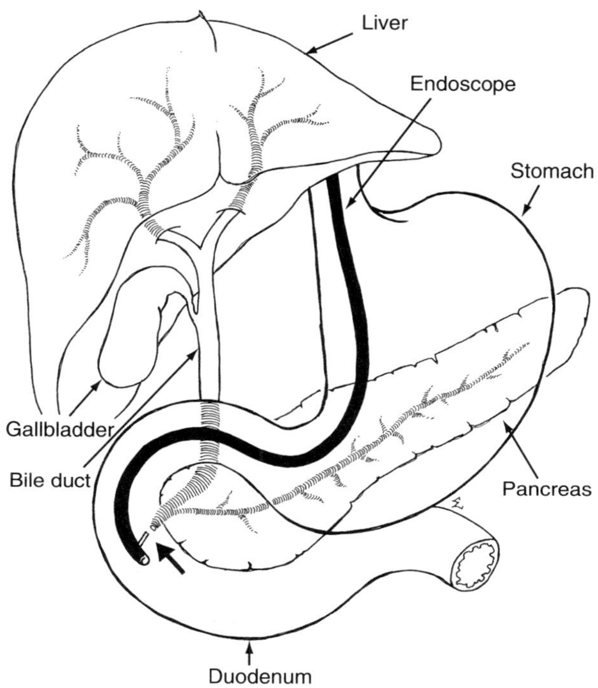

Figure 1. The endoscope is placed in the mouth and advanced down the esophagus into the stomach and then to the duodenum. The tip of the endoscope is positioned just opposite the opening of the bile duct, and a short side arm is extended from it, facing the opening. A very thin plastic tube coming from the side arm *(bold arrow)* can then be placed into the bile duct. Dye is injected through this tube into the bile ducts, and x-rays are taken as it flows throughout the duct.

The bile ducts start inside the liver, and when they reach the outside they combine as a main duct (the *common bile duct*) that is about as big around as a pencil. This duct goes down about another inch and gives off a small side duct that connects with the gallbladder. The common duct continues along about 2 more inches and empties into the first part of the small intestine called the *duodenum*. Just where the common bile duct enters the duodenum is a circular muscle *(sphincter of Oddi)* that acts as a valve.

Nearby is the *pancreas*. One thing the pancreas does is make juices to help you digest the fats and proteins you eat. These juices empty from the pancreas through a tube or duct that also drains into the duodenum. The duct that drains the pancreas and the bile duct join and enter the duodenum at the same spot.

CONDITIONS THAT MAY NEED ERCP

- There is some type of blockage of the bile duct.
- There is a stone in the bile duct that needs to be removed.
- There is a certain type of jaundice (yellow skin and eyes).
- The sphincter of Oddi at the end of the bile duct is too tight.
- The common duct is blocked by some type of growth.
- There is some type of blockage of the pancreas duct.
- There might be leakage of fluid from the bile duct or pancreas duct.

After careful consideration of all the factors relating to your problem, it is recommended that you have an ERCP.

PREPARATION FOR ERCP

- You will have an examination of your blood.
- Do not eat or drink anything for 8 hours before the procedure.
- Shower as usual on the morning of the procedure.
- You will be given medicine that will make you feel drowsy before you are brought to the procedure room.

□ OPERATION

- The ERCP is done with an *endoscope*. This is a long, smooth, flexible, instrument about as big around as the tip of your little finger. It has lenses as well as a light at its tip. Also, very thin cables with tiny instruments attached to them can be passed through the endoscope to come out at its tip. These instruments can be used to work on the tissue in front of the tip of the endoscope.
- Your mouth and throat will be sprayed with an anesthetic to make them numb. Also, you will be given some medicine to make you relaxed and sleepy just before the procedure is started. The endoscope will be lubricated and then gently inserted into your throat and passed down the esophagus into the stomach. There, the endoscope will be passed into the duodenum just to the spot where the common bile duct and pancreas duct empty into it.
- A very thin tube will then be pushed out of the end of the endoscope and advanced up the common bile duct or pancreas duct. Dye will be injected through this thin tube and x-ray pictures taken of the ducts. Sometimes it may not be possible to get pictures of the ducts this way.
- A number of things can now be done, depending on what is found to be the problem:
  - Stones can be removed.
  - The sphincter of Oddi can be cut to loosen it.
  - Sometimes a tube can be left in place to make it possible for juices to get past a blocked area or to fix areas of leakage.

- Some problems that might be found cannot be corrected with the endoscope.

The entire procedure takes about 1 hour. However, because of the medicines given, many patients remember little of the procedure and think it took just a few minutes.

POSTOPERATIVE CARE

- You will wake up in a recovery room. When your blood pressure, pulse, and breathing are stable and you are completely alert, you should be able to go home that same day with a responsible adult. If it is necessary to cut some muscle fibers to loosen the sphincter of Oddi, you may need to stay overnight.
- Wait until the numbness in your throat is gone completely (about 1–2 hours) before you eat anything. Otherwise, fluid or food might go down your windpipe and lungs.
- You will have some pain in the back of your throat with swallowing for several days.
- As with any operation, complications are always possible. Although they are uncommon with this type of operation, they can include damage to your esophagus, stomach, intestine, or bile duct. There may be a flare-up of your liver, pancreas, or bile duct problem. There can be bleeding or infection.

✚ HOME CARE

- Resume your usual activities.
- You may eat as you did before the operation.

✆ CALL OUR OFFICE IF

- You develop abdominal pain, feel nauseated, or vomit.
- You develop any unusual signs or symptoms.
- You develop a temperature higher than 100°F.
- You have any questions.

WHAT IS AN ESOPHAGOSCOPY?

An *esophagoscopy* is looking directly down the esophagus with a special instrument (an *esophagoscope*). Esophagoscopy is a very important procedure used to find out what is actually wrong when a person has a problem with the esophagus. The esophagus is about 11 inches long. Most often the esophagus is examined along with the stomach and duodenum.

HOW CAN ESOPHAGOSCOPY HELP?

The following are some of the ways esophagoscopy can be helpful:

- Determine the cause of difficult or painful swallowing.
- Determine whether narrowing of the esophagus is from scar tissue or from some problem with its muscles.
- Determine the cause of inflammation that may be present as heartburn.
- Look for the cause of bleeding.
- Remove an accidentally swallowed foreign body that is stuck in the esophagus.
- Investigate a possible tear in the esophagus.
- Help verify the diagnosis of hiatal hernia.

PREPARATION FOR AN ESOPHAGOSCOPY

- A detailed history and a thorough physical examination will be done.
- For most examinations, there should be no drinking or eating for 8 hours before the procedure. If there is serious narrowing and fluid cannot get by easily or may still be there, you should not drink or eat anything for a longer period.
- Before the esophagoscopy, an x-ray of the esophagus with barium in it will be taken for a general look.

INSTRUMENTS

There are two types of esophagoscope.

- **Flexible esophagoscope:** This is an optical instrument with a light at its tip that is smooth, flexible, and about as big around as the tip of your little finger.

Its advantages are as follows:

  - It is flexible so that it can bend around curves more easily.
  - It is thinner and easier to use.

Its disadvantages are the following:

  - It does not stretch a narrowed esophagus quite as well as a rigid esophagoscope.

- **Rigid esophagoscope:** This is a rigid tube about as thick around as your index finger with a light at its tip.

Its advantages are as follows:

  - Things can be seen more directly.
  - Narrowed areas can be stretched more easily and safely.

Its disadvantages are the following:

  - It cannot go around curves.
  - It requires greater skill to use.
  - It potentially has a greater risk of injury.

The doctor doing your esophagoscopy will know which type of instrument to use and how to use it.

THE ESOPHAGOSCOPY

- Some fluids will be started in your vein.
- You will be given some medicine that will make you feel drowsy before you are brought into the endoscopy room.
- Your mouth and throat will be sprayed with an anesthetic to make them numb.
- You will be given some medicine through the vein to keep you drowsy during the procedure.
- The esophagoscope will be placed gently into your mouth and down your esophagus. It will examine everything carefully as it travels down and back up your esophagus. If anything suspicious is seen, a small piece of it (a *biopsy*) can be taken for examination in the laboratory.
- Unless there is a specific reason not to do so, the esophagoscope customarily is advanced into the stomach and (if a flexible esophagoscope is used) just past it into the duodenum so that they too can be examined for any unsuspected problem.
- When the examination is complete, the esophagoscope is removed.
- The medicine that kept you drowsy will be stopped, and you should become alert again quickly.
- The entire procedure takes about 30 minutes. Most patients remember very little of it.
- When your blood pressure, pulse, and breathing are stable and you are completely alert, you should be able to go home with a responsible adult.
- As with any operation, complications are always possible, some of them serious. With this type of operation, they can include injury or even perforation of the esophagus.

✚ HOME CARE

- Be certain that all the numbness in your mouth is gone (usually in 1–2 hours) before you start eating. Otherwise, food or fluid may go down the wrong way into your trachea.
- Resume your usual activities.

✆ CALL OUR OFFICE IF

- You continue to have severe pain with swallowing.
- You have pain in your chest or abdomen.
- You develop a temperature higher than 100°F.
- You have any questions.

△ GENERAL INFORMATION

This is an outpouching (a *diverticulum*) of the lining of the esophagus in the area of the neck. There actually are two problems:

- The diverticulum itself.
- The muscle fibers that surround the esophagus in this area that permit the lining of the esophagus to squeeze between them to the outside to form the diverticulum.

The diverticulum can be as small as a cranberry or as large as a chicken egg (Fig. 1).

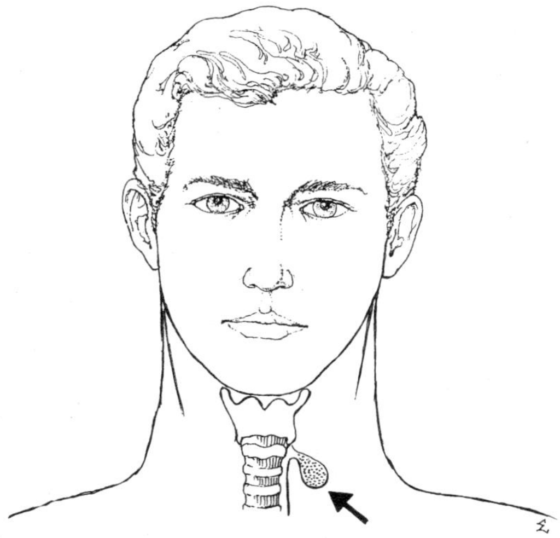

Figure 1. This illustrates a modest diverticulum with a narrow opening communicating with the esophagus. The size of the diverticulum and of its opening into the esophagus can vary significantly.

COMMON SIGNS AND SYMPTOMS

- Food has some difficulty in passing down past the neck area.
- Without warning, the person may bring up food or pills that were swallowed hours before. This is food that falls into the diverticulum and sits there, and sometimes without warning it comes up into the mouth.
- There's a gurgling sensation from the neck during swallowing. This is caused by food and liquid that fill the diverticulum.
- There may be choking, because the diverticulum fills with food and then presses on the esophagus from the outside, preventing food from going down easily.
- Some of the liquid that is brought up into the throat may then go down into the *trachea* (the windpipe), causing infection.

DIAGNOSIS

- If anyone has the above history or symptoms, there should be concern about their having a diverticulum of the esophagus.
- *Esophagogram*: You will be given barium to swallow. X-rays will be taken as it goes down the esophagus and into the diverticulum. This will demonstrate the location and size of the diverticulum.
- *Esophagoscopy*: This is done with an optical instrument as big around as the tip of your little finger that is smooth, flexible, and has a light at its tip. You will be given some medicine that will make you feel drowsy before you are brought into the endoscopy room. Your mouth and throat will be sprayed with an anesthetic to make them numb. The instrument will be placed gently down your esophagus, and the esophagus and diverticulum will be examined thoroughly.
- Do not eat until the sensation in your mouth and throat has returned completely. Otherwise, food and fluid may go down the wrong way into your trachea.

○ TREATMENT

A diverticulum of this type and in this location should be operated on before there are any complications. This means removing the diverticulum and working on the muscle fibers through which this happened.

PREOPERATIVE PREPARATION

- You will have an examination of your blood, urine, heart (EKG), and lungs (chest x-ray).
- Do not eat or drink anything for 8 hours before the operation.
- Shower (and shave) as usual on the morning of the operation.
- You may be given medicine that will make you feel drowsy before you are brought to the operating room.

□ OPERATION

- You will be asleep for the operation.
- There will be a cosmetic incision in a skin crease of your neck.
- You will not need a blood transfusion.
- The incision will be closed in a cosmetic manner.
- The operation usually takes about 1½ hours.

POSTOPERATIVE CARE

- You will be taken to a recovery room and observed. When your blood pressure, pulse, and breathing are stable, you will be taken to a regular hospital room.
- That evening you will be helped to sit up in bed and on the next day to get out of bed.
- There will be a small, soft rubber drain coming from the incision for a day or two.
- Pain will be controlled with medicine.
- You will be given liquids as you tolerate them and then will advance to mushy foods.
- As with any operation, complications are always possible. With your type of operation they can include leakage from the incision and infection, among others.
- You should be able to go home in about 2 days.
- Arrangements will be made for your medicine, follow-up office visit, and stitch removal.

✚ HOME CARE

- You may resume your usual activities.
- You may walk about as you wish, even climb stairs.
- Follow the diet schedule suggested for you.
- Take medicine as prescribed for your pain.
- You may shower as you wish and with any dressings on or off.
  - There may be narrow strips of tape across the incision. It's all right if they get wet; they will be removed in the doctor's office.
  - After you dry yourself, replace any dressings with clean, dry ones.
- You may return to work when you feel up to it.

✆ CALL OUR OFFICE IF

- You develop any unusual signs or symptoms.
- The incision becomes red or swollen, or there is drainage from it.
- You develop a temperature higher than 100°F.
- You have any questions.

ESOPHAGUS CANCER: Abdominal Approach

△ GENERAL INFORMATION

The *esophagus* is a muscular tube about as big around as a mop handle. It goes from just below the back of your throat down to the neck and then through the chest to enter the stomach in the upper abdomen. Important structures are around it along the way. Cancer can be found in any area of the esophagus and occurs mostly in older males.

COMMON SIGNS AND SYMPTOMS

- Initially, it is slightly difficult to swallow solid foods; later to swallow soft, mushy foods; and finally even to get liquids past the blockage.
- Swallowing is painful.
- Lung infection occurs.
- There is weight loss.

DIAGNOSIS

- A detailed history and a thorough physical examination can strongly suggest the diagnosis, but you will need some or all of the following tests to confirm it:
- *Esophagogram*: You will be given some barium to swallow (it has the consistency of buttermilk). As it goes down the esophagus, x-ray pictures will be taken to determine the location and extent of the problem.
- *Esophagoscopy*: This is done with an optical instrument (an *esophagoscope*) that has a light at its tip and is smooth, flexible, and as big around as the tip of your little finger. Your mouth and throat will be sprayed with an anesthetic to make them numb. Also, you will be given medicine to make you feel very drowsy. The esophagoscope will be placed gently down your esophagus and into your stomach so they can be examined thoroughly. Several tiny pieces of the tumor will be removed (a *biopsy*) for laboratory examination.
- *Bronchoscopy*: This procedure is the same as that for an esophagoscopy except that the instrument (a *bronchoscope*) is used to examine the trachea and some of its branches that are just in front of the esophagus.
- *CT scan (computed tomography scan)*: The x-rays are taken as thin slices through the esophagus and the upper abdomen. This makes it possible to see the fine details in the esophagus, stomach, liver, and pancreas, as well as the surrounding tissue.

○ TREATMENT

The cancer in your esophagus is best treated by an operation. The specific technique of the operation depends on a number of factors, a very important one being the location of the cancer in the esophagus. The most common operations are done through an incision in the abdomen, through an incision in the chest, or through incisions in both the abdomen and the neck. Each of these three techniques has advantages in specific situations.

After careful consideration of all factors, the recommendation is that you have your operation through an incision in your abdomen. X-ray therapy or chemotherapy—or even both—in addition to the operation may be helpful. If this is so in your case, it will be explained to you.

PREOPERATIVE PREPARATION

- In addition to other tests, you will have examinations of your blood, heart (EKG), lungs (chest x-ray), kidneys (urine examination), and liver.
- Any other medical problems will be cleared as much as possible before the operation.
- Do not eat or drink anything for 8 hours before the operation.

□ OPERATION

- You will be asleep for the operation.
- Every effort will be made to remove that portion of your esophagus with the cancer in it and to reconnect the cut ends by making an incision in your abdomen only (Figs. 1 and 2).
- You will not receive a blood transfusion unless it is absolutely necessary.
- The operation usually takes about 3 to 4 hours.

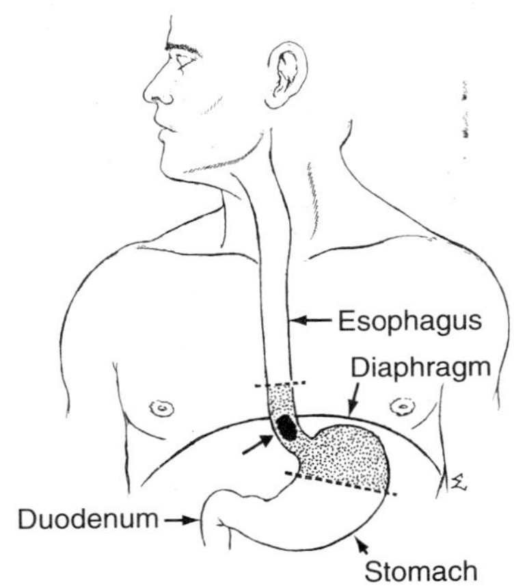

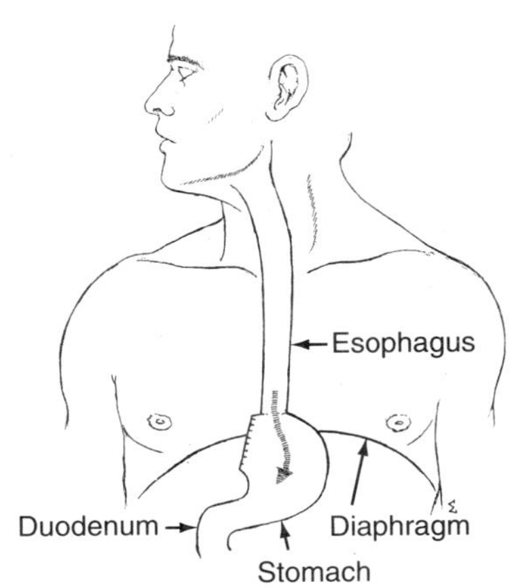

Figures 1 and 2. When a cancer is low in the esophagus, (*bold arrow*, Fig. 1) it often can be removed and the cut ends reconnected entirely through an abdominal incision (Fig. 2). This is possible because several inches of the lower esophagus are actually in the abdominal cavity. The incisions across the esophagus and stomach are shown by the dashed line. The area typically removed is stippled.

POSTOPERATIVE CARE

- You will be taken to a recovery room and observed. When your blood pressure, pulse, and breathing are stable, you will be taken to a regular hospital room.
- You will have a thin plastic tube in your nose. It goes down to your stomach to suck up the air you swallow. It will be removed when the new connection in your esophagus is healed well enough and when your bowels start working, usually in about 5 days.
- During the operation, you will have a thin plastic tube (a J tube) placed in your small intestine and brought through the skin to the outside. It will be used to help give you nourishment until you can do this completely by mouth.
- That evening you will be helped to sit up in bed and on the next day to get out of bed.
- Pain will be controlled with medicine.
- You should be able to go home in about 1 week.
- As with any operation, complications are always possible, some of them serious. With this type of operation, they can include bleeding, leaking of the new connection of your esophagus, pneumonia, heart problems, wound infection, and possibly others.
- Arrangements will be made for your medicines, follow-up office visit, and stitch or clip removal.

✚ HOME CARE

- You may walk about as you wish, even climb stairs, but don't overdo things.
- Follow the diet suggested for you. Avoid beef for several weeks. Chew your food slowly and thoroughly; it should be mushy before you swallow it. Avoid large pills.
- Take the medicines prescribed for you.
- Unless instructed otherwise, you may shower if you wish and with any dressings on or off. Be certain to keep the J tube taped so that it will not fall out. After you dry yourself, replace any dressings with clean, dry ones.
- Do not drive a car or return to work until we first discuss it during your follow-up office visit.

✆ CALL OUR OFFICE IF

- You have difficulty swallowing or breathing.
- The incision becomes red or swollen, or there is drainage from it.
- You develop a temperature higher than 100°F.
- You have any questions.

△ GENERAL INFORMATION

The *esophagus* is a muscular tube about as big around as a mop handle. It goes from just below the back of your throat down to the neck and then through the chest to enter the stomach in the upper abdomen. Important structures are around it along the way. Cancer can be found in any area of the esophagus and occurs mostly in older males.

COMMON SIGNS AND SYMPTOMS

- Initially, it is slightly difficult to swallow solid foods; later to swallow soft, mushy foods; and finally even to get liquids past the blockage.
- Swallowing is painful.
- Lung infection occurs.
- There is weight loss.

DIAGNOSIS

- A detailed history and a thorough physical examination can strongly suggest the diagnosis, but you will need some or all of the following tests to confirm it:
- *Esophagogram*: You will be given some barium to swallow (it looks and flows like buttermilk). As it goes down the esophagus, x-ray pictures will be taken to determine the location and extent of the problem.
- *Esophagoscopy*: This is done with an optical instrument (an *esophagoscope*) that has a light at its tip and is smooth, flexible, and as big around as the tip of your little finger. Your mouth and throat will be sprayed with an anesthetic to make them numb. Also, you will be given medicine to make you feel very drowsy. The esophagoscope will be placed gently down your esophagus and into your stomach so they can be examined thoroughly. Several tiny pieces of the tumor will be removed (a *biopsy*) for laboratory examination.
- *Bronchoscopy*: This procedure is the same as that for an esophagoscopy except that the instrument (a *bronchoscope*) is used to examine the trachea and some of its branches that are just in front of the esophagus.
- *CT scan (computed tomography scan)*: The x-rays are taken as thin slices through the esophagus and the upper abdomen. This makes it possible to see the fine details in the esophagus, stomach, liver, and pancreas, as well as the surrounding tissue.

○ TREATMENT

The cancer in your esophagus is best treated by an operation. The specific technique of the operation depends on a number of factors, a very important one being the location of the cancer in the esophagus. The most common operations are done through an incision in the abdomen, through an incision in the chest, or through incisions in both the abdomen and the neck. Each of these three techniques has advantages in specific situations.

After careful consideration of all factors, the recommendation is that you have your operation through an incision in your abdomen and in your neck (Figs. 1 and 2). X-ray therapy or chemotherapy—or even both—in addition to the operation may be helpful. If this is so in your case, it will be explained to you.

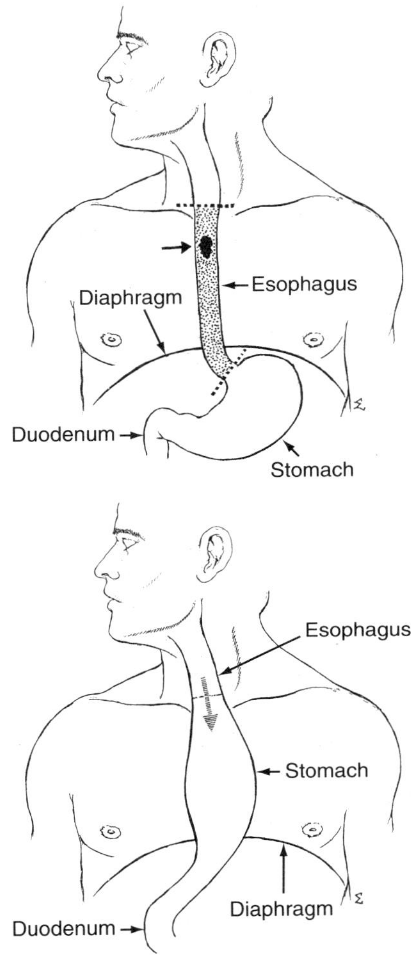

Figures 1 and 2. When a cancer is in the upper part of the esophagus (*bold arrow*, Fig. 1), it often can be removed and the cut ends reconnected without having to make an incision in the chest wall. This is done by making an abdominal incision to be able to dissect the stomach face. The esophagus with the cancer in it is then dissected free from below (the abdomen) by widening a natural opening in the diaphragm and from above through a short incision in the neck. The esophagus is cut across the dashed lines and removed (see stippled area). The stomach is then brought up through the chest and into the neck area, and the open ends are reconnected (Fig. 2).

PREOPERATIVE PREPARATION

- In addition to other tests, you will have examinations of your blood, heart (EKG), lungs (chest x-ray), kidneys (urine examination), and liver.
- Any other medical problems will be cleared as much as possible before the operation.
- Do not eat or drink anything for 8 hours before the operation.

☐ OPERATION

- You will be asleep for the operation.
- Every effort will be made to remove that portion of your esophagus with the cancer in it and to reconnect the cut ends by making the incisions in your abdomen and neck only.
- You will not receive a blood transfusion unless it is absolutely necessary.
- The operation usually takes about 3 to 4 hours.

POSTOPERATIVE CARE

- You will be taken to a recovery room and observed. When your blood pressure, pulse, and breathing are stable, you will be taken to a regular hospital room.
- You will have a thin plastic tube in your nose for a few days.
- During the operation, you will have a thin plastic tube (a J tube) placed in your small intestine and brought through the skin to the outside. It will be used to help give you nourishment until you can do this completely by mouth.
- That evening you will be helped to sit up in bed and on the next day to get out of bed.
- Pain will be controlled with medicine.
- You may be given an incentive spirometer. Breathing into this as you are instructed will help expand your lungs and reduce the risk of developing pneumonia.
- While the tube is in your nose and stomach, you will be fed by vein. After that you will be started on a liquid diet. This will be supplemented by a liquid diet given through the J tube.
- You should be able to go home in about 1 week.
- As with any operation, complications are always possible, some of them serious. With this type of operation, they can include leaking of the new connection of your esophagus, pneumonia, heart problems, wound infection, and possibly others.
- Arrangements will be made for your medicines, follow-up office visit, and stitch or clip removal.

✚ HOME CARE

- You may walk about as you wish, even climb stairs, but don't overdo things.
- Follow the diet suggested for you. Avoid beef for several weeks. Chew your food slowly and thoroughly; it should be mushy before you swallow it. Avoid large pills.
- Take the medicines prescribed for you.
- Unless instructed otherwise, you may shower if you wish and with any dressings on or off. Be certain to keep the J tube taped so that it will not fall out. After you dry yourself, replace any dressings with clean, dry ones.
- Do not drive a car until we first discuss it.
- You may return to work when you feel up to it.

✆ CALL OUR OFFICE IF

- You have difficulty swallowing or breathing.
- The incision becomes red or swollen, or there is drainage from it.
- You develop a temperature higher than 100°F.
- You have any questions.

△ GENERAL INFORMATION

The *esophagus* is a muscular tube about as big around as a mop handle. It goes from just below the back of your throat down to the neck and then through the chest to enter the stomach in the upper abdomen. Important structures are around it along the way. Cancer can be found in any area of the esophagus and occurs mostly in older males.

COMMON SIGNS AND SYMPTOMS

- Initially, it is slightly difficult to swallow solid foods; later to swallow soft, mushy foods; and finally even to get liquids past the blockage.
- Swallowing is painful.
- Lung infection occurs.
- There is weight loss.

DIAGNOSIS

- A detailed history and a thorough physical examination can strongly suggest the diagnosis, but you will need some or all of the following tests to confirm it:
- *Esophagogram*: You will be given some barium to swallow (it looks and flows like buttermilk). As it goes down the esophagus, x-ray pictures will be taken to determine the location and extent of the problem.
- *Esophagoscopy*: This is done with an optical instrument (an *esophagoscope*) that has a light at its tip and is smooth, flexible, and as big around as the tip of your little finger. Your mouth and throat will be sprayed with an anesthetic to make them numb. Also, you will be given medicine to make you feel very drowsy. The esophagoscope will be placed gently down your esophagus and into your stomach so they can be examined thoroughly. Several tiny pieces of the tumor will be removed (a *biopsy*) for laboratory examination.
- *Bronchoscopy*: This procedure is the same as that for an esophagoscopy except that the instrument (a *bronchoscope*) is used to examine the trachea and some of its branches that are just in front of the esophagus.
- *CT scan (computed tomography scan)*: The x-rays are taken as thin slices through the esophagus and the upper abdomen. This makes it possible to see the fine details in the esophagus, stomach, liver, and pancreas, as well as the surrounding tissue.

○ TREATMENT

The cancer in your esophagus is best treated by an operation. The specific technique of the operation depends on a number of factors, a very important one being the location of the cancer in the esophagus. The most common operations are done through an incision in the abdomen, through an incision in the chest, or through incisions in both the abdomen and the neck. Each of these three techniques has advantages in specific situations.

After careful consideration of all factors, the recommendation is that you have your operation through an incision in your chest (Figs. 1 and 2). X-ray therapy or chemotherapy—or even both—in addition to the operation may be helpful. If this is so in your case, it will be explained to you.

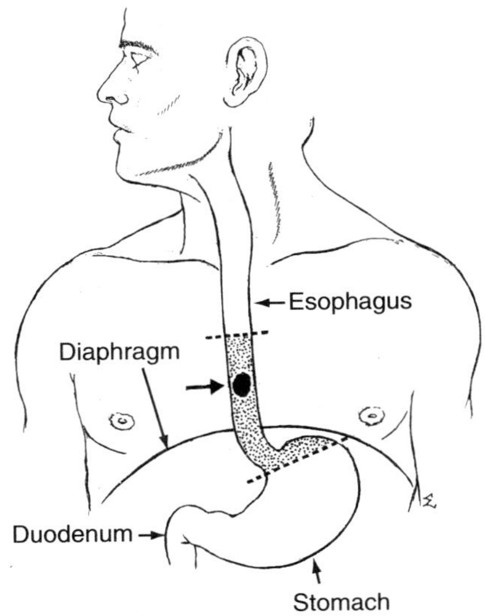

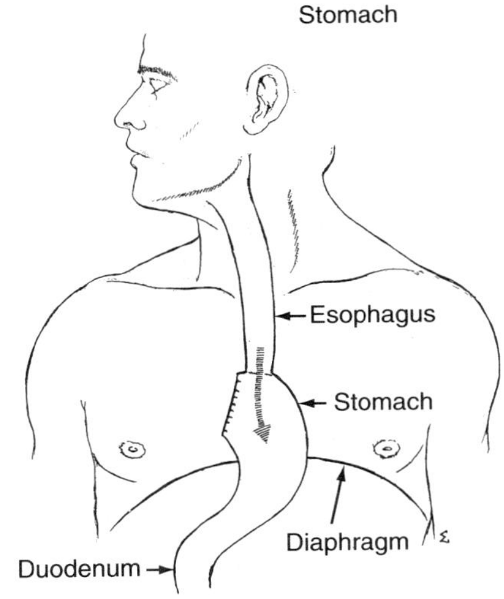

Figures 1 and 2. When a cancer is in the middle part of the esophagus (*bold arrow*, Fig. 1), removing it and reconnecting the cut ends often is done through an opening in the right side of the chest. The incisions made across the esophagus and the stomach are shown by the dashed line. The area typically removed is stippled. Part of the stomach needs to be brought up into the chest to reconnect the open ends (Fig. 2). For this reason often an abdominal incision also needs to be made to free the stomach and make it possible for it to be brought up into the chest.

PREOPERATIVE PREPARATION

- In addition to other tests, you will have examinations of your blood, heart (EKG), lungs (chest x-ray), kidneys (urine examination), and liver.
- Any other medical problems will be cleared as much as possible before the operation.
- Do not eat or drink anything for 8 hours before the operation.

☐ OPERATION

- You will be asleep for the operation.
- Usually the incision is on the right side of the chest.
- You will not receive a blood transfusion unless it is absolutely necessary.
- The operation usually takes about 3 to 4 hours.

POSTOPERATIVE CARE

- You will be taken to a recovery room and observed. When your blood pressure, pulse, and breathing are stable, you will be taken to a regular hospital room.
- There will be one or two plastic tubes coming to the outside from your chest and a thin plastic tube in your nose. Both will be removed in a few days.
- During the operation, you will have a thin plastic tube (a J tube) placed in your small intestine and coming through the skin to the outside. It will be used to help give you nourishment until you can do this completely on your own.
- That evening you will be helped to sit up in bed and on the next day to get out of bed.
- Pain will be controlled with medicine.
- You may be given an incentive spirometer. Breathing into this as you are instructed will help expand your lungs and reduce the risk of developing pneumonia.
- While the tube is in your nose and stomach, you will be fed by vein. After that you will be started on a liquid diet. This will be supplemented by a liquid diet given through the J tube.
- You should be able to go home in about 1 week.
- As with any operation, complications are always possible, some of them serious. With this type of operation, they can include leaking of the new connection of your esophagus, pneumonia, heart problems, wound infection, and possibly others.
- Arrangements will be made for your medicines, follow-up office visit, and stitch or clip removal.

✚ HOME CARE

- You may walk about as you wish, even climb stairs, but don't overdo things.
- Follow the diet suggested for you. Avoid beef for several weeks. Chew your food slowly and thoroughly; it should be mushy before you swallow it. Avoid large pills.
- Take the medicines prescribed for you.
- Unless instructed otherwise, you may shower if you wish and with any dressings on or off. Be certain to keep the J tube taped so that it will not fall out. After you dry yourself, replace any dressings with clean, dry ones.
- Do not drive a car until we first discuss it.
- You may return to work when you feel up to it.

✆ CALL OUR OFFICE IF

- You have difficulty swallowing or breathing.
- The incision becomes red or swollen, or there is drainage from it.
- You develop a temperature higher than 100°F.
- You have any questions.

EXPLORATORY OPERATION (EXPLORATORY LAPAROTOMY)

△ GENERAL INFORMATION

This used to be a very common operation because there were so few other ways to "look at" organs inside the abdomen (and even these few were not so good). Surgeons had to open up the abdomen to explore the inside.

"EXPLORATION"

Now there are a number of ways to explore—or look inside—the abdomen without actually having to open it up.

A few of these newer methods are the following:

- **Ultrasound:** Harmless sound waves are aimed at your abdomen. The sound waves bouncing back (the echoes) from this area are seen as a picture on a screen. This is a convenient, painless, and harmless way to examine organs and tissues inside your abdomen.
- **CT Scan (Computed Tomography Scan):** These pictures are taken by a special x-ray machine shaped like a huge doughnut. You will lie on the table inside the hole in the "doughnut." The x-rays are taken as very thin slices through any area of the body. This makes it possible to see the fine details in the area being examined.
- **MRI (Magnetic Resonance Imaging):** No x-rays are used with this technique. Instead, magnetic fields and radio waves are used. A computer develops the pictures to show organs from several angles. It is especially valuable for examining blood vessels and nerve tissue.
- **PET Scan (Positron-Emission Tomography Scan):** This is one of the latest and most sophisticated ways of looking at tumors. This technique not only can locate tumors but also can show how active they are *biologically*.
- **Colonoscopy:** This is done with an optical instrument called a *colonoscope*. It is smooth, flexible, and as big around as your little finger and has a light at its tip. You will be given medicine that will make you feel drowsy during the procedure. The tip of the instrument will be lubricated and then gently inserted into your anus. It can be used to inspect your entire large bowel.
- **Laparoscopy:** This method uses a rigid optical instrument called a *laparoscope*. It is as big around as the tip of your little finger and has a light at its tip. With the patient asleep, the laparoscope is inserted into the abdomen through a very small incision in the navel so the inside of the abdomen can be examined directly. If something suspicious is seen, a tiny piece (a *biopsy*) can be removed for laboratory examination.
- **ERCP (Endoscopic Retrograde Choledocho-pancreatography).** This is an optical instrument (an *endoscope*) that has a light at its tip and is smooth, flexible, and about the size of your little finger. After the mouth and throat are sprayed to make them numb, the patient is given medicine and is put into a "twilight sleep." The instrument is inserted through the mouth, down the esophagus, past the stomach, and to the duodenum, where the bile duct empties its juices. A special tube (thinner than a toothpick) is then passed out of the instrument into the bile ducts coming from the liver. Pictures of the bile ducts can be taken to look for stones or other problems. Often the problems found can be taken care of at the same time.
- **Peritoneal Lavage:** This is most often used in persons who have had an injury to the abdomen and often to other areas as well. Sometimes it is difficult to know if there is bleeding or infection inside the abdomen. Although this is an important question, there may be injuries to other areas of the body that need prompt attention. Which should be taken care of first? A very thin plastic tube is inserted into the abdomen, and through this plastic tube a bottle of salt solution is instilled into the abdomen. After a short while, the salt solution is removed through the same tube and examined for any red blood cells, white blood cells, bacteria, or chemicals. This procedure may provide information about what may be happening inside the abdomen.

These and other modern techniques help doctors "see" inside the abdomen. This does not mean that the abdomen does not need to be opened to make the diagnosis and take care of the problem. What it does mean is the following:

- The abdomen does not *always* need to be opened to find out what is wrong.
- Sometimes biopsy and observation not only can make the diagnosis but also can show that the problem does not require specific care—it will get well by itself. Or the problem can be taken care of with medicine and x-rays rather than with a formal operation.
- The surgeon can know what is wrong beforehand and so can make plans to take care of the problem without any surprises. Also, the patient knows what to expect.
- Sometimes a laparoscope can be used to both make the diagnosis and to take care of the problem.
- It can spare a patient with multiple injuries, and possible but unknown injuries to the abdomen, an unnecessarily wide opening of the abdomen to determine whether anything is actually wrong. This then allows the doctor to take care of the other injuries without worrying about missing something serious in the abdomen.

Now an exploratory abdominal operation can be more focused. The surgeon more often knows what is there and what needs to be done. These new techniques and a number of other associated advances are the reasons that abdominal operations are now more appropriate, safer, and more effective.

△ GENERAL INFORMATION

The eye and brow region are the most attractive, expressive units of the face. The mobility of the eyebrow is an important component of facial expression. The eyebrows are considered a frame for the eyes, and the location of the brow contributes to the appearance of a youthful, attractive eye. Any detraction from these features can be quite noticeable. For this reason, surgical rejuvenation of the upper third of the face is a vitally important part of aesthetic facial surgery.

With modern medical and technical advances, a number of operations are available for correcting conditions that affect the eyebrows. When choosing a facial or general plastic surgeon, it is wise to look for one who has a continuing interest, specific training, appropriate experience, and demonstrated skills in this cosmetic operation.

CANDIDATES FOR EYEBROW LIFT

By far, most persons have this procedure for cosmetic improvement. Significant drooping of the eyebrows and consequent hooding over the eyes may portray an incorrect communication about your age, mood, or feelings to others. Downward displacement of the medial (inner third) of the eyebrows makes a person appear older, angry, or annoyed. Lateral drooping of the brows might produce a tired, sad, or older appearance. For this reason, it is *you* who should decide that you want the operation, not someone else who wants you to have it.

- Getting an opinion from two facial or general plastic surgeons is appropriate.
- An in-depth consultation between patient and surgeon with a history and facial evaluation is essential.
- You should have realistic expectations and a full understanding of the healing process.
- Finally, you should know the possible complications that may accompany the procedure.

○ TREATMENT

- There are a number of operative techniques to correct eyebrow hooding. The best technique for your particular problem will be decided after you are examined. It will be thoroughly discussed with you.

PREOPERATIVE PREPARATION

- You will have a detailed history and physical examination as it pertains to your eyebrows.
- The surgeon will need to have assurance that you are not troubled with any significant illness.
- Certain laboratory tests will be done.
- A number of photographs will be taken of you with special attention to the eye and eyebrow area.
- Do not take aspirin or aspirin-containing compounds, vitamin E, garlic, or mood-altering drugs; drink alcohol; or smoke for 1 week before the operation.
- Shower or bathe on the morning of the operation.
- Remove all facial makeup completely, especially mascara.
- You may be given medicine that will make you feel drowsy before you are brought to the operating room.

□ OPERATION

- The procedure will be performed under local or general anesthesia. For local anesthesia, the affected area will be made numb by injecting an anesthetic into it with a fine needle. Also, you will be given medicine to keep you in a drowsy condition.
- During the operation, you may feel some tugging but no pain.
- The operation usually takes about 1 hour.
- You will be taken to a recovery room. When your blood pressure, pulse, and breathing are stable and you are completely alert, you should be able to go home that same day with a responsible adult.
- Arrangements will be made for your medicine and follow-up office visit.

✣ HOME CARE

- For the first 2 days, apply an ice compress over the eyebrows every 2 hours for about 20 minutes.
- You may eat as you did before the operation.
- During the first week, sleep with your head elevated on two or three pillows.
- Do not get your sutures wet.
- Take the medicines prescribed for you.
- Do not tweeze your eyebrows for 1 month.
- The sutures are dissolvable.
- Do not use aspirin or products containing aspirin, codeine, or antihistamines for 10 days after the operation.
- You may return to work when you feel up to it.

✆ CALL OUR OFFICE IF

- You develop any unusual signs or symptoms.
- The incision becomes red or swollen, or there is drainage from it.
- You develop a temperature higher than 100°F.
- You have any questions.

FACE LIFT (RHYTIDECTOMY)

△ GENERAL INFORMATION

Thousands of women and men have cosmetic surgery of the face and for a number of reasons: to remove wrinkles; to improve sagging skin that makes them look older than they truly are; to remove features that make them look different, such as a tired or sad appearance; or to correct a specific undesirable feature. Thus, it is obvious that *face lift* is often a general term that might not apply to all of the concerns a patient may have about facial appearance.

A face lift usually involves only the tailoring and repositioning of the skin of the face and neck. A number of specific areas of the face often require attention in addition to the face lift, however, namely, the forehead, eyelids, nose, cheeks, ears, and chin. For this reason, these areas may be operated on at the same time that the face lift is done.

With modern medical and technologic advances, a number of operations are available for a face lift. Therefore, when choosing a plastic surgeon for a face lift, it is wise to look for one who has continuing interest, specific training, appropriate experience, and demonstrated clinical skills in performing this operation.

CANDIDATES FOR FACE LIFT

Most persons have this operation for cosmetic improvement. It is important to remember that *you* are the one who should want the operation, not someone else who thinks you should have it. Getting an opinion from two plastic surgeons is appropriate. The surgeon and you should discuss at least the following:

- The problem as it is perceived by you. Also, it should be clear to you the degree to which the surgeon agrees with you.
- The planned operation.
- The expected (not guaranteed) results. Also, you should have a realistic expectation of the results.
- The possibility that both your expectations and the surgeon's will not be realized.
- The possible complications.

○ TREATMENT

There are a number of concerns with a face lift, and each of them requires a different operative technique to correct it. Your particular problem—or combination of problems—will be pointed out to you as well as the method necessary to correct it.

PREOPERATIVE PREPARATION

- A detailed history will be taken and a physical examination will be done that covers your face and neck.
- Your personal doctor must provide assurance that you do not have any significant illness that might affect your ability to have this operation safely.
- A number of photographs will be taken of your face and neck and from several angles.
- You may be shown a gallery of photos of other patients to give you an idea *(only)* of the possible results in you.
- Do not take aspirin or medicines with aspirin in them, alcohol, or mood-altering drugs for 1 week before the operation. Do not smoke for 1 week before the operation.
- Shower or bathe as usual on the morning of the operation.
- Completely remove all makeup on the morning of the operation.
- You will be given medicine that will make you feel drowsy before you are brought to the operating room.

□ OPERATION

The type of anesthesia used will depend on how extensive a face lift is planned. If it is to be done under local anesthesia, you will be given medicine that will make you feel drowsy. A very fine needle will be used to inject an anesthetic in the area to be operated on so that it will be numb. In addition, you will be given some medicine by vein throughout the operation to keep you in a twilight sleep. During the operation, you may feel some tugging but not pain. Many patients who have this operation done under local anesthesia with sedation have very little recollection of the operation itself after it is completed.

- You will be taken to a recovery room and observed until your blood pressure, pulse, and breathing are stable. If it was a short operation, it may be possible for you to go home that same day with a responsible adult. Otherwise, you will be taken to a regular hospital room.
- You will have on a large, snug, bulky dressing that covers your entire face except the eyes, nose and the mouth.
- You will be given liquid nourishment.
- The bulky dressing will be removed in 24 hours and replaced with a smaller dressing, over which will be placed a facial support garment.
- As with any operation, there are side effects and possible complications. With this operation, they can include swelling of the tissue, bruised areas, and decreased sensation of the skin, which usually is minimal and almost always goes away but occasionally is permanent. Also, there can be bleeding, nerve damage, infection, skin loss, some loss of hair, abnormal scars, and possibly others.
- You will be continued on the antibiotics started before the operation.
- Arrangements will be made for your medicine, follow-up office visit, and stitch removal.

✣ HOME CARE

- You should have a very responsible adult with you for the first 24 hours.
- You should engage in very limited activity and do only what is essential.
- Have a liquid to soft diet.
- For the first 3 days, lie down as much as possible with your head elevated on two pillows.
- Continue with the preoperative antibiotics.

- This operation can cause discomfort, but if there is pain, notify the surgeon, as there may be bleeding or the dressings may be too tight.
- Because of all of the above, you may find it difficult to sleep. If this is the case, medicine can be prescribed for you.
- If you have discomfort after the first few days, it generally means that you have been overactive.
- Gradually increase the amount of your walking.
- Do not engage in any physical exercise or driving for 2 weeks.

✆ CALL OUR OFFICE IF

- You develop any unusual signs or symptoms.
- You develop a temperature higher than 100°F.
- You have any questions.

△ GENERAL INFORMATION

The spine is composed of a number of bones that are stacked one on top of the other like toy building blocks. Sidearms of bone called *facets* stick out and touch similar facets above and below (Fig. 1). The facets are smooth in the areas they touch each other. These are called the *facet joints*.

Nerves go right past these facet joints—almost touching them. These nerves carry sensations (including pain) from all parts of the body to the spinal cord. From the spinal cord, these sensations (of pain) are carried to the brain.

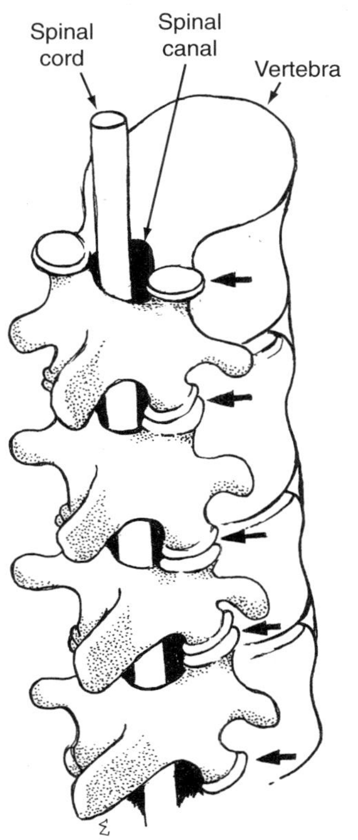

Figure 1. Variously shaped knobs of bone stick out of the sides and back of each vertebra and glide against each other to help steady vertebrae as they move. The areas that glide against each other are called *facets (arrows)*. These facets can be injected with medicine when they are inflamed and painful.

COMMON SIGNS AND SYMPTOMS

If the facet joint becomes inflamed or irritates the nerves that pass close by or touch the area, the nerve that is irritated sends this information to the brain as pain—often very severe pain.

- When the pain is severe enough or is present long enough, it can set up a "pain cycle" in the following manner: the irritated nerve sends a signal to the spinal cord, which normally carries it to the brain. With the pain cycle, however, some of the pain signals sent to the spinal cord are sent right back to the nerve. This irritates the nerve even more, and the nerve responds by sending more signals to the cord. The cycle can go on, making it difficult for the pain to stop; the pain feeds on itself, so to speak.
- The areas of the spine most commonly affected are those that normally have a lot of motion in them, namely, the neck and the middle of the back.

DIAGNOSIS

The diagnosis begins by taking a detailed history of the pain in addition to doing a thorough physical and neurologic examination.

- Typically the pain is about one-half inch to the left or right side of the midline of the back. The pain usually lessens if you bend forward and is worse if you bend backward, especially if you also twist side-to-side. This bending backward and twisting causes the facet joints to rub against each other the most.
- A number of tests may need to be done, including some of the following:
  - X-rays of the spine, with special attention to the facet joints, looking for signs of damage.
  - CT scan (computed tomography scan): These special x-rays are taken by a machine that is shaped like a huge doughnut. You will lie on a table inside the hole in the "doughnut." The x-rays are taken as very thin slices through the area of the spine that is hurting. This makes it possible to see the fine details in the facet joints.
  - MRI (magnetic resonance imaging): No x-rays are used with this technique. Instead, it is done with harmless magnetic fields and radio waves. A computer develops the pictures to show organs from several angles. It is especially valuable for examining the relationship of bone tissue to nerves.
- The above test results may be normal, even though the person is having problems with the facet joints. The reason probably is the small size of the joint. Not too much has to be wrong with it to produce pain.

○ TREATMENT

- This can consist of avoiding movements that trigger pain.
- Wearing a brace to limit motion of the affected part of the spine can give some relief.
- Taking nonsteroidal anti-inflammatory medicine.
- Injecting the facet joint with a local anesthetic as well as a small amount of steroid.

After careful consideration of all factors, the recommendation may be that you have an injection of your affected facet joint.

PREOPERATIVE PREPARATION

- Do not eat or drink anything for 8 hours before the procedure.
- You may have an examination of your blood, urine, heart (EKG), and lungs (chest x-ray), depending on your age and your medical condition.
- You may be given medicine that will make you feel drowsy before you are brought to the operating room.

PROCEDURE

- You will be lying on your stomach during the procedure.
- The area over the affected facet joint will be swabbed with an antiseptic solution and surrounded with sterile towels.
- You will be given additional medicine to keep you feeling drowsy.
- A fine needle will be used to inject an anesthetic in the skin to make it numb.
- A special needle will then be placed through the numbed skin and down to the facet joint (see Fig. 1).
- An x-ray will be taken of the needle in place to be certain it is in the correct position.
- An anesthetic solution with a small amount of steroids will be injected into the facet joint and the needle withdrawn.

POSTOPERATIVE CARE

- You will be taken to a recovery room and observed until your blood pressure, pulse, and breathing are stable and you are completely alert.
- You will be examined to determine the effect of the facet joint injection.
- You then will be free to go home with a responsible adult.
- Because you were given medicine to keep you drowsy, many patients barely remember the actual procedure.

HOME CARE

- Lie down for the day.
- Any relief of pain may last only 3 or 4 hours and then return. That's the anesthetic wearing off. The steroid, however, often has a delayed action and may take 3 or 4 days before it starts working.
- Do not do any exercising or engage in strenuous activity for 1 week.
- The procedure may give relief of pain, but in a week or two the pain returns. In such a situation, the injection can be repeated with a more permanent treatment that can be effective for 6 months or even longer.

CALL OUR OFFICE IF

- Your leg or arm becomes numb.
- Your pain is getting worse.
- You cannot control urine or bowel movements.
- You develop a fever higher than 100°F.
- You develop a headache that gets worse on sitting and is relieved by lying down.

FEMOROPOPLITEAL BYPASS

△ GENERAL INFORMATION

The *aorta* comes off the heart and travels down through the chest and into the lower abdomen, giving off branches all along the way. At just below the umbilicus, it divides into the left and the right *iliac arteries*. In the groins and thighs, iliac arteries become the left and right *femoral* arteries. At the knee area, the femoral arteries become the *popliteal* arteries.

Sometimes, one or both femoral arteries become partially blocked by cholesterol deposits (called *atheromas*) that prevent enough blood from getting to the legs.

COMMON SIGNS AND SYMPTOMS

- Cramping pain in the calves, thighs, and buttocks when walking.
- Pain in the toes and feet, most prominent at night, that gets better with sitting or standing.
- Very slow healing of any sore on the leg or foot.
- Thin, shiny skin over the legs with loss of some hair.
- Pale legs.
- Weak or almost absent pulses at the ankles.

○ TREATMENT

- Many patients can be treated medically.
  - Stop smoking.
  - Take off excess weight.
  - Start an exercise program.
- An operation is strongly advised in the following circumstances:
  - There is severe disability from the cramping pain.
  - There is pain while resting, particularly at night while in bed.
  - There is a nonhealing ulcer on the leg.
- You will have an examination of your blood, urine, heart (EKG), and lungs (chest x-ray).
- Special attention will be given to the aorta for the presence of an aneurysm that would indicate any weakness and widening in the wall. Also the vessels to the brain, the *carotid arteries*, will be examined for any evidence of blockage.
- Arteriography: The skin in your back will be painted with an antiseptic solution. An area will be injected with an anesthetic to make it numb. A fine needle will be inserted through the numbed skin into your aorta, and dye contrast liquid will be injected. X-ray pictures will be taken as the contrast passes down to the arteries of your pelvis and legs. This will show the location and extent of the blockage.
- Stop smoking. Smoking decreases the chance of successful therapy.
- Shower (and shave) as usual on the morning of the operation.
- You may be given medicine that will make you feel drowsy before you are brought to the operating room.

□ OPERATION

- You will be given an appropriate anesthetic. Usually you are put to sleep. At times a spinal anesthetic will be offered.
- After you are asleep, your abdomen and legs will be scrubbed with antiseptic solution and draped.
- The aim of the operation is to use an artificial vessel or a vein from nearby in your body to bridge over the blocked area of the artery (Fig. 1). This will restore a better flow of blood to the area beyond the blockage.

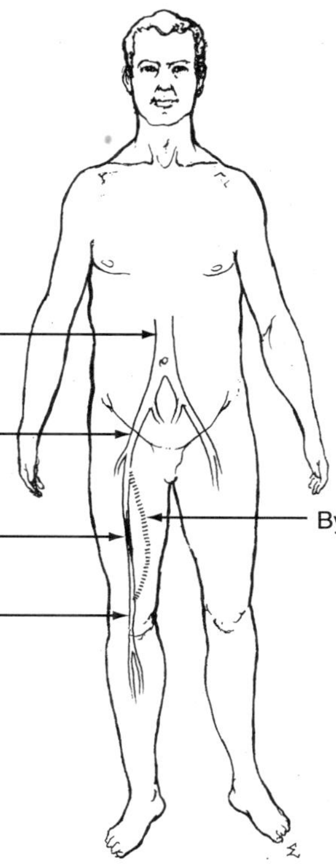

Figure 1. The pertinent anatomy and a typical bypass are shown.

- Incisions will be made over the artery in the groin at an area above and another below the blockage. One end of a graft will be sewed to the femoral artery above the blocked area; the lower end of the graft will be sewed to the artery at a spot below the blockage. This, then, bypasses the blocked area and increases the flow of blood to the leg and foot.
- When adequate circulation is ensured, the incisions are closed.
- You will not receive a blood transfusion unless it is absolutely necessary.
- The operation generally takes 2 hours.

POSTOPERATIVE CARE

- You will be taken to a recovery room. When your blood pressure, pulse, and breathing are stable, you will be taken to a regular hospital room.
- The circulation to your legs will be watched very carefully.
- The next day you will be helped to stand at the bedside.

- Pain can be controlled with medicine.
- As with any operation, complications are always possible, some of them serious. With your type of operation, they can include reclotting of the artery; sometimes it simply cannot be corrected. There can be bleeding, heart problems, infection, and even gangrene of tissue.
- You should be able to go home in 4 to 5 days.

HOME CARE

- Continue with the program started while you were in the hospital.
- You may walk about as you wish, even climb stairs, but don't overdo things.
- You may eat as you did before the operation.
- You may shower if you wish and with any dressings on or off.
  - There may be narrow strips of tape across the incision. It's all right if they get wet; they will be removed in the doctor's office.
  - After you dry yourself, replace any dressings with clean, dry ones.
- It is important to remember not to cross your legs and not to sit for long periods. These positions tend to reduce the flow of blood through the arteries and encourage clot formation. Also, your feet and lower legs can swell and become uncomfortable.
- Driving your car may be important to you, but when you can do this safely depends on the operation you had, the medicines you are taking, and your condition in general. During the follow-up visit, let's talk about when you can resume driving and return to work.
- You may resume sexual activity whenever you choose.

CALL OUR OFFICE IF

- You develop increasing pain in the toes or foot, they have changed color, or you cannot move them.
- The incisions become red or swollen, or there is drainage from them.
- You develop a temperature higher than 100°F.
- You have any questions.

△ GENERAL INFORMATION

The forearm is the part between the wrist and the elbow. Within it are two long bones, the *radius* and the *ulna*, that run alongside each other. One or both bones may break after a hard fall or from a direct blow.

COMMON SIGNS AND SYMPTOMS

- There is pain and swelling between the wrist and elbow.
- The forearm may be visibly crooked.
- There is pain with use of the hand or arm.
- There may be weakness of the hand or arm.

DIAGNOSIS

- Usually, the diagnosis can be made by taking a detailed history and doing a thorough physical examination, but the surest way is to take an x-ray of the forearm that includes the elbow and wrist.

○ TREATMENT

In All Instances

- If the bones are straight and the skin is not cut by the fractured bone, a cast extending from the hand to the shoulder is applied and usually is sufficient. If the skin was cut by the bone when it broke, the wound will need to be washed thoroughly in the operating room to help prevent infection.

Adults and Older Teenagers

- Usually, the broken bones are crooked, and an operation is needed. The broken bones are straightened, and then stainless steel plates are applied to them.

Children and Younger Teenagers

- If the bones are crooked, they need to be straightened. This is attempted without an open operation. It is not harmful if the bones still are a little crooked after such straightening, because a child's bones will straighten as they grow.
- To ease the pain during straightening of the broken bones, an anesthetic usually is necessary. The decision on which type to use will be discussed with you beforehand.
- If the bones are still too crooked, an operation may be necessary to put in stainless steel plates, as is commonly done with adults and older teenagers.

After careful consideration of all factors, it is recommended that your fracture be treated by an open operation.

PREOPERATIVE PREPARATION

- Usually, there will be an examination of your blood, urine, heart (EKG), and lungs (chest x-ray).
- A healthy person usually has this operation promptly. A person with serious health problems, however, may need these problems corrected as much as possible before the operation.
- Do not eat or drink anything for 8 hours before the operation.
- A delay of a week or longer usually is not harmful.

THE OPERATION

- You either will be asleep for the operation or have a nerve block that makes only the arm numb. The choice will be discussed with you beforehand.
- One or two long incisions will be made lengthwise along the forearm.
- The bones will be straightened, and one or two steel plates several inches long will be attached to the straightened bones with screws to keep them in that position as they heal (Fig. 1).

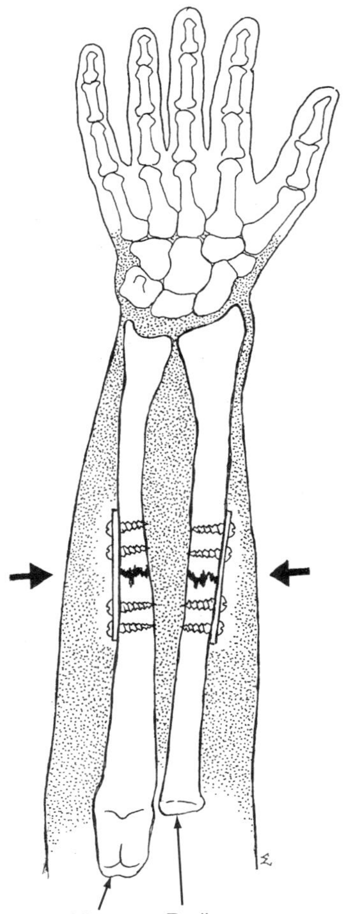

Figure 1. An example of a way that plates and screws *(arrows)* can be used to hold straightened broken bones in a correct position while they heal.

- If the elbow or wrist was injured at the same time as the forearm, this may need to be fixed during the same operation.
- The operation usually takes about 2 hours.

POSTOPERATIVE CARE

- You will be taken to a recovery room and observed. When your blood pressure, pulse, and breathing are stable, you will be taken to a regular hospital room.
- You may or may not have a cast on your arm.

- The condition of the blood vessels and nerves of your forearm will be checked closely to be certain they are working properly.
- Pain will be controlled with medicine.
- Your diet will be as you tolerate it.
- You should be able to go home in about 2 days.
- Arrangements will be made for your medicine, follow-up office visit, and stitch removal.
- As with any operation, complications are always possible. With this type of operation, they can include infection, the plates coming loose, nerve or blood vessel injury, and possibly others.

✣ HOME CARE

- You may walk about as you wish, even climb stairs.
- Keep the cast completely dry. Placing a small plastic bag over the entire arm and sealing the top with tape help keep the cast from getting wet while you bathe.
- You will need to be very careful for many months after the operation. Even though the forearm feels stable, the steel plates can break or pull out of the bone if you do heavy activity with the arm.
- After the bones are healed, you can do whatever you like. Generally, the plates do not need to be removed unless they bother you.
- You will probably lose a little motion of the forearm, but on the whole your arm should function very well.

✆ CALL OUR OFFICE IF

- You develop any unusual signs or symptoms.
- The incision becomes red or swollen, or there is drainage from it.
- You develop a temperature higher than 100°F.
- You have any questions.

△ GENERAL INFORMATION

The liver makes bile that is the color and consistency of thin motor oil. It leaves the liver through the bile ducts on its way to the intestine. Along the way, some of it is stored in the gallbladder that is located under the liver, where it is concentrated and becomes as thick as diesel oil. Shortly after a meal, the gallbladder squeezes down to get an extra amount of concentrated bile into the intestine, where it helps digest fats and other foods we eat.

Sometimes, stones form in the gallbladder. A stone starts off as a tiny particle. There may be only one stone or many of them. They grow in size, usually to that of a pea, but often get much larger.

COMMON SIGNS AND SYMPTOMS

The symptoms produced by gallstones depends on their location (Fig. 1):

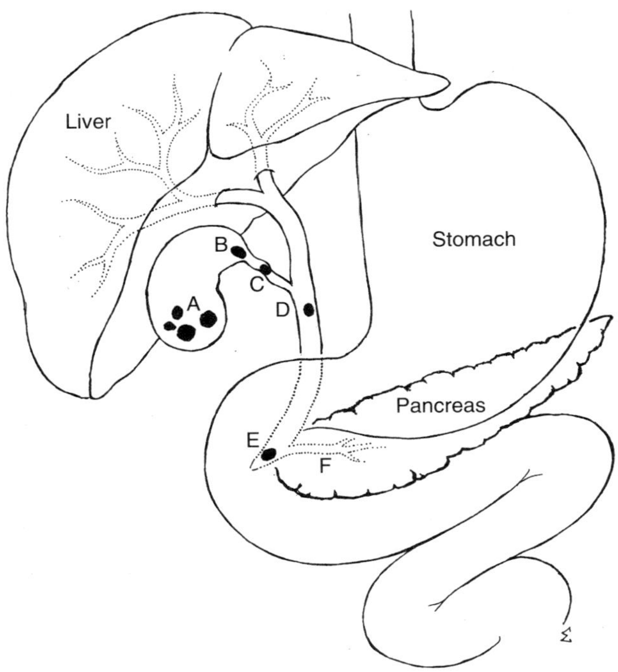

Figure 1.

- **Stones in the Gallbladder.** The stones may be in the gallbladder only (position A). This is called *cholelithiasis*. These stones may not produce any symptoms or may cause indigestion, especially after eating. If a stone gets stuck in the opening of the gallbladder and plugs it (position B), a sharp, severe pain in the right side of the upper abdomen is produced as the gallbladder squeezes to get the bile out. This is a gallbladder colic. If the stone remains stuck long enough, the gallbladder becomes infected, resulting in *acute cholecystitis*. Often, the stones fall back into the gallbladder, relieving the blockage, the pain, and the infection. This can happen again and again, producing what is called *chronic cholecystitis*.
- **Stone in the Cystic Duct.** Sometimes the stone gets stuck in the small duct (the *cystic duct*) that carries the bile from the gallbladder to the main channel (the *common duct*) (position C). The stone cannot go forward or backward. In such an instance, the attack will not let up and requires early treatment.
- **Stone in the Common Bile Duct.** Sometimes the stone is small enough to pass out of the gallbladder and into the *common bile duct* (position D). If such a stone does not interfere with the flow of bile, it may just sit there and cause little trouble. Often, however, it will drift downward and can plug the common duct (position E). This will produce pain because all of the bile ducts are blocked and stretched; the bile cannot come out, so it backs up into the tissues of the body causing the skin to become yellow (called *jaundice*). Such patients often get shaking chills and high fever, a condition that is called *cholangitis*. Cholangitis is a serious problem that requires immediate attention.
- **Pancreas Duct Obstruction.** In some persons, the duct that drains the pancreas juices (they also help digest foods we eat) connects to the common bile duct and from there pancreas and bile juices empty into the intestine. In such a patient, a stone in position E blocks the pancreas juices, forcing them back into the pancreas gland itself, causing considerable inflammation (called *acute pancreatitis*). This is a most serious problem.

DIAGNOSIS

- Usually, the diagnosis can be made by taking a detailed history, doing a thorough physical examination, and considering the laboratory reports.
- There is an examination of the blood with particular attention to the function of the liver and pancreas. In addition, there is an examination of the urine, heart (EKG), and lungs (chest x-ray).
- Gallbladder scan: A special dye is injected into the vein. It circulates in the blood stream and leaves the body through the liver, bile ducts, and gallbladder. X-ray pictures are taken to see if the dye is in these locations. If the gallbladder is acutely infected, it will not take up the dye, helping establish the diagnosis of an acute problem there.
- Ultrasound: Harmless sound waves are aimed at the area of the gallbladder. The sound waves bouncing back (the echoes) from this area are seen as a picture on a screen. Ultrasound is a painless and convenient way to examine the gallbladder to see if there are any stones in it.

○ TREATMENT

- A person with gallstones that produce symptoms needs to have the problem corrected. The best treatment for a diseased symptom-producing gallbladder is to remove it. This can be done by one of two techniques:

- **Open**: An incision is made in the abdomen over the gallbladder, and the gallbladder is removed.
- **Laparoscopic**: This is done with instruments (called *laparoscopes*) that are as thick as the tip of your little finger. They have lenses and a built-in light as well as the capability to perform many functions necessary to operate on an organ. Three or four tiny abdominal incisions are made, the laparoscopes are inserted into the abdomen, and the gallbladder is removed.

  Both of these operations, when properly selected and performed, have very low risk.

How all of this applies to you will be discussed with you in great detail before anything is recommended, planned, or done.

△ GENERAL INFORMATION

Practically all moving joints have lubricating fluid in them that is clear and almost like mineral oil in consistency. This fluid is kept inside the joint space by a thin but tough tissue around the joint. Sometimes, however, this tissue weakens and balloons out with joint fluid in it. This is called a *ganglion cyst* (Fig. 1). In some persons, a ganglion is associated with some type of repetitive strain on the wrist. In most persons, however, the cause is not known.

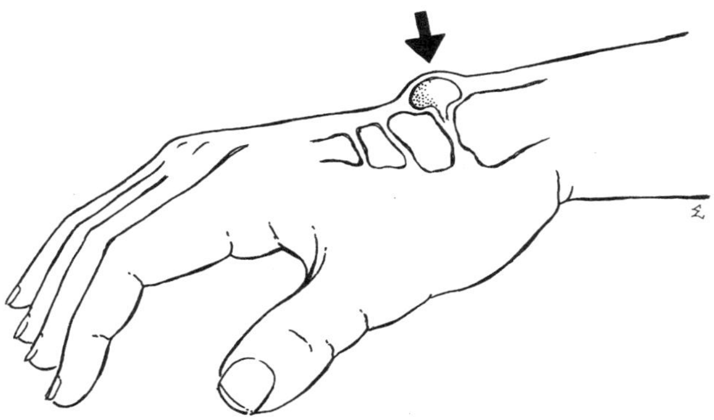

Figure 1. A ganglion arises from between the joints of the wrist bones. Precise and meticulous technique is necessary to remove the deepest part of the cyst lining.

COMMON SIGNS AND SYMPTOMS

- There is a domed, smooth swelling under the skin over the back or front of the wrist. The mass does not move but the skin over it moves freely.
- A ganglion may be a little uncomfortable; most are harmless. They frequently become larger or smaller over time as they fill up with or lose joint fluid.
- Usually the diagnosis can be made by taking a detailed history, doing a thorough physical examination, and considering the laboratory reports carefully.

○ TREATMENT

- An x-ray of the wrist is taken if there is any question about the diagnosis.
- Once the diagnosis is made, patients have two options. One is to simply live with the cyst (it is benign); the other is to have it removed surgically.
- A ganglion can be aspirated (fluid removed with a needle). Generally, however, it will come back because the cyst originates off a stalk from the joint capsule.

After careful consideration, it is recommended that you have an operation.

PREOPERATIVE PREPARATION

- Do not eat or drink anything for 8 hours before the operation.
- You may need an examination of your blood, urine, heart (EKG), and lungs (chest x-ray).
- You will be given medicine that will make you feel drowsy before you are brought to the operating room.

□ OPERATION

- The operation is performed under general anesthesia or by injecting an anesthetic solution into your armpit to numb the entire arm.
- A tourniquet will be placed around your upper arm. This is to prevent the tissue from bleeding during the operation so that all the structures can be seen very clearly as they are dissected.
- During the operation you should feel no pain.
- The operation usually takes less than 1 hour.

POSTOPERATIVE CARE

- You will be taken to a recovery room.
- There will be a snug bandage around your wrist, often with an internal splint to immobilize it.
- After your blood pressure, pulse, and breathing are stable and you are completely alert, you should be able to go home with a responsible adult.
- Arrangements will be made for your medicine, follow-up office visit, and stitch removal.
- As with any operation, complications are always possible. Although they are uncommon with this type of operation, they can include a local infection, bleeding, separation of the skin incision, some stiffness of the wrist and possibly others.

✙ HOME CARE

- Continue with your usual activities.
- Take medicine as prescribed for your pain.
- Keep the arm elevated for several days on pillows while you are sitting or asleep. The wrist will feel more comfortable when it is elevated. It is important to move your fingers as much as possible following surgery so they do not become stiff.
- You will be given instructions on how to take care of the dressings.
- You may shower if you wish, but the dressings should be protected by placing your arm in a small plastic bag and sealing it with tape.
- Physical therapy may be prescribed for you so your wrist does not become stiff. It may take several weeks to regain all of your wrist motion.
- When you return to work depends on how much you can use your wrist. Let's talk about it during your follow-up office visit.

✆ CALL OUR OFFICE IF

- Your fingers turn pale or blue.
- You have pain in your hand without any letup, and it keeps getting worse.
- You develop a temperature higher than 100°F.
- You have any questions.

GASTROESOPHAGEAL REFLUX DISEASE: Laparoscopic Repair

△ GENERAL INFORMATION

Gastro (stomach) *esophageal* (esophagus) *reflux* (flowing back) is a disease in which acid and bile in the stomach flow back up the esophagus. Some flowing back is normal; belching and burping, especially after a meal, are examples of this. However, it is abnormal and can cause trouble if it happens after *every* meal as well as *between* meals. Partial causes can be that the opening in the diaphragm for the esophagus to pass from the chest into the abdomen is too large (a *hiatal hernia*) or that the valve at the end of the esophagus is not working well.

COMMON SIGNS AND SYMPTOMS

- There is heartburn and even pain that begins low in the breast bone and travels upward.
- Food or sour liquid is felt to come up the esophagus when stooping over or lying down, especially immediately after a meal.
- Swallowed food may not go down easily.
- While sleeping, a few drops of stomach fluid can come up the esophagus and go down the windpipe, possibly causing lung problems.

DIAGNOSIS

It will be necessary for you to have some or even all of these tests:

- *Upper gastrointestinal (GI) x-ray series*: You will be given liquid barium to swallow (it is the color and consistency of buttermilk). X-rays will be taken as it goes down the esophagus, into the stomach, and then out into the duodenum to see whether any of it backs up into the esophagus and, if so, the possible reason for this.
- *Esophagoscopy*: This is done with an esophagoscope that is smooth, flexible, and almost as big around as your little finger and has a light at its tip. Your mouth and throat will be sprayed with an anesthetic to make them numb, and you will be given medicine to make you feel very drowsy. The esophagoscope will be placed gently down your esophagus and then into your stomach and duodenum, which will be examined thoroughly.
- *Esophageal pressure studies*: A thin, soft, flexible tube is swallowed so that it goes down the entire length of your esophagus. Inside this tube are tiny gauges that measure what the pressures are along the way as you swallow. This helps determine the cause of the reflux. There may be measurements of how far the acid from your stomach travels back up the esophagus.

○ TREATMENT

The initial treatment for gastroesophageal reflux should be medical.

- Use gravity to help keep the stomach and bile juices inside the stomach where they belong: Use blocks to raise the head of the bed 6 inches, avoid bedtime eating, avoid lying down soon after eating, and avoid stooping.
- Reduce the harm from the juices that come up the esophagus: Take antacid medicine or medicine that helps empty your stomach, or both.
- Reduce the pressure in or on the stomach: Eat small amounts at a time, take off any excess weight, avoid tight clothing, and stop smoking and drinking.

After careful consideration of all factors, it is recommended that you have an operation performed with laparoscopes. (This technique is less painful and the recovery is faster.) The laparoscopes are as big around as the tip of your little finger. Three or four laparoscopes will be placed in your abdomen through very short incisions, and the entire operation is performed using them. Occasionally, however, when everything inside is examined with the laparoscope, conditions are such that it is not possible to do the operation this way. If that is the case with you, an open incision will have to be made.

PREOPERATIVE PREPARATION

- In addition to your other tests, you will have an examination of your blood, urine, heart (EKG), and lungs (chest x-ray).
- Do not eat or drink anything for 8 hours before the operation.

□ OPERATION

- You will be asleep for the operation.
- The X's show common locations of placement of the laparoscopes (Fig. 1).
- The lower part of your esophagus will be wrapped by the upper part of the stomach. In this way, the opening in the diaphragm for passage of the esophagus will be made snug (Fig. 2).
- The operation usually takes about 2 hours.

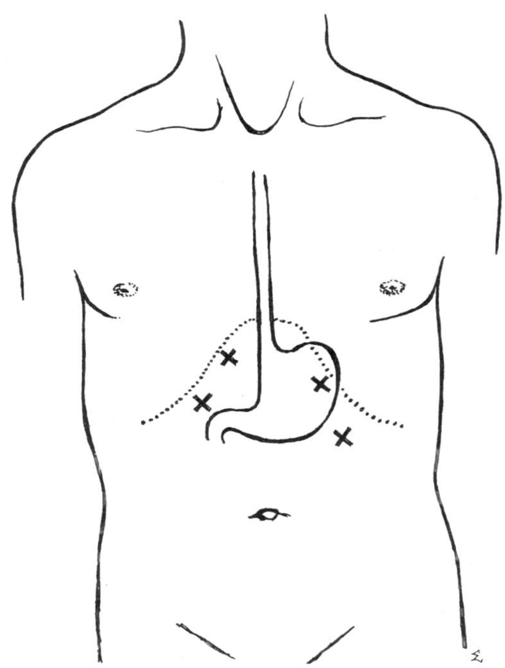

Figure 1.

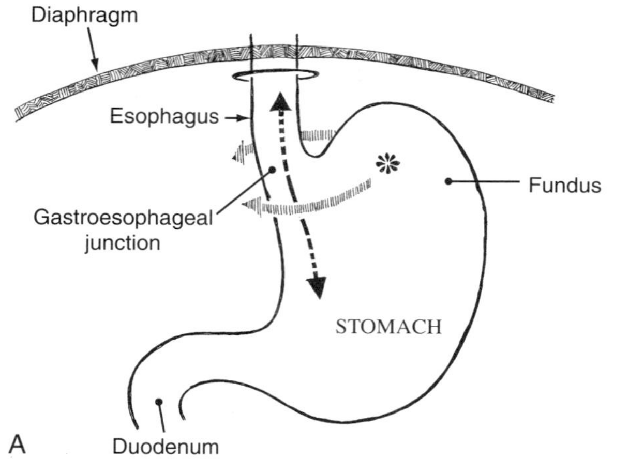

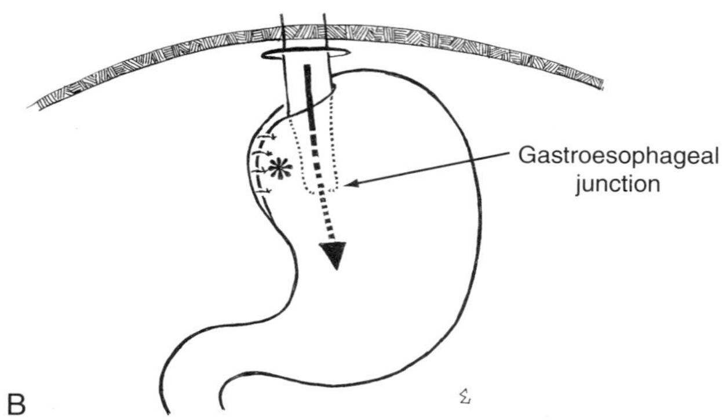

Figure 2. *A*, In gastroesophageal reflux disease, food goes into the stomach but also can easily come back up (reflux) into the esophagus. An important part of this operation to correct the problem is to fold the front and back part of the fundus *(asterisk)* around the esophagus. *B*, Some of the fundus is now located around the other side of the esophagus *(asterisk)*. This wrapped-around bulk of tissue gently squeezes the lower esophagus, hindering food from refluxing up the esophagus (arrow now shows food going only one way).

POSTOPERATIVE CARE

- You will be taken to a recovery room and observed. When your blood pressure, pulse, and breathing are stable, you will be taken to a regular hospital room.
- You will have a thin plastic tube in your nose. It goes down to your stomach to suck up the air you swallow and will be removed when your bowels start working.
- Pain will be controlled with medicine.
- That evening you will be helped to sit up in bed and on the next day to get out of bed.
- After the tube in your nose is removed, you will be started on a liquid diet that will be increased as you tolerate it.
- As with any operation, complications are always possible. With this type of operation, they can include bleeding, injury to your esophagus or spleen, pneumonia, infection, blood clots, and possibly others.
- You should be able to go home in about 5 days.
- Arrangements will be made for your medicine, follow-up office visit, and stitch removal.

✚ HOME CARE

- You may walk about as you wish, even climb stairs, but don't overdo things.
- Follow the diet outlined for you when you were in the hospital.
- Take medicine as prescribed for your pain.
- Unless instructed otherwise, you may return to work when you feel up to it.

✆ CALL OUR OFFICE IF

- You have any difficulty swallowing or develop any unusual signs or symptoms.
- The incision becomes red or swollen, or there is drainage from it.
- You develop a temperature higher than 100°F.
- You have any questions.

GASTROESOPHAGEAL REFLUX DISEASE: Open Abdominal Repair

△ GENERAL INFORMATION

Gastro (stomach) *esophageal* (esophagus) *reflux* (flowing back) is a disease in which acid and bile in the stomach flow back up the esophagus. Some flowing back is normal; belching and burping, especially after a meal, are examples of this. However, it is abnormal and can cause trouble if it happens after *every* meal as well as *between* meals. Partial causes can be that the opening in the diaphragm for the esophagus to pass from the chest into the abdomen is too large (a *hiatal hernia*) or that the valve at the end of the esophagus is not working well.

COMMON SIGNS AND SYMPTOMS

- There is heartburn and even pain that begins low in the breast bone and travels upward.
- Food or sour liquid is felt to come up the esophagus when stooping over or lying down, especially immediately after a meal.
- Swallowed food may not go down easily.
- While sleeping, a few drops of stomach fluid can come up the esophagus and go down the windpipe, possibly causing lung problems.

DIAGNOSIS

It will be necessary for you to have some or even all of these tests:

- *Upper gastrointestinal (GI) x-ray series*: You will be given liquid barium to swallow (it is the color and consistency of buttermilk). X-rays will be taken as it goes down the esophagus, into the stomach, and then out into the duodenum to see whether any of it backs up into the esophagus and, if so, the possible reason for this.
- *Esophagoscopy*: This is done with an esophagoscope that is smooth, flexible, and almost as big around as your little finger and has a light at its tip. Your mouth and throat will be sprayed with an anesthetic to make them numb, and you will be given medicine to make you feel very drowsy. The esophagoscope will be placed gently down your esophagus and then into your stomach and duodenum, which will be examined thoroughly.
- *Esophageal pressure studies*: A thin, soft, flexible tube is swallowed so that it goes down the entire length of your esophagus. Inside this tube are tiny gauges that measure what the pressures are along the way as you swallow. This helps determine the cause of the reflux. There may be measurements of how far the acid from your stomach travels back up the esophagus.

○ TREATMENT

The initial treatment for gastroesophageal reflux should be medical.

- Use gravity to help keep the stomach and bile juices inside the stomach where they belong: Use blocks to raise the head of the bed 6 inches, avoid bedtime eating, avoid lying down soon after eating, and avoid stooping.
- Reduce the harm from the juices that come up the esophagus: Take antacid medicine or take medicine that helps empty your stomach, or both.
- Reduce the pressure in or on the stomach: Eat small amounts at a time, take off any excess weight, avoid tight clothing, and stop smoking and drinking alcoholic beverages.

After careful consideration of your condition, and especially the fact that it has not responded satisfactorily to medical therapy, it is recommended that you have it corrected with an operation performed through an open incision in your abdomen.

PREOPERATIVE PREPARATION

- In addition to your other tests, you will have an examination of your blood, urine, heart (EKG), and lungs (chest x-ray).
- Do not eat or drink anything for 8 hours before the operation.

□ OPERATION

- You will be asleep for the operation.
- The dashed line shows a common location of the abdominal incision (Fig. 1).
- The lower part of your esophagus will be wrapped by the upper part of the stomach. In this way the opening in the diaphragm for passage of the esophagus will be made snug (Fig. 2).
- The operation usually takes about 2 hours.

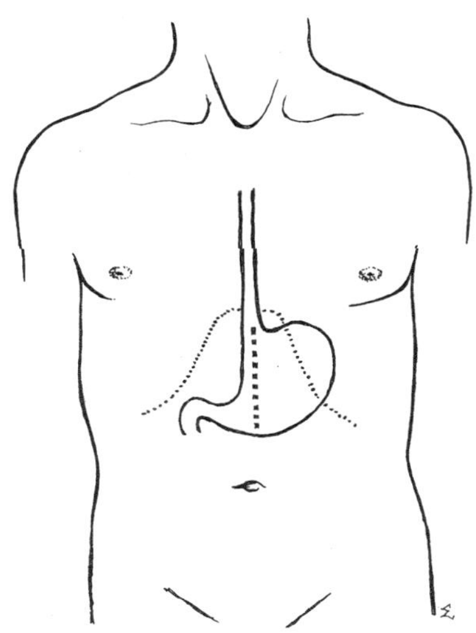

Figure 1.

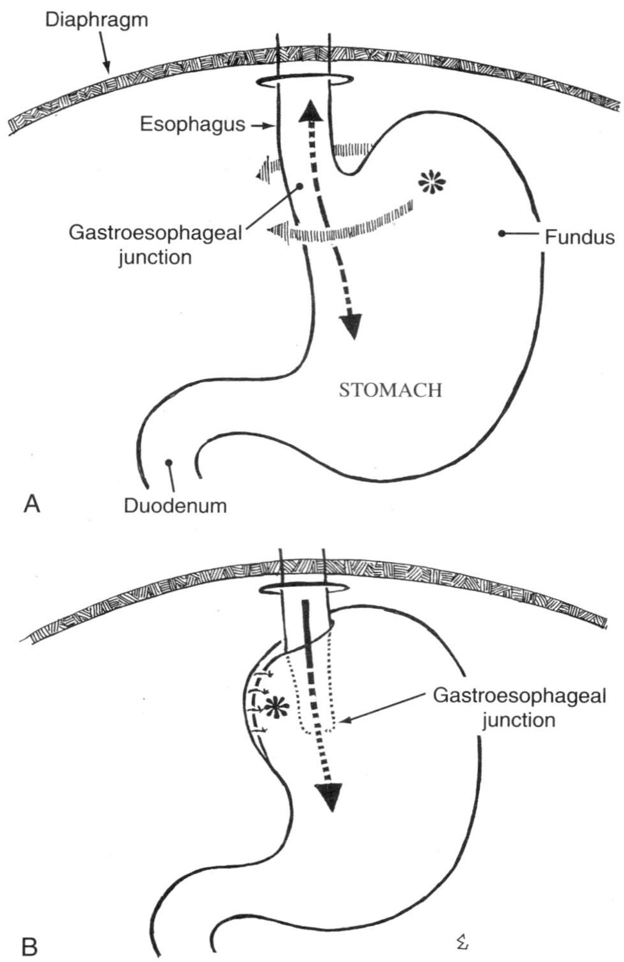

Figure 2. *A*, In gastroesophageal reflux disease, food goes into the stomach but also can easily come back up (reflux) into the esophagus. An important part of this operation to correct the problem is to fold the front and back part of the fundus *(asterisk)* around the esophagus. *B*, Some of the fundus is now located around the other side of the esophagus *(asterisk)*. This wrapped-around bulk of tissue gently squeezes the lower esophagus, hindering food from refluxing up the esophagus (arrow now shows food going only one way).

POSTOPERATIVE CARE

- You will be taken to a recovery room and observed. When your blood pressure, pulse, and breathing are stable, you will be taken to a regular hospital room.
- You will have a thin plastic tube in your nose. It goes down to your stomach to suck up the air you swallow and will be removed when your bowels start working.
- Pain will be controlled with medicine.
- That evening you will be helped to sit up in bed and on the next day to get out of bed.
- After the tube in your nose is removed, you will be started on a liquid diet that will be increased as you tolerate it.
- As with any operation, complications are always possible. With this type of operation, they can include bleeding, injury to your esophagus or spleen, pneumonia, infection, blood clots, and possibly others.
- You should be able to go home in about 5 days.
- Arrangements will be made for your medicine, follow-up office visit, and stitch removal.

HOME CARE

- You may walk about as you wish, even climb stairs, but don't overdo things.
- Follow the diet outlined for you when you were in the hospital.
- Take medicine as prescribed for your pain.
- Unless instructed otherwise, you may shower as you wish and with any dressings on or off. After you dry yourself, replace any dressings with clean, dry ones.
- Do not drive a car until we first discuss it during your follow-up visit.
- You may return to work when you feel up to it.

CALL OUR OFFICE IF

- You have any difficulty with swallowing or develop any unusual signs or symptoms.
- The incision becomes red or swollen, or there is drainage from it.
- You develop a temperature higher than 100°F.
- You have any questions.

GASTROESOPHAGEAL REFLUX DISEASE:
Thoracic Repair

△ GENERAL INFORMATION

Gastro (stomach) *esophageal* (esophagus) *reflux* (flowing back) is a disease in which acid and bile in the stomach flow back up the esophagus. Some flowing back is normal; belching and burping, especially after a meal, are examples of this. However, it is abnormal and can cause trouble if it happens after *every* meal as well as *between* meals. Partial causes can be that the opening in the diaphragm for the esophagus to pass from the chest into the abdomen is too large (a *hiatal hernia*) or that the valve at the end of the esophagus is not working well.

COMMON SIGNS AND SYMPTOMS

- There is heartburn and even pain that begins low in the breast bone and travels upward.
- Food or sour liquid is felt to come up the esophagus when stooping over or lying down, especially immediately after a meal.
- Swallowed food may not go down easily.
- While sleeping, a few drops of stomach fluid can come up the esophagus and go down the windpipe, possibly causing lung problems.

DIAGNOSIS

It will be necessary for you to have some or even all of these tests:

- *Upper gastrointestinal (GI) x-ray series*: You will be given liquid barium to swallow (it is the color and consistency of buttermilk). X-rays will be taken as it goes down the esophagus, into the stomach, and then out into the duodenum to see whether any of it backs up into the esophagus and, if so, the possible reason for this.
- *Esophagoscopy*: This is done with an esophagoscope that is smooth, flexible, and almost as big around as your little finger and has a light at its tip. Your mouth and throat will be sprayed with an anesthetic to make them numb, and you will be given medicine to make you feel very drowsy. The esophagoscope will be placed gently down your esophagus and then into your stomach and duodenum, which will be examined thoroughly.
- *Esophageal pressure studies*: A thin, soft, flexible tube is swallowed so that it goes down the entire length of your esophagus. Inside this tube are tiny gauges that measure what the pressures are along the way as you swallow. This helps determine the cause of the reflux. There may be measurements of how far the acid from your stomach travels back up the esophagus.

○ TREATMENT

The initial treatment for gastroesophageal reflux should be medical.

- Use gravity to help keep the stomach and bile juices inside the stomach where they belong: Use blocks to raise the head of the bed 6 inches, avoid bedtime eating, avoid lying down soon after eating, and avoid stooping.
- Reduce the harm from the juices that come up the esophagus: Take antacid medicine or take medicine that helps empty your stomach, or both.
- Reduce the pressure in or on the stomach: Eat small amounts at a time, take off any excess weight, avoid tight clothing, and stop smoking and drinking.

After careful consideration of your condition, and especially the fact that it has not responded satisfactorily to medical therapy, it is recommended that you have it corrected with an operation performed through the chest.

PREOPERATIVE PREPARATION

- In addition to your other tests, you will have an examination of your blood, urine, heart (EKG), and lungs (chest x-ray).
- Do not eat or drink anything for 8 hours before the operation.

□ OPERATION

- You will be asleep for the operation.
- The incision will be in your left chest (Fig. 1).
- The lower part of your esophagus will be wrapped by the upper part of the stomach. In this way, the opening in the diaphragm for passage of the esophagus will be made snug (Fig. 2).
- The operation usually takes about 2 hours.

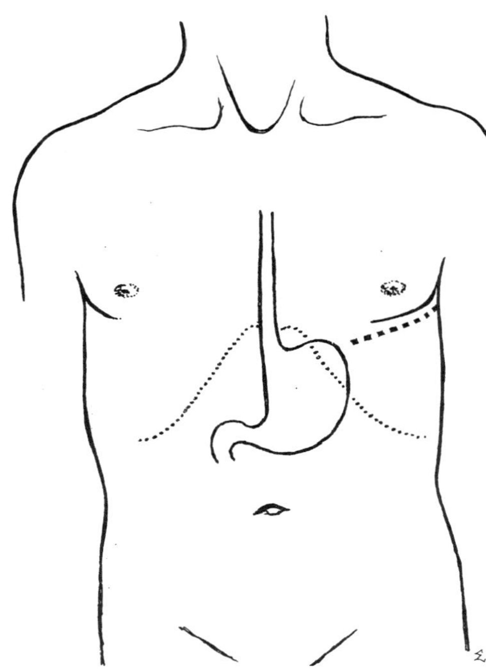

Figure 1.

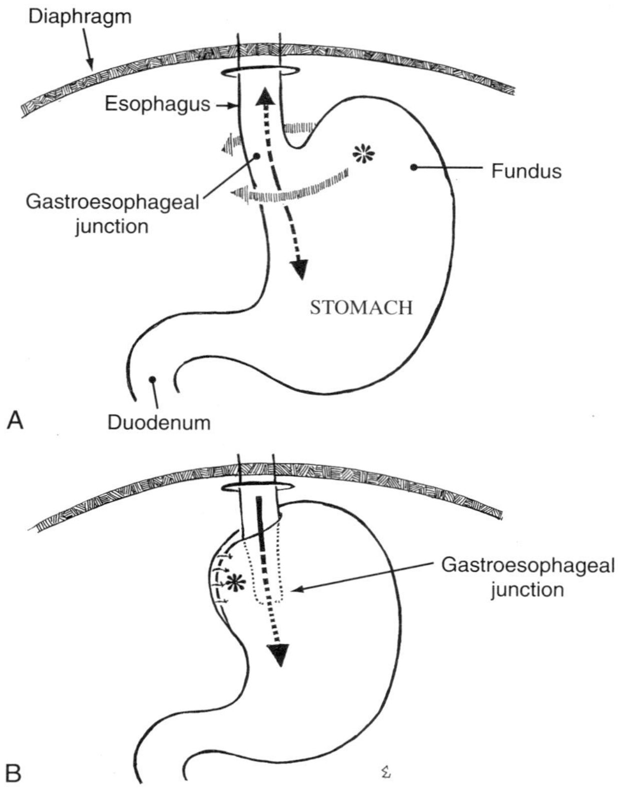

Figure 2. *A*, In gastroesophageal reflux disease, food goes into the stomach but also can easily come back up (reflux) into the esophagus. An important part of this operation to correct the problem is to fold the front and back part of the fundus *(asterisk)* around the esophagus. *B*, Some of the fundus is now located around the other side of the esophagus *(asterisk)*. This wrapped-around bulk of tissue gently squeezes the lower esophagus, hindering food from refluxing up the esophagus (arrow now shows food going only one way).

POSTOPERATIVE CARE

- You will be taken to a recovery room and observed. When your blood pressure, pulse, and breathing are stable, you will be taken to a regular hospital room.
- You will have one or two plastic tubes coming out of your chest and a thin plastic tube in your nose. Both will be removed in several days.
- Pain will be controlled with medicine.
- That evening you will be helped to sit up in bed and on the next day to get out of bed.
- You may be given an incentive spirometer. Breathing into this as you are instructed will help expand your lungs and reduce the risk of developing pneumonia.
- After the tube in your nose is removed, you will be started on a liquid diet that will be increased as you tolerate it.
- As with any operation, complications are always possible. With this type of operation, they can include bleeding, injury to your esophagus or spleen, pneumonia, infection, blood clots, and possibly others.
- You should be able to go home in about 5 days.
- Arrangements will be made for your medicine, follow-up office visit, and stitch removal.

✙ HOME CARE

- You may walk about as you wish, even climb stairs, but don't overdo things.
- Follow the diet outlined for you when you were in the hospital.
- Take the medicines prescribed for you.
- Unless instructed otherwise, you may shower as you wish and with any dressings on or off. After you dry yourself, replace any dressings with clean, dry ones.
- Do not drive a car until we first discuss it during your follow-up visit.
- You may return to work when you feel up to it.

✆ CALL OUR OFFICE IF

- You have any difficulty with swallowing or develop any unusual signs or symptoms.
- The incision becomes red or swollen, or there is drainage from it.
- You develop a temperature higher than 100°F.
- You have any questions.

△ GENERAL INFORMATION

Gastroscopy is looking down your stomach with a special instrument called a *gastroscope.* Gastroscopy is done for several reasons, including the following:

- Something was seen in your stomach on x-ray examination.
- Something is suspected of being in your stomach.

This is a very common procedure, and it has been explained to you why you need one. It is part of a follow-up to medical therapy or an operation.

DIAGNOSIS

There are several ways to investigate the stomach. Only with gastroscopy, however, can the inside of the stomach be seen directly.

PREOPERATIVE PREPARATION

- Do not eat or drink anything for 8 hours before the procedure.
- A needle will be placed in your vein and some fluids started.
- You will be given some medicine by vein that will make you feel drowsy, and your throat will feel dry.

THE PROCEDURE

- The gastroscope is an instrument with lenses in it and a light at its tip. It is smooth, flexible, and almost as big around as your little finger.
- Your mouth and throat will be sprayed to make them numb.
- You will be positioned on a comfortable table.
- Next, you will be given medicine to continue keeping you drowsy during the procedure.
- The gastroscope will be introduced gently into your mouth and then into your throat and down your esophagus, which also will be examined on the way down to the stomach.
- When in the stomach, the tip of the gastroscope can be turned in all directions and the wall of the stomach can be examined thoroughly.
- The gastroscope will be advanced through the exit of the stomach and into the duodenum for about 6 inches.
- If anything suspicious is seen, a tiny piece will be taken (a *biopsy*) for examination in the laboratory.
- When the examination is complete, the gastroscope is removed.
- The medicine that made you feel drowsy will be stopped, and you should become alert again quickly.
- The entire procedure takes around 30 minutes.
- Most patients remember very little of the procedure and think it took only a few minutes.
- When your blood pressure, pulse, and breathing are stable and you are completely alert, you should be able to go home with a responsible adult.
- Your attending physician will discuss the results of the gastroscopy with you.

✣ HOME CARE

- Be certain that all the numbness in your mouth is gone (usually in 1–2 hours) before you start eating. Otherwise, food or fluid may go down the wrong way into your trachea.
- Resume your normal activities.

✆ CALL OUR OFFICE IF

- You develop pain in the chest or abdomen.
- You develop any unusual signs or symptoms.
- You develop a temperature higher than 100°F.
- You have any questions.

GASTROSTOMY: Endoscopic-Guided

△ GENERAL INFORMATION

Gastrostomy is the placement of a thin plastic tube into the stomach straight through the skin from the outside (Fig. 1). Most of the time it is done to allow food directly into the stomach, bypassing the esophagus.

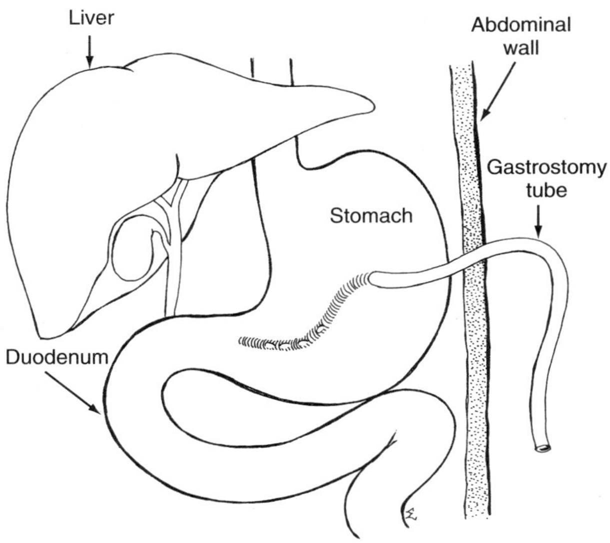

Figure 1.

REASONS FOR GASTROSTOMY TUBE PLACEMENT

- Inability to swallow food.
- Blockage of esophagus.
- Swallowing disorders that cause pneumonia.
- Inability to swallow enough food to meet one's calorie requirements because of severe weakness, illness, or lack of appetite.
- A recent operation on the esophagus so that food temporarily cannot be permitted to cross the stitches.

○ TREATMENT

If you have any of the above conditions, several treatment options are available.

Medical

- Drinking a special liquid diet that is rich in calories and can go past areas of partial blockage. If blockage is not a problem, this liquid simply goes down without any chewing required.
- Passing a very thin, smooth plastic tube through the nose, down the esophagus (past any partial blockage, if that's the problem), and into the stomach. Liquid food can then be passed through this tube. Swallowing is not required when a feeding tube is in place.

Surgical

- A short incision is made on the skin, and one end of the tube is placed directly into the stomach and the other end brought out through the skin.

After taking all facts into consideration, it is recommended that you have this operation.

PREOPERATIVE PREPARATION

- Do not eat or drink anything for 8 hours before the operation.
- Shower as usual on the morning of the operation.
- You may be given medicine that will make you feel drowsy before you are brought to the operating room.

□ OPERATION

- The operation is usually performed in the endoscopy suite at the hospital.
- The skin over the stomach will be painted with an antiseptic solution, draped with towels, and injected with an anesthetic to make it numb.
- Next, a *gastroscope* is used. This is an optical instrument with a light at its tip that is smooth, flexible, and as thick as your little finger.
- After your mouth and throat are sprayed to make them numb, you will be given medicine that will make you feel very drowsy.
- The gastroscope will then be passed into the stomach.
- The gastroscope will be used to watch from the inside as things begin to happen from the outside. The light from the tip of the gastroscope can be seen through the skin. A very short incision will be made directly over the light. The tip of the stomach tube will be placed directly through the skin into the stomach, and the other end of the tube will remain on the outside.
- The gastrostomy tube is now in position.
- The operation usually takes about 1 hour.

POSTOPERATIVE CARE

- You will be taken to a recovery room. When your blood pressure, pulse, and breathing are stable and you are completely alert, you should be able to go home that same day accompanied by a responsible adult. (Of course, if you are already a hospitalized patient, you will be returned to your regular room.)
- Arrangements will be made for your medicine, follow-up office visit, plans for your liquid nourishment, and stitch removal.
- As with any operation, complications are always possible. With this type of operation, they can include infection, leakage, bleeding, and possibly others.

✣ HOME CARE

- Resume your usual activities.
- You may walk about as you wish, even climb stairs.

- The gastrostomy tube can be used in 24 hours.
- You will be shown how to take care of the tube; it's not difficult.
- Arrangements can be made for a home visiting nurse if one is needed.

✆ CALL OUR OFFICE IF

- The area around the tube becomes red and swollen, or there is pus draining from it.
- You develop a temperature higher than 101°F.
- You develop abdominal pain other than where the tube goes in.
- You have any questions.
- If the tube falls out, it will have to be replaced immediately because the hole tends to close soon. This can be done at home by your home care nurse, in your doctor's office, or in the emergency room of the hospital.

△ GENERAL INFORMATION

Gastrostomy is the placement of a thin plastic tube into the stomach straight through the skin from the outside (Fig. 1). Most of the time it is done to allow food to pass directly into the stomach, bypassing the esophagus.

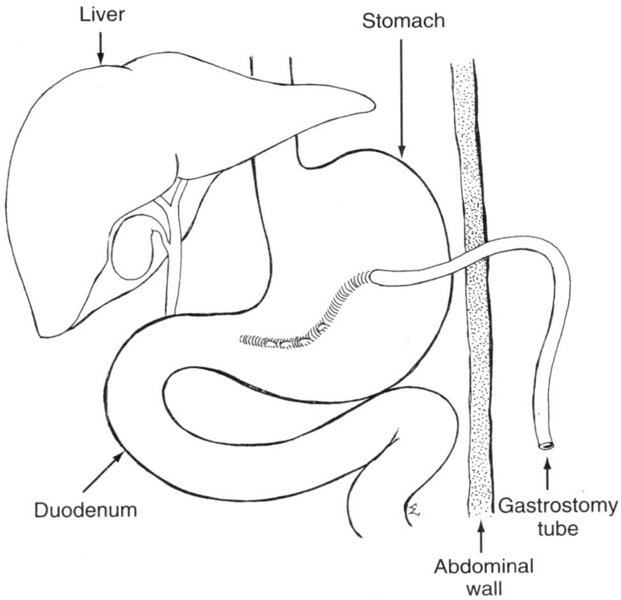

Figure 1. Although open gastrostomy is commonly done on frail, malnourished patients, it is a safe operation when done with attention to detail. It can be used to give nourishment within 24 hours.

REASONS FOR GASTROSTOMY TUBE PLACEMENT

- Inability to swallow food.
- Blockage of esophagus.
- Swallowing disorders that cause pneumonia.
- Inability to swallow enough food to meet one's calorie requirements because of severe weakness, illness, or lack of appetite.
- A recent operation on the esophagus so that food temporarily cannot be permitted to cross the stitches.

○ TREATMENT

If you have any of the above conditions, several treatment options are available.

Medical

- Drinking a special liquid diet that is rich in calories and can go past areas of partial blockage. If blockage is not a problem, this liquid simply goes down without any chewing required.
- Passing a very thin, smooth plastic tube through the nose, down the esophagus (past any partial blockage, if that's the problem), and into the stomach. Liquid food can then be passed through this tube. Swallowing is not required when a feeding tube is in place.

Surgical

- A short incision is made on the skin, and one end of the tube is placed directly into the stomach and the other end brought out through the skin.

After taking all facts into consideration, it is recommended that you have this operation done through a short incision on your abdomen.

PREOPERATIVE PREPARATION

- Do not eat or drink anything for 8 hours before the operation.
- Shower as usual on the morning of the operation.
- You may be given medicine that will make you feel drowsy before you are brought to the operating room.

□ OPERATION

- Your abdomen and lower chest will be painted with an antiseptic solution and properly draped.
- An area on the skin over the middle of the upper abdomen will be made numb with an anesthetic. A short incision will be made. One end of the tube will be placed in the stomach and the other end brought to the outside through the skin.
- During the operation, you may feel some tugging but not pain.
- The operation usually takes about 1 hour.

POSTOPERATIVE CARE

- You will be taken to a recovery room. When your blood pressure, pulse, and breathing are stable and you are completely alert, you should be able to go home that same day accompanied by a responsible adult. (Of course, if you are to be hospitalized, you will be returned to your regular room.)
- Arrangements will be made for your medicine, follow-up office visit, plans for your liquid nourishment, and stitch removal.
- As with any operation, complications are always possible. Although they are uncommon with this type of operation, they can include infection, leakage, and possibly others.

✣ HOME CARE

- Resume your usual activities.
- You may walk about as you wish, even climb stairs.
- The gastrostomy tube can be used in 24 hours.
- You will be shown how to take care of the tube; it's not difficult.
- Arrangements can be made for a home visiting nurse if one is needed.

✆ CALL OUR OFFICE IF

- The incision becomes red or swollen, or there is drainage from it.
- You develop a temperature higher than 101°F.
- You have any questions.
- The tube falls out. It is important to let your doctor know about this immediately. If the doctor cannot be reached, go to the emergency room, where the tube will be reinserted, or call the home care nurse. Often the home nurse is able to reinsert the tube.

GOITER (THYROID GOITER)

△ GENERAL INFORMATION

The thyroid gland is located in the neck on each side of the *trachea* (windpipe), just below the *larynx* (voicebox). It manufactures hormones that regulate how slow or fast many areas in your body work.

Sometimes the cells in the thyroid gland don't work as well as they should; they are weak. The body has the thyroid make more cells, expecting that having more cells will make up for the fact that they are weak. The result is that the thyroid gland becomes large. This is called a *goiter* (Fig. 1). The reason these cells are weak may be unknown, or the weakness can be an inherited trait, or there may not be enough iodine in the diet (rare).

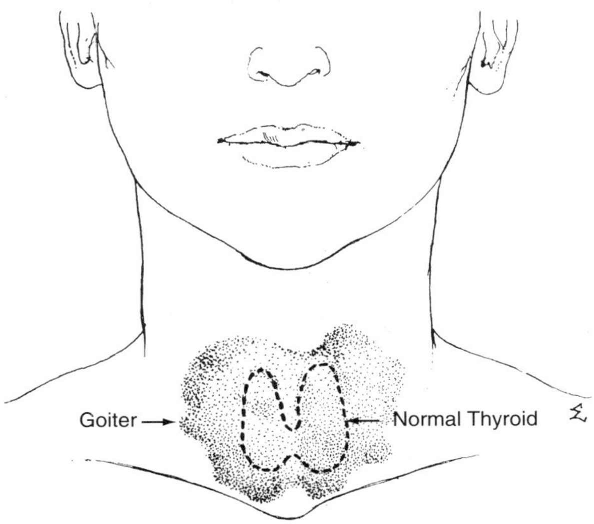

Figure 1. A goiter can assume many shapes inside the neck and can come close to vital structures such as the recurrent laryngeal nerves that supply the larynx (voice box), the parathyroid glands that regulate calcium metabolism, and the trachea (windpipe). These structures must not be damaged during the operation.

COMMON SIGNS AND SYMPTOMS

- Some difficulty with breathing or swallowing.
- A change in the character of the voice.
- The veins in the neck stand out.

DIAGNOSIS

The diagnosis can be determined by taking a detailed history, doing a thorough physical examination, and considering the laboratory reports carefully. Some or all of the following tests may be done:

- You will have an examination of your blood, urine, heart (EKG), and lungs (chest x-ray).
- Ultrasound: Harmless sound waves are aimed at the area of your thyroid gland. The sound waves bouncing back (the echoes) from this area are seen as a picture on a screen. Ultrasound is a convenient and painless way to examine fine details in your thyroid gland.
- CT scan (computed tomography scan): These special x-rays are taken as very thin slices through the neck and upper chest. This makes it possible to see more accurately how large the gland is, how much it surrounds and presses on the trachea and esophagus, and whether it extends down into the chest.

○ TREATMENT

The treatment of a goiter depends a lot on the cause of the goiter.

- Inherited difficulty with making thyroid hormone: Give the hormone (thyroxin).
- Rarely, there is not enough iodine in the diet: Supply the iodine or give hormone.
- Stop any medicines that prevent the thyroid from making hormone.

An operation to remove most of the thyroid is recommended in the following circumstances:

- The goiter responds poorly or not at all to other treatments.
- The symptoms (pain, difficulty with swallowing or breathing, voice change) continue.
- There are many lumps in the thyroid. This type doesn't respond well to medical therapy.
- The person with the goiter simply wants it removed because it is unsightly.

PREOPERATIVE PREPARATION

- Do not eat or drink anything for 8 hours before the operation.
- Shower (and shave) as usual on the morning of the operation.

□ OPERATION

- You will be asleep for the operation.
- A cosmetic incision will be made crosswise in a crease in your lower neck.
- The operation usually takes about 2 hours.

POSTOPERATIVE CARE

- You will be taken to a recovery room and observed. When your blood pressure, pulse, and breathing are stable, you will be taken to a regular hospital room.
- Pain will be controlled with medicine.
- You may be a little hoarse for a few days.
- That evening you will be helped to sit up in bed and on the next day to get out of bed.
- You will advance from drinking liquids to eating solids within 24 hours of the operation.
- You should be able to go home in 1 or 2 days.
- As with any operation, complications are always possible. With this type of operation, they can include bleeding, low calcium, and hoarseness. The hoarseness is usually temporary, but very rarely it can be permanent. There are ways to treat this.
- Arrangements will be made for your medicine, follow-up office visit, and stitch removal.

✣ HOME CARE

- You may walk about as you wish, even climb stairs.
- Unless instructed otherwise, you may shower if you

wish and with any dressings on or off. After you dry yourself, replace any dressings with clean, dry ones.

- Don't drive a car unless you can move freely and without pain and you are not taking medicines that decrease your alertness.
- You may return to work when you feel up to it but let's first talk about it during your follow-up office visit.

✆ CALL OUR OFFICE IF

- You develop any tingling of the fingers, toes, or around your lips, or you develop cramps or spasms of your hands or feet.
- The incision becomes red or swollen, or there is drainage from it.
- You develop a temperature higher than 100°F.
- You have any questions.

△ GENERAL INFORMATION

The groin has many lymph nodes ("glands") in it. These lymph nodes strain the fluid (called *lymph*) that passes through them as it comes from the leg, the external sex organs, and the anus. The nodes can trap different types of cells that pass through them, including cancer cells coming from these areas.

COMMON SIGNS AND SYMPTOMS

- There is no set number of lymph nodes in the groin (or in any location), just as there is no set number of hairs on your scalp.
- Most of the time, lymph nodes are small; sometimes, a few can be felt even though there is nothing wrong with them. At other times they can get larger and be felt easily. This can happen for no apparent reason or because the nodes are reacting to an infection or are involved with cancer. These enlarged lymph nodes can get to be the size of an olive or larger. There may be only one or many of them.
- Normal lymph nodes and nodes involved with cancer are usually not painful. On the other hand, infected nodes can be quite tender. However, there are exceptions to this rule.

DIAGNOSIS

If a person has a current or past history of a cancer in the area that drains into the groin with enlarged lymph nodes, obtaining a sample of the node (a *biopsy*) is recommended.

- *Needle aspiration biopsy*: This is performed by making the skin over the lymph node numb and inserting a needle through the numbed skin into the lymph node to obtain tissue for laboratory examination.
- *Open biopsy*: The skin is made numb, and a short incision is made over the lymph node to obtain all or a piece of it.

○ TREATMENT

- If a biopsy shows the presence of cancer in the lymph nodes, a groin dissection is recommended.

PREOPERATIVE PREPARATION

- You will first need to have some or all of these tests performed:
  - An examination of your blood, urine, heart (EKG), and lungs (chest x-ray).
  - Bone scan: A fine needle is used to inject a solution with a tiny amount of a harmless radioactive material into your vein. The solution circulates throughout your entire body and attaches itself to any bone that has anything wrong with it. You will then lie on a table, and a special recording machine will pass over your entire body taking a photograph (a *scan*) of all the bones from your skull to your toes. A specialist will examine the scan for any abnormalities.
  - CT scan (computed tomography scan): These special x-rays are taken as very thin slices through the area of the groin. This makes it possible to see fine details in the tissues of the groin.
- Do not eat or drink anything for 8 hours before the operation.
- You will be instructed on how to clean out your bowels if necessary.

□ OPERATION

- You will be asleep for the operation.
- The operation will be done through an incision in your groin area. The fatty tissue that contains your lymph nodes will be removed (see stippled area in Fig. 1).
- The operation usually takes about 2 hours.

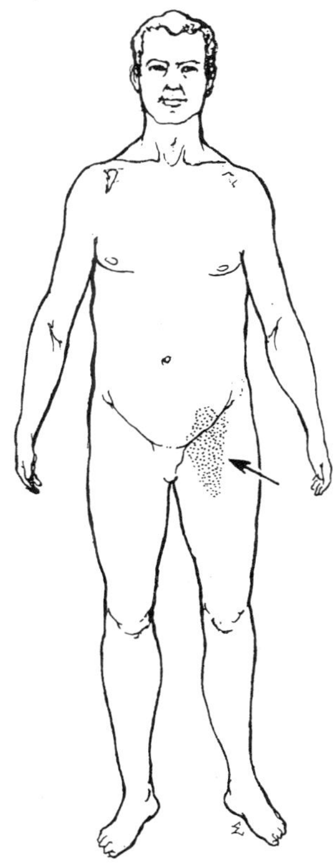

Figure 1. The tissue removed in a groin dissection is indicated by the stippled area. In selected instances, tissue above the groin crease is also removed.

POSTOPERATIVE CARE

- You will be taken to a recovery room and observed. When your blood pressure, pulse, and breathing are stable, you will be taken to a regular hospital room.
- A thin plastic tube that is connected to a small plastic container may be coming from the wound to drain any excess fluid.
- That evening you will be helped to get out of bed.
- When lying in bed or sitting, your leg will be elevated on pillows.
- Pain will be controlled with medicine.

- Your diet will be as you tolerate it.
- You should be able to go home in about 3 or 4 days.
- As with any operation, complications are always possible. With this type of operation, they can include bleeding, infection, collection of fluid in the wound, and possibly others.
- An estimate of your chances of cure can be made only after all the test results are back.
- Arrangements will be made for your medicine, follow-up office visit, and stitch removal.

✚ HOME CARE

- Rest frequently by lying down with your operated leg on a pillow.
- Take medicine as prescribed for your pain.
- If you have on an elastic bandage or stocking, remove and reapply it as you were shown.
- Include plenty of roughage and liquids in your diet to avoid constipation.
- Do not drive a car until we first discuss it.
- Let's discuss when it would be advisable for you to return to work.

✆ CALL OUR OFFICE IF

- The incision becomes red or swollen, or there is drainage from it.
- You develop a temperature higher than 100°F.
- Your leg swells and stays that way, even when you get up in the morning.
- You have any questions.

△ GENERAL INFORMATION

Gynecomastia is the abnormal enlargement of one or both breasts in an adolescent male. This condition is fairly common in boys between the ages of 11 and 15 years. The cause is thought to be hormonal stimulation as a male goes through puberty.

COMMON SIGNS AND SYMPTOMS

- The breast is noticeably enlarged under the nipple.
- It is smooth, rubbery, moves freely and is sometimes tender to the touch. It is not reddened or inflamed, and there is no discharge from the nipple.
- More often, only one breast is involved.

DIAGNOSIS

- The appearance and the feel of the breast tissue are characteristic.
- Some boys are simply obese, and breast enlargement is caused by abundant, soft, fatty tissue in this area.
- All boys with gynecomastia should have their testicles examined to be certain that no tumor is present. Sometimes such tumors produce female hormones that cause the breasts to enlarge.
- There are some illnesses, medicines, or drugs, such as marijuana, that can produce enlargement of the breasts.

○ TREATMENT

- The problem of true gynecomastia sometimes corrects itself in a year or two, and one can wait to see what happens.
- Most often, however, an adolescent boy has an acute psychological and social concern about his appearance and peer acceptance.
- Under most circumstances, it is reasonable to remove the enlarged breast tissue to restore the adolescent's normal physique and self-image.

PREOPERATIVE PREPARATION

- There will be a routine examination of the blood and urine.
- Do not eat or drink anything for 8 hours before the operation.
- You may be given some medicine that will make you feel drowsy before you are brought into the operating room.

□ OPERATION

- The operation is easier and faster if it is done under general anesthesia, especially if both breasts are to be reduced.
- The incision usually is made in the dark part of the nipple so that it will barely show.
- The incision will be closed in a cosmetic manner with fine sutures.
- There may be an injection of local anesthetic in the skin around the incision to help with relief of postoperative pain.
- The operation generally takes about 1 hour.

POSTOPERATIVE CARE

- You will wake up in a recovery room, and when your blood pressure, pulse, and breathing are stable and you are completely alert and tolerating liquids, you should be able to go home the same day with a responsible adult.
- Arrangements will be made for your pain medicine, follow-up office visit, and stitch removal.

✚ HOME CARE

- Walk about and eat as you wish.
- You may shower if you wish and with any dressings on or off.
  - There may be narrow strips of tape across the incision. It's all right if they get wet; they will be removed in the doctor's office.
  - After you dry yourself, replace any dressings with clean, dry ones, if requested by your surgeon.
- You may return to school at any time.
- Avoid contact sports for 3 weeks.

✆ CALL OUR OFFICE IF

- The incision becomes red or swollen, or there is drainage from it.
- You develop a fever higher than 101°F.
- You have any questions.

△ GENERAL INFORMATION

This is the enlargement of one or both breasts in an adult male to an abnormal size.

- It is seen in men being treated for cancer using female hormones.
- It also occurs in persons with liver disease, especially cirrhosis, and a number of other diseases.
- Also, gynecomastia can result from taking certain medicines.
- Marijuana abuse can cause breast enlargement.
- In older men, cancer of the breasts can manifest as an enlargement of the breast.
- Finally, certain tumors of the testicle can produce female hormones that make the breasts (usually both) become larger.

COMMON SIGNS AND SYMPTOMS

- More commonly, both breasts are enlarged.
- The breast tissue feels somewhat nodular. If the enlargement is on one side only and if the breast tissue is firm to hard, cancer should definitely be considered as a possible diagnosis, even though cancer of the breast in men is not at all common.

DIAGNOSIS

- A careful history and a thorough physical examination will be done to be certain some general disease or medicines that you may be taking are not responsible for the breast enlargement.
- The testicles will be examined for the presence of a tumor.
- Many persons who are obese have enlarged breasts. Examination shows the enlargement of the breasts to be simply soft, fatty tissue in this area. It's easy to tell the difference.
- Enlargement of only one breast needs to be looked at very carefully, especially if the enlargement is firm and off to the side of the nipple.
- Mammography: This can be helpful but is not foolproof.
- Needle biopsy: The skin over the mass will be painted with an antiseptic solution. A fine needle will be used to inject an anesthetic to make the area numb. A needle will be placed through the numb skin and into the mass, and cells or tissue will be removed (a *needle aspiration* or *core biopsy*) for examination in the pathology laboratory.
- Open biopsy: The skin is prepared as for a needle biopsy. Here, a short incision is made in the skin down to the mass and a small piece of the mass is removed for examination in the laboratory. This is a simple outpatient procedure.

○ TREATMENT

- Most often, close observation of the breast mass every 4 months is reasonable under the following circumstances:
  - There is no concern about cancer.
  - There is a general illness, or medicines are being taken that are known to cause breast enlargement.
  - There is serious concern about appearance.
- The medicines can be changed if this is thought to be the cause.
- The breast tissue can be removed for cosmetic reasons.
- If a biopsy shows that cancer is present, then a different and more radical operation is necessary. It will not be described or discussed here now because we don't yet know the diagnosis.

PREOPERATIVE PREPARATION

- You will have routine examination of the blood, urine, heart (EKG), and lungs (chest x-ray).
- Do not eat or drink anything for 8 hours before the operation.
- You may be given some medicine that will make you feel drowsy before you are brought into the operating room.

□ OPERATION

- The operation can be performed under local anesthesia with sedation or with you asleep. The choice will be discussed with you beforehand.
- The operation generally takes about 1 hour.
- You will not need a blood transfusion.

POSTOPERATIVE CARE

- You will wake up in a recovery room. When your blood pressure, pulse, and breathing are stable and you are completely alert, you will be taken to your hospital room.
- That evening, you will be helped to get out of bed.
- You should be able to go home the next morning.
- Pain can be controlled with medicine.
- Arrangements will be made for your pain medicine, follow-up office visit, and stitch removal.
- As with any operation, complications are always possible. With your type of operation, they can include bleeding, infection, and possibly others.

✚ HOME CARE

- You may walk about as you wish, even climb stairs.
- Eat as you wish.
- You may shower if you wish and with any dressings on or off.
  - There may be narrow strips of tape across the incision. It's all right if they get wet; they will be removed in the doctor's office.
  - After you dry yourself, replace any dressings with clean, dry ones.
- Driving a car with an automatic shift is not too

demanding. But if you suddenly have to slam on the brakes or twist to turn a wheel, you may strain the sutures or tear something. During the follow-up visit, let's discuss when you can resume driving.

- You may return to work when you feel up to it.

✆ CALL OUR OFFICE IF

- The incision becomes red or swollen, or there is drainage from it.
- You develop a temperature higher than 100°F.
- You have any questions.

HEART CATHETERIZATION AND CORONARY ANGIOGRAPHY

△ GENERAL INFORMATION

In many situations, it is necessary to know more about a patient's heart than the information that can be gathered from an ordinary physical examination. There are two noninvasive ways to examine the heart. In a *treadmill stress test,* the person is connected to an electrocardiogram (EKG) machine and then walks on a treadmill as the function of the heart is recorded. In an *echocardiogram,* harmless sound waves are directed toward the heart. The waves bouncing back (the echoes) are seen as pictures on a screen. This is a convenient and painless way to examine the heart, its chambers, and the blood flowing through them. If the results of one of these studies are abnormal, however, then further information can be obtained through the performance of a cardiac catheterization and coronary arteriography.

With *cardiac catheterization,* the pressures inside the heart chambers are measured, as is the amount of blood the heart muscle pumps each time it squeezes. In *coronary arteriography,* dye is injected into the coronary artery to see whether there are any obstructions or serious narrowings within the coronary arteries. The items that are looked at during cardiac catheterization and coronary arteriography procedures are as follows:

- How well the heart muscle is pumping.
- Whether there are narrowings or leaking of any of the heart valves.
- Whether there are any abnormal communications between the heart chambers.
- Whether there are any narrowings in the coronary arteries and, if so, how serious they are.
- If abnormalities are present, what may be the best way to correct them.

The cardiologist then takes the results from these studies and combines them with other additional information: the patient's history, the findings on physical examination, the evidence of any recent serious episodes of chest pain, and the presence of any other illnesses.

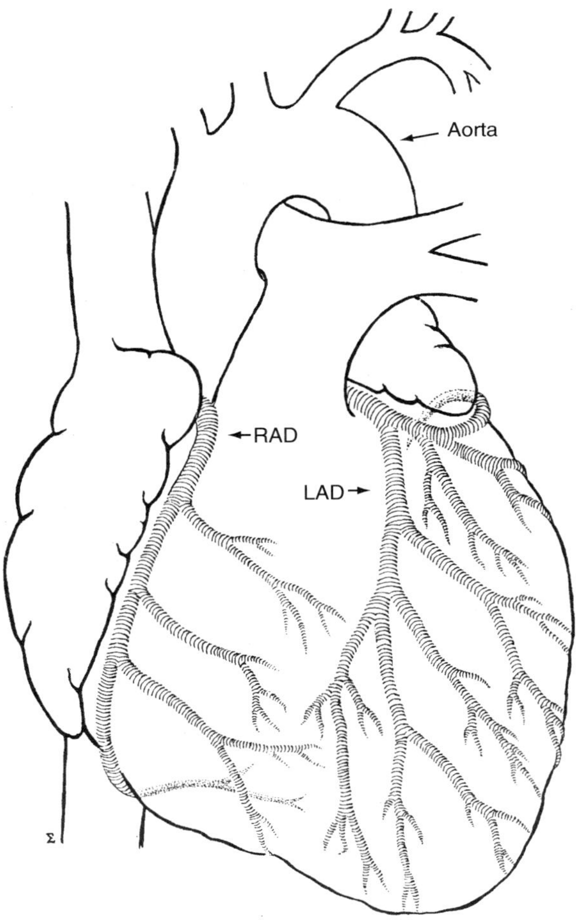

Figure 1. Typical distribution of coronary arteries as seen from the outside of the heart. LAD, Left anterior descending coronary artery; RAD, right anterior descending coronary artery.

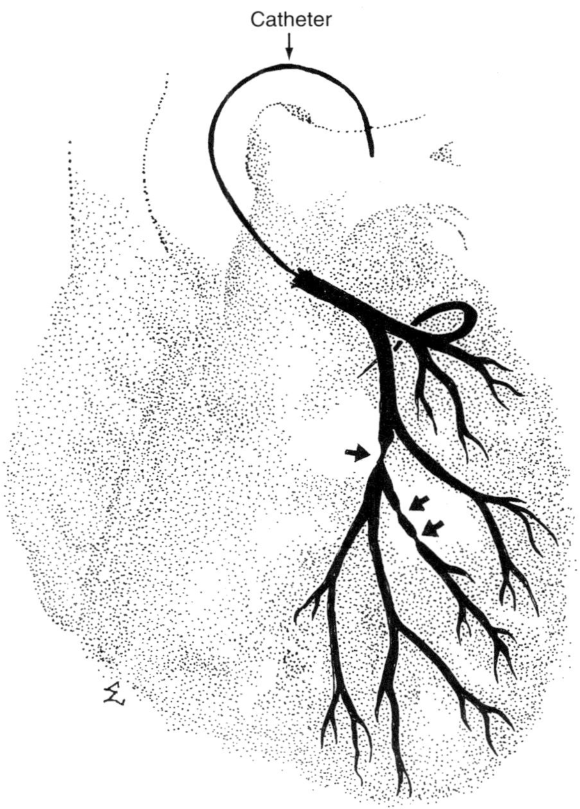

Figure 2. A thin catheter is placed in the aorta (through the groin area) and advanced upward to the beginning of the aorta, the main vessel from the heart. A special dye is injected into one of the coronary arteries (the LAD) that slants at this point. X-rays are taken as the dye flows through this artery, making it possible to see abnormalities in the artery. Three areas of marked narrowing are indicated by the short arrows.

All this information taken together helps the cardiologist make the proper decision about the condition of a person's heart and any necessary therapy.

PREPARATION FOR THE PROCEDURE

- You will have an examination of your blood, urine, heart (EKG), and lungs (chest x-ray).
- Do not eat or drink anything for 8 hours before the procedure.

THE ANGIOGRAPHY

- When an angiogram is performed by an experienced, skilled cardiologist in a laboratory that does a large number of them, the risk of the procedure is low.
- You will be placed on a special padded table with very sophisticated equipment around you.
- The groin area, where the femoral vessels are located, will be painted with an antiseptic solution. A fine needle will be used to inject an anesthetic solution in the skin over the femoral vessels to make this area numb. A very thin plastic tube, no larger than the size of angel hair spaghetti, will be placed in the femoral vessel and advanced into the main blood vessel of the body (the *aorta*) and then into the heart chambers. Various pressure measurements as well as blood samples will be taken. The catheter will be placed next at the opening of the coronary arteries. Dye will be injected through the catheter into the coronary arteries, and multiple pictures will be taken of them (Figs. 1 and 2).
- You will be awake but drowsy during the procedure. Little or no pain is involved.

AFTER THE ANGIOGRAPHY

- The catheter will be removed, and a firm pressure will be held for 20 minutes over the puncture site.
- You will be taken to a hospital room with a firm bandage over the groin area and will be expected to remain fairly flat for approximately 6 hours.
- You should be able to go home later that day or early the next morning with a responsible adult.
- As with any procedure, complications are always possible. With this type of procedure, they can include bleeding from the site where the catheter was inserted into the femoral vessels, injury to the femoral vessels, a loss of rhythm of the heart, a heart attack, and possibly others. **Note:** Very rarely, the coronary artery becomes plugged during the angiography. This requires an immediate open heart operation by a cardiac surgeon to prevent the heart muscle from dying. That is why, during angiography, a heart surgeon is available in the event such a blockage develops.

CALL THE CARDIOLOGIST IF

- There is any swelling, tenderness, or discharge in the area where the catheter was inserted.
- There is any pain in the leg, around the knee, or in the calf area.
- You develop a temperature higher than 100°F.
- You have any questions.

△ GENERAL INFORMATION

The heart has four chambers (Fig. 1). They are as follows:

- Blood from the entire body (A) goes to a small chamber on the right side (the *atrium*, B) and then through a one-way valve (C) to the larger chamber under it (the *right ventricle*, D). From there the blood goes through a one-way valve (E) to the lungs (F), where it gives off waste carbon dioxide and picks up fresh oxygen.
- Blood from the lungs (G) goes to the left *atrium* (H) and then through a one-way valve (I) to the *left ventricle* (J) just below it. From here, the blood is pumped through a one-way valve (the *aortic* valve, K) into the aorta (L) and then to all areas of the body (M).

All of the above processes take place at the same time with every heartbeat, day after day.

Sometimes the valves between the chambers become diseased and don't work properly. The heart is very good at overcoming some of these problems by itself or with the help of medicines. For some persons, however, a heart valve no longer responds to medicines, and an operation is necessary to replace the diseased heart valve.

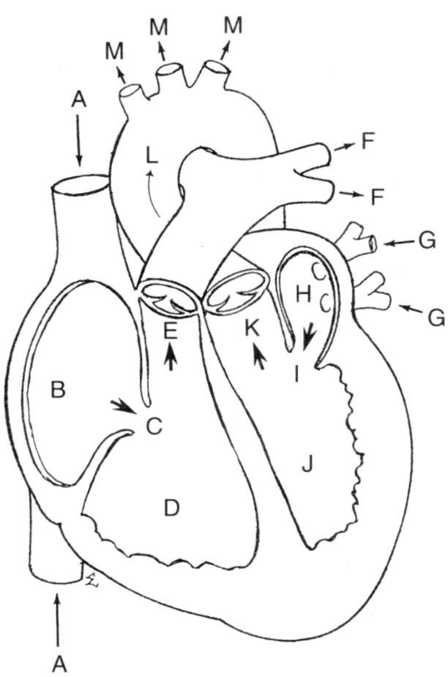

Figure 1.

COMMON SIGNS AND SYMPTOMS

The symptoms vary a lot, depending on a number of things:

- Which valve is involved, whether it is loose and leaking or too tight and the blood not flowing through it properly, how seriously it is involved, how long the condition has been present, and how rapidly the condition has been getting worse.
- Whether other organs such as the lungs, kidney, and liver are affected by this problem.
- Whether other illnesses are also present.
- The condition of the heart muscle in general.

DIAGNOSIS

- Usually the diagnosis can be made by taking a detailed history, doing a thorough physical examination, and considering the laboratory reports carefully. Although a diagnosis may be strongly suspected, a number of tests still need to be done.
- Electrocardiogram (EKG): This is a simple test yet one that can give a lot of information about your heart. Also, the results can be compared with those of EKGs you had in the past to see what changes may have developed in the meantime.
- Heart catheterization: You will lie on a table that is surrounded by very sophisticated machinery and will be given some medicine that will make you feel drowsy. The area of your groin will be painted with an antiseptic solution, surrounded with sterile towels, and made numb with an anesthetic solution. A very small catheter (tube) will be inserted into the artery in the groin area and advanced up to the heart. A special solution will be injected through the catheter into the heart, and x-ray pictures will be taken of it as it travels through the heart chambers. A number of pictures and measurements will be taken of the chamber and the valves to determine how well they work.

○ TREATMENT

All this information has been evaluated very carefully, and the recommendation is that you have one of your heart valves replaced (Fig. 2).

PREOPERATIVE PREPARATION

- If any important associated problems are found in any of your other organs, they will be corrected as much as possible before the operation.
- Do not eat or drink anything for 8 hours before the operation.
- You will be given medicine that will make you feel drowsy before you are brought to the operating room.

□ OPERATION

- After you are asleep, wires from recording machines will be taped to certain areas of your body so that your heart rate, breathing, levels of oxygen in your blood, and other important functions can be followed continuously during the operation.

- The incision will be down the center of your breastbone, the valve replaced and the chest closed.
- The operation usually takes about 4 hours.

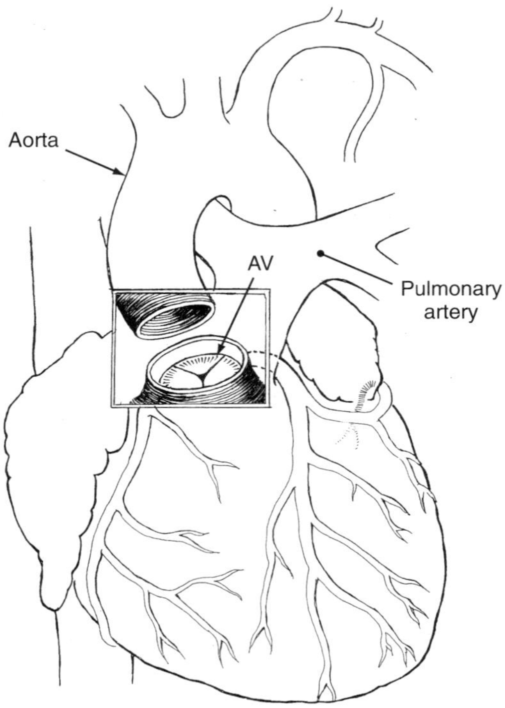

Figure 2. A window has been cut out of the upper part of the heart to show the inside of the aorta and the aortic valve (AV). The aortic valve is one that commonly needs replacement.

POSTOPERATIVE CARE

- You will be taken to the Surgical Intensive Care Unit, where the doctors and nurses are very experienced in taking care of patients like yourself. As soon as you are coming along well enough, you will be transferred to a regular hospital room.
- You may have a tube down your throat to help you with your breathing. You will be drowsy and not uncomfortable from this.
- Pain will be controlled with medicine.
- There will be several plastic drainage tubes coming out next to the lower part of the incision.
- You will be gotten out of bed as soon as possible.
- You may be given an incentive spirometer. Breathing into this as you are instructed will help expand your lungs and reduce the risk of developing pneumonia.
- Your diet will be as you tolerate it.
- You should be able to go home in about 4 to 7 days.
- Arrangements will be made for your medicine, follow-up office visit, and stitch removal.
- As with any operation, complications are always possible. With this type of operation, they can include bleeding, pneumonia, stroke, heart attack, disturbed heart rhythm, infection, and possibly others.

✚ HOME CARE

- You will be given specific instructions about your activities.
- Take medicine as prescribed for your pain.
- Sponge bathe until the stitches are removed. You then may shower or tub bathe.
- Include plenty of roughage and liquids in your diet to help prevent constipation.
- Do not drive a car or return to work until we first discuss it during your follow-up visit.

✆ CALL OUR OFFICE IF

- The incision becomes red or swollen, or there is drainage from it.
- You develop a temperature higher than 100°F.
- You have any questions.

△ GENERAL INFORMATION

Hemorrhoids are congested, swollen veins that are called *internal hemorrhoids* when they are just inside the anus. They are called *external hemorrhoids* when they are at the anal opening. There are many causes of hemorrhoids, including the following: chronic constipation, a job that requires a lot of sitting, pregnancy, liver disease, loss of muscle strength in the anal area with advancing age, and obesity.

COMMON SIGNS AND SYMPTOMS

There can be a number of symptoms, sometimes more than one at the same time.

- Rectal bleeding.
- Protrusion of the hemorrhoids on the outside.
- Pain in the anus with external hemorrhoids.
- Itching in and around the anus.
- Blood in the stool.
- External hemorrhoids that are clotted and very painful.

DIAGNOSIS

- Usually, the diagnosis can be made by taking a detailed history and doing a thorough physical examination.
- A painful, clotted hemorrhoid on the outside of the anus is easy to see.
- Anoscopy: This examination is done with a hollow instrument as long and as thick as your finger. It is lubricated and inserted into the anus gently so that the entire area can be inspected.
- Flexible sigmoidoscopy: This is done with a smooth, flexible instrument as thick as your little finger. It has lenses in it and light coming out of its tip. The instrument is passed through the anus and is used to inspect the inside of the lower 20 inches of the bowel.

○ TREATMENT

Managing hemorrhoids requires a number of approaches:

Avoidance

- Avoid constipation: Include enough roughage and plenty of liquids in your diet. Use stool softeners, if necessary.
- Avoid sitting on the toilet longer than is necessary.
- If your job involves sitting a lot, get up and walk around when you can.
- Reduce your weight if you are overweight.

Nonoperative Treatment

- Sitz baths: Sit in a bathtub with enough warm (not hot) water just to cover your anal area. Do this for 15 minutes three times a day and after each bowel movement, if possible. Or you can use a pan that holds 2 quarts of warm water with 1 tablespoon of epsom salts in it.
- You can buy various preparations without prescription to soothe swelling or itching.

Operation

Most patients with hemorrhoids do not require an operation. An operation is necessary, however, in the following circumstances:

- The hemorrhoids are large and stick out.
- It is very difficult to keep your anal area clean.
- The hemorrhoids don't get better with other treatment.
- The hemorrhoids bleed too often or clot more than one time and are very painful.

There are several operations, as listed below, for correcting a hemorrhoidal problem.

Internal Hemorrhoids

- Placing a special type of rubberband around the hemorrhoid and strangling it.
- Injecting the hemorrhoid area with a solution that causes it to scar down.
- Burning the hemorrhoid with laser. This causes the hemorrhoid to shrivel to a scar.
- Removing the hemorrhoid.

External Hemorrhoids (Clotted)

- A very fine, short needle is used to inject an anesthetic in the area to make it entirely numb. For a clotted hemorrhoid, a short incision is made over it and the clot removed. If there is a lot of extra tissue hanging there, it will be trimmed.

After careful consideration of all factors, the recommendation is that you have an operation to correct your hemorrhoid problem.

PREOPERATIVE PREPARATION

- You may have an examination of your blood and urine, as well as an examination of your heart (EKG) and lungs (chest x-ray). The number of tests will be determined by the extent of the operation and your condition in general.
- Do not eat or drink anything for 8 hours before the operation.
- No laxatives, enemas, or any other bowel preparation is necessary before the operation.
- You may be given medicine that will make you feel drowsy before you are brought to the operating room.

□ OPERATION

The type of anesthesia you have will be determined by the location of your hemorrhoids and their size. The choice will be discussed with you beforehand.

- The operation generally lasts from half an hour to an hour and a half, depending on how extensive the problem is and what needs to be done.

POSTOPERATIVE CARE

If no anesthesia is used (this usually is the case with rubberbanding of internal hemorrhoids; it is an office procedure), you should be able to go home directly after the operation. Generally, you should be able to go home that same day with a responsible adult if the operation involved the following:

- Removing or evacuating an external hemorrhoid.
- Removing one area of internal hemorrhoid.
- Rubberbanding of internal hemorrhoids.

Generally, following an operation more involved than the above, you will need to stay in the hospital for a day or two.

- That afternoon you will be helped to get out of bed and walk about.
- Pain will be controlled with medicine.
- Your diet will be as you tolerate it.

✜ HOME CARE

- You may walk about as you wish, even climb stairs, but don't overdo things.
- You may shower as you wish in the usual fashion.
- Take a sitz bath for 15 minutes two to three times a day and after a bowel movement. Do this as long as you have discomfort.
- Take medicine as prescribed for your pain.
- Include enough roughage and plenty of liquids in your diet to help avoid constipation. You may need some help with a mild laxative (example: milk of magnesia).

✆ CALL OUR OFFICE IF

- You have any bleeding from the anus after the first bowel movement.
- You develop a temperature higher than 100°F.
- You have any questions.
- You do not have a bowel movement for 48 hours.

△ GENERAL INFORMATION

A *femoral hernia* is a bulge of weakened tissue just below the crease in the groin. Its name comes from the opening through which the vessels (*femoral artery* and *vein*) go to and from the leg. There is an opening in the groin just large enough for the blood vessels to come out of the abdomen on the way to and from the leg (Fig. 1). In some persons, however, this opening relaxes or becomes larger. Because of this, some intestine or fatty tissue goes into this area to produce the bulge. These types of hernias are most commonly seen in older people.

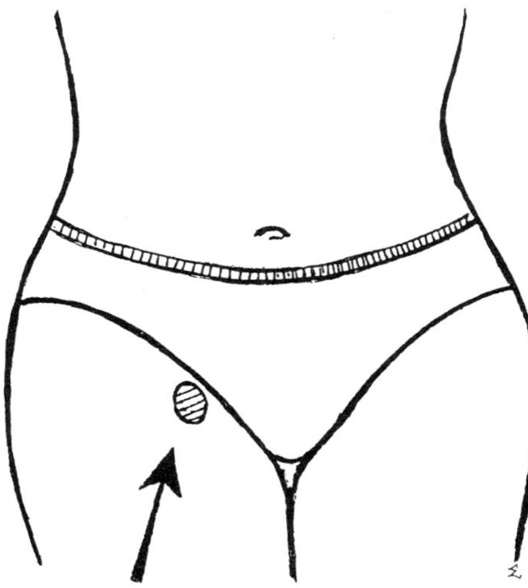

Figure 1.

COMMON SIGNS AND SYMPTOMS

- Sometimes there is a bulge, but it does not produce any symptoms.
- At other times there is pain in the area, especially if there is tissue caught *(incarcerated)* in the hernia sac.
- Occasionally, the tissue in the hernia may become strangulated. This is an emergency. Unless the bowel is released, it will become gangrenous, if it has not already done so.

DIAGNOSIS

- Usually the diagnosis can be made by taking a detailed history, doing a thorough physical examination, and considering the laboratory reports carefully.

○ TREATMENT

- The treatment for a femoral hernia is to correct it by an operation, even if there are no symptoms. Otherwise, there is a risk that it might become strangulated.
- If the hernia appears incarcerated or strangulated, the operation must be done as an emergency.

After careful consideration of all factors, the recommendation is that you have an operation to correct your hernia. The reasons for this have been explained to you.

PREOPERATIVE PREPARATION

- There will be an examination of your blood, urine, heart (EKG), and lungs (chest x-ray).
- Do not eat or drink anything for 8 hours before the operation.
- Shower or bathe as usual on the morning of the operation.
- You may be given medicine that will make you feel drowsy before you are brought to the operating room.

□ OPERATION

- There are several ways to repair a femoral hernia. The technique chosen depends on several things.
  - Whether the operation is done as an emergency.
  - The size of the hernia.
  - Your general physical condition.
- The anesthesia can be local with sedation, general, or a spinal type, depending on the size of the hernia, the repair technique that is used, and your general condition. This will be discussed with you beforehand.
- The operation usually takes 1 to 2 hours.

POSTOPERATIVE CARE

- You will be taken to a recovery room and observed. When your blood pressure, pulse, and breathing are stable and you are completely alert, a decision will be made as to whether you are able to go home that same day with a responsible adult. On occasion one must stay in the hospital for a day or two.
- That evening you will be helped to sit up in bed and on the next day to get out of bed.
- Pain will be controlled with medicine.
- Your diet will be as you tolerate it.
- Arrangements will be made for your pain medicines, postoperative office visit, and stitch or clip removal.

✣ HOME CARE

- You may walk about as you wish, even climb stairs.
- You may eat as you did before the operation.
- Take medicine as prescribed for your pain.
- Be careful that you do not become constipated.
  - Include enough roughage and plenty of liquids in your diet.
  - You may need a mild laxative (example: milk of magnesia).
- You may shower as you wish and with any dressings on or off.
  - There may be narrow strips of tape across the incision. It's all right if they get wet; they will be removed in the doctor's office.
  - After you dry yourself, replace any dressings with clean, dry ones.
- Take medicine as prescribed for your pain.
- Don't lift anything heavier than 5 pounds. Ask someone to do it for you.
- Driving a car with an automatic shift is not too demanding. But if you suddenly have to slam on the brakes or twist to turn a wheel, you may strain the

sutures or tear something. Remind me during the follow-up visit to discuss with you when you can resume driving.
- You may resume sexual activity whenever you choose.
- You may return to work when you feel up to it, but let's talk about it first during a follow-up office visit.

✆ CALL OUR OFFICE IF

- There is redness or swelling of the incision, or there is drainage from it.
- You develop a temperature higher than 100°F.
- You have any questions.

△ GENERAL INFORMATION

The *diaphragm* is a thin sheet of muscle that separates the chest and the abdomen. The esophagus, which is almost as big around as a dust mop handle, passes through a hole (the *hiatus*) in the diaphragm on its way to the stomach (Fig. 1). Sometimes, tissue around the hiatus weakens, so the hiatus stretches and the weakened tissue bulges into the chest *(hiatal hernia)*. Sometimes a part of the stomach is inside the bulge into the chest (Fig. 2).

The exact cause of hiatal hernia is not known.

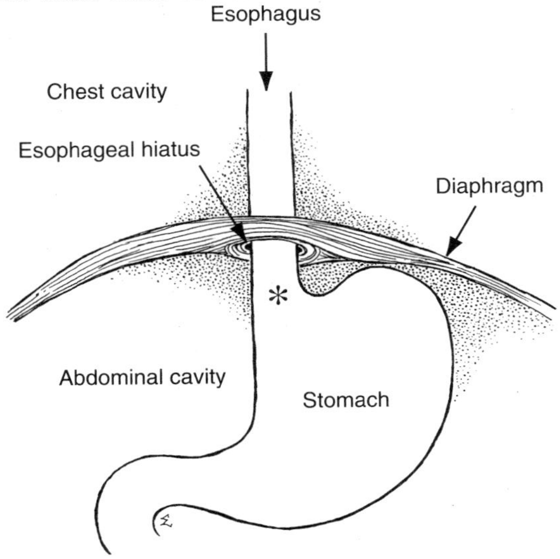

Figure 1. Normal situation: The hole in the diaphragm (the *esophageal hiatus*) permits the esophagus to enter the abdominal cavity. Where the esophagus meets the stomach is the esophagogastric junction *(asterisk)*.

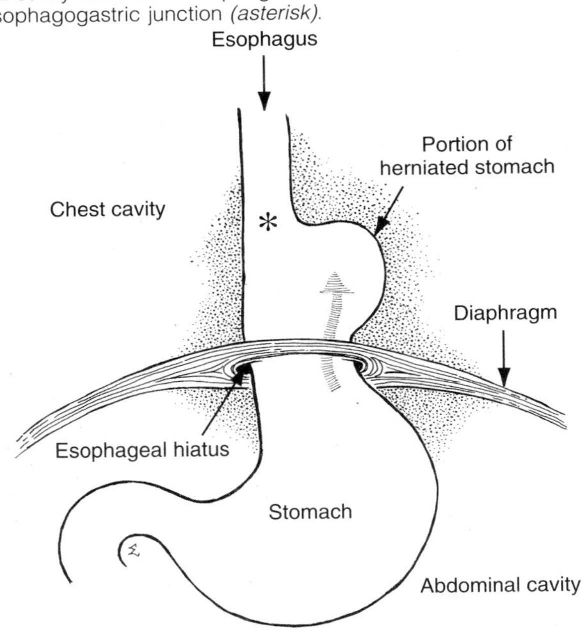

Figure 2. The esophageal hiatus has relaxed and become larger, so that some of the stomach has herniated into the chest. The aim of the operation is to bring the esophageal junction *(asterisk)* and stomach back into the abdominal cavity.

COMMON SIGNS AND SYMPTOMS

- Often, there is heartburn. This is the acid from the stomach backing up into the esophagus.
- Sometimes there's the feeling of regurgitation of food. This is made worse when stooping or lying flat; it gets better when standing. This is because the valve between the esophagus and stomach is weak, and food backs up into the esophagus easily but much less so if you are standing.
- Occasionally, you have difficulty swallowing because of spasm of the irritated esophagus.
- Often, there is pain under the *sternum* (breastbone) from the inflammation in the esophagus.
- Many times there's a sense of something sticking in the throat. Spasm from the irritation doesn't let the muscles relax and work smoothly enough to carry the food down easily.

DIAGNOSIS

- Usually the diagnosis can be made by taking a detailed history, doing a thorough physical examination, and considering the laboratory reports carefully.
- Esophagogram: You will be given liquid barium to swallow (it looks and flows like buttermilk). X-rays of the barium will be taken as it goes down your esophagus and into your stomach. This will show any hernia, or possibly other problems.
- Special tests may be done to see how the esophagus squeezes down and relaxes normally.
- Esophagoscopy: This is done with an optical instrument called an *esophagoscope* that has a light at its tip, is smooth, flexible, and as big around as your little finger. Your mouth and throat will be sprayed with an anesthetic to make them numb. Also, you will be given medicine that will make you feel drowsy. The esophagoscope will then be placed gently down your esophagus so that the esophagus can be examined thoroughly. After this, the esophagoscope will be passed into your stomach so that it too can be inspected.

○ TREATMENT

- If the hernia does not produce any symptoms, then no treatment is necessary.
- If there are symptoms, medical therapy should be tried first. An operation is considered only if medical therapy fails.
- There are three ways to repair such a hernia:
  - Through an opening in the abdomen.
  - Through an opening in the chest.
  - Using four instruments *(laparoscopes)* that are as big around as your little finger. They are placed in the abdomen through four tiny incisions, and the operation is done through these incisions.

After very careful consideration of all factors, the recommendation is that you have an operation through an abdominal incision to repair your hernia.

PREOPERATIVE PREPARATION

- You will have an examination of your blood, urine, heart (EKG), and lungs (chest x-ray).
- Do not eat or drink anything for 8 hours before the operation.

□ OPERATION

- You will be asleep for the operation.
- The incision will be in the upper part of the abdomen.
- The operation usually takes about 2 hours.

POSTOPERATIVE CARE

- You will be taken to a recovery room and observed. When your blood pressure, pulse, and breathing are stable, you will be taken to a regular hospital room.
- You will have a thin plastic tube in your nose for a few days. It will be removed when your bowels start working.
- That evening you will be helped to sit up in bed and on the next day to get out of bed.
- Pain will be controlled with medicine.
- When the tube from your nose is removed, you will be started on a liquid diet that will be increased to more solid food as you tolerate it.
- As with any operation, complications are always possible. With this type of operation, they can include bleeding, infection, difficulty getting food down, blood clots, and possibly others.
- You should be able to go home in about 3 to 5 days.
- Arrangements will be made for your medicine, follow-up office visit, and stitch or clip removal.

✚ HOME CARE

- Chew your food well to the consistency of oatmeal before you swallow it.
- For the first few weeks, you may feel a little soreness in your esophagus when eating or a sense that the food is sticking. This feeling should improve.
- Take the medicine prescribed for you.
- Unless instructed otherwise, you may shower if you wish and with any dressings on or off. After you dry yourself, replace any dressings with clean, dry ones.
- Let's discuss when you may drive a car or return to work at the follow-up visit.

✆ CALL OUR OFFICE IF

- Your food truly seems not to go down and sticks in your esophagus, or you even vomit.
- The incision becomes red or swollen, or there is drainage from it.
- You develop a temperature higher than 100°F.
- You have any questions.

△ GENERAL INFORMATION

The *diaphragm* is a thin sheet of muscle that separates the chest and the abdomen. The esophagus, which is almost as big around as a dust mop handle, passes through a hole (the *hiatus*) in the diaphragm on its way to the stomach (Fig. 1). Sometimes, tissue around the hiatus weakens, so the hiatus stretches and the weakened tissue bulges into the chest (a *hiatal hernia*). Sometimes a part of the stomach is inside the bulge into the chest (Fig. 2).

The exact cause of hiatal hernia is not known.

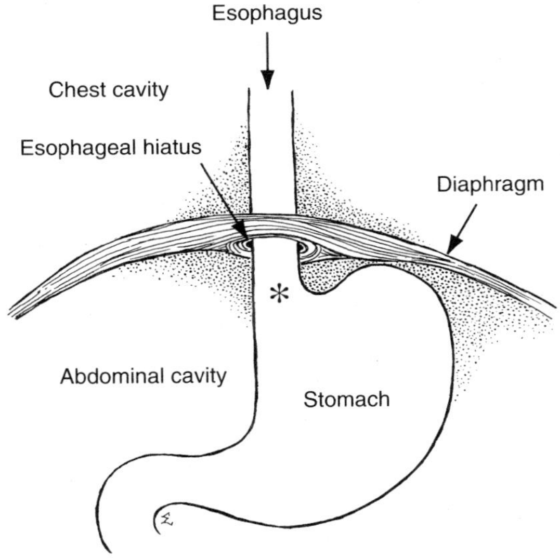

Figure 1. Normal situation: The hole in the diaphragm (the *esophageal hiatus*) permits the esophagus to enter the abdominal cavity. Where the esophagus meets the stomach is the esophagogastric junction *(asterisk)*.

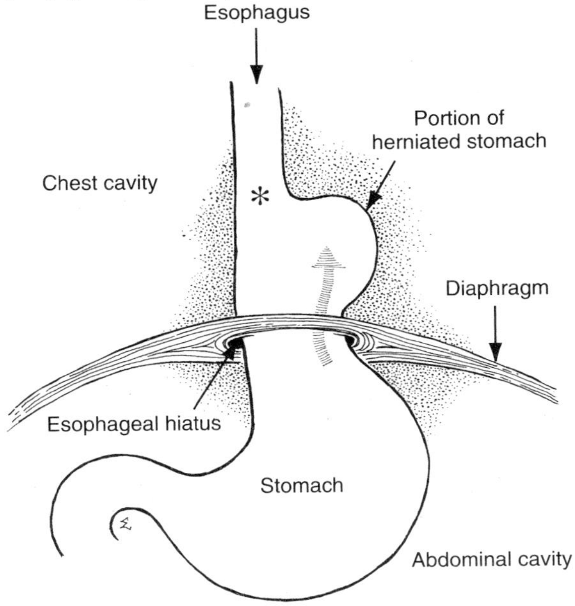

Figure 2. The esophageal hiatus has relaxed and become larger, so that some of the stomach has herniated into the chest. The aim of the operation is to bring the esophageal junction *(asterisk)* and stomach back into the abdominal cavity.

COMMON SIGNS AND SYMPTOMS

- Often, you feel heartburn. This is the acid from the stomach backing up into the esophagus.
- Sometimes there's the feeling of regurgitation of food. This is made worse when stooping or lying flat; it gets better when standing. This is because the valve between the esophagus and stomach is weak, and food backs up into the esophagus easily but much less so if you are standing.
- Occasionally, you have difficulty swallowing because of spasm of the irritated esophagus.
- Often, there is pain under the *sternum* (breastbone) from the inflammation in the esophagus.
- Many times there's a sense of something sticking in the throat. Spasm from the irritation doesn't let the muscles relax and work smoothly enough to carry the food down easily.

DIAGNOSIS

- Usually the diagnosis can be made by taking a detailed history, doing a thorough physical examination, and carefully considering the laboratory report.
- Esophagogram: You will be given liquid barium to swallow (it looks and flows like buttermilk). X-rays of the barium will be taken as it goes down your esophagus and into your stomach. This will show any hernia, or possibly other problems.
- Special tests may be done to see how the esophagus squeezes down and relaxes normally.
- Esophagoscopy: This is done with an optical instrument called an *esophagoscope* that has a light at its tip and is smooth, flexible, and as big around as your little finger. Your mouth and throat will be sprayed with an anesthetic to make them numb. Also, you will be given medicine that will make you feel drowsy. The esophagoscope will then be placed gently down your esophagus so that the esophagus can be examined thoroughly. After this, the esophagoscope will be passed into your stomach so that it too can be inspected.

○ TREATMENT

- If the hernia does not produce any symptoms, then no treatment is necessary.
- If there are symptoms, medical therapy should be tried first. An operation is considered only if medical therapy fails.
- There are three ways to repair such a hernia:
  - Through an opening in the abdomen.
  - Through an opening in the chest.
  - Using four instruments *(laparoscopes)* that are as big around as your little finger. They are placed in the abdomen through four tiny incisions, and the operation is done through these incisions.

After consideration of all factors, the recommendation is that you have a laparoscopic operation to repair your hernia. There is less pain and an earlier recovery with this technique.

PREOPERATIVE PREPARATION

- You will have an examination of your blood, urine, heart (EKG), and lungs (chest x-ray).
- Do not eat or drink anything for 8 hours before the operation.

☐ OPERATION

- You will be asleep for the operation.
- There will be three or four tiny incisions in the upper part of the abdomen.
- The operation usually takes about 2 hours.

POSTOPERATIVE CARE

- You will be taken to a recovery room and observed. When your blood pressure, pulse, and breathing are stable, you will be taken to a regular hospital room.
- You will have a thin plastic tube in your nose for a day or two.
- The evening of the operation you will be helped to sit up in bed and on the next day to get out of bed.
- Pain will be controlled with medicine.
- When the tube from your nose is removed, you will be started on a liquid diet that will be increased to more solid food as you tolerate it.
- As with any operation, complications are always possible. With this type of operation, they can include bleeding, infection, difficulty getting food down, blood clots, and possibly others.
- You should be able to go home in about 2 to 4 days.
- Arrangements will be made for your medicine, follow-up office visit, and stitch or clip removal.

✚ HOME CARE

- Chew your food well to the consistency of oatmeal before you swallow it.
- For the first few weeks, you may feel a little soreness in your esophagus when eating or a sense that the food is sticking. This feeling should improve.
- Take the medicine prescribed for you.
- Unless instructed otherwise, you may shower if you wish.
- During your follow-up office visit, let's discuss when you may drive a car and return to work.

✆ CALL OUR OFFICE IF

- Your food truly seems not to go down and sticks in your esophagus, or you even vomit.
- The incision becomes red or swollen, or there is drainage from it.
- You develop a temperature higher than 100°F.
- You have any questions.

△ GENERAL INFORMATION

The *diaphragm* is a thin sheet of muscle that separates the chest and the abdomen. The esophagus, which is almost as big around as a dust mop handle, passes through a hole (the *hiatus*) in the diaphragm on its way to the stomach (Fig. 1). Sometimes, tissue around the hiatus weakens, so the hiatus stretches and the weakened tissue bulges into the chest (a *hiatal hernia*). Sometimes a part of the stomach is inside the bulge into the chest (Fig. 2).

The exact cause of hiatal hernia is not known.

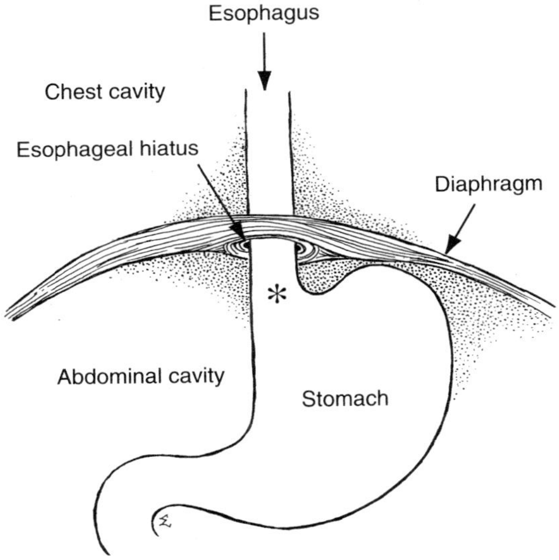

Figure 1. Normal situation: The hole in the diaphragm (the *esophageal hiatus*) permits the esophagus to enter the abdominal cavity. Where the esophagus meets the stomach is the esophagogastric junction *(asterisk)*.

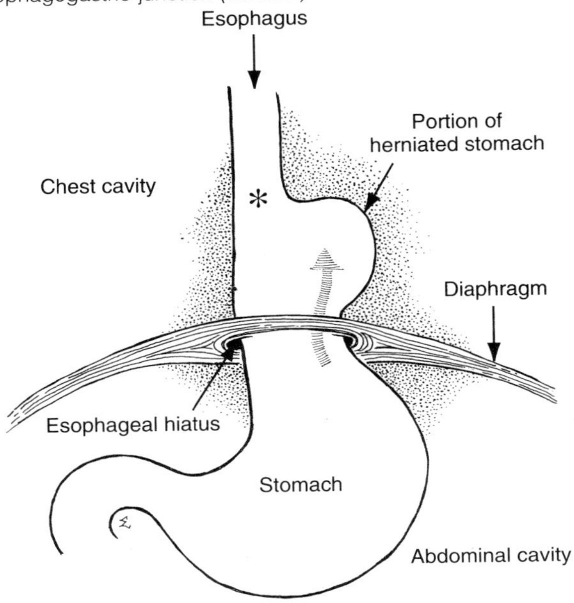

Figure 2. The esophageal hiatus has relaxed and become larger, so that some of the stomach has herniated into the chest. The aim of the operation is to bring the esophageal junction *(asterisk)* and stomach back into the abdominal cavity.

COMMON SIGNS AND SYMPTOMS

- Often, there is heartburn. This is the acid from the stomach backing up into the esophagus.
- Sometimes there's the feeling of regurgitation of food. This is made worse when stooping or lying flat; it gets better when standing. This is because the valve between the esophagus and stomach is weak, and food backs up into the esophagus easily but much less so if you are standing.
- Occasionally, you have difficulty swallowing because of spasm of the irritated esophagus.
- Often, there is pain under the *sternum* (breastbone) from the inflammation in the esophagus.
- Many times there's a sense of something sticking in the throat. Spasm from the irritation doesn't let the muscles relax and work smoothly enough to carry the food down easily.

DIAGNOSIS

- Usually the diagnosis can be made by taking a detailed history, doing a thorough physical examination, and considering the laboratory reports carefully.
- Esophagogram: You will be given liquid barium to swallow (it looks and flows like buttermilk). X-rays of the barium will be taken as it goes down your esophagus and into your stomach. This will show any hernia, or possibly other problems.
- Special tests may be done to see how the esophagus squeezes down and relaxes normally.
- Esophagoscopy: This is done with an optical instrument called an *esophagoscope* that has a light at its tip and is smooth, flexible, and as big around as your little finger. Your mouth and throat will be sprayed with an anesthetic to make them numb. Also, you will be given medicine that will make you feel drowsy. The esophagoscope will then be placed gently down your esophagus so that the esophagus can be examined thoroughly. After this, the esophagoscope will be passed into your stomach so that it too can be inspected.

○ TREATMENT

- If the hernia does not produce any symptoms, then no treatment is necessary.
- If there are symptoms, medical therapy should be tried first. An operation is considered only if medical therapy fails.
- There are three ways to repair such a hernia.
  - Through an opening in the abdomen.
  - Through an opening in the chest.
  - Using four instruments *(laparoscopes)* that are as big around as your little finger. They are placed in the abdomen through four tiny incisions, and the operation is done through these incisions.

After very careful consideration of all factors, the recommendation is that you have an operation through a chest incision to repair your hernia.

PREOPERATIVE PREPARATION

- You will have an examination of your blood, urine, heart (EKG), and lungs (chest x-ray).
- Do not eat or drink anything for 8 hours before the operation.

□ OPERATION

- You will be asleep for the operation.
- The incision will be in the left side of your chest.
- The operation usually takes about 2 hours.

POSTOPERATIVE CARE

- You will be taken to a recovery room and observed. When your blood pressure, pulse, and breathing are stable, you will be taken to a regular hospital room.
- You will have a thin plastic tube in your nose for a day or so.
- There will be a plastic tube coming from your chest for a day.
- That evening you will be helped to sit up in bed and on the next day to get out of bed.
- Pain will be controlled with medicine.
- You will be given an incentive spirometer. Breathing into this as you are instructed will help expand your lungs and reduce the risk of developing pneumonia.
- You will be started on a liquid diet that will be increased to more solid food as you tolerate it.
- As with any operation, complications are always possible. With this type of operation, they can include bleeding, pneumonia, difficulty getting food down, blood clots, and possibly others.
- You should be able to go home in about 3 to 5 days.
- Arrangements will be made for your medicine, follow-up office visit, and stitch or clip removal.

✚ HOME CARE

- Chew your food well to the consistency of oatmeal before you swallow it.
- For the first few weeks, you may feel a little soreness in your esophagus when eating or a sense that the food is sticking. This feeling should improve.
- Take the medicine prescribed for you.
- Unless instructed otherwise, you may shower if you wish.
- During your follow-up office visit let's discuss when you may drive a car or return to work.

✆ CALL OUR OFFICE IF

- Your food truly seems not to go down and sticks in your esophagus, or you even vomit.
- The incision becomes red or swollen, or there is drainage from it.
- You develop a temperature higher than 100°F.
- You have any questions.

△ GENERAL INFORMATION

This is a bulge in tissue that has been *incised* (cut) during a previous operation but that has not healed to its original strength. The weak tissue now bulges. Most incisional hernias are on the abdominal wall (Fig. 1). Incisional hernias occur more commonly in older, obese persons. Of the known causes, infection in the surgical incision is the most common.

Fortunately, the intestine that can be found inside the hernia does not often become *strangulated* (twisted).

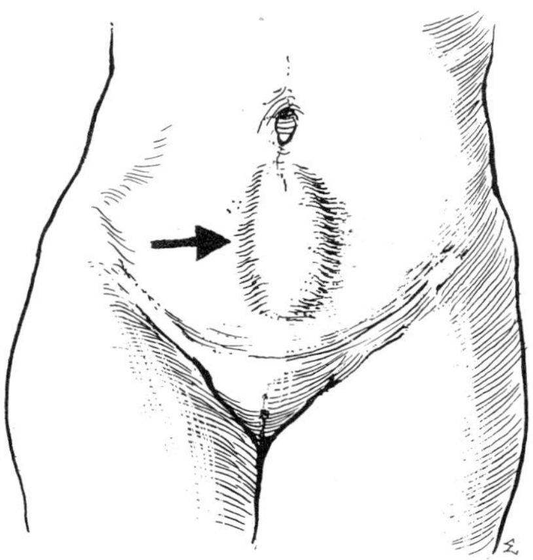

Figure 1. A ventral hernia can appear practically anywhere in the abdominal wall and can be small or large. It can be a simple sac, or it can have a number of compartments to it. A typical example is shown.

COMMON SIGNS AND SYMPTOMS

- There is a bulge in the area of a previous incision. It may be small or as large as a football.
- The rim of the hernia may ache as it is suddenly stretched with coughing.
- Persons with lung problems may have difficulty coughing well. The force of the cough is wasted in pushing out the hernia instead of pushing the mucus out of the lung.

○ TREATMENT

- Many hernias do not produce symptoms and can be kept reasonably flat with a girdle or a similar garment.
- The only way to repair a hernia is by operating.
- Many persons wish to have their hernias repaired because they consider them unsightly, or because they truly interfere with the ability to dress properly.

After careful consideration of all factors, the recommendation is that you have an operation to repair your incisional hernia.

PREOPERATIVE PREPARATION

- You will have an examination of your blood, urine, heart (EKG), and lungs (chest x-ray).
- If you have a coughing problem, it should be corrected as much as possible beforehand.
- Just as obesity is a common cause of an incisional hernia, it also is a common reason for a hernia repair to fail. If you are obese, a serious effort must be made to take off some weight.
- Men with prostate trouble who strain a lot when urinating may need to deal with this problem before the hernia is repaired. Otherwise the same straining may be harmful to the repair.

□ OPERATION

- Most repairs of a ventral hernia are done under general anesthesia. However, if the hernia is small, it can be repaired under local anesthesia along with medicine to make you very drowsy. The choice will be discussed with you beforehand.
- There are several techniques of repairing an incisional hernia: *A small hernia with a strong rim:* The edges of the rim are brought together and stitched with strong permanent suture material. *A large hernia with a weak rim:* These often are repaired by pushing the intestines back in and stitching a sheet of extremely strong synthetic mesh over both the hernia and the weak tissue around it.

POSTOPERATIVE CARE

- You will be taken to a recovery room and observed. When your blood pressure, pulse, and breathing are stable and you are completely alert and if the operation was not extensive, you may be able to go home the same day. Otherwise you will need to stay in the hospital as necessary.
- That evening you will be helped to sit up in bed and on the next day to get out of bed.
- Pain will be controlled with medicine.
- Your diet will be as you tolerate it.
- Arrangements will be made for your medicine, follow-up office visit, and stitch or clip removal.

✚ HOME CARE

- You may walk about as you wish, even climb stairs, but don't overdo things.
- You may eat as you wish.
- Take medicine as prescribed for your pain.
- You may shower as you wish and with any dressings on or off. There may be narrow strips of tape across the incision. It's all right if they get wet; they will be removed in the doctor's office. After you dry yourself, replace any dressings with clean, dry ones.
- Don't lift anything heavier than 5 pounds. Ask someone to do it for you.
- Include plenty of roughage and liquids in your diet to help prevent constipation.
- Your incision and the muscles of the abdomen may ache, especially at the end of the day and after you have been standing for a long period. You can

support your abdomen by wearing a girdle or similar garment that is snug.
- When you may drive a car or return to work depends on the size and characteristics of your hernia, how it was repaired, your general condition, and your job. Let's discuss all this during your follow-up office visit.

✆ CALL OUR OFFICE IF

- The incision becomes red or swollen, or there is drainage from it.
- You develop a temperature higher than 100°F.
- You have any questions.

HERNIA, INGUINAL: Infant or Child

△ GENERAL INFORMATION

Some months before a baby boy is born, his testicles are located near the kidneys. A short while before birth, the testicles descend and travel through an opening in the groin that leads to the scrotum. As they drop down, they drag some of the lining tissue of the inner abdomen with them. Normally, the sac of tissue around the testicle fuses and the opening in the groin closes. If it fails to close completely, there is a space in the groin and scrotum that can fill with fluid or intestine and that looks like a lump (Fig. 1).

In girls, this sac exists and goes from the inner abdomen through the opening in the groin and attaches in the labia below the pubic bone. In girls, if the sac does not close at birth, fluid, intestine, or, more commonly, an ovary can pop into the sac and look like a swelling or a lump.

This lump in the groin area is called an *inguinal hernia.* It occurs on both sides in 10 to 15% of the cases.

COMMON SIGNS AND SYMPTOMS

- A swelling in the groin that comes and goes as the child strains, cries, coughs, or is standing upright.
- The hernia can be pushed back into the abdomen; it is easier if the child is not crying or grunting.
- If the hernia lump becomes hard and tender and cannot be pushed back into the abdomen easily, then the intestine or ovary may be stuck. This is an emergency requiring prompt attention.

DIAGNOSIS

- Usually, the diagnosis can be made by taking a detailed history and doing a thorough physical examination.

○ TREATMENT

- The treatment is an operation to repair the hernia and close the sac completely.
- Hernias should be repaired soon after they are discovered, even in very young infants, to prevent the bowel or an ovary from getting stuck or twisted in the sac.

PREOPERATIVE PREPARATION

- If your child is younger than 6 months of age, he or she may have milk or solids until 4 hours before the operation and clear liquids up to 2 hours before the operation.
- If your child is older than 6 months of age, he or she may have milk or solids up to 6 hours (8 hours in some hospitals) before surgery and clear liquids up to 3 hours before surgery.
- Clear liquids means water, apple juice, or an electrolyte solution.

□ OPERATION

- The child will have a general anesthetic for the operation.
- After the child is asleep, it is common to use an injection of local anesthetic in the wound to help relieve pain when the child is awake.
- The operation usually takes about 1 hour.

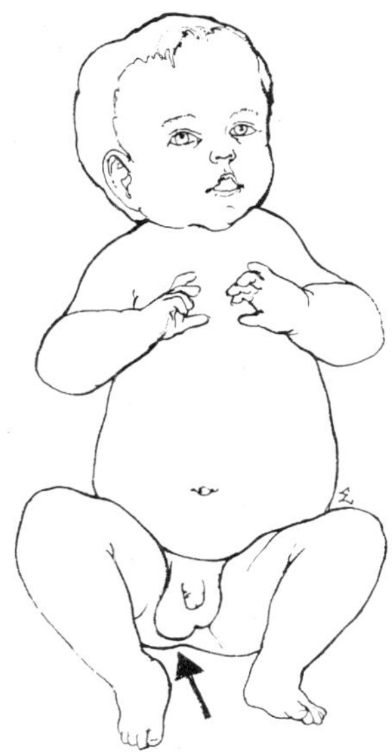

Figure 1. The incision is made in a cosmetic fashion, and the hernia is closed. Usually, no dissection and strengthening of the muscles is necessary, as is common in adults, because no muscle weakness exists.

POSTOPERATIVE CARE

- The child will be taken to the recovery room.
- After the blood pressure, pulse, and breathing are stable and the child is awake, alert, and tolerating liquids by mouth, he or she should be able to go home the same day.

✚ HOME CARE

- Arrangements will be made for a follow-up office visit.
- The surgeon will discuss with you when to resume the child's normal diet, activities, and bathing; wound care; and administration of pain medication.

✆ CALL OUR OFFICE IF

- The incision becomes red or swollen, or there is drainage from it.
- Your child develops a fever higher than 101°F.
- You have any questions.

HERNIA, INGUINAL (GROIN HERNIA): Laparoscopic Repair

△ GENERAL INFORMATION

An inguinal hernia is a bulging out of the tissue in the groin area. One type, an indirect hernia, is a bulge through the stretched, natural opening in the groin through which blood vessels and other structures pass on the way to the *testicle* in the *scrotum.*

The bulge associated with a hernia is from the intestines and some fatty tissue that has slipped into the hernia sac. Sometimes the intestine or fatty apron gets stuck in the sac. This is called an *incarcerated hernia.* Occasionally the tissues in the hernia become twisted. This is called a *strangulated hernia;* it can develop gangrene.

COMMON SIGNS AND SYMPTOMS

- Occasionally, there is a bulge but no symptoms, or just a vague aching in the area.
- Most of the time, the bulge can be pushed back, or it goes back on its own when the person lies down.
- If there is something caught in the sac, the bulge can be painful when handled. If there is strangulated tissue in the hernia, the pain is intense and fever, abnormal laboratory findings, and other signs of infection are present.

DIAGNOSIS

The diagnosis usually can be made by taking a detailed history and doing a thorough physical examination.

○ TREATMENT

The safest, and so the best, treatment for an inguinal hernia is to repair it by an operation. There are several ways to treat an inguinal hernia:

Open Operation. Until a few years ago, practically the only technique was to make an incision over the bulge and then dissect the tissue over this bulge until the hernia was reached. The hernia sac is then repaired and the overlying tissues brought together again.

The advantages of this technique are that it has been used by surgeons on hundreds of thousands of patients and that it most often can be done under local anesthesia. The disadvantages of this technique are that most of the pain and disability associated with this technique are from the cutting and dissection necessary to reach the hernia, rather than from the suturing of the hernia sac itself.

Laparoscopic Technique. More recently, and in appropriate patients, repair of the hernia is being done from inside the abdomen with a *laparoscope.* This instrument is about as big around as the tip of your little finger and has lenses in it and a light at its tip.

- The operation is done under general anesthesia.
- Three such instruments are introduced into the abdominal cavity through tiny incisions (Fig. 1).
- The hernia is repaired from the inside and the instruments withdrawn.

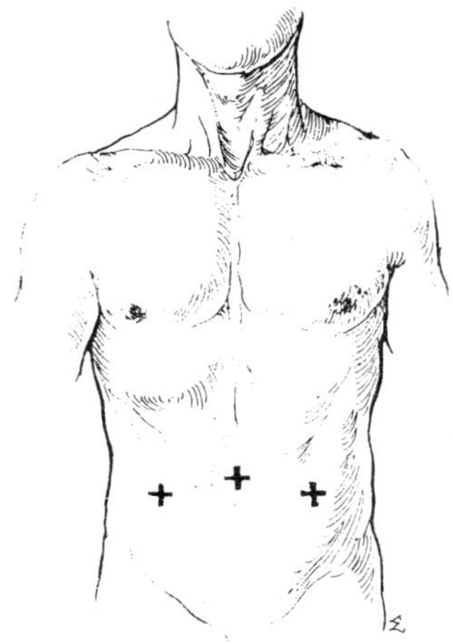

Figure 1. When repairing an inguinal (groin) hernia by laparoscopy, three instruments (laparoscopes) are used. They are introduced inside the abdomen through three tiny incisions. The typical locations of the incisions are indicated by the Xs.

Advantages of the Laparoscopic Technique

- Less pain and disability are present after the operation and thus an earlier return to daily activities.
- It is more suitable for a person with a recurrent hernia in whom there is a lot of scar tissue that would need to be cut through to repair the hernia from the outside.
- It can be suitable in persons who are overweight and have a lot of fatty tissue that would need to be cut through to reach the hernia.

Disadvantages of the Laparoscopic Technique

- You need to be asleep for the operation.
- There's a little more likelihood that you will need to stay in the hospital at least overnight.

After careful consideration of all factors, the recommendation is that you have a laparoscopic hernia repair.

PREOPERATIVE PREPARATION

- Any associated problems that might affect the success of the operation will be corrected as much as possible before the operation.
- If you smoke, *stop* or cut down drastically. This will help your lungs during and after the operation. Also, any coughing (as from smoking) strains the stitches.
- Do not eat or drink anything for 8 hours before the operation.
- Shower or bathe as usual on the morning of the operation.
- You may be given medicine that will make you feel drowsy before you are brought to the operating room.

□ OPERATION

- You will be asleep for the operation.
- The operation usually takes about 1 hour.

POSTOPERATIVE CARE

- You will be taken to a recovery room and observed. When your blood pressure, pulse, and breathing are stable and you are completely alert, you may be able to go home that same day with a responsible adult. Otherwise, you will stay in the hospital until the next day.
- That evening, you will be helped to get out of bed and walk around.
- Pain will be controlled with medicine.
- Arrangements will be made for your medicine, follow-up office visit, and stitch or clip removal.
- As with any operation, complications are always possible. With this type of operation, they can include bleeding, infection, and possibly others.

✣ HOME CARE

- You may walk about as you wish, even climb stairs.
- Inactivity is not good for you, but neither is overdoing it. Don't try to do too much too soon.
- Don't lift anything heavier than 5 pounds. Ask someone to do it for you.
- Eat as you wish.
- You may shower as you wish.
- Be careful that you do not become constipated.
  - Include enough roughage and plenty of liquids in your diet.
  - You may need some help with a mild laxative (example: milk of magnesia).
- You may resume sexual activity whenever you choose.
- You may return to work when you feel up to it, but let's talk about it first during a follow-up office visit.

✆ CALL OUR OFFICE IF

- You develop any unusual signs or symptoms:
- Your scrotum swells and continues to do so.
- The incisions become red or swollen, or there is drainage from them.
- You develop a temperature higher than 100°F.
- You have any questions.

HERNIA, INGUINAL (GROIN HERNIA): Open Repair

△ GENERAL INFORMATION

An *inguinal* hernia is a bulging out of the tissue in the groin area. One type, an indirect hernia, is a bulge through the stretched, natural opening in the groin through which blood vessels and other structures pass on the way to the *testicle* in the *scrotum* (Fig. 1).

The bulge associated with a hernia is from the intestines and some fatty tissue that has slipped into the hernia sac. Sometimes the intestine or fatty apron gets stuck in the sac. This is called an *incarcerated hernia.* Occasionally, the tissues in the hernia become twisted. This is called a *strangulated hernia;* it can develop gangrene.

COMMON SIGNS AND SYMPTOMS

- Occasionally, there is a bulge but no symptoms, or just a vague aching in the area.
- Most of the time, the bulge can be pushed back, or it goes back on its own when the person lies down.
- If there is something caught in the sac, the bulge can be painful when handled. If there is strangulated tissue in the hernia, the pain is intense and fever, abnormal laboratory findings, and other signs of infection are present.

DIAGNOSIS

The diagnosis usually can be made by taking a detailed history and doing a thorough physical examination.

○ TREATMENT

The safest, and so the best, treatment for an inguinal hernia is to repair it by an operation. There are several ways to treat an inguinal hernia:

Open Operation. Until a few years ago, practically the only technique was to make an incision over the bulge and then dissect the tissue over this bulge until the hernia was reached. The hernia sac is then repaired and the overlying tissues brought together again.

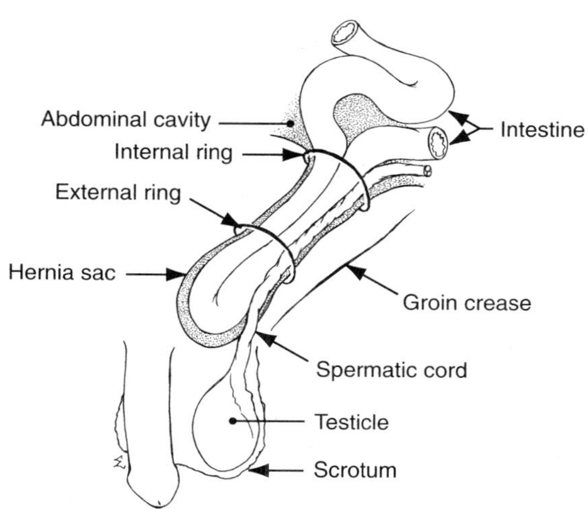

Figure 1. The incision is made in a natural crease, if possible. This results in a less obvious scar.

Advantages of the Open Technique
- It has been used by surgeons on hundreds of thousands of patients.
- It most often can be done under local anesthesia.

Disadvantages of the Open Technique
- Most of the pain and disability associated with this technique are from the cutting and dissection necessary to reach the hernia, rather than from the suturing of the hernia sac itself.

Laparoscopic Technique. More recently, and in appropriate patients, repair of the hernia is being done from inside the abdomen with a *laparoscope.* This instrument is about as big around as the tip of your little finger and has lenses in it and a light at its tip.
- The operation is done under general anesthesia.
- Three such instruments are introduced into the abdominal cavity through tiny incisions.
- The hernia is repaired from the inside and the instruments withdrawn.

Advantages of the Laparoscopic Technique
- There is less pain and disability after the operation and thus an earlier return to daily activities.
- It is more suitable for a person with a recurrent hernia in whom there is a lot of scar tissue that would need to be cut through to repair the hernia from the outside.
- It can be suitable in persons who are overweight and have a lot of fatty tissue that would need to be cut through to reach the hernia.

Disadvantages of the Laparoscopic Technique
- You need to be asleep for the operation.
- There's a little more likelihood that you will need to stay in the hospital at least overnight.

After careful consideration of all factors, the recommendation is that you have an open hernia repair from the outside.

PREOPERATIVE PREPARATION

- Any associated problems that might affect the success of the operation will be corrected as much as possible before the operation.
- If you smoke, *stop* or cut down drastically. This will help your lungs during and after the operation. Also, any coughing (as from smoking) strains the stitches.
- Do not eat or drink anything for 8 hours before the operation.
- Shower or bathe as usual on the morning of the operation.
- You may be given medicine that will make you feel drowsy before you are brought to the operating room.

□ OPERATION

- The operation will be done by injecting a local anesthetic in the groin area to make it completely numb. Also, you will be given medicine to keep you drowsy.

- The operation may be done under general anesthesia. The choice will be discussed with you beforehand.
- The operation usually takes about 1 hour.

POSTOPERATIVE CARE

- You will be taken to a recovery room and observed. When your blood pressure, pulse, and breathing are stable and you are completely alert, you probably will be able to go home that same day with a responsible adult. Otherwise, you will stay in the hospital until the next day.
- That evening, you will be helped to get out of bed and walk around.
- Pain will be controlled with medicine.
- Arrangements will be made for your medicine, follow-up office visit, and stitch or clip removal.
- As with any operation, complications are always possible. With this type of operation, they can include bleeding, infection, and possibly others.

✚ HOME CARE

- You may walk about as you wish, even climb stairs, but don't overdo things.
- Don't lift anything heavier than 5 pounds. Ask someone to do it for you.
- Eat as you wish. Be careful that you do not become constipated.
  - Include enough roughage and plenty of liquids in your diet.
  - You may need some help with a mild laxative (example: milk of magnesia).
- You may shower if you wish and with any dressings on or off.
  - There may be narrow strips of tape across the incision. It's all right if they get wet; they will be removed in the doctor's office.
  - After you dry yourself, replace any dressings with clean, dry ones.
- You may resume sexual activity whenever you choose.
- You may return to work when you feel up to it, but let's talk about it first during a follow-up office visit.

✆ CALL OUR OFFICE IF

- You develop any unusual signs or symptoms.
- Your scrotum swells and continues to do so.
- The incisions become red or swollen, or there is drainage from them.
- You develop a temperature higher than 100°F.
- You have any questions.

△ GENERAL INFORMATION

Immediately after a child is born, the umbilical cord is clamped and divided. In several weeks the stump of the umbilical cord dries and falls off, leaving behind the *umbilicus* (navel). Because this drying umbilicus has a lot of scar tissue in it, there always is some weakness there. As one becomes older, this tissue relaxes even more. If the tissue in this area relaxes enough, it can bulge, forming an *umbilical hernia.*

Umbilical hernias in adults are seen more commonly in women, especially women who have had multiple pregnancies. Also, they are seen more commonly in those who are overweight.

COMMON SIGNS AND SYMPTOMS

- Sometimes the bulge is very minimal: A finger used to push the bulge back can feel the opening. It can be as small as a penny. If the person is obese, the bulge might not be visible, but it can be felt through the fat overlying it (Fig. 1).

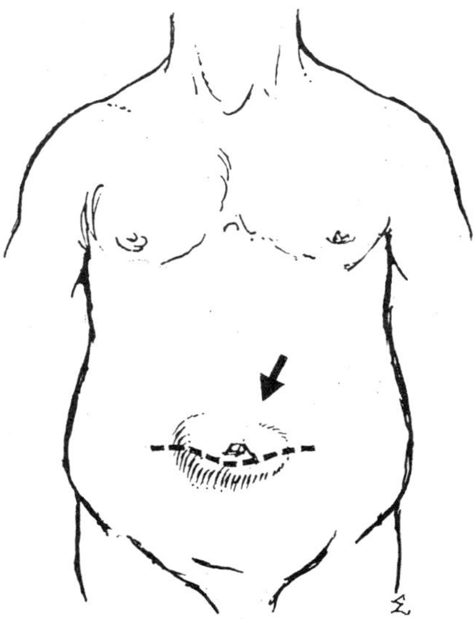

Figure 1. An umbilical hernia in an adult can have an opening as small as a nickel and no protrusion or symptoms, or it can be huge and require an operation—sometimes an emergency operation. A common incision is shown.

- More often there is a smooth bulge. It can be the size of your thumb or as big as a grapefruit.
- Most umbilical hernias will go back into the abdomen when they are pushed gently, or when a person lies down.
- If tissue from inside the abdomen becomes caught in the hernia, the hernia cannot be pushed back into the abdomen. This is called an *incarcerated umbilical hernia.*
- The intestine or fatty tissue in the hernia can even become twisted and its blood supply cut off. The bulge becomes very painful. Peritonitis may develop. This is a *strangulated umbilical hernia.*

DIAGNOSIS

- The diagnosis usually can be made from taking a detailed history of the symptoms and doing a thorough physical examination.

○ TREATMENT

- An umbilical hernia in an adult should be corrected even when it does not produce symptoms because there is the risk that the tissue in it will become strangulated.

After careful consideration of all factors, it is recommended that you have an operation to repair your umbilical hernia.

PREOPERATIVE PREPARATION

- You will have an examination of your blood, urine, heart (EKG), and lungs (chest x-ray).
- Do not eat or drink anything for 8 hours before the operation.
- Shower as usual on the morning of the operation.
- You may be given medicine that will make you feel drowsy before you are brought to the operating room.

□ OPERATION

- The type of anesthesia used can be local, general, or a type of spinal (epidural). This will depend on your symptoms, the size of the hernia, how long it has been present, and your condition in general. If the operation is done under local anesthesia, a fine needle will be used to inject an anesthetic into the tissue around the hernia to make it completely numb. Also, during the operation, you will be given medicine to make you feel very drowsy.
- During the operation, you may feel some tugging but not pain.
- Occasionally, the hernia is so large that the tissue cannot be brought together. In such a situation, the hernia will be repaired by using a strong synthetic mesh to cover the opening.
- The operation usually takes 1 to 2 hours, depending on the size of the hernia and the technique needed to repair it.

POSTOPERATIVE CARE

- You will be taken to a recovery room and observed until your blood pressure, pulse, and breathing are stable. If the hernia was small and done under local anesthesia, you may be able to go home that same day with a responsible adult. If the hernia was large or if you had a repair with mesh, you will be taken to a regular hospital room.
- That evening you will be helped to sit up in bed and on the next day to get out of bed.
- Pain will be controlled with medicine.
- Your diet will be as tolerated.
- As with any operation, complications are always possible. With this type of operation, they can include bleeding, infection, and possibly others.

- Arrangements will be made for your medicine, follow-up office visit, and stitch removal.

✣ HOME CARE

- You may walk about as you wish, even climb stairs.
- You may eat as you did before the operation. Be careful that you do not become constipated.
  - Include enough roughage and plenty of liquids in your diet.
  - You may need a mild laxative (example: milk of magnesia).
- You may shower as you wish and with any dressings on or off.
  - There may be narrow strips of tape across the incision. It's all right if they get wet; they will be removed in the doctor's office.
  - After you dry yourself, replace any dressings with clean, dry ones.
- Your incision and the muscles of the abdomen may ache, especially at the end of the day and after you have been standing for a long period. You can support them and be more comfortable by wearing a girdle or similar garment that is snug (but not too tight). Wearing it over a cotton undergarment is easier on your incision and the stitches.
- Driving a car with an automatic shift is not too demanding. But if you have to slam on the brakes suddenly or twist to turn the steering wheel, you may get into an accident or you may strain the sutures or tear something. During your follow-up visit, let's discuss when you can resume driving.
- You may resume sexual activity whenever you choose.
- You may return to work when you feel up to it.

✆ CALL OUR OFFICE IF

- The incision becomes red or swollen, or there is drainage from it.
- You develop any unusual signs or symptoms.
- You develop a temperature higher than 100°F.
- You have any questions.

△ GENERAL INFORMATION

Before being born, an infant is attached to the mother's womb by the umbilical cord that is about as big around as your little finger. The umbilical cord has two arteries, a vein, and a tiny cord-like structure connected to the urinary bladder. Protective tissue covers all these structures and all of them go through an opening in the abdominal wall.

A few minutes after the child is born, the cord is clamped close to the skin and divided. The stump of the cord begins to dry up and falls off in about 2 weeks. The scar that remains is the *umbilicus* or navel ("belly button").

The hole in the abdominal wall through which the umbilical cord passes usually closes as the abdominal muscles grow together during the child's development in the womb. Sometimes, however, the hole does not close completely although it is always covered by skin. This skin-covered defect in the muscles of the navel is called an *umbilical hernia.*

COMMON SIGNS AND SYMPTOMS

- Most commonly, a soft, smooth lump is present. It is the size of the end of your thumb and sticks out of the navel. It bulges more when the infant cries (Fig. 1).

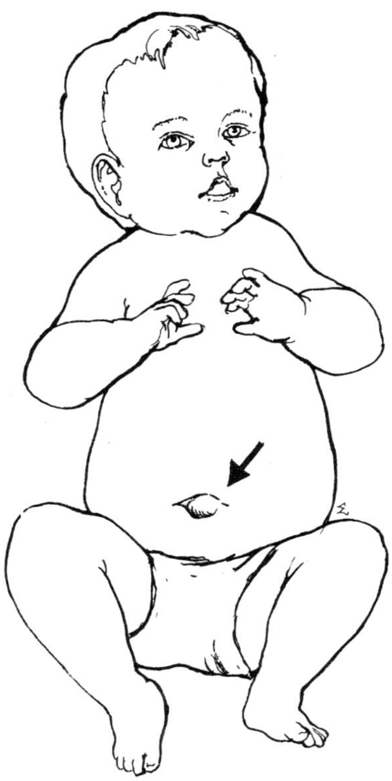

Figure 1. An umbilical hernia in an infant typically sticks out like a marble, doesn't cause symptoms, and usually disappears by the time the infant reaches 1 year of age. An operation is advisable if the hernia sticks out more than the usual ("elephant trunk"), if it is still present and unchanged at 1 year of age, or if the hole in the abdominal wall is sizable.

- The inside of the lump contains part of the small intestine.
- Using a fingertip, one can push the lump back inside the abdomen and feel the edges of the hernia opening.
- Very infrequently, instead of the lump being somewhat small, it sticks out and is almost as long and fat as your entire thumb.

DIAGNOSIS

- The diagnosis can usually be made from the history and physical examination.

○ TREATMENT

- Most of these hernias will close on their own over time. For this reason, the preferred treatment is to be patient and wait until the child reaches 4 years of age.
- If the umbilical hernia has not closed by itself by age 4 years, then it should be repaired with an operation.
- The exceptions to this approach are hernias that have an "elephant-trunk" appearance. These may be repaired surgically at a slightly earlier age.
- It is unusual for the intestine to get stuck in an umbilical hernia in a child.

PREOPERATIVE PREPARATION

- Do not feed the child liquids or solids for 6 hours before the operation.

□ OPERATION

- The operation will be done under quick-acting general anesthesia.
- The operation involves removing the hernia sac, closing the hole in the abdominal wall with stitches, and sometimes removing excess skin.
- The operation usually takes about 1 hour.
- There may be an injection of a local anesthetic around the incision to help with relief of postoperative pain.

POSTOPERATIVE CARE

- The child will awake in the recovery room. When the blood pressure, pulse, and breathing are stable and the child is alert and tolerating liquids by mouth, you may take your child home the same day.
- Arrangements will be made for a follow-up office visit.

✚ HOME CARE

- Resume the usual activities and diet.
- There will be a discussion with you on when to resume bathing, how to care for the wound, and what medications to give for pain relief.

✆ CALL OUR OFFICE IF

- The incision becomes red or swollen, or there is drainage from it.
- The child develops a temperature higher than 101°F.
- You have any questions.

△ GENERAL INFORMATION

The spine is made up of a number of bones called *vertebrae.* In the lower back they look roughly like big marshmallows with a knob that sticks out the back and from the left and right sides. The vertebrae sit atop one another from the skull down to the pelvis and are held together by very tough tissue that goes all the way around their edges. This tissue is called the *anulus fibrosus.* Between the vertebrae is a soft substance (something like bubble gum in consistency) that acts as a cushion between the vertebrae. This is the *nucleus pulposus* or disk.

Behind the vertebrae and disks is a tunnel. The spinal cord goes through this tunnel from the brain down to just below the waist. Along the way, the spinal cord gives off nerve branches at regular intervals. These nerves carry the signals from the brain that make muscles move. Other nerves carry pain sensations back to the brain.

The anulus fibrosus sometimes becomes weakened or tears (especially in the waist area) and allows the nucleus pulposus to squeeze out (like bubble gum out of the mouth). This is called a *herniated disk* (a herniated nucleus pulposus) (Figs. 1 and 2). The part that is squeezed out can pinch one of the nerves nearby that is branching from the spinal cord.

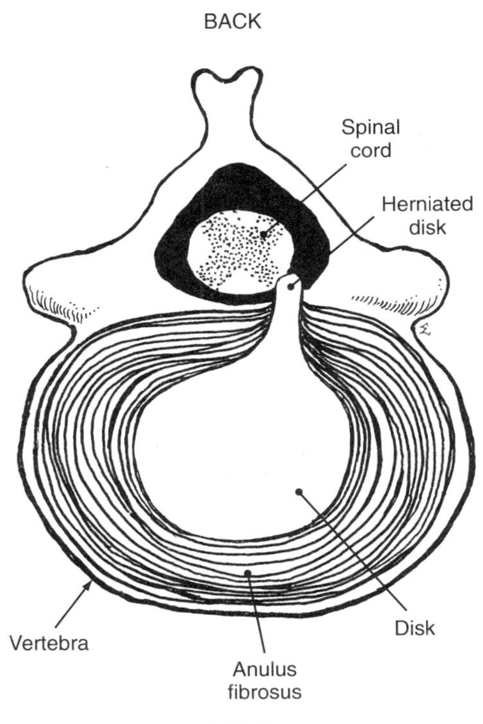

Figure 1. A single vertebra seen from the top, showing the relationship of the spinal cord to the herniated disk that is pressing on it.

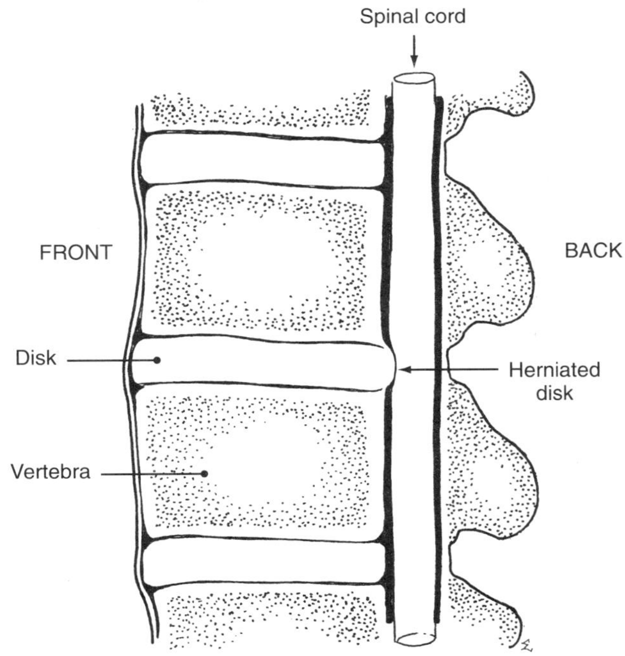

Figure 2. Side view of spine, showing a herniated disk pressing on the spinal cord.

COMMON SIGNS AND SYMPTOMS

- The signs and symptoms depend on the location of the herniated disk, the nerve the herniated disk is pinching, and how fast the herniation is growing.
- The signs and symptoms produced include pain in the area where the nerve goes, "pins and needles" sensation in the foot, and spasm of the muscles of the low back.
- While lying down, a person cannot raise the leg while it is straight—that is, not bent at the knee.

DIAGNOSIS

- Usually, a preliminary diagnosis can be made by taking a detailed history and doing a thorough physical examination with special emphasis on the neurologic examination. Several other examinations can be very useful.
- X-rays of the spine can give important information to help make the diagnosis.
- MRI (magnetic resonance imaging): No x-rays are used with this technique. Instead, it is done with harmless magnetic fields and radio waves. A computer develops pictures from several angles, showing the vertebrae, the nucleus pulposus, the spinal cord, and the nerves to and from the spinal cord. In this manner, abnormalities can be seen accurately.
- CT scan (computed tomography scan): These special x-rays are taken and shown as very thin slices of the area being studied, making it possible to see very fine details in the spine.

○ TREATMENT

- An early operation is advised if the pinching of the nerve is severe enough to cause paralysis of the muscles. If this is neglected, the symptoms can become permanent, even if there is an operation later and the herniated disk is corrected.
- Otherwise, the initial treatment for slipped disk should be strict bedrest for a few days, mild cervical traction, and pain and anti-inflammatory medicines.
- If a person does not get better in a few weeks or if the person gets better but attacks recur frequently, then an operation is advised.

After careful consideration of all factors, the recommendation is that you have an operation on your cervical disk.

PREOPERATIVE PREPARATION

- You will have an examination of your blood, urine, heart (EKG), and lungs (chest x-ray).
- Do not eat or drink anything for 8 hours before the operation.

□ OPERATION

- Your entire neck and one side of your hip area will be painted with an antiseptic solution and surrounded with sterile drapes.
- The incision will be on one side of your neck.
- The herniated disk that is pinching the nerve will be removed.
- A small wedge of bone will be taken from your hip area and inserted in the space from which the disk was removed. This will help stabilize (fuse) this part of the spine. This will not affect your walking, but the area will hurt for a few weeks.
- The operation usually takes about 2 hours.

POSTOPERATIVE CARE

- You will be taken to a recovery room and observed. When your blood pressure, pulse, and breathing are stable, you will be taken to a regular hospital room.
- You will have on a cervical collar. This helps stabilize your spine until the bones fuse. You will be shown how to handle the cervical collar.
- Pain will be controlled with medicine.
- Your diet will be as you tolerate it.
- As with any operation, complications are always possible. With this type of operation, they can include bleeding, infection, injury to a nerve, blood clots, and possibly others.
- You should be able to go home several days following the operation.
- Arrangements will be made for your medicine, follow-up office visit, and stitch removal.

✣ HOME CARE

- At the beginning, walking is the only exercise needed. A rehabilitation exercise program will be outlined for you.
- Do not do any lifting. Ask someone to do it for you.
- Eat as you wish.
- During your follow-up office visit, let's discuss when you may drive a car, resume sexual activity, and return to work.

✆ CALL OUR OFFICE IF

- The incision becomes red or swollen, or there is drainage from it.
- You develop a temperature higher than 100°F.
- You have any questions.

HERNIATED DISK (SLIPPED DISK): Lumbar (Back)

△ GENERAL INFORMATION

The spine is made up of a number of bones called *vertebrae.* In the lower back they look roughly like big marshmallows with a knob that sticks out the back and from the left and right sides. The vertebrae sit atop one another from the skull down to the pelvis and are held together by very tough tissue that goes all the way around their edges. This is called the *anulus fibrosus.* Between the vertebrae is a soft substance (something like bubble gum in consistency) that acts as a cushion between the vertebrae. This is the *nucleus pulposus* or disk.

Behind the vertebrae and disks is a tunnel. The spinal cord goes through this tunnel from the brain down to just below the waist. Along the way, the spinal cord gives off nerve branches at regular intervals. These nerves carry the signals from the brain that make muscles move. Other nerves carry pain sensations back to the brain.

The anulus fibrosus sometimes becomes weakened or tears (especially in the waist area) and allows the nucleus pulposus to squeeze out (like bubble gum out of the mouth). This is called a *herniated disk* (a herniated nucleus pulposus) (Fig. 1). The part that is squeezed out can pinch one of the nerves nearby that is branching from the spinal cord.

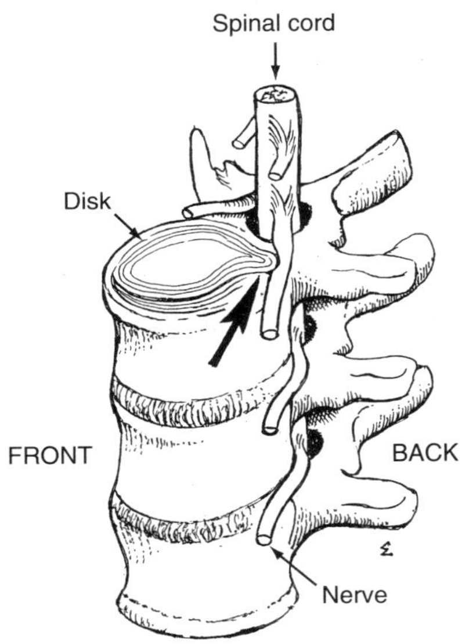

Figure 1. Three vertebrae from the lumbar (waist area) of the spine. The disk has broken through (herniated) the ligament holding it in place and is pinching the nerve *(arrow).*

COMMON SIGNS AND SYMPTOMS

- The signs and symptoms depend on the location of the herniated disk, the nerve the herniated disk is pinching, and how fast the herniation is growing.
- The signs and symptoms produced include pain in the area where the nerve goes, "pins and needles" sensation in the foot, and spasm of the muscles of the low back.
- While lying down, a person cannot raise the leg while it is straight—that is, not bent at the knee.

DIAGNOSIS

- Usually, a preliminary diagnosis can be made by taking a detailed history and doing a thorough physical examination with special emphasis on the neurologic examination. Several other examinations can be very useful.
- X-rays of the spine can give important information to help make the diagnosis.
- MRI (magnetic resonance imaging): No x-rays are used with this technique. Instead, it is done with harmless magnetic fields and radio waves. A computer develops pictures from several angles, showing the vertebrae, the nucleus pulposus, the spinal cord, and the nerves to and from the spinal cord. In this manner, abnormalities can be seen accurately.
- CT scan (computed tomography scan): These special x-rays are taken and shown as very thin slices of the area being studied, making it possible to see very fine details in the spine.

○ TREATMENT

- An early operation is advised if the pinching of the nerve is severe enough that the muscles involved become paralyzed or there is some loss of control of the bladder or bowel. If such symptoms are allowed to persist, they can become permanent, even if there is an operation later and the herniated disk itself is corrected.
- Other than the above exception, the *initial* treatment for a slipped disk should be strict bedrest for a few days and pain and anti-inflammatory medicines.
- If a person does not get better in a few weeks or if the person gets better but attacks recur frequently, then an operation is advised.

After careful consideration of all factors, the recommendation is that you have an operation on your back to try to correct your pain problem.

PREOPERATIVE PREPARATION

- You will have an examination of your blood, urine, heart (EKG), and lungs (chest x-ray).
- Do not eat or drink anything for 8 hours before the operation.

□ OPERATION

- You will be asleep for the operation.
- After you are asleep, you will be turned on your abdomen because the incision will be along the middle of your lower back.
- The operation usually takes about 2 hours.

POSTOPERATIVE CARE

- You will be taken to a recovery room and observed. When your blood pressure, pulse, and breathing are stable, you will be taken to a regular hospital room.
- Pain will be controlled with medicine.

- The nurse and the hospital team, including the physical therapist, will help you get out of bed and sit in a chair. They also will teach you how to get up and about by yourself.
- Your diet will be as you tolerate it.
- As with any operation, complications are always possible. With this type of operation, they can include bleeding, infection, injury to a nerve, blood clots, and possibly others.
- You should be able to go home several days after the operation.
- Arrangements will be made for your medicine, follow-up office visit, and stitch removal.

HOME CARE

- At the beginning, walking is the only exercise needed. A rehabilitation exercise program will be outlined for you.
- Do not do any lifting. Ask someone to do it for you.
- You may shower as you wish and with any dressings on or off. After you dry yourself, have someone replace any dressing with a clean, dry one.
- Eat as you wish. Include plenty of roughage and liquids in your diet to help avoid constipation. You may need some help with a mild laxative.
- During your follow-up office visit, let's discuss when you may drive a car, resume sexual activity, and return to work.

✆ CALL OUR OFFICE IF

- The incision becomes red or swollen, or there is drainage from it.
- You develop a temperature higher than 100°F.
- You have any questions.

△ GENERAL INFORMATION

The body has two types of sweat glands. *Eccrine* glands are found virtually all over the body and produce the ordinary, clear sweat when the body becomes warm. About 99% of this type of sweat is water. The other type of glands are the *apocrine*. They develop during puberty and are found mostly in the armpits and groin, around the genitals, and around the anus. They put out a thicker, cloudy fluid that has a slight odor (it's the one for which so many persons use deodorants).

Sometimes the apocrine glands become plugged and infected. The reason for this is not clear in most instances. Some persons, however, seem to get an infection if they use antiperspirants. Antiperspirants do their job by plugging the sweat pores: no sweat, no odor. This is different from the way deodorants work; they let the sweat come out and then try to mask its odor.

COMMON SIGNS AND SYMPTOMS

- The affected skin has one or many infected pockets; some may be draining pus.
- The infected areas can be painful or limit motion of the arm or leg.
- There usually is a foul odor.

DIAGNOSIS

- Usually, the diagnosis can be made by taking a detailed history and doing a thorough physical examination.

○ TREATMENT

- Whenever possible, the treatment is medical. This may include the following:
  - Applying warm, moist packs to the affected area.
  - Taking antibiotics to fight the infection.
  - Using antibiotic soap.
  - Losing weight if one is obese.
  - Nicking the skin over the pus pockets to let out the pus.

Although most patients respond reasonably well to the above treatment, other persons keep getting worse in spite of everything. For such an individual an operation is advisable.

- There are several operations for this condition. An operation may be rather minor, or it may be extensive. In certain situations, all the affected skin needs to be removed. If the edges of the incision are too far apart and cannot be brought together, then a skin graft may need to be used.
- Which operation is chosen depends on at least the following:
  - The part of the body involved.
  - How large an area is affected.
  - Whether the infection is acute or chronic.

After careful consideration of all factors, the recommendation is that you have an operation to try to correct your condition. The specific operation that is proposed will be discussed with you.

PREOPERATIVE PREPARATION

- Do not eat or drink anything for 8 hours before the operation.
- An examination of your blood, urine, heart (EKG), and lungs (chest x-ray) will be done.
- Shower as usual on the morning of the operation.
- You may be given medicine that will make you feel drowsy before you are brought to the operating room.

□ OPERATION

- You will be asleep for the operation.
- If a skin graft is necessary, it will be taken from your abdomen.
- The duration of the operation depends on how much tissue has to be removed and whether a skin graft is necessary.
- You will not need a blood transfusion.

POSTOPERATIVE CARE

- You will be taken to a recovery room and observed. When your blood pressure, pulse, and breathing are stable, you will be taken to a regular hospital room.
- That evening you will be helped to sit up in bed and on the next day to get out of bed.
- Pain will be controlled with medicine.
- Your diet will be as you tolerate it.
- As with any operation, complications are always possible. With this type of operation, they can include infection, blood clots, an ineffective skin graft, a thick scar in the area from which the skin graft was taken, and possibly others.
- When you go home depends on the extent of your operation.
- Arrangements will be made for your medicine, follow-up office visit, and any stitch removal.

✣ HOME CARE

- You may walk about as you wish, even climb stairs.
- You may eat as you did before the operation.
- If there is no skin graft, you may shower as you wish.
  - There may be narrow strips of tape across the incision. It's all right if they get wet; they will be removed in the doctor's office.
  - After you dry yourself, replace any dressings with clean, dry ones.
- If a skin graft is in place, the surgeon will instruct you on when you may start bathing or taking a shower and how to take care of the incision.
- You may return to work when you feel up to it, but let's talk about it first during a follow-up office visit.

✆ CALL OUR OFFICE IF

- The incision becomes red or swollen, or there is drainage from it.
- You develop a temperature higher than 100°F.
- You have any questions.

△ GENERAL INFORMATION

Total replacement of the hip (*arthroplasty*) is a method used to relieve the pain and disability caused by problems around the hip, most often hip arthritis or hip fracture. Hip replacement involves replacing parts of the joint that actually move past one another. The surfaces of these joints are covered in white, shiny cartilage material that normally makes it possible to have smooth, pain-free movement of the hip. When this cartilage is damaged, movement of the joint is painful and limited.

COMMON SIGNS AND SYMPTOMS

Pain and limitation of the joint are the most common symptoms. There may be difficulty in walking or putting on socks or shoes. The presence of a limp is commonly noted. In case of fracture, the signs and symptoms are more acute. Some type of fall is almost always noted, with severe pain and inability to walk.

DIAGNOSIS

- Most often, the diagnosis can be made by taking a detailed history and having x-ray pictures taken of the hip, which usually show damage to the hip joint.
- When the x-ray pictures don't clearly demonstrate the problem, additional imaging studies such as a bone scan may be done. Computed tomography scans (CT scans) and magnetic resonance imaging (MRI) can be critical in demonstrating a fracture that is not seen by other means.

○ TREATMENT

If the symptoms are caused by arthritis, the initial treatment includes the following:

- Anti-inflammatory and pain-relieving medicines.
- Modification of activity.
- Assistive devices for walking.
- Physical therapy to strengthen muscles around the hip.

If the above methods do not bring enough pain relief or return of function in an arthritic hip, then hip joint replacement may be the most effective treatment. Also, some cases of fracture of the hip are best treated by replacement. Such treatment is almost always used in the elderly, in whom fracture healing is less reliable and the prolonged rehabilitation necessary with fracture fixation can be a severe burden.

After careful consideration of all factors, the recommendation is that you have a total hip replacement.

PREOPERATIVE PREPARATION

- You will have an examination of your blood, urine, heart (EKG), and lungs (chest x-ray).
- Be certain your medical doctors are aware of any medications you are now taking and of any prior operations.
- It is important to know of any history of blood clots, infections, or complications with prior operations. Be sure to inform the doctors and nurses of any allergies, including those to medicines, tape, iodine, or latex.
- The operation may involve loss of blood, making it necessary to give you a transfusion. Let's discuss your donating some of your own blood 10 to 15 days before the operation. This blood is then stored, and in the meantime, your body will make more blood. The blood you donated can be transfused back to you if needed during or after the operation.
- Stop taking aspirin or similar medicines at least 10 days before the operation. Be certain to let the surgeon know if you are on any type of blood thinner.
- Do not eat or drink anything for 8 hours before the operation.

□ OPERATION

- You will be asleep for the operation or be offered a spinal type of anesthesia.
- Wires connected to recording machines will be taped to areas of your skin to keep track of your blood pressure, pulse, and breathing and the levels of oxygen in your blood.
- The diseased hip joint will be removed and replaced with a new one (Figs. 1–3).

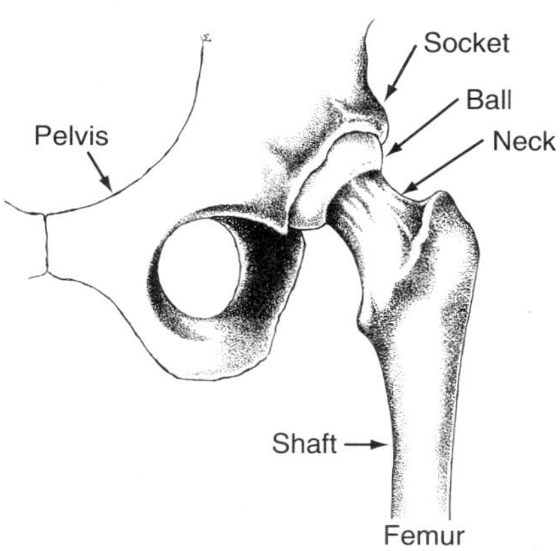

Figure 1. Normal hip.

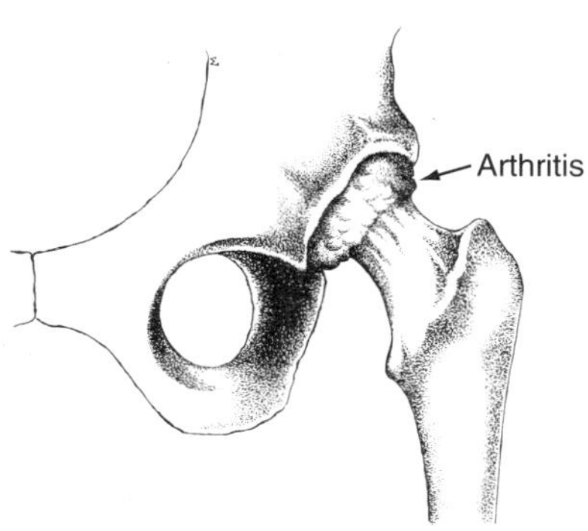

Figure 2. Hip with marked arthritis.

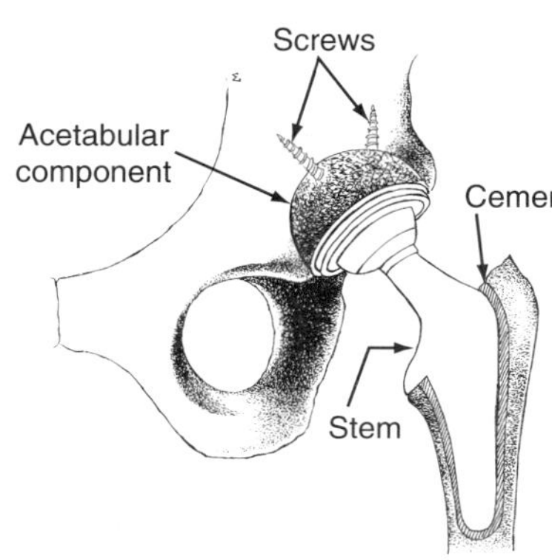

Figure 3. New hip joint.

- The entire operation takes from 1 to 3 hours, depending on the circumstances of your particular case.

POSTOPERATIVE CARE

- You will be taken to a recovery room and observed. When your blood pressure, pulse, and breathing are stable, you will be taken to a regular hospital room.
- Pain will be controlled with medicine.
- You will be encouraged to follow a routine that will allow you to recover from the operation and return to normal function as rapidly as is safely possible.
- Your diet will be as you tolerate it.
- Getting you up and about is a standard goal after hip replacement. You will have a customized therapy program, and the particulars of therapy will be explained to you before you leave the hospital.
- Leaving the hospital requires that you are feeling well enough to transfer to a suitable facility (home, skilled nursing unit), that you are eating and drinking well, that your discomfort is well managed by oral pain medicines, and that your wounds are clean and dry.
- As with any operation, complications are always possible, some of them serious. With this type of operation, they can include infection of the operated area, blood clots of the legs or the lungs, bleeding, pneumonia, heart problems, and possibly others.

✚ HOME CARE

- Continue with the program started while you were in the hospital.
- Arrangements will be made for a visiting nurse or therapist to assist you on a scheduled basis. The therapy you do at home will be similar to the exercises you did in the hospital and will allow you to recover muscle function.
- Keep the wound dry until the stitches or staples are removed.
- Driving and other more stressful activity will be discussed with you during your follow-up office visit.

✆ CALL OUR OFFICE IF

- The incision becomes red or swollen, or there is drainage from it.
- You develop a temperature higher than 101°F.
- The pain in the operative area increases.
- You have any questions.

△ GENERAL INFORMATION

Fracture of the hip is very common among the elderly, especially among women. Fracture of the hip itself is unfortunate, but it's the problems that can go with it that are the serious threats. The most common cause of a fracture is a fall or a twisting of the leg. If your bones have osteoporosis, it is easier for them to break even though the fall is not really serious.

Older people who lie in bed for long periods have a higher chance of getting pneumonia and other breathing problems. They often have heart problems and other problems with their circulation that can get worse if they lie in bed too long. The kidneys may not be in the best condition and not able to handle any additional stress.

COMMON SIGNS AND SYMPTOMS

- You have severe pain in the hip or groin area.
- You cannot move the leg, and you cannot stand up.
- If you are on your back after the injury, the foot of the broken leg points outward.

You will need to be taken to the hospital in an ambulance.

DIAGNOSIS

- X-rays will be taken of your hip to confirm you have a fracture and to see the exact location of the fracture.
- Usually the diagnosis can be made by taking a detailed history, doing a thorough physical examination, and considering the x-rays and laboratory reports carefully.

○ TREATMENT

- The first priority for doctors, nurses, and the rest of the hospital team is to get your fracture fixed and to get you up and about as soon as possible. This involves an operation to put the broken bone together and to hold it in that position as it heals.
- A hip fracture really is a fracture of the upper part of your thigh bone (the *femur*). The type of operation that needs to be done and the chances that it will be successful depend a lot on exactly which part of the hip is fractured. That's why several types of x-rays of your hip will be taken.
- On average, you will regain most but not all of the hip function that you had before the fracture.

PREOPERATIVE PREPARATION

- You will have an examination of your blood, urine, heart (EKG), and lungs (chest x-ray).
- Do not eat or drink anything for 8 hours before the operation.
- You may be given medicine that will make you feel drowsy before you are brought to the operating room.

□ OPERATION

- You will be asleep for the operation or be offered a spinal type of anesthetic.
- The exact operation to be performed on your hip depends on whether the bones are apart and twisted or just cracked but together. Thus, the operation can include some special plates or screws to hold the cracked pieces together, or the broken part of the joint may need to be replaced with an artificial part (Fig. 1).
- You will not receive a blood transfusion unless it is absolutely necessary.
- The operation usually takes around 2 hours.

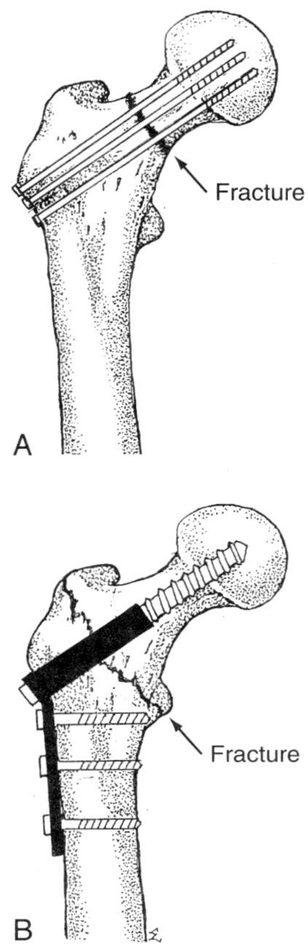

Figure 1. *A* and *B*, Two examples of the many ways a fracture of the hip can be repaired.

POSTOPERATIVE CARE

- You will be taken to a recovery room and observed. When your blood pressure, pulse, and breathing are stable, you will be taken to a regular hospital room.
- There will be pain in the hip area, but this can be controlled with medicines.
- There will be a pillow between your legs to help keep them properly separated.
- Often, special stockings—called "boots"—will be placed on your legs. They will help the blood in your veins circulate properly so that they don't develop blood clots.
- The nurses and the physical therapist will help you get out of bed and then sit in a chair. Also, you will be helped to learn to walk and to climb stairs.

- Once you have learned to move about and your medical condition is stable, you will be able to go home. Possibly, you may wish to go to a rehabilitation facility for a short while before going directly home.
- Arrangements will be made for your medicine, follow-up office visit, and stitch removal.
- You will be given blood thinners for several weeks after the surgery to help prevent blood clots.

✣ HOME CARE

- Continue with the program started while you were in the hospital, possibly with home physical therapist or nurse visits.
- Be careful that you do not become constipated.
  - Include enough roughage and plenty of liquids in your diet.
  - You may need a mild laxative (example: milk of magnesia).

✆ CALL OUR OFFICE IF

- The incision becomes red or swollen, or there is drainage from it.
- The pain in your hip is getting worse.
- You develop a temperature higher than 100°F.
- You have any questions.

HUMERUS: Fracture at Elbow (Lower Third)

△ GENERAL INFORMATION

Fractures involving the lower one-third of the humerus and elbow are often complex and difficult to treat in spite of modern advances in fracture fixation (Fig. 1). In younger persons, these fractures commonly are caused by a severe, direct blow to the area of the elbow. In older persons, they usually are the result of a fall and either landing on the outstretched arm or striking the elbow directly.

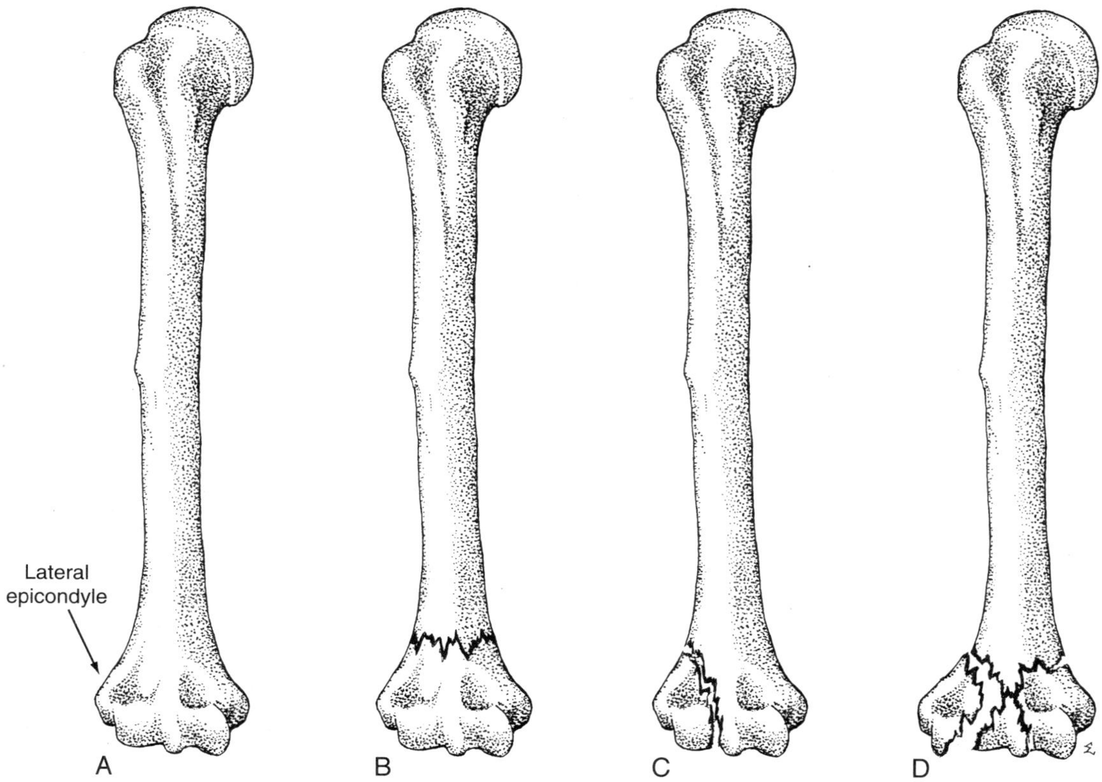

Figure 1. *A*, Normal humerus. *B–D*, Several examples of fractures of the elbow area.

COMMON SIGNS AND SYMPTOMS

- There is severe pain in the elbow, especially when the elbow is moved.
- Because the nerves that progress into the forearm and hand are near this part of the humerus, there may also be numbness, tingling, or an inability to use the muscles that move the wrist, hand, and fingers.
- The fractured bone may penetrate the skin (a *compound fracture*).

DIAGNOSIS

- The diagnosis often is suspected after taking a detailed history and performing a thorough physical examination. The diagnosis is confirmed by x-rays of the entire arm. Special x-ray views may be necessary to help plan treatment. Because these fractures commonly enter into the elbow joint itself, several additional tests may be performed.
- CT scan (computed tomography scan): These special x-rays are taken as very thin slices through the area of the elbow. They allow an analysis of the exact nature of the fracture and provide important information that is useful in planning treatment.
- If the blood supply to the forearm or hand appears to be affected, x-rays of the blood vessels may be taken (an *arteriogram*).
- The fracture fragments may actually pinch or directly injure the nerves that progress past the elbow joint, and thus a person can lose the ability to move the wrist, hand, and fingers.

○ TREATMENT

- Many fractures that involve the lower humerus or elbow joint require an operation to obtain the best results because the elbow bones have many angles and curves. In particular, an operation is recommended for active patients. An operation is absolutely necessary for patients with fractures that penetrate the skin and fractures associated with injury to the nerves or blood vessels.
- Even fractures with many pieces *(comminuted fractures)* can be treated successfully using modern techniques.
- Sometimes the fracture involving the elbow joint involves so many pieces that it is not possible to put

all the fragments together properly. In such an instance, the fracture can be treated in a splint for 2 weeks, and then a gentle mobilization program is begun. Sometimes it is best to do a total elbow replacement.

The plan of treatment that is most suitable for you will be explained in full detail before anything is planned or done.

PREOPERATIVE PREPARATION

- You will have an examination of your blood, urine, heart (EKG), and lungs (chest x-ray).
- Do not eat or drink anything for 8 hours before the operation.

☐ OPERATION

- The aim of the operation is as follows: to stabilize the fracture fragments in the correct position so that you can have early range of motion of your elbow joint, to minimize any injury to the muscles and nerves around the fracture, and to encourage the most rapid healing of the fracture.
- You will be asleep for the operation.
- Metal plates and screws are used to fix the fracture fragments. A complex array of these fixation devices may be necessary to repair this fracture, depending on the nature of the fracture fragments. These techniques have been developed worldwide for the treatment of these complex fractures.
- Occasionally, some bone chips (a bone graft) are needed to speed up the healing. Such bone chips most often are taken from the waist-hip area. This does not affect the strength of your bones that are required for walking or moving.
- The operation usually takes about 3 to 4 hours, depending on the complexity of the fracture.

POSTOPERATIVE CARE

- You will be taken to a recovery room and observed. When your blood pressure, pulse, and breathing are stable, you will be taken to a regular hospital room.
- Pain will be controlled with medicines.
- Your arm will be in a splint and sling for protection of the fracture site and for comfort.
- That evening you will be helped to sit up in bed and on the next day to get out of bed.
- The doctors will observe closely your ability to feel and move your wrist, hand, and fingers.
- Arrangements will be made for your medicine, follow-up office visit, and stitch removal.
- The seriousness of the fracture will influence when you are started on elbow motion.

POSSIBLE COMPLICATIONS

- As with any operation, complications are always possible. With this operation, they can include bleeding injury to the nerves close to the fracture, infection, poor wound healing, and possibly others.
- In spite of appropriate fixation, some fractures may not heal and may require additional surgery.

✚ HOME CARE

- You may walk about as you wish, even climb stairs, but don't overdo things.
- Take the medicines prescribed for you.
- Unless instructed otherwise, keep the dressing and splint on at all times.
- If you choose to bathe, the entire arm can be placed in a plastic trash bag and sealed at the top with tape.
- Move your fingers, hand, and wrist as much as your dressings will allow after the operation to help reduce swelling and stiffness.

✆ CALL OUR OFFICE IF

- The incision becomes red or swollen, or there is drainage from it.
- You experience severe or unexpected pain that is unrelieved by your prescription medication.
- You develop a temperature higher than 100°F.
- You have numbness and tingling in the arm or hand.
- You have any questions.

HUMERUS: Fracture at Neck (Upper Third)

△ GENERAL INFORMATION

The *humerus* is the bone of the upper arm. Most fractures of the upper one-third of the humerus (called the *neck* of the humerus) occur after a fall on the arm from a standing height (Fig. 1).

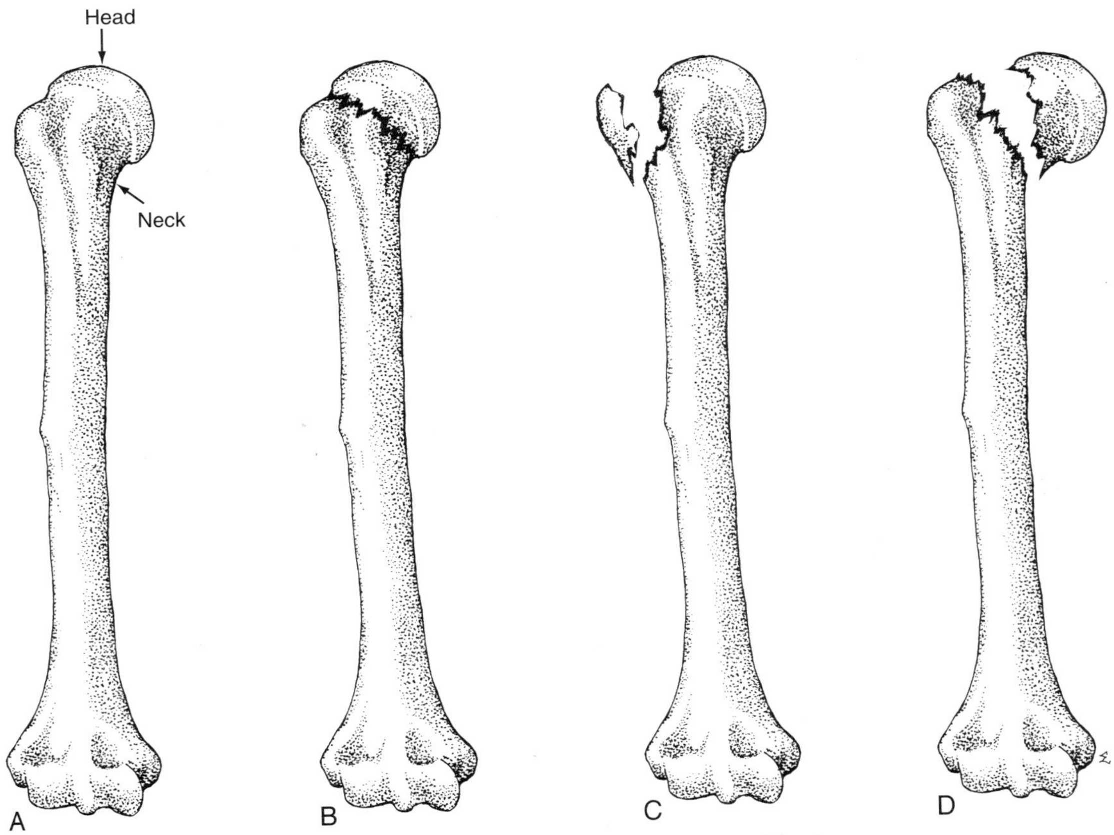

Figure 1. *A,* Normal humerus. *B–D,* Typical types of fractures.

COMMON SIGNS AND SYMPTOMS

- The arm cannot be lifted.
- Rotation of the arm causes pain.
- Significant swelling and bruising are seen at 24 to 72 hours following the injury.
- The pain generally is constant and is not relieved well by immobilizing the arm in a sling or in a shoulder immobilizer.

DIAGNOSIS

- The diagnosis is strongly suspected from a detailed history and careful physical examination of the shoulder region. X-rays of the arm can confirm the diagnosis and help to plan treatment.
- A neurologic examination is performed to evaluate the function of the arm nerves that go past the upper end of the humerus and that might be damaged.
- CT scan (computed tomography scan): These special x-rays are taken as very thin slices through the area of the humerus. They make it possible to see the fine details in the humerus and can be valuable in evaluating the fracture pattern and in planning for an operation on a complex fracture.

○ TREATMENT

- Most often the fractured bones are not out of line, or are minimally so, and can be treated with pain medicine and immobilization for a period of 3 to 4 weeks followed by a program of gradual return of range of motion.
- Fractures that are too much out of line require an operation to realign the bone fragments properly and then to stabilize them in that position. Such stabilization can be accomplished with a number of different techniques. The use of pins can be sufficient in less complex fractures. Wires and sutures and plates and screws can be employed as well. In a very severely damaged upper humerus, a shoulder replacement device may be necessary.

After careful consideration of all factors, the recommendation is that you have an operation for your humerus fracture.

PREOPERATIVE PREPARATION

- You will have an examination of your blood, urine, heart (EKG), and lungs (chest x-ray).
- Do not eat or drink anything for 8 hours before the operation.

☐ OPERATION

- You will be asleep during the operation.
- Although a plan will be developed before the operation, the complexity of the fracture when it is exposed at operation will determine the technique used.
- If bone chips (a bone graft) need to be placed to help with healing of the fracture, they most commonly are taken from the waist-hip area. This does not affect the strength of your bones that are used for walking or moving.

POSTOPERATIVE CARE

- You will be taken to a recovery room and observed. When your blood pressure, pulse, and breathing are stable, you will be taken to a regular hospital room.
- There will be a bandage on your shoulder, and your arm will be in a sling.
- Your doctors and nurses will observe carefully your ability to feel your shoulder, arm, forearm, and hand and to move the muscles that control your elbow, wrist, and hand.
- You will be assisted to sit up as well as get out of bed.
- Pain will be controlled with medicine.
- You should be able to leave the hospital in 2 or 3 days.
- Arrangements will be made for your medicines, follow-up visit, and stitch removal.
- As with any operation, complications are always possible. With this type of operation, they can include bleeding, injury to the nerves that are close to the fracture, infection, poor wound healing, and possibly others. In some patients, the fracture may not heal or the fixation may not be satisfactory and additional surgery may be necessary.

✚ HOME CARE

- Unless instructed otherwise, keep the sling or immobilizer on at all times.
- You may bathe as you wish; however, the entire area should be covered so that the surgical site does not get wet.
- Take the medicines prescribed for you.
- Move your fingers, hand, and wrist as much as possible to help reduce swelling as well as to minimize stiffness of the fingers and hand.
- A physical rehabilitation program will be outlined for you.
- Do not drive until you have easy and painless use of both arms and are not taking medicines that reduce your alertness.
- You may return to work when you feel comfortable, but let's first talk about it during your follow-up office visit.

✆ CALL OUR OFFICE IF

- There is swelling, redness, or drainage from the surgical area.
- You have pain that is severe, unexpected, or increasing and that is not relieved by your prescription medication.
- You develop a temperature higher than 100.5°F.
- You have numbness or tingling of the arm or hand.
- You have any questions or develop other unusual signs or symptoms.

HUMERUS: Fracture at Shaft (Middle Third)

△ GENERAL INFORMATION

The *humerus* is the bone of the upper arm. Fractures of the middle part of the humerus (the shaft) are most commonly the result of a fall on the arm (Fig. 1).

- The fractured bone has pierced the skin.
- The blood vessels are injured.
- There are associated multiple injuries to the arm.
- The nerve is being pinched by the fractured bones.

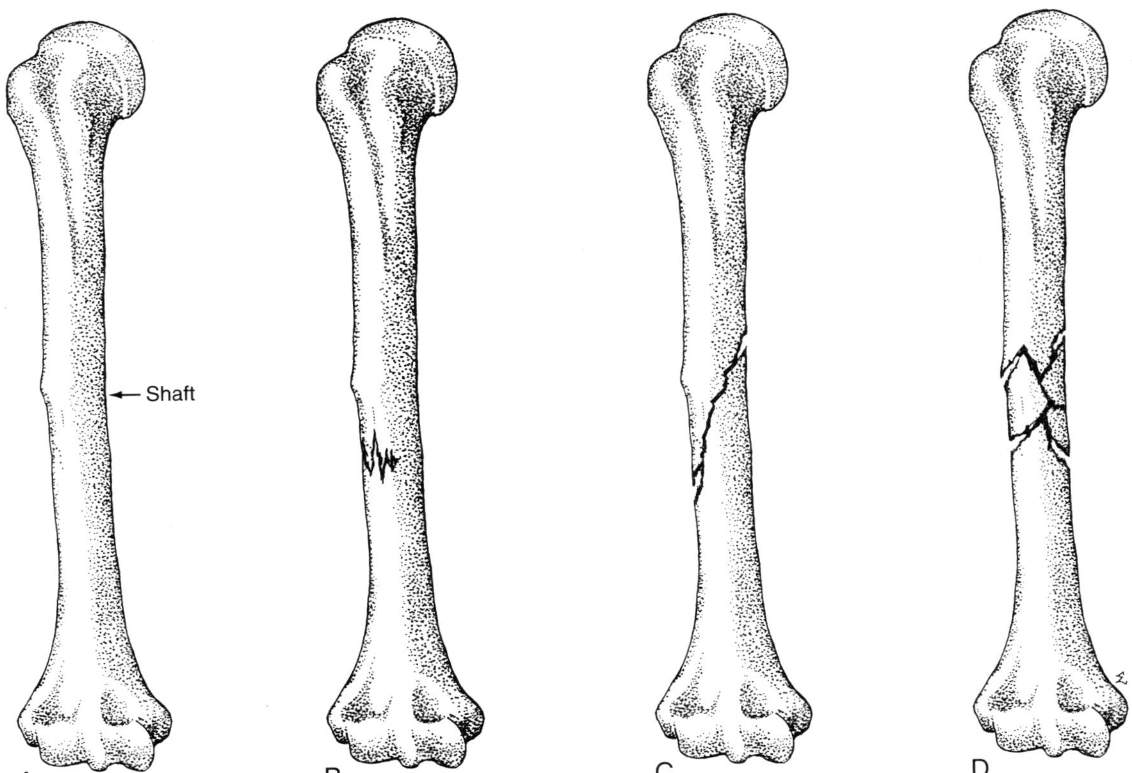

Figure 1. *A*, Normal humerus. *B–D*, Examples of fractures.

COMMON SIGN AND SYMPTOMS

- There is severe pain with inability to use the arm for any activity.
- Because nerves of the arm run very close to the shaft, there may be numbness and tingling or inability to use some of the muscles of the arm.

DIAGNOSIS

- The diagnosis can be suspected after taking a history and performing a physical examination. The diagnosis is confirmed by x-rays of the entire arm.
- If the blood vessels in the area appear to be affected, x-ray pictures of the artery (an *arteriogram*) may be necessary.

○ TREATMENT

- Most fractures of the shaft of the humerus are treated initially by immobilization with a plaster splint held in a sling that is around the neck and attached to the wrist.
- An operation is necessary in the following circumstances:
- Less frequent problems requiring an operation may include the following:
  - Inability to reduce the fracture to an acceptable position by closed manipulation.
  - Fractures involving multiple limbs.
  - Non-union of the fracture.

After careful consideration of all factors, the recommendation is that you have an operation to fix your fracture.

PREOPERATIVE PREPARATION

- You will have an examination of your blood and urine, heart (EKG), and lungs (chest x-ray).
- Do not eat or drink anything for 8 hours before the operation.

□ OPERATION

- The aim of the operation is as follows:
  - To stabilize the fracture fragments in a normal position.
  - To minimize any injury to the muscles and nerves around the fracture.

- To encourage the most rapid healing of the fracture.
- Two well-accepted methods of fixation of fractures of the humerus are (1) placing a metal plate across the fracture and holding it in position with multiple screws and (2) lining up the broken humerus and placing a thin metal rod inside of it to hold it in position.

The choice of technique will be discussed with you beforehand.

- You will be asleep for the operation.
- Occasionally, some bone chips (a bone graft) are needed to help with the healing of the fracture. These bone chips are usually gotten from the hip-waist area. This does not affect the bones that are required for walking or moving.
- The operation usually takes about 2½ hours.

POSTOPERATIVE CARE

- You will be taken to a recovery room and observed. When your blood pressure, pulse, and breathing are stable, you will be taken to a regular hospital room.
- There will be a bandage around your arm, and your arm will be in a sling.
- Your ability to feel and move all parts of your arm will be checked frequently.
- You will be assisted to sit up in bed as well as get out of bed to sit in a chair.
- Pain will be controlled with medicine.
- You should be able to go home the next day.
- Arrangements will be made for your medicine, follow-up office visit, and stitch removal.
- As with any operation, complications are always possible. With this operation they can include bleeding, injury to the nerves in the area, infection, poor wound healing, and possibly others. Very infrequently, the fracture does not heal and may require additional surgery.

✚ HOME CARE

- Unless instructed otherwise, keep the sling or immobilizer on at all times.
- If you bathe, the entire area should be properly covered.
- Take the medicines prescribed for you.
- Move your fingers, hand, and wrist as much as possible to help reduce swelling as well as to minimize stiffness of the fingers and hand.
- Do not resume driving or return to work until we first discuss it during your office visit.

✆ CALL OUR OFFICE IF

- The incision becomes red or swollen, or there is drainage from it.
- You have unexpected or increased pain or pain that is not relieved by your medicine.
- You have a temperature higher than 100.5°F.
- You experience numbness and tingling in your arm or hand.
- You have any questions.

HYDROCELE: Adult

△ GENERAL INFORMATION

The two testicles each lie in separate pockets in the *scrotum* (the sac). Each testicle is always making a little fluid that is absorbed by the lining of the sac. If, for some reason, the fluid is not absorbed fast enough, it begins to build up and the scrotum on one side becomes swollen. This swelling can be just a little or fairly large—sometimes the size of a grapefruit. This condition is called a *hydrocele* (Fig. 1).

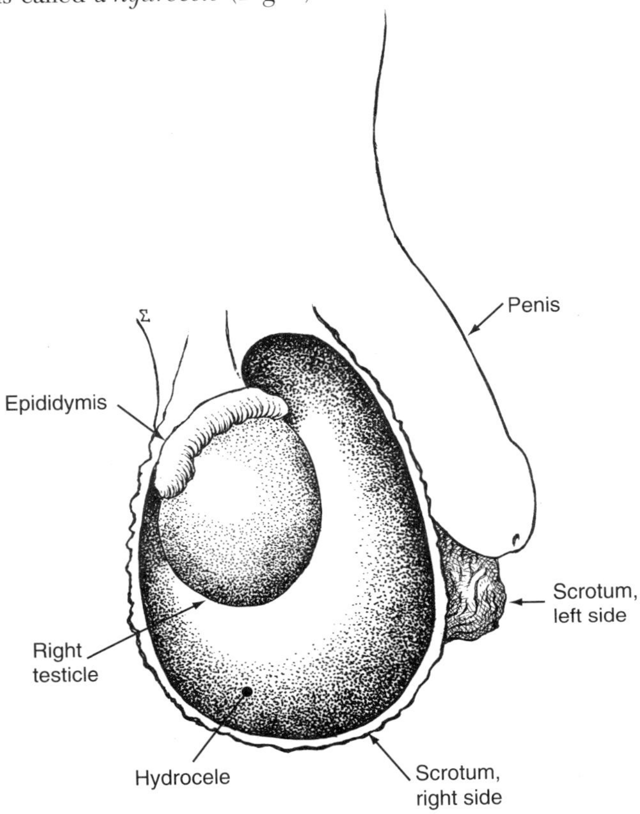

Figure 1. In this operation, the hydrocele is opened and the fluid removed. The sac of the hydrocele is excised almost entirely, and the remainder of it is sutured so that a hydrocele cannot reform.

COMMON SIGNS AND SYMPTOMS

- There is a swelling of one side of the scrotum that is smooth, does not hurt, and feels like a balloon filled with water.

DIAGNOSIS

- Usually, the diagnosis can be made by taking a detailed history and doing a thorough physical examination.
- Ultrasound: Harmless sound waves are aimed at the scrotum. The sound waves bouncing back (the echoes) from this area are seen as a picture on a television screen. This is a convenient, painless, and harmless way to examine the testicles and the other tissues inside the scrotum. This test is done to make certain the testicle is normal and that the swelling is fluid, not a cancerous growth.

○ TREATMENT

- The treatment is an operation to prevent the buildup of fluid.
- The fluid should never just be removed with a needle because of the following:
  - It will just reaccumulate.
  - It may become infected. This would greatly complicate matters.

PREOPERATIVE PREPARATION

- An examination of your blood, urine, heart (EKG), and lungs (chest x-ray) will be done.
- Do not eat or drink anything for 8 hours before the operation.
- Shower (and shave) as usual on the morning of the operation.
- You may be given medicine that will make you feel drowsy before you are brought to the operating room.

□ OPERATION

- You will be asleep for the operation.
- Your genitals will be scrubbed with an antiseptic solution and draped.
- You will not need a blood transfusion.
- The operation usually takes about 1 hour.

POSTOPERATIVE CARE

- You will wake up in a recovery room. When your blood pressure, pulse, and breathing are stable, you will be taken to a regular hospital room and should be able to go home with a responsible adult. Occasionally, it may be necessary for you to remain in the hospital overnight.
- There will be a snug bandage around your scrotum. This may make it look as large as before the operation; don't be concerned.
- That evening you will be helped to sit up in bed and on the next day to get out of bed.
- Pain can be controlled with medicine.
- As with any operation, complications are always possible. Although they are uncommon with your type of operation, they can include bleeding and infection, among others.
- Arrangements will be made for your medicine and follow-up office visit.

✚ HOME CARE

- Walk about as you wish, but lie down 10 minutes every hour or so, if you can. This will help reduce any swelling and also make you feel more comfortable.
- Take medicine as prescribed for your pain.
- You may shower as you wish and with any dressings on or off.
  - There may be narrow strips of tape across the incision. It's all right if they get wet. They will be removed in the doctor's office.

- After you dry yourself, replace any dressings with clean, dry ones.
- Wearing jockey-type rather than boxer-type shorts is more comfortable and a good way to hold dressings in place.
- You may drive your car as you wish, provided you are not on any medicines that reduce your alertness.
- You may return to work when you feel up to it.
- The swelling from the operation may not go down appreciably for 4 to 6 months. Do not be alarmed.

✆ CALL OUR OFFICE IF

- The incision becomes red or swollen, or there is drainage from it.
- You develop a temperature higher than 100°F.
- You have any questions.

△ GENERAL INFORMATION

A *hydrocele* is a condition in which fluid accumulates in the *scrotum* (the sac) around the testicle. A hydrocele does not communicate with the abdominal cavity. Because of this, there is no risk that intestines from within the abdominal cavity might enter the hydrocele.

The cause of hydrocele is not known.

COMMON SIGNS AND SYMPTOMS

Hydrocele typically is seen in a healthy infant whose mother or pediatrician notices a swelling of the scrotum.

- The infant or child is not in distress and typically is eating and behaving normally.
- The lump or swelling should not be tender. It may have a slightly purplish discoloration.
- There may be some slight daily difference in the size of the swelling.

DIAGNOSIS

- The diagnosis can almost always be made simply by taking a detailed history and performing a thorough physical examination (Fig. 1).
- It may be difficult to distinguish a hydrocele (especially one that comes on within a short period) from a hernia in which intestine is stuck in the hernia sac. In these circumstances, a scrotal ultrasound or an abdominal x-ray may be helpful.
  - *Scrotal ultrasound*: Sound waves (they are very much like sonar) are aimed at the scrotum. The sound waves bouncing back (the echoes) are seen as pictures on a screen. This is a convenient, harmless, and painless way to see what is inside the scrotum.
  - *Abdominal x-ray*: The x-ray can help show if the swelling in the scrotum is intestine.

○ TREATMENT

- A hydrocele in an infant should simply be observed, as in many cases it will go away by itself by the age of 1 year.
- A hydrocele that persists past 1 year of age, or first appears in a child older than 1 year of age, should be repaired by an operation.
- A hydrocele that changes greatly in size from day to day means that a hernia also is present. In such a situation, a prompt operation is necessary regardless of the age of the child.

PREOPERATIVE PREPARATION

- Do not give the child anything to eat or drink for 4 hours before the scheduled operation.

□ OPERATION

- The child will be asleep for the operation.
- A short incision will be made in the groin area. The hydrocele will be corrected. Sometimes, there is a pinpoint opening into the abdominal cavity (actually a hernia). If so, this too will be corrected.
- The incision will be closed with dissolving stitches.
- The operation usually takes about 1 hour.

POSTOPERATIVE CARE

- The child will be taken to a recovery room.
- When the blood pressure, pulse, and breathing are stable and the child is fully awake and able to tolerate liquids, you should be able to take your child home.
- Arrangements will be made for any medicines and the follow-up visit.

✆ CALL OUR OFFICE IF

- The incision becomes red or swollen, or there is drainage from it.
- The scrotum swells.
- The child develops a temperature higher than 101°F.
- You have any questions.

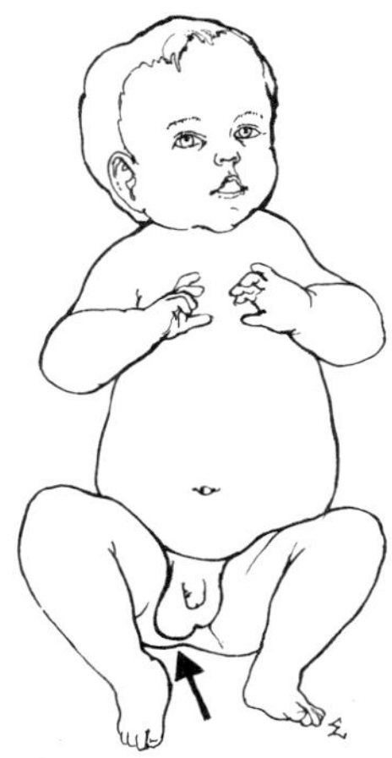

Figure 1. Generally, the hydrocele is associated with a hernia, and both are corrected through the hernia incision.

HYPERPARATHYROIDISM

△ GENERAL INFORMATION

The *parathyroid glands* are four glands in your neck that are the size and shape of lentils. They are right next to the thyroid gland (Fig. 1). They regulate the calcium level in your blood. Sometimes, one or more of these glands does not work properly, and your calcium level rises above normal.

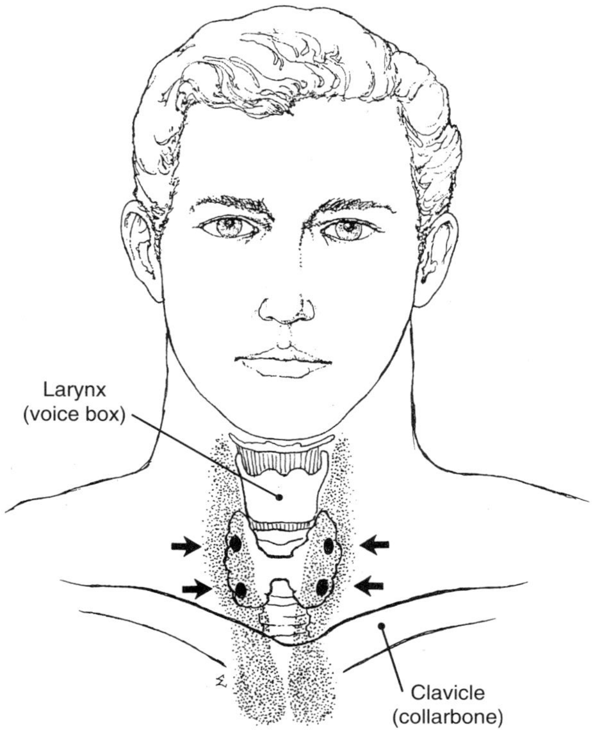

Figure 1. Two each of the four parathyroid glands *(arrows)* are located on either side of the thyroid gland. Sometimes there are five or only three glands. Although most often they are located in the areas indicated by the four arrows, they can be found throughout the stippled area. Note that the stippled area extends behind the sternum (breastbone) inside the chest.

COMMON SIGNS AND SYMPTOMS

- Your muscles may feel weak.
- There is a tendency to form kidney stones.
- Some persons develop constipation.
- There is the need to pass urine more often.
- There is increased nervousness.
- The joints become sore.

DIAGNOSIS

- There may not be any symptoms at all to concern anyone. A high calcium level is discovered on a routine blood examination.
- The blood tests are done at least twice to be certain that the calcium level is really elevated.
- The parathyroid hormone level in the blood will be measured; usually it is elevated.
- Ultrasound: Harmless sound waves are aimed at the neck. The sound waves bouncing back (the echoes) from this area are seen as a picture on a screen. This is a convenient, painless, and harmless way to examine organs and tissues in the neck.

A high level of calcium can cause serious problems with the way your nerves work. Such a high calcium level can also cause problems with your kidneys, bones, and blood vessels, among others.

The reason for the abnormal function of the parathyroid gland is usually not known.

○ TREATMENT

- An operation to remove the one or more diseased glands is the only treatment that can cure this condition.

After careful consideration of your symptoms and physical and laboratory findings, the recommendation is that you have a parathyroid operation.

PREOPERATIVE PREPARATION

- You may have an examination of your blood, urine, heart (EKG), and lungs (chest x-ray).
- Do not eat or drink anything for 8 hours before the operation.
- Shower (and shave) as usual on the morning of the operation.
- You may be given medicine that will make you feel drowsy before you are brought to the operating room.

□ OPERATION

- You will be asleep for the operation.
- The incision will be made in a cosmetic fashion in a skin crease in your lower neck.
- The parathyroid glands sometimes are not where they are supposed to be, so the operation can be arduous. Even so, it is not a dangerous operation.
- You will not need a blood transfusion.
- There will be a cosmetic closure.
- The operation usually takes about 2 hours.
- There always is a small possibility that the diseased parathyroid gland will not be found in your neck because in up to 5% of persons, the abnormal gland is really located under the upper part of the *sternum* (the breastbone) and not in the neck. This will be discussed with you further before the operation.

POSTOPERATIVE CARE

- You will wake up in a recovery room. When your blood pressure, pulse, and breathing are stable, you will be taken to a regular hospital room.
- There will be a dressing over your incision.
- You will have a sore throat for a day or so.
- There is not much pain, and it can be controlled with medicine.
- That evening you will be helped to get out of bed with assistance.
- Your level of calcium will be followed very closely to see how well it adjusts to a normal level.

- You will be fed as soon as you feel hungry.
- You should be able to go home the next day.
- As with any operation, complications are always possible. Although they are uncommon with your type of operation, they can include bleeding, infection, or injury to your vocal cord. Sometimes the amount of parathyroid gland left behind is not able to regulate your calcium properly. This may make it necessary for you to take medicine for a number of months. In addition, there is the possibility that the abnormal gland cannot be found.
- Arrangements will be made for your medicine, follow-up office visit, and stitch removal.

HOME CARE

- Resume your usual activities.
- You may walk about as you wish, even climb stairs.
- Your diet can be as before the operation.
- You may shower as you wish and with any dressings on or off.
- Driving a car with an automatic shift is not too demanding. But if you suddenly have to slam on the brakes or twist to turn the steering wheel, you might get into an accident or strain the sutures or tear something. During your follow-up visit, let's discuss when you can resume driving.
- You may resume sexual activity whenever you choose.
- You may return to work when you feel up to it.

CALL OUR OFFICE IF

- You have tingling or spasm of your fingers or toes.
- You develop any unusual signs or symptoms.
- The incision becomes red or swollen, or there is drainage from it.
- You develop a temperature higher than 101°F.
- You have any questions.

△ GENERAL INFORMATION

The thyroid gland is located in the neck on each side of the *trachea* (windpipe), just below the *larynx* (voice box). The thyroid gland makes hormones that regulate how slow or fast many of the body functions work. Sometimes, the thyroid makes too much hormone so that the body functions go into high gear. This is called *hyperthyroidism.*

COMMON SIGNS AND SYMPTOMS

- Extreme irritability.
- Weight loss even with increased eating.
- Intolerance to heat.
- Episodes of emotional instability.
- Enlargement of the thyroid gland to some degree.
- Bulging of the eyes (called *exophthalmos*).

DIAGNOSIS

- Usually the diagnosis can be made by taking a detailed history, doing a thorough physical examination, and performing some laboratory tests.

○ TREATMENT

There are three ways to treat hyperthyroidism. Each way has some advantages and disadvantages:

Control with Antithyroid Drugs

This involves taking medicine that slows down the thyroid gland.

Advantages

- No operation is necessary. Sometimes when the medicines are stopped, the hyperthyroidism does not return.

Disadvantages

- If the medicine is not taken every day, most of the time the hyperthyroidism returns.
- Sometimes the medicine causes a rash and fever.
- About one in 100 persons develops a serious blood problem.
- It can be difficult (or even dangerous) to use this medicine in pregnant women.

Destruction of the Thyroid Gland with Radioiodine

This involves combining a radioactive material with iodine. The person drinks this "atomic cocktail," and the iodine (along with the radioactive material) is taken up by the thyroid gland. The radioactivity slowly kills the thyroid tissue.

Advantages

- No operation is necessary.
- There is no risk of injuring the parathyroid glands or the nerve to the voice box.

Disadvantages

- It takes a number of weeks for this treatment to work.
- It is very difficult to calculate the exact amount of radioiodine necessary to kill the correct amount of thyroid tissue. Because of this, too much or too little of the gland may be destroyed, necessitating additional therapy.
- If an operation must be done after this, there is greater risk to the parathyroids or to the nerve.
- It cannot be used in pregnant women.

Surgical Removal of Most of the Thyroid Gland

Advantages

- It quickly stops the hyperthyroidism.
- There are no late side effects.
- There is less risk of permanent hypothyroidism.
- It can be used in pregnant women.

Disadvantages

- An operation is necessary.
- There is a 1 to 2% risk of injury to the nerve to the larynx, which causes hoarseness, or to the nearby parathyroid glands that control your calcium metabolism (Fig. 1).

After careful consideration of all factors, it is recommended that you have an operation to remove most of your thyroid gland.

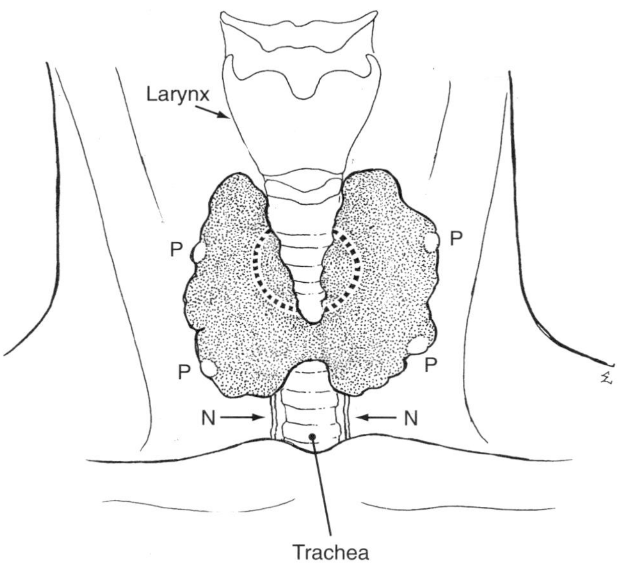

Figure 1. In this operation, the three important aims are to remove just the right amount of tissue (everything outside the circular dashed line), to safeguard the important four parathyroid glands (P), and not to injure the nerve (N) to the larynx (the voice box).

PREOPERATIVE PREPARATION

- You will have an examination of your blood, urine, heart (EKG), and lungs (chest x-ray).
- You will be placed on an antithyroid medicine to slow your metabolism before the operation. This will make your operation safer.
- Do not eat or drink anything for 8 hours before the operation.
- You may be given medicine that will make you feel drowsy before you are brought to the operating room.

☐ OPERATION

- You will be asleep for the operation.
- A cosmetic incision will be made side to side in a crease in your lower neck.
- The operation usually takes about 2 hours.

POSTOPERATIVE CARE

- You will be taken to a recovery room and observed. When your blood pressure, pulse, and breathing are stable, you will be taken to a regular hospital room.
- There may be a drain coming through the incision. It will be removed the next morning.
- That evening you will be able to get out of bed with assistance.
- Pain will be controlled with medicine.
- Your diet will be as you tolerate it.
- You should be able to go home the next day.
- Arrangements will be made for your medicine, follow-up office visit, and stitch removal.
- As with any operation, complications are always possible. With this type of operation they can include bleeding, hoarseness, injury to the parathyroid glands, and possibly others.

✚ HOME CARE

- Resume your usual activities.
- You may walk about as you wish, even climb stairs, but don't overdo things.
- You may eat as you wish.
- You may shower if you wish with any dressings removed. After you dry yourself, replace any dressings with clean, dry ones.
- Do not drive your car unless you can move your neck freely and without pain.
- You may return to work when you feel up to it.

✆ CALL OUR OFFICE IF

- You develop any unusual signs or symptoms.
- The incision becomes red or swollen, or there is drainage from it.
- You develop a temperature higher than 101°F.

HYPERTROPHIC PYLORIC STENOSIS

△ GENERAL INFORMATION

Hypertrophic (overgrown) *pyloric* (muscle valve at the outlet of the stomach) *stenosis* (narrowing) is just that. The muscle valve at the end of the stomach is thickened and elongated so that food and liquid cannot empty from the stomach. The condition is seen in infants usually between the ages of 3 and 12 weeks. It occurs most commonly in first-born males but can occur in females and is often seen in families.

The exact cause is not known.

COMMON SIGNS AND SYMPTOMS

- The infant begins to vomit part or all of the feedings.
- The vomitus is curdled milk, and there is no bile in it.
- As the blockage gets worse the vomiting becomes more frequent and so forceful that it seems to shoot out of the child's mouth.
- After vomiting, the child is very hungry and wants to eat again.
- If the vomiting continues long enough, the infant becomes very low on fluids (dehydrated) and body chemicals.
- The child may lose weight and become listless.

DIAGNOSIS

- If within the first 2 to 3 months of life the infant has a history of vomiting material that has no bile in it and vomiting that shoots out, there should be concern about hypertrophic pyloric stenosis.
- Usually, the diagnosis can be made by taking a detailed history, doing a thorough physical examination, and considering the laboratory reports carefully.
- Often the pylorus muscle can be felt through the abdominal wall by an experienced physician. It feels like an "olive" and is located in the right upper abdomen.
- Ultrasound: Harmless sound waves are aimed at the area of the stomach. The sound waves that bounce back (echoes) from this area are seen as a picture on a screen. This is a convenient and painless way to examine the stomach and pylorus.
- An x-ray of the stomach may be obtained after the child has swallowed barium. Although this test has been replaced by ultrasound, it still is useful to look at the anatomy of esophagus, stomach, and the area of the pylorus.

○ TREATMENT

- The treatment is an operation called a *pyloromyotomy,* which means opening up the muscle of the pylorus and relieving the blockage (Fig. 1).

PREOPERATIVE PREPARATION

- It is important to correct any imbalances in the child's body fluids and chemicals before performing the operation; this makes the operation much safer. This is done with fluids and salts given by vein and not by mouth.
- Your child may require a small tube, which goes from the nose into the esophagus and stomach. This will drain fluid from the stomach and help prevent recurrent vomiting.

□ OPERATION

- Your child will have a general anesthetic.
- The incision is usually on the right side of the upper abdomen.
- The operation usually takes about 1 hour.
- Frequently, there will be some anesthetic injected into the skin around the incision to help with relief of postoperative pain.

POSTOPERATIVE CARE

- Within 24 hours after the operation, the child will be given liquids by mouth. Occasionally, an infant will continue to have some minor "spitting-up," but it won't be as much or as forceful as it was before the operation.
- The infant is usually ready for discharge 1 to 3 days after the operation.
- Arrangements will be made for the first postoperative visit.

✚ HOME CARE

- You will be given instructions regarding feedings, bathing, care of the wound, and pain medication.
- Feed the infant slowly, and make sure the child burps.

✆ CALL OUR OFFICE IF

- The infant continues to have significant vomiting ("wet-burps" or minor spitting-up is acceptable).
- The incision becomes red or swollen, or there is drainage from it.
- The infant develops a temperature higher than 101°F.
- You have any questions.

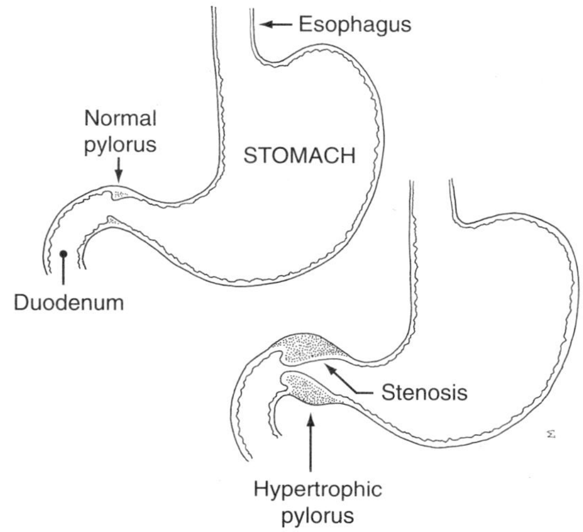

Figure 1. The thickened, overgrown blocking part of the outlet of the stomach (the *hypertrophic pylorus*) is reached and corrected through a very short incision directly over the lesion in the right side of the upper abdomen.

△ GENERAL INFORMATION

The stomach empties its food into the duodenum and then into the small intestine. The first half of the small intestine is called the *jejunum* and the second half is the *ileum*. Food in the ileum (by now it is stool) has the consistency of applesauce. This liquid-to-mushy stool empties into the large bowel, where water is absorbed from it. It becomes the firm stool that is passed through the anus when you have a bowel movement.

Sometimes it is necessary to bring the ileum straight through the skin to the outside. This is called an *ileostomy*. The stool from the ileostomy will then empty into a special bag attached to the skin.

REASONS FOR ILEOSTOMY

There are several possible reasons for an ileostomy.

- The colon needs to be removed because of the following:
  - There has been long-standing ulcerative colitis that is steadily getting worse and has reached the point where it is a constant and serious disability.
  - The ulcerative colitis has flared up and is bleeding dangerously, despite all efforts to stop it. Death is likely if the large bowel is not removed.
  - There is such severe infection of the ulcerated large bowel that the bowel is about to burst and produce peritonitis, unless it is removed.
  - There are several separate areas of cancer in the colon. The rest of the colon is felt to be at high risk for developing additional cancers. Removal is advised because of the cancer risk.

To temporarily bypass the colon:

- The stool needs to be detoured to the outside temporarily. Part of the colon has been removed and the ends have to be reconnected. The reconnection heals more safely if stool does not pass across it for a few days.

After careful consideration of all factors, the recommendation is that you have an ileostomy.

PREOPERATIVE PREPARATION

- You will have an examination of your blood, urine, heart (EKG), and lungs (chest x-ray).
- Do not eat or drink anything for 8 hours before the operation.
- Shower or bathe as usual on the morning of the operation.
- You may be given medicine that will make you feel drowsy before you are brought to the operating room.

□ OPERATION

- You will be asleep for the operation.
- Your entire abdomen will be swabbed with an antiseptic solution and surrounded with sterile draping.
- The ileostomy opening will be in the lower right side of your abdomen.
- You will not receive a blood transfusion unless it is absolutely necessary.
- The operation usually takes several hours, depending on what else besides the ileostomy may need to be done at the same time.

POSTOPERATIVE CARE

- You will be taken to a recovery room and observed. When your blood pressure, pulse, and breathing are stable, you will be taken to a regular hospital room.
- You may have a thin plastic tube in your nose. It goes down to your stomach to suck up the air you swallow. It will be removed when your ileostomy starts working.
- Pain can be controlled with medicine. The nurse will give it to you, or you can give yourself a preset amount of pain medicine when you feel you need it. This is done with a device called patient-controlled analgesia (PCA) that is connected to the tubing giving you intravenous fluids.
- The evening after the surgery you will be helped to sit up in bed and on the next day to get out of bed.
- The hospital support team of doctors and nurses will start working with you early to give you close supervision on how to learn to take care of your ileostomy.
- The dietitian will work with you on how to manage your diet so that the ileostomy will work in the best way.
- As with any operation, complications are always possible, and some of them are serious. With your type of operation, these complications include abscess, wound infection, leakage of the ileal pouch, and bowel obstruction, among others.
- You should be able to go home in about 1 week.
- Arrangements will be made for your medicine, follow-up office visit, and stitch or clip removal.

✙ HOME CARE

- Continue with the program that was started while you were in the hospital.
- You may walk about as you wish, even climb stairs.
- Follow the diet recommendations that were arranged for you.
- You may shower as you wish, with any dressings on or off.
  - There may be narrow strips of tape across the incision. It's all right if they get wet; they will be removed in the doctor's office.
  - After you dry yourself, replace any dressings with clean, dry ones.
- Arrangements can be made for a home visiting nurse if one is needed.
- Driving a car with an automatic shift may not seem to be too demanding, but you may have to slam on

the brakes or twist to turn the steering wheel and end up straining the sutures or tearing something. So during your follow-up visit, let's discuss when you can resume driving.

- You may resume sexual activity whenever you choose.
- You may return to work when you feel up to it, but let's first talk about it during your follow-up visit.

✆ CALL OUR OFFICE IF

- You develop any unusual signs or symptoms.
- Nothing comes out of the ileostomy for 12 hours.
- The incision becomes red or swollen, or there is drainage from it.
- You develop a temperature higher than 100°F.
- You have any questions.

IMPOTENCE SURGERY: Inflatable Prosthesis

△ GENERAL INFORMATION

Impotence is a condition in which a man usually cannot get an erection of the penis that is rigid enough and lasts long enough to complete sexual intercourse. It is a common and treatable problem. Men with erection problems often still have other sexual functions; they may still have sexual desire and may still be able to have orgasm and ejaculate semen.

It may help if first you understand how an erection occurs:

The shaft of the penis has a *corpus cavernosum* on each side. These are spongy tissues filled with arteries that bring blood to the penis and veins that drain the blood. Usually, the vessels in the corpus cavernosa are collapsed, so the penis is soft.

When a man is sexually aroused, the brain sends nerve signals to the penis that make all the arteries open up, allowing blood to rush in. As the penis swells it tends to squeeze the veins, preventing the blood from easily leaving the penis. This causes the penis to become rigid and ready for intercourse.

Erection is the result of physical as well as psychologic factors and usually takes place differently in younger, middle-aged, and older men. Conditions that can interfere with the mechanism of erection include the following:

- Diseases that cause hardening of the arteries or otherwise affect arteries.
- Diseases that affect the nervous system.
- Diabetes (it affects both the vessels and the nervous system).
- Heavy smoking and heavy drinking.
- A number of drugs, including those given to treat high blood pressure.
- Psychologic causes that can include stress and anxiety due to marital, financial, or other external problems. Anxiety about the ability to perform well during intercourse can in itself be a common cause of impotence.

DIAGNOSIS

- Essential to making a diagnosis is a medical, detailed psychologic, and sexual history.
- There will be a thorough examination of the genitalia.
- You will have an examination of your blood, urine, heart (EKG), and lungs (chest x-ray).
- Ultrasound: Harmless sound waves are aimed at the area of your penis. The sound waves bouncing back (the echoes) from this area are seen as a picture on a screen. Ultrasound is a convenient and painless way to examine tissues inside the penis. This test will be done before and after medicine is given to you to make the vessels in your penis enlarge to see if anything might be wrong with this mechanism.
- Injecting a medicine into the penis that normally stimulates an erection and then observing the response.
- A test to determine whether you have an erection when asleep. Performing this test during sleep reduces the effect of psychologic factors.

○ TREATMENT

When having the conference with the urologist, it is important that you discuss the following issues in a frank and honest manner:

- The degree of motivation to correct the problem.
- The degree of the partner's support and involvement in this whole process.
- The willingness to learn the necessary techniques so that they can be performed properly.

The following types of treatment are available:

- Substituting medicines you are taking that are known to cause impotence.
- Taking hormones if they are in short supply in your body.
- Proper counseling and therapy, which can have excellent results.
- Repair of faulty blood vessels if this is found to be the cause.
- Drug therapy. Some very promising medicines are now available to treat impotence. Such treatment should almost always be a first consideration. If you try these medicines and they do not work, then other treatments can be considered.

Vacuum Constriction Device (VCD): This consists of a plastic cylinder, a vacuum pump, and an elastic constriction band. The five steps are as follows:

- Lubricant is applied to the penis.
- The cylinder is placed over the penis.
- Air is pumped out of the cylinder to create a vacuum, which causes an erection.
- The constriction band is transferred to the base of the erect penis to maintain erection.
- The cylinder is removed. The constriction band can safely be left on the penis for half an hour.

Penile Injection Therapy: Medicine is injected into the penis that causes expansion of arteries and relaxation of penile tissue. Blood flow then increases into the two erection chambers, helping to cause the erection.

Penile Prosthesis: Two types of prostheses are (1) a *semirigid* malleable rod that is placed in the shaft of the penis and can be straightened to an erect position as desired and (2) an *inflatable* soft prosthesis that is placed in the shaft of the penis and can be inflated to a rigid shape as desired.

After careful consideration of all the factors, the recommendation is that you have an inflatable prosthesis placed in the shaft of your penis.

PREOPERATIVE PREPARATION

- You will have an examination of your blood, urine, heart (EKG), and lungs (chest x-ray).
- Do not eat or drink anything for 8 hours before the operation.

☐ OPERATION

- You will be asleep for the operation.
- An incision will be on the underside of the shaft of the penis; another will be made on the side of the *scrotum* (the sac) and another one several inches above the base of the penis (Fig. 1).
- The operation takes about 2 hours.

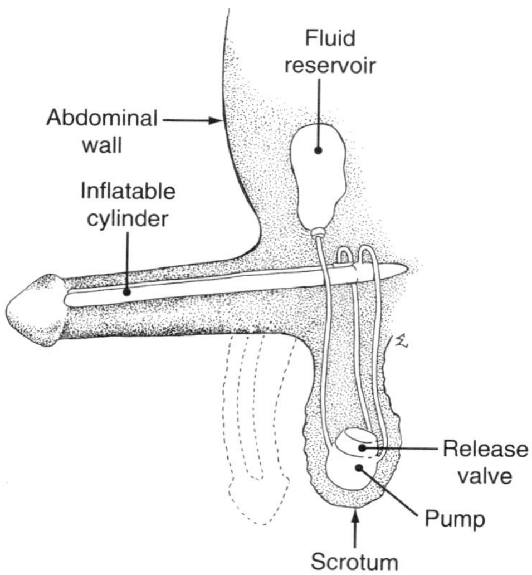

Figure 1. In this operation, the prosthesis has three parts: (1) the inflatable prosthesis in the penis, (2) the valve in the scrotum, and (3) the reservoir bag of fluid in the soft tissue several inches above the base of the penis.

POSTOPERATIVE CARE

- You will be taken to a recovery room and observed. When your blood pressure, pulse, and breathing are stable, you will be taken to a regular hospital room.
- You should be able to go home in a day or two.
- Arrangements will be made for your medicine, follow-up office visit, and stitch removal.
- As with any operation, complications are always possible. With this type of operation, complications can include bleeding, infection, malfunctioning of the prosthesis, and possibly others.

✚ HOME CARE

- Resume your usual activities, increasing them gradually as tolerated over the next few weeks.
- Take medicines as prescribed.
- You may shower as usual starting on the second day after the operation.
- Do not attempt to inflate or deflate your prosthesis or engage in intercourse until you have first been examined by the urologist and it has been determined that the tissue has healed properly.

✆ CALL OUR OFFICE IF

- You develop any unusual signs or symptoms.
- Any of the incisions become red or swollen, or there is drainage from them.
- You develop a temperature higher than 100°F.
- You have any questions.

IMPOTENCE SURGERY: Semirigid Malleable Prosthesis

△ GENERAL INFORMATION

Impotence is a condition in which a man usually cannot get an erection of the penis that is rigid enough and lasts long enough to complete sexual intercourse. It is a common and treatable problem. Men with erection problems often still have other sexual functions; they may still have sexual desire and may still be able to have orgasm and ejaculate semen.

It may help if first you understand how an erection occurs:

The shaft of the penis has a *corpus cavernosum* on each side. These are spongy tissues filled with arteries that bring blood to the penis and veins that drain the blood. Usually, the vessels in the corpus cavernosa are collapsed, so the penis is soft.

When a man is sexually aroused, the brain sends nerve signals to the penis that make all the arteries open up, allowing blood to rush in. As the penis swells it tends to squeeze the veins, preventing the blood from easily leaving the penis. This causes the penis to become rigid and ready for intercourse.

Erection is the result of physical as well as psychologic factors and usually takes place differently in younger, middle-aged, and older men. Conditions that can interfere with the mechanism of erection include the following:

- Diseases that cause hardening of the arteries or otherwise affect arteries.
- Diseases that affect the nervous system.
- Diabetes (it affects both the vessels and the nervous system).
- Heavy smoking and heavy drinking.
- A number of drugs, including those given to treat high blood pressure.
- Psychologic causes that can include stress and anxiety due to marital, financial, or other external problems. Anxiety about the ability to perform well during intercourse can in itself be a common cause of impotence.

DIAGNOSIS

- Essential to making a diagnosis is a medical, detailed psychologic, and sexual history.
- There will be a thorough examination of the genitalia.
- You will have an examination of your blood, urine, heart (EKG), and lungs (chest x-ray).
- Ultrasound: Harmless sound waves are aimed at the area of your penis. The sound waves bouncing back (the echoes) from this area are seen as a picture on a screen. Ultrasound is a convenient and painless way to examine tissues inside the penis. This test will be done before and after medicine is given to you to make the vessels in your penis enlarge to see if anything might be wrong with this mechanism.
- Injecting a medicine into the penis that normally stimulates an erection and then observing the response.
- A test to determine whether you have an erection when asleep. Performing this test during sleep reduces the effect of psychologic factors.

○ TREATMENT

When having the conference with the urologist, it is important that you discuss the following issues in a frank and honest manner:

- The degree of motivation to correct the problem.
- The degree of the partner's support and involvement in this whole process.
- The willingness to learn the necessary techniques so that they can be performed properly.

The following types of treatment are available:

- Substituting medicines you are taking that are known to cause impotence.
- Taking hormones if they are in short supply in your body.
- Proper counseling and therapy, which can have excellent results.
- Repair of faulty blood vessels if this is found to be the cause.
- Drug therapy. Some very promising medicines are now available to treat impotence. Such treatment should almost always be a first consideration. If you try these medicines and they do not work, then other treatments can be considered.

Vacuum Constriction Device (VCD): This consists of a plastic cylinder, a vacuum pump, and an elastic constriction band. The five steps are as follows:

- Lubricant is applied to the penis.
- The cylinder is placed over the penis.
- Air is pumped out of the cylinder to create a vacuum, which causes an erection.
- The constriction band is transferred to the base of the erect penis to maintain erection.
- The cylinder is removed. The constriction band can safely be left on the penis for half an hour.

Penile Injection Therapy: Medicine is injected into the penis that causes expansion of arteries and relaxation

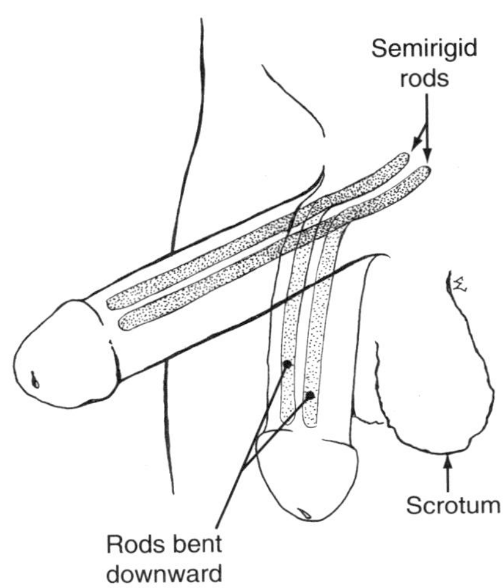

Figure 1. The malleable rods within the penis need to be bent to the desired shape as necessary.

of penile tissue. Blood flow then increases into the two erection chambers, helping to cause the erection.

Penile Prosthesis: Two types of prostheses are (1) a *semirigid* malleable rod that is placed in the shaft of the penis and can be straightened to an erect position as desired (Fig. 1) and (2) an *inflatable* soft prosthesis that is placed in the shaft of the penis and can be inflated to a rigid shape as desired.

After careful consideration of all the factors, the recommendation is that you have an operation in which a semirigid prosthesis is placed in the shaft of your penis.

PREOPERATIVE PREPARATION

- You will have an examination of your blood, urine, heart (EKG), and lungs (chest x-ray).
- Do not eat or drink anything for 8 hours before the operation.

□ OPERATION

- You will be asleep for the operation.
- The incisions will be on the underside of the shaft of the penis and the prostheses inserted.
- The operation takes about 2 hours.

POSTOPERATIVE CARE

- You will be taken to a recovery room and observed. When your blood pressure, pulse, and breathing are stable, you will be taken to a regular hospital room.
- You should be able to go home in a day or two.
- Arrangements will be made for your medicine, follow-up office visit, and stitch removal.
- As with any operation, complications are always possible. With this type of operation, complications can include bleeding, infection, malfunctioning of the prosthesis, and possibly others.

✚ HOME CARE

- Resume your usual activities, increasing them gradually as tolerated over the next few weeks.
- Take medicines as prescribed.
- You may shower as usual, starting on the second day after the operation.
- Do not engage in sexual activity for about 6 weeks and then only if the incision is well healed.
- Do not drive a car if you are taking medicines that reduce your alertness.

✆ CALL OUR OFFICE IF

- You develop any unusual signs or symptoms.
- Any of the incisions become red or swollen, or there is drainage from them.
- You develop a temperature higher than 100°F.
- You have any questions.

△ GENERAL INFORMATION

An ingrown toenail can produce a lot of pain. Actually, it is *not* the toenail growing *in*; the nail just grows straight ahead as it should. Instead, it's the flesh that is *pushed in front* of the growing toenail.

The toenail should be allowed to grow as in Figure 1*A*. It should *not* be cut as in Figure 1*B*. Otherwise, the flesh is pushed in front of the sharp edge of the toenail. The toenail then grows, and pretty soon it simply cuts into the flesh, which gets irritated and infected (Fig. 1*C*). This is a condition that is called *ingrown toenail.*

Some of the things that make this happen are the following:

- Cutting the nail too short (arrow in *B*) so that the flesh is in front of the growing nail at the sides of the toe.
- Wearing pointed shoes that are too snug at the toes. The shoe pushes the flesh of the big toe into the sharp edge of the growing toenail.
- Feet that are too warm and sweaty, making the skin softer. It then is easier for the irritated toe to become infected.
- Trauma from kicking or bumping.

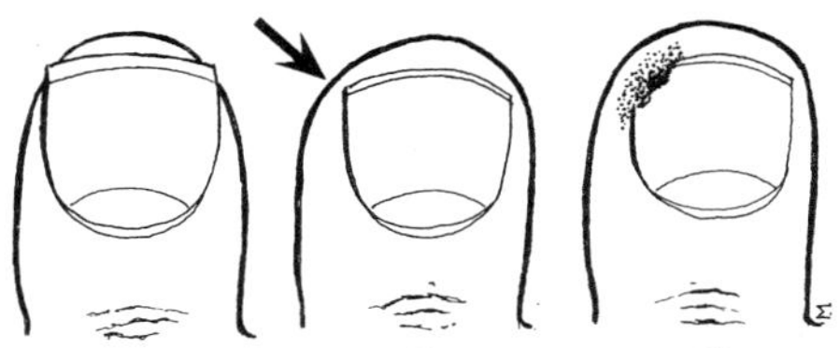

Figure 1. The degree of inflammation and infection associated with an ingrown toenail can vary considerably. However, the principles of treatment remain the same.

COMMON SIGNS AND SYMPTOMS

- Any toe can be involved, but most commonly it is the tip of the big toe.

DIAGNOSIS

- Usually the diagnosis can be made by taking a detailed history and thoroughly examining the toe.

○ TREATMENT

- **Medical:** If the condition is seen and treated early, you can try to keep the flesh away from the sharp cutting corner of the toenail until the toenail can grow over the flesh. For this you will need a fine tweezer, a little cotton, and some ordinary rubbing alcohol.
  - If you like, take some over-the-counter pain medicine before you start.
  - Take a tiny bit of cotton and dip it in the alcohol.
  - Very gently push the cotton under the edge of the sharp cutting edge of the toenail. Just leave it there. At first, this may seem impossible, but with patience, it can be done. Perhaps the doctor can do it for you the first time. This will shrink the tissue a bit and make it easier to do it again the next day.
  - Repeat this every day until the nail grows *over* the skin of the toe, as it should.
- **Surgical:** If the condition is too advanced for the above treatment, then a portion of the toenail needs to be removed so that it does not continue to dig into the flesh (see Fig. 1*C*).

PREOPERATIVE PREPARATION

- Do not eat or drink anything for 8 hours before the operation.

□ OPERATION

- The front part of the foot will be painted with an antiseptic solution and draped.
- A very fine, short needle will be used to inject an anesthetic into the nerves of the toe. This will make the entire toe numb.
- The involved side of the toenail will be removed so that all of the infected soft tissue can heal. The toenail will slowly heal back to the shape it was before, but this time it will grow *over* the tissue.
- You should be able to go home directly after the operation.
- Arrangements will be made for your medicine, follow-up office visit, and first dressing change.

POSTOPERATIVE CARE

- Walk about as you wish, but at the beginning you will need some type of open-toed shoe. It will hurt too much to wear a regular shoe. Besides, there will be a large bandage on the toe, and it will not fit inside a shoe with a closed toe.
- Take medicine as prescribed for your pain.
- There will be less pain if every hour or two you lie down with the leg elevated on a pillow.
- The first dressing will be changed at the doctor's office. At that time, you will be shown how to change it yourself.
- After the first dressing change, you can take a shower or bath with the dressing in place. After you dry yourself, remove the wet dressing (it will come off more easily when wet) and replace it with a new one.

✆ CALL OUR OFFICE IF

- The toe becomes red and more swollen than before the operation.
- You develop a temperature higher than 100°F.
- You have any questions.

△ GENERAL INFORMATION

The *pancreas* is located in the upper part of your abdomen and just behind the stomach. It makes several things, such as the pancreas juices that help to digest the food you eat. Also, it has cells called *beta cells*. These cells make *insulin,* which regulates the level of sugar in your blood. Sometimes these beta cells form into a tumor (ranging in size from a cranberry to a walnut), which is called an *insulinoma.* The insulinoma can produce dramatic increases in the amount of insulin in your blood. This in turn can seriously lower the level of your blood sugar.

Most insulinomas are benign. Some, however, are cancerous or suspicious of being cancerous. Insulinomas are seen mostly in persons 40 to 70 years of age.

COMMON SIGNS AND SYMPTOMS

Most symptoms are brought about by the low level of sugar in the blood.

- Symptoms can vary a lot, but they include the following: sweating, hunger, weakness, and a fast pulse. Other symptoms are headache, mental confusion, eyesight problems, convulsions, and even unconsciousness.
- Some people are so afraid that their blood sugar will be too low that they constantly eat a lot of carbohydrates, and so they become obese.

DIAGNOSIS

The diagnosis can be strongly suspected with the following:

- An attack of symptoms after fasting or engaging in hard work (and burning up of sugar).
- The blood sugar is extremely low at such times.
- The symptoms go away when the person eats some form of sugar.

A number of tests will be done to make certain there is not another cause for your low sugar level and symptoms.

- *CT scan (computed tomography scan):* These special x-rays are taken by a machine that is shaped like a huge doughnut. You will lie on the table inside the hole in the "doughnut." The x-rays are taken as very thin slices through the pancreas. This makes it possible to see the fine details in the pancreas.
- *MRI (magnetic resonance imaging):* No x-rays are used with this technique. Instead, it is done with harmless magnetic fields and radio waves. A computer develops the pictures to show organs from several angles. This technique is especially valuable for examining your blood vessels and nerve tissue.
- *PET scan (positron emission tomography scan):* A solution containing chemicals that are used by growing tumors is mixed with a tiny amount of radioactive material. The solution then is injected into your vein, and it goes to the tumor. You will lie on a table, and the area of the suspected tumor will be looked at closely to see if any of the radioactive material is there. This will indicate how fast or slowly the tumor is using the solution, which identifies it as a fast- or slow-growing tumor.

○ TREATMENT

- The treatment is an operation to remove the insulinoma. After careful consideration, the recommendation is that you have such an operation.

PREOPERATIVE PREPARATION

- You will be admitted to the hospital at least 1 day before the operation to be as certain as possible that the sugar levels and other chemicals in your blood are brought to and kept at a level that is as ideal as possible.
- You will have an examination of your blood, urine, heart (EKG), and lungs (chest x-ray).
- Do not eat or drink anything for 8 hours before the operation.
- Shower as usual on the morning of the operation.
- You may be given medicine that will make you feel drowsy before you are brought to the operating room.

□ OPERATION

- You will be asleep for the operation.
- The incision will be across your upper abdomen.
- The part of the pancreas with the insulinoma in it will be removed.
- You will not receive a blood transfusion unless it is absolutely necessary.
- It is not always possible to find the insulinoma. It can be as small as a cranberry; it can be buried inside the pancreas and not visible. Or, it can be buried in tissue near the pancreas, rather than in the pancreas itself.
- The operation usually takes about 3 hours.

POSTOPERATIVE CARE

- You will be taken to the Surgical Care Unit, where the doctors and nurses are very experienced in taking care of patients with your condition. As soon as you are coming along well enough, you will be transferred to a regular hospital room.
- You will have a thin plastic tube in your nose. It goes down to your stomach to suck up the air you swallow. It will be removed when your bowels start working.
- Pain will be controlled with medicine.
- The evening after the surgery you will be helped to sit up in bed and on the next day to get out of bed.
- Your blood sugar and insulin levels will be watched carefully.
- As with any operation, complications are always possible. With your type of operation, they can include bleeding, pneumonia, peritonitis, and blood clots, among others.
- You should be able to go home in about 7 to 10 days.
- Arrangements will be made for your medicine, follow-up office visit, and stitch or clip removal.

✣ HOME CARE

- Continue with the program started while you were in the hospital.
- You may walk about as you wish, even climb stairs.
- Follow the diet schedule arranged for you while you were in the hospital.
- Be certain to take the medicines as prescribed for you.
- You may shower as you wish, with any dressings on or off.
  - There may be narrow strips of tape across the incision. It's all right if they get wet; they will be removed in the doctor's office.
  - After you dry yourself, replace any dressings with clean, dry ones.
- Driving your car may be important to you, but when you can do this safely depends on the operation you had, the medicines you are taking, and your condition in general. During your follow-up visit, talk with your doctor about when you can resume driving.
- You may resume sexual activity whenever you choose.
- You may return to work when you feel up to it.

✆ CALL OUR OFFICE IF

- You develop any unusual signs or symptoms.
- The incision becomes red or swollen, or there is drainage from it.
- You develop a temperature higher than 100°F.
- You have any questions.

INTUSSUSCEPTION

△ GENERAL INFORMATION

This is a condition in which the intestine telescopes into itself. The likely cause is some thickening or lump in the wall of the intestine. Food passing by tries to push along this thickening or lump, but because the lump is attached to the wall of the intestine, it pulls the intestine along with it, causing the intestine to telescope on itself (Fig. 1).

One type of lump that can do this is lymph tissue in the wall of the lower part of the small intestine (especially in children) that becomes swollen after a virus infection. Other types can be tumors, either benign or malignant.

Intussusception can occur at any age but is most common between the ages of 2 months and 2 years.

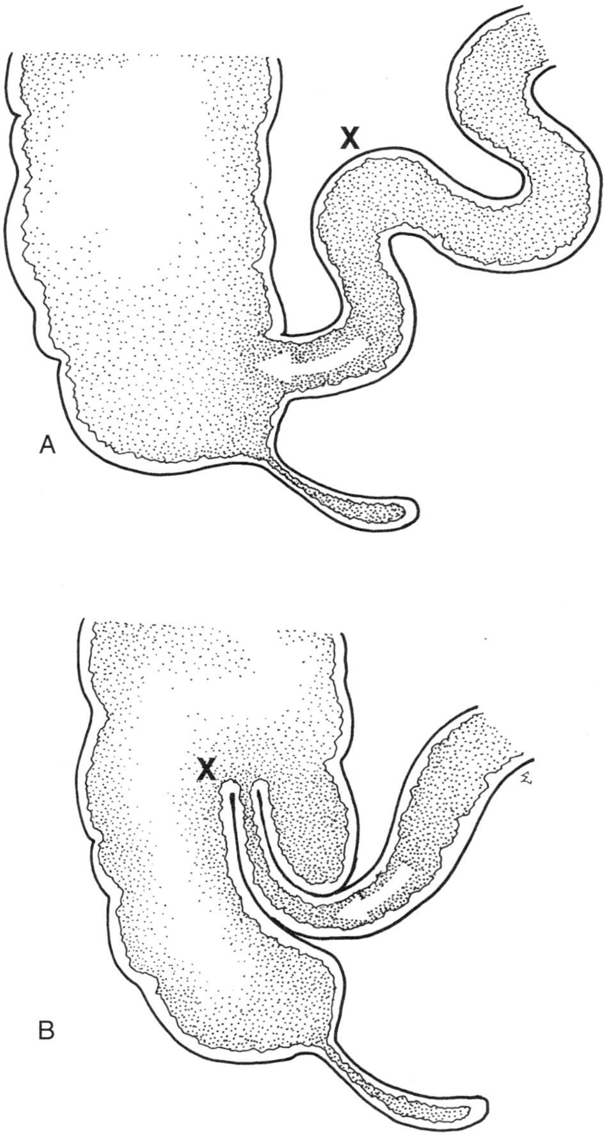

Figure 1. *A*, This demonstrates the normal anatomy of the ileum (distal small bowel) and the colon. The arrow indicates the direction of the flow of food. *B*, With intussusception, part X in *A* telescopes into the colon ahead of it and advances to the new position shown here.

COMMON SIGNS AND SYMPTOMS

- Typically, a healthy infant develops abdominal pain that comes and goes. With each attack of pain, the infant cries and bends the legs against the abdomen.
- Later, the abdomen swells and there may be vomiting.
- There may be some stool, but this is more like pink Jell-O because of a little bleeding that can occur with a congested, telescoped intestine.
- Sometimes, the telescoped part of the intestine can be felt.

DIAGNOSIS

- Usually, the diagnosis can be made by taking a detailed history, doing a thorough physical examination, and carefully considering the laboratory reports.
- An x-ray of the abdomen shows a distended bowel, but not necessarily in the first few hours.
- Barium enema: Liquid barium is carefully given as an enema (just like a regular enema) and watched as it goes up to the telescoped part of the intestine. This gives a typical picture, which can make the diagnosis.

○ TREATMENT

- The treatment is to reduce the obstruction caused by the intussusception. This can be attempted without an operation if the intussusception is seen early.

Medical Treatment

- Complete blood counts will be done and fluids started by vein.
- With the surgeon standing by, an experienced radiologist (x-ray doctor) will start the barium enema and watch as the barium goes up to the blocked area. Then, very gently and carefully, the radiologist will continue to put in more barium and build up the pressure, hoping to push back the telescoped bowel. This can be done successfully about 60% of the time. If so, the child is returned to the hospital room and permitted to recover. This usually takes a day or so.

Surgical Treatment

- If the above method is not successful, then an immediate operation is necessary.

□ OPERATION

- The operation is done under general anesthesia.
- With the abdomen open, it is usually possible to push back the telescoped intestine.
- If it is not possible to safely push back the telescoped intestine, then that part of the intestine will be resected and the healthy ends reconnected.

POSTOPERATIVE CARE

- The child will be taken to a recovery room and observed. When the blood pressure, pulse, and respirations are stable, your child will be taken to a regular hospital room.
- There may be a small plastic tube in the child's nose going down to the stomach for a day or two until the bowels start working.
- After the tube from the nose is removed, liquids will be given by mouth, and the child will be advanced quickly to a normal diet.
- The child should be ready to go home in 3 to 5 days.
- Arrangements will be made for medicine, follow-up office visit, and stitch removal.

✚ HOME CARE

- Resume the usual activities and diet.
- Sponge-bathe the child (with the dressings on or off) but without too much soaking. There may be narrow strips of tape across the incision. It's all right if they get wet; they will be removed in the doctor's office. After drying, replace any dressings with clean, dry ones.
- Change diapers as soon as possible after they become soiled.

✆ CALL OUR OFFICE IF

- There are any unusual signs or symptoms.
- The child does not have a bowel movement on any one day.
- The incision becomes red or swollen, or there is drainage from it.
- The child develops a temperature higher than 100°F.
- You have any questions.

IVP (INTRAVENOUS PYELOGRAM)

△ GENERAL INFORMATION

Your kidneys are located deep in your back just below the last ribs. The fleshy part of the kidneys makes urine that runs into a shallow collecting area on the middle side of the kidney. It then runs down the *ureters* (they are tubes the size and consistency of boiled macaroni) and into the bladder. The urine collects in the bladder until you get the urge to urinate.

If you were to lie on an x-ray table just as you are and have a picture taken of your abdomen, very little of your kidneys would show up. No details could be seen. But, if dye were mixed with the urine, much more could be seen of the kidneys, the ureters, and bladder. This is called an intravenous pyelogram (IVP).

It has been determined that you need an IVP to get a better look at your kidneys, ureters, and bladder and what might be the problem there.

PREPARATION

- Some people are allergic to x-ray dyes (used for this test) because they contain iodine. If you have an allergy to iodine or products that contain it, be sure to let the x-ray technician know. You may need some medicine before the test can be done.
- If you are diabetic and on Glucophage, you should stop taking that medication at least 24 hours before this test.
- Your bowel will need to be as clean as possible because stool in the bowel can blur the details in the kidneys. At 4:00 P.M. on the day before the IVP, drink a 10-ounce bottle of citrate of magnesia.
- Drink more liquids than usual.
- Eat a light supper.
- Do not eat anything after midnight. If, however, you are diabetic or have a kidney problem or otherwise must take liquids or medicine that morning, check with the doctor on this.
- About 3 hours before the IVP, use a Dulcolax rectal suppository as directed on the package.

Note: If you are having a lower gastrointestinal (GI) examination (barium enema) the same morning as the IVP, follow the bowel preparation instructions given to you for the barium enema.

THE EXAMINATION

- You will lie on an x-ray table.
- First, ordinary x-rays of your abdomen will be taken to look for any kidney stones in your kidneys, ureters, or bladder.
- Next, a special dye used for the IVP will be injected into your vein. You might feel a warm sensation and have a metallic taste in your mouth. This is common and will not harm you. Both will go away in a few minutes.
- The dye will circulate in the blood, and when it gets to the kidney it will come out with the urine.
- X-ray pictures will be taken of the dye as it travels through your kidneys, ureter, and bladder. These x-ray pictures will be taken from several angles to be certain that the best possible views and details are obtained (Fig. 1).

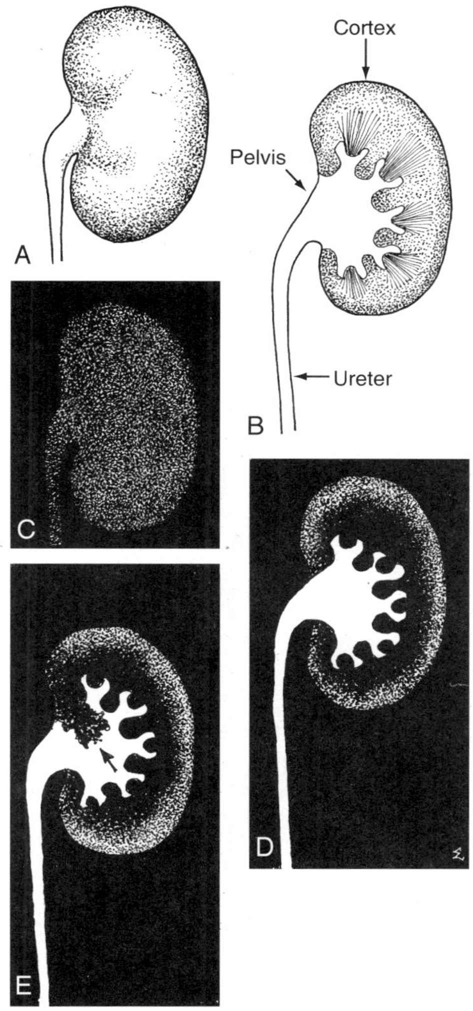

Figure 1. Appearance of left kidney. *A*, From outside. *B*, When cut lengthwise. *C*, When x-ray is taken of it through abdomen. *D*, Following injection into a vein of special liquid that is excreted through the kidneys. X-rays cannot pass through this liquid, so it appears white. *E*, Same procedure as in *D*. Example of tumor growing into pelvis of kidney *(arrow)*.

- At the end of the procedure, you are free to go and to conduct your affairs as usual.
- All of the x-rays will be assembled and examined by a specialist.
- The results will be reported to your personal physician.

△ GENERAL INFORMATION

This is an operation in which a small plastic tube is placed directly from the skin to the inside of your small intestine (the *jejunum*) (Fig. 1). This is the part of the intestine that is past the stomach. The feeding tube is used to give liquid nourishment to a person who cannot eat in the normal way. The feeding tube can be used temporarily or permanently.

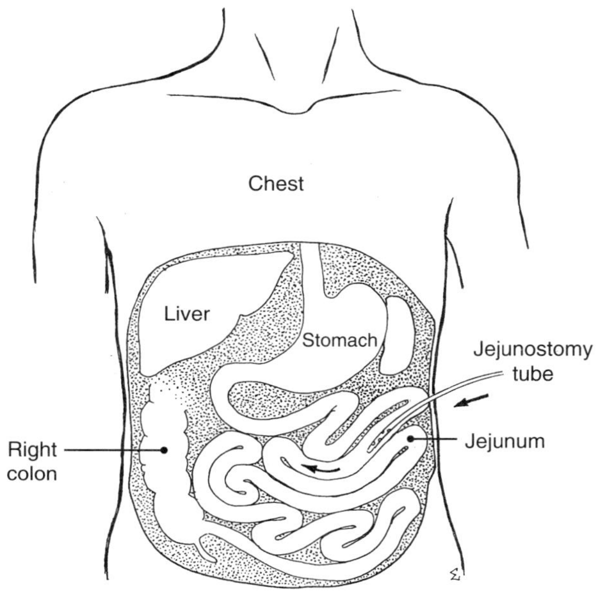

Figure 1.

PREOPERATIVE PREPARATION

- You will have an examination of your blood, urine, heart (EKG), and lungs (chest x-ray).
- Your red blood cell count will be looked at carefully because severe anemia can slow down the healing of an incision. It is possible that you will require blood transfusions to bring your red blood count closer to normal.
- The protein level in your blood may be very low. This also affects healing. You may be given intravenous albumin and other products through your vein to help this situation.
- You may be low on the amount of fluid in your system, probably because you have not been drinking enough. If so, you will be given fluids through your vein to correct this.
- Certain chemicals in your blood may be low. They can be added to the fluids you get by vein.
- Do not eat or drink anything for 8 hours before the operation.
- You may be given medicine that will make you feel drowsy before you are brought to the operating room.

ANESTHESIA

The anesthesia used will depend on a number of things, including your diagnosis and your general condition.

- **Local anesthesia:** The skin over your abdomen will be painted with an antiseptic solution. Surgical drapes will cover your body. The skin over the area where the tube will go in will be injected with an anesthetic solution to make it numb.
- During the operation, you will be given medicine that will make you feel drowsy.
- During the operation, you may feel tugging or pressure, but not pain.
- **General anesthesia:** You will be put to sleep with quick-acting anesthesia. When the operation is over, you will wake up quickly in the recovery room.

□ OPERATION

- A short incision will be made in your upper abdomen. The tip of a plastic tube approximately the size of a pencil will be placed inside the jejunum. The other end of the tube will remain to outside of your abdomen.
- The operation usually takes about 1 hour.

POSTOPERATIVE CARE

- You will wake up in a recovery room. When your blood pressure, pulse, and breathing are stable, you will be taken to a regular hospital room.
- The evening after the surgery you will be encouraged to walk about in your room with assistance.
- Pain can be controlled with medicine.
- The tube often is ready for use within 24 to 48 hours.
- You and a member of your family will be shown how to use the tube for feeding; it is not difficult.
- You will be given information on special liquids you can place in the tube. They have all the necessary calories, minerals, and vitamins that you will need and that will help you.
- You will be given information on how to select the proper foods and how to prepare them so that they can also be given through the tube.
- Finally, you will be shown how to take care of the tube to keep it clean. Again, this is not difficult.
- As with any operation, complications are always possible. With this type of operation, complications can include infection, leakage of the tube, pneumonia, heart problems, and possibly others.
- Arrangements will be made for your medicine, follow-up office visit, and stitch removal.
- Arrangements can be made for a home visiting nurse if one is needed.

✚ HOME CARE

- You may walk about as you wish and even climb stairs.
- Follow the suggestions on what nourishment to place in the jejunostomy and how to do it.
- You may shower as you wish and with any dressings on or off.

- There may be narrow strips of tape across the incision. It's all right if they get wet; they will be removed in the doctor's office.
- The jejunostomy tube is securely anchored in place with stitches and should be safe. Just the same, don't pull on it. It is often wise to attach the dangling end of the tube to your skin with a piece of tape until you are through with your shower.
- After you dry yourself, replace any dressings with clean, dry ones.

✆ CALL OUR OFFICE IF

- The tube falls out. The hole can close quickly. So, if you cannot reach your doctor right away, go to the nearest hospital emergency room so that the tube can be put back again in a safe manner.
- The incision becomes red or swollen, or there is drainage from it.
- You develop a temperature higher than 101°F.
- You have any questions.

LONG-TERM CARE

This type of tube can be left in place as long as necessary. When the tube is no longer needed, it's a simple matter for the doctor or nurse to snip the stitch holding it in place and slip the tube right out. The hole closes completely by itself in a day or two. The tube can be removed at home by a home care nurse or in the surgeon's office.

△ GENERAL INFORMATION

Kaposi's sarcoma is a disease that was first described in a few old white men 125 years ago. It was a condition of the skin, predominantly in the lower legs. The lesions were bluish red and flat or slightly raised. The tumor was slow growing, and, after time, the affected leg became swollen and firm.

Just 15 years ago there were only 100 or so new cases reported each year in the United States. Now, it is very often associated with AIDS (acquired immunodeficiency syndrome), a disease in which a person does not have enough of the cells that help with *immunity* (protection) against disease.

With the increasing number of patients with AIDS, the incidence of Kaposi's sarcoma has reached epidemic proportions in the United States and elsewhere, particularly in Central Africa.

COMMON SIGNS AND SYMPTOMS

- There are several different types of skin bumps:
  - General skin involvement.
  - A lesion that grows inward into the tissue.
  - Involvement of other areas in the body such as the lymph nodes, mouth, and intestine.
- The type of Kaposi's sarcoma seen before 1980 was slow growing, and the lesions were mostly raised and in the legs. The Kaposi's sarcoma seen at present is more often associated with AIDS, grows more swiftly, and involves many other types of tissue besides the skin.

DIAGNOSIS

- If anyone has the history or symptoms described above, there should be concern about Kaposi's sarcoma.
- The diagnosis can usually be made by taking a detailed history, doing a thorough physical examination, and considering the laboratory reports carefully.
- For an exact diagnosis, a small piece of a lesion needs to be taken (a *biopsy*) for examination in the laboratory.

○ TREATMENT

- Basically, the treatment for the general involvement type of Kaposi's sarcoma is with multiple drugs. In addition, an important part of treatment is supportive therapy for associated problems.
- If a lesion is full-grown but is somewhat localized and is the principle lesion causing the trouble, radiation therapy may be helpful.
- The role of surgery can be to help with the diagnosis (as in performing a biopsy) or to give relief of symptoms in lesions that are ulcerated and painful.

PREOPERATIVE PREPARATION

- An important part of the preparation is to see that any associated conditions are controlled as much as possible. This will help make the operation as safe as possible.

□ OPERATION

Local Anesthesia

- A very fine needle will be used to inject the anesthetic around the involved area to make it completely numb.
- During the operation you may feel some tugging but no pain.
- You should be able to go home directly after the operation.

General Anesthesia

- You may be given medicine that will make you feel drowsy before you are brought to the operating room.
- There will be special precautions to prevent complications from any of your associated problems.
- The length of time the operation takes depends on what needs to be done.
- You will be taken to a recovery room and observed. When your blood pressure, pulse, and breathing are stable, you should be able to go home with a responsible adult. Otherwise, you will be transferred to a regular hospital room.
- The evening after the surgery you will be helped to get out of bed and walk.
- Pain can be controlled with medicine.
- As with any operation, complications are always possible, some of them serious. With your type of operation, they can include infection, bleeding, and breakdown of the operative wound, and possibly others.
- Arrangements will be made for your medicine, follow-up office visit, and stitch removal.

✚ HOME CARE

- Resume your usual activities.
- You may shower as you wish, with any dressings on or off.
  - There may be narrow strips of tape across the incision. It's all right if they get wet; they will be removed in the doctor's office.
  - After you dry yourself, replace any dressings with clean, dry ones.
- You may eat as you did before the operation.
- Be certain to take the medicines prescribed for you.

✆ CALL OUR OFFICE IF

- You develop any unusual signs or symptoms.
- The incision becomes red or swollen, or there is drainage from it.
- You develop a temperature higher than 100°F.
- You have any questions.

△ GENERAL INFORMATION

When an incision is made on the skin and then stitched together, the body starts the process of healing very quickly. Certain chemicals and tissues are involved in this healing. One of these tissues, *collagen*, forms scar. The body, however, keeps the collagen formation in check and gradually takes some of it away. That's one reason an incision heals and then becomes less obvious with time.

In some people, however, the body does not keep check on the collagen, so it continues to grow and grow and forms a much bigger scar than is normal. This is called a *keloid*.

Keloids occur more commonly in people with darker skin and in certain areas of the body, especially the front of the chest and the shoulders in young women.

COMMON SIGNS AND SYMPTOMS

- There is a thick, shiny, raised scar that is wider and darker than expected.
- The scar often itches severely. It can also be quite painful.

DIAGNOSIS

- Usually, the diagnosis can be made by taking a detailed history and doing a thorough physical examination.

○ TREATMENT

- There may not be any treatment; the keloids can simply be tolerated and observed. Most keloids get somewhat better with time.
- There is no foolproof therapy to prevent the keloid from forming or to take care of it once it has formed.
- Pressure garments are often used to lessen the size of a keloid or to slow down its growth. For example, a keloid on an earlobe may be improved with a specially made clip-on earring.
- Some skin lubricants may help with the itching, or to soften the scar.
- A bandage made of silicone is sometimes placed on the keloid to soften it and to reduce the degree of redness.
- Injecting the keloid with cortisone-like medicine can help reduce the itching. It doesn't do much to make the keloid smaller.
- Simply cutting out the scar and resuturing the incision does not work. Another keloid forms just like it did before; sometimes this keloid is even worse than before.
- Excising the keloid and resuturing the incision while at the same time giving some radiation treatment to the incision to slow down the healing (scarring) process has been known to help. Unfortunately, the long-term effects can be harmful, so few surgeons use this method.
- From the standpoint of appearance and itching, one of the more successful methods is a multiple-part operation.

After very careful consideration of all factors, including possible complications, the recommendation is to proceed with an operation.

PREOPERATIVE PREPARATION

- Do not eat or drink anything for 8 hours before the operation.
- Shower (and shave) as usual on the morning of the operation.
- You may be given medicine that will make you feel drowsy before you are brought to the operating room.

□ OPERATION

- The operation will be done under local anesthesia; the affected area will be made numb. Also, you will be given medicine that will make you feel very drowsy.
- During the operation you may feel some tugging but no pain.
- The operation will consist of the following:
  - The keloid will be carefully excised with very gentle handling of the tissue.
  - Cortisone will be injected into the surrounding tissue. This will tend to hold back the healing tissue from coming in too fast and too abundantly (which is what leads to the tendency to form keloid).
  - The incision will be closed in a cosmetic fashion.
  - Extra precautions will be taken that the wound does not become infected.
- You should be able to go home directly after the operation.
- You will be given specific instructions on how to help take care of the incision.
- The doctor will discuss with you how to go about taking your usual shower or bath.
- Arrangements will be made for your medicine, follow-up office visit, and stitch removal.

✆ CALL OUR OFFICE IF

- The incision becomes red or swollen, or there is drainage from it.
- You develop a temperature higher than 100°F.
- You have any questions.

KIDNEY BIOPSY: Needle Aspiration

△ GENERAL INFORMATION

There are situations in which it is necessary to know the condition of the kidney. Some examples are as follows:

- There is an acute illness in the kidneys, and they are not making enough or the proper type of urine.
- There is a chronic kidney problem, and exact and accurate information about it is needed because major therapy may be needed.
- An individual has had a kidney transplant, and it is important to know exactly how well the transplanted kidney is working.

The most accurate and reliable way to know the status of a kidney is to examine a small piece of it under the microscope. The easiest and safest way to do this is to remove a small piece of the kidney (a *biopsy*) with a needle.

It has been recommended that you have a kidney biopsy.

PREPARATION FOR THE BIOPSY

- Do not eat or drink anything for 8 hours before the operation.
- Shower (and shave) as usual on the morning of the operation.
- You will be given medicine that will make you feel drowsy before you are brought to the operating room.

THE BIOPSY

- You will be helped to lie down on a comfortable table.
- The skin over the area of the kidney will be painted with an antiseptic solution and draped with sterile towels.
- A thin needle will be used to inject an anesthetic into the skin over the kidney. The entire area will become numb.
- The needle will be passed through the numbed skin and guided by ultrasonography. This involves harmless sound waves (ultrasound) aimed at the kidney. The sound waves bouncing back (the echoes) show the kidney as a picture on a screen. This is a harmless, painless, and convenient way to see the kidney. The tip of the needle is placed in the kidney, and a small piece is removed. This part of the procedure should not take longer than 1 minute.
- The specimen will be sent to the pathology laboratory for complete examination.

RECOVERY AFTER THE BIOPSY

- You will be asked to remain flat on a small bed for 2 hours. During this time, your blood pressure, pulse, and breathing will be checked. You should be able to go home that same day with a responsible adult.
- You are not permitted to drive on the day of the biopsy or on the following day.

✚ HOME CARE

- Take it easy for the day. Lie down at every opportunity, preferably most of the day.
- Eat as you wish.
- Be careful that you do not become constipated.
  - Include enough roughage and liquid in your diet.
  - You may need a mild laxative (example: milk of magnesia).
- Don't lift anything heavier than 5 pounds. Ask someone to do it for you.
- You may shower or bathe as you wish.
- You may resume sexual activity whenever you choose.
- Return to work when you feel up to it.

✆ CALL OUR OFFICE IF

- You develop any unusual signs or symptoms—especially abdominal, back, or flank pain or nausea.
- There is blood in your urine. The first time you pass urine, it is rather common for some blood to be present. The urine usually clears after this. Just the same, call our office if you see blood even the first time you urinate.
- You develop a temperature higher than 100°F.
- You have any questions.

△ GENERAL INFORMATION

Cancer of the kidney can occur in both men and women but is seen more often in men between the ages of 40 and 60 years. The cause is not known.

COMMON SIGNS AND SYMPTOMS

Cancer of the kidney very often does not produce any symptoms at all. When there are symptoms, they can manifest in a variety of ways.

- Pain that may be steady and low grade or severe because of blocked urine.
- Blood in the urine; it can be caused by a growing tumor in the kidney.
- A large tumor sometimes can be felt if it is in the lower part of the kidney.
- Other symptoms may include weight loss, *anemia* (low blood count), fever, and high blood pressure.

DIAGNOSIS

- The diagnosis can often be made by taking a detailed history, doing a thorough physical examination, and considering the results of the laboratory tests carefully.
- *IVP (intravenous pyelogram)*: A special clear liquid that is eliminated by the kidney and shows up well on x-rays is injected into the vein. The x-rays taken can show details of the inside of the kidneys and their drainage tubes *(ureters)*.
- *Cystoscopy*: By this technique, a special hollow instrument (a *cystoscope*) with a lens in it and a light at its tip is used to look inside your bladder. The cystoscope is as big around as the tip of your little finger. You will lie on a table and the urologist will squirt anesthetic medicine in your urethra (the opening of the bladder) to make it numb. The cystoscope will be passed gently into the urethra and into the bladder to examine it thoroughly.
- *Ultrasound*: Harmless sound waves are aimed at the area of the kidney. The sound waves bouncing back (the echoes) from the kidneys are seen as a picture on a screen. This is a convenient and painless way to examine the kidney and the tissue around it.
- *CT scan (computed tomography scan)*: This technique uses a special x-ray machine that is shaped like a huge doughnut. You will lie on the table inside the hole in the "doughnut." X-rays are taken as very thin slices through the kidneys. This makes it possible to see the fine details in the kidneys and surrounding tissue.
- *MRI (magnetic resonance imaging)*: No x-rays are used with this technique. Instead, harmless magnetic fields and radio waves are used. A computer develops the pictures to show the kidneys from several angles. This technique is especially valuable for examining the blood vessels coming from the kidneys to see if any tumor is present in them.

○ TREATMENT

- The best treatment is to remove the cancerous kidney along with the surrounding fat and lymph nodes. Being left with one normal kidney does not require any change in diet or lifestyle.

After careful consideration of all factors, the recommendation is that you have your cancerous kidney removed.

PREOPERATIVE PREPARATION

- You will have an examination of your blood, urine, heart (EKG), and lungs (chest x-ray).
- Do not eat or drink anything for 8 hours before the operation.

□ OPERATION

- You will be asleep during the operation.
- The kidney, ureter, and surrounding lymph nodes will be removed (Fig. 1).
- You will not receive a blood transfusion unless it is absolutely necessary.
- The operation usually takes about 3 hours.

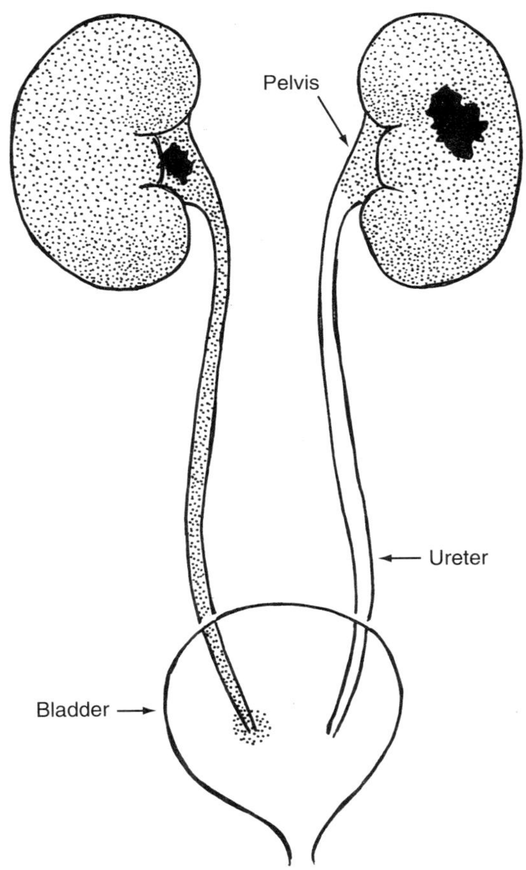

Figure 1. Tissue removal is indicated by the stippled area. For cancer of the kidney itself *(right)*, this includes the kidney, the kidney pelvis, and the surrounding fat and lymph nodes. For cancer of the pelvis *(left)*, the tissue removed is the same plus the entire ureter, along with a small button of bladder tissue.

POSTOPERATIVE CARE

- You will be taken to a recovery room and observed. When your blood pressure, pulse, and breathing are stable, you will be taken to a regular hospital room.
- Pain will be controlled with medicine.
- You may have a thin plastic tube in your nose. It goes down to your stomach to suck up the air you swallow. It will be removed when your bowels start working.
- There will be a catheter coming from your bladder. This is to make it easier to accurately measure the amount of urine you are making.
- The evening after the surgery you will be helped to sit up in bed and on the next day to get out of bed.
- You should be able to go home in about 3 to 5 days.
- Arrangements will be made for your medicine, follow-up office visit, and stitch removal.
- Your condition can be cured. An estimate of your chances can be made only after all the test results are back.
- As with any operation, complications are always possible. Although they are uncommon with your type of operation, they can include infection, blood clots, bleeding, pneumonia, and some others.

✣ HOME CARE

- You may walk about as you wish, even climb stairs, but don't overdo things.
- Take medicine as prescribed for your pain.
- Your diet can be the same as before the operation.
- Unless otherwise instructed, you may shower if you wish, with any dressings on or off. After you dry yourself, replace any dressings with clean, dry ones.
- Do not drive a car unless you can move freely and without pain and are not taking medicine that reduces your alertness.
- You may resume sexual activity whenever you choose.
- You may return to work when you feel up to it.

✆ CALL OUR OFFICE IF

- You develop any unusual signs or symptoms.
- The incision becomes red or swollen, or there is drainage from it.
- You develop a temperature higher than 100°F.
- You have any questions.

△ GENERAL INFORMATION

The kidney is shaped like a kidney bean (which is how the bean got its name) and is about as big as your fist. There is a kidney deep inside each side of your back. The main function of the kidneys is to eliminate waste products from your body through the urine.

A number of things can affect the kidneys. One of these is cysts. A cyst is a hollow cavity in the shape of a sphere that is filled with fluid. The cause of most cysts is a birth defect.

COMMON SIGNS AND SYMPTOMS

Most cysts do not cause symptoms. They are found when the abdomen is examined for some other reason. A cyst may cause symptoms if it suddenly becomes larger—usually because of bleeding into it.

DIAGNOSIS

When a mass is suspected or seen on a kidney, it is necessary to find out what the mass is. It may be something that is not important, or it may be something serious.

- A detailed history and a thorough physical examination will be done.
- *CT scan (computed tomographic scan)*: This technique uses a machine that is shaped like a huge doughnut to take special x-rays. You will lie on a table inside the hole in the "doughnut." The x-rays are taken as very thin slices through the area of the kidneys. This makes it possible to see the fine details in the kidneys.
- *Ultrasound*: Harmless sound waves are aimed at the area of your kidneys. The sound waves bouncing back (the echoes) from this area are seen as a picture on a screen. Ultrasound is a convenient and painless way to examine organs and tissues, and especially cysts, inside this area of your body.

CT and ultrasound may show the following: There may be one cyst or many. The cyst may be as small as a pea or as large as a tennis ball, or even larger. There can be many in separate locations in the kidney, or they can be touching each other. If they are touching each other, they may connect with each other, or not.

These findings can indicate several things, including the following:

- A group of benign cysts of the kidney that are not harmful.
- A kidney cancer that has formed some cavities (cysts) in it.
- An ordinary kidney cancer.
- A number of other possible diseases, including an abscess (a cavity filled with pus), a blood clot in the kidney, a sarcoma (a special type of cancer), and others.

The urologist gathers all this information, including information from the history and physical examination as well as the laboratory findings, in an effort to try to narrow down the diagnosis. For example, with no fever, an abscess is not a likely diagnosis; with no trauma to the kidney, it is unlikely that it could be a blood clot; sarcoma is found mostly in children; and so forth.

○ TREATMENT

- If it is confirmed that the mass represents a benign condition, then the patient's condition is just followed carefully.
- If there is a chance that the kidney *might* be cancerous, then it is appropriate to remove a tiny piece of it (a *biopsy*) for examination in the laboratory.
- If the diagnosis is *most likely* cancer, then an operation is necessary to remove that cancer.

After careful consideration of all factors, the recommendation is that a biopsy specimen be taken from your lesion to determine its true nature. This will make it possible to plan proper further therapy.

PREPARATION FOR THE BIOPSY

- Do not eat or drink anything for 8 hours before the operation.
- Shower or bathe on the morning of the operation.
- You may be given medicine that will make you feel drowsy before you are brought to the operating room.

THE NEEDLE ASPIRATION

- You will lie on a table face down.
- The area of the back that is over the suspected cyst will be swabbed with an antiseptic solution and surrounded with sterile towels.
- A fine needle will be used to inject anesthetic in the skin to make it completely numb.
- A special needle will be inserted through the numbed skin.
- As everything is watched by ultrasonography, the special needle is placed inside the suspected cyst. If it is a cyst, the fluid will be removed for examination. If it is solid, a small piece (called a biopsy) is removed for laboratory examination (Fig. 1).

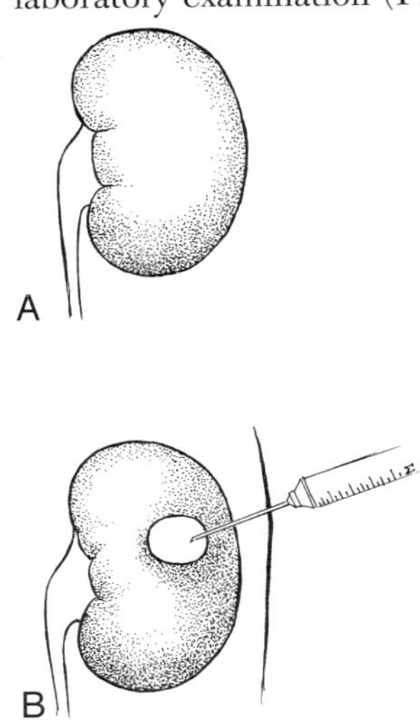

Figure 1. *A*, Normal kidney. *B*, Cyst being aspirated.

POSTOPERATIVE CARE

- You will be taken to a recovery room and observed. You should be able to go home that same day with a responsible adult, after your blood pressure, pulse, and breathing are stable and you are completely alert.
- Arrangements will be made for your medicine, follow-up office visit, and discussion of the laboratory results.
- As with any procedure, complications are always possible. With this type of operation, complications can include hemorrhage, bruising of the kidney, injury to other organs, not obtaining enough tissue, and possibly others.

✣ HOME CARE

- Take it easy for the first day. Lie down except when you need to go to the bathroom.
- Do not engage in exercises or strenuous activity for 2 days, or until your urine is not bloody.
- Eat as you wish.
- You may return to work after a day or two if there is no blood in your urine.

✆ CALL OUR OFFICE IF

- You pass red blood in your urine after 24 hours of bedrest.
- You develop any unusual signs or symptoms.
- You develop a temperature higher than 100°F.
- You have any questions.

△ GENERAL INFORMATION

Kidney stones are common, both in men and women, mostly in persons older than 25 years of age. The cause of your kidney stones cannot be identified.

COMMON SIGNS AND SYMPTOMS

The signs and symptoms produced by a kidney stone depend, in part, on where it is located in the body (Fig. 1).

The kidney (K) makes urine that collects in the *renal pelvis* (RP), a small cavity that is part of the kidney. The urine then flows down the ureter (U), a soft tube the size of macaroni, and into the bladder (B). It collects there and when there is the urge to urinate, it comes to the outside through the *urethra* (UR).

If the stone is simply lying in the center of the renal pelvis (A), there are few symptoms. If it settles at the opening of the renal pelvis (B), the urine is blocked, causing a deep aching pain in the flank. If it passes into the ureter (C), there may be no symptoms or there may be severe pain. If it gets stuck at the bottom end of the ureter (D) (it is narrower there), the symptoms are a steady or colicky pain. If the stone reaches the bladder, there usually are few serious symptoms. There may be blood in the urine, fever, and pain that shoots to the groin.

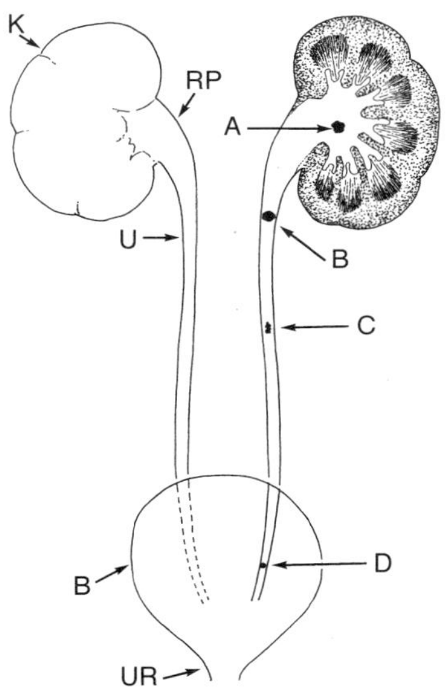

Figure 1.

DIAGNOSIS

Usually, the diagnosis can be made by taking a detailed history, doing a thorough physical examination, and considering the laboratory report.

Necessary tests may include some, or even all, of the following:

- *Abdominal x-ray*: An x-ray of the abdomen may show the stone if it has calcium in it.
- *IVP (intravenous pyelogram)*: A special dye is injected into the vein. It quickly leaves the body with the urine. X-rays are taken of it to see if the stone blocks the urine.
- *Ultrasound*: Harmless sound waves are aimed at the area of the kidneys, ureters, and bladder. The sound waves bouncing back (the echoes) are seen as a picture on a screen. This is a convenient, painless way to examine this area of your body for stones.
- *CT scan (computed tomography scan)*: This technique uses special x-rays that are taken as very thin slices through the area of the kidneys, ureters, and bladder. CT scans make it possible to see the fine details, including stones, in these organs.

○ TREATMENT

The treatment of kidney stones can consist of one or several of the following:

- No treatment if you have no symptoms.
- Modification of your diet if the stones are caused by certain foods you eat.
- Medicines to cancel out the effects of certain foods you eat that cause stone formation.
- An operation to remove the stones.
- Passing of a fine wire instrument into the bladder and then up and into the ureter to pull out the stone.
- Lithotripsy: This is crushing of a stone with shock waves that are generated hundreds of times per second. This is how it works and is used (Fig. 2):
  - If shock waves of the correct type strike something soft, not much happens to it, just like striking a pillow with a paddle. If, however, the shock waves repeatedly strike something hard and brittle, it will eventually break into tiny pieces.

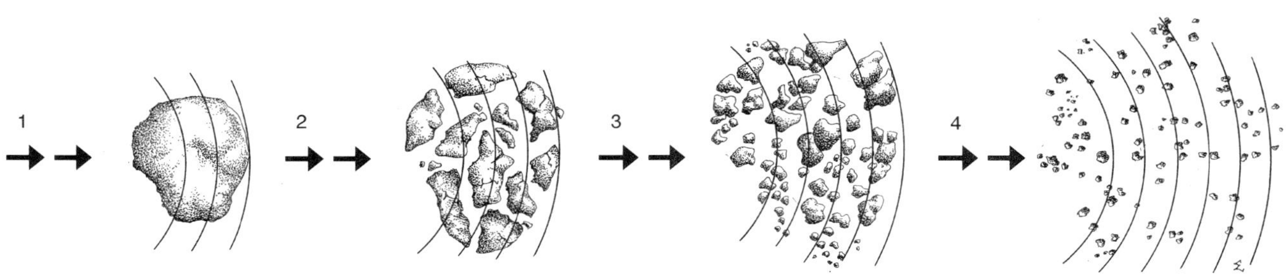

Figure 2. Progressive fragmentation of stone subjected to shock waves.

- Shock waves are aimed at the stone until it breaks into tiny pieces. The tiny stones can now pass out with the urine.
- As with any operation, lithotripsy is not always successful. How this might apply will be explained to you.

PREOPERATIVE PREPARATION

- Do not eat or drink anything for 8 hours before the operation.
- You will have an examination of your blood, urine, heart (EKG), and lungs (chest x-ray).
- Stop taking aspirin or aspirin-containing products for 1 week before the lithotripsy.
- If you are on anticoagulants (blood thinners), arrangements will need to be made for you to be off such medicines before you have lithotripsy.
- If you are pregnant or think you might be pregnant, be certain to tell the doctor because lithotripsy cannot be used on pregnant women.

☐ OPERATION

- The procedure can be done with you asleep or on medicine to keep you drowsy and relaxed, possibly along with some pain medicine. The choice will be discussed with you beforehand.
- You will lie face down on a special table.
- At the completion of the lithotripsy, you will be taken to a recovery room and observed until you are stable. You then should be able to go home that same day with a responsible adult.
- Arrangements will be made for your medicines and follow-up office visit.

✣ HOME CARE

- You may walk about as you wish, even climb stairs, but don't overdo things.
- You may eat as you did before the operation.
- Include plenty of roughage and liquids in your diet to avoid constipation.
- You may return to work when you feel up to it.

✆ CALL OUR OFFICE IF

- You develop flank pain that is becoming progressively worse.
- You pass red blood in your urine.
- You develop a temperature higher than 101°F.
- You have any questions.

△ GENERAL INFORMATION

Kidney transplants are done for patients whose own kidneys are no longer working properly.

○ TREATMENT

The most common treatment for kidney failure is dialysis, which is the mechanical removal of waste products from the body. This can be done in two ways: *Hemodialysis* involves removing the blood, passing it through a cleaning machine, and then returning it to the patient. *Peritoneal dialysis* involves placing a special fluid in the abdominal cavity. The waste products of the body find their way into this fluid, which is then removed. Neither form of dialysis is as efficient as having a properly working kidney. A major advantage of successful kidney transplantation is that the waste products are cleared better, and quality of life is considerably improved.

A large number of things are taken into consideration in deciding whether to perform a transplant or to continue with dialysis.

- The cause of the kidney damage.
- The age of the person.
- How the person's general health might affect the success of an operation.
- How swiftly the condition of the kidneys is getting worse.
- The lifestyle and support system of the individual.
- The availability of a kidney and its condition.

After the most careful consideration of all factors as well as the detailed conversations with you, the recommendation is that you have a kidney transplant.

PREOPERATIVE PREPARATION

A very detailed workup needs to be done to make as certain as possible that there is a good chance of recovery from the operation and to determine the likelihood that you will be able to tolerate the transplant medicines.

The necessary tests or procedures will include some and possibly all of the following:

- *Echocardiogram*: You will lie on a comfortable table as harmless, painless sound waves (that you cannot hear) are directed toward your heart. The sound waves bouncing back (the echoes) are transformed by a computer into pictures that can be seen on a screen and by which the condition of your heart can be evaluated.
- *Ultrasound of the abdomen*: Harmless sound waves are aimed at your abdomen. The sound waves bouncing back (the echoes) from this area are seen as a picture on a screen. Ultrasound is a convenient and painless way to look for any unexpected abnormalities inside the abdomen.
- *Prostate examination*: This is done to be certain there will be no blockage to urine flow.
- *Infection*: Tests will be done to evaluate for the potential of infection.

WAITING FOR A KIDNEY TRANSPLANT

If a kidney is being donated by a living donor, the transplant can usually be done within 3 months after the initial visit to the transplant team. Most patients, however, receive their new kidney from a person who has just died. Available kidneys are distributed primarily according to the blood type of the recipient and the length of time that person has been on the waiting list.

It is very important that the transplant team be able to reach you at all times while you are on the waiting list.

- When a kidney becomes available, the transplant team will call to have you come promptly to the hospital. Usually the transplantation is done within 6 to 18 hours from the time that you come into the hospital.
- The transplant team will tell you which medicines to take and other more specific preparations to make before coming to the hospital.
- You will be asleep for the operation.
- The new kidney will be placed in the side of your pelvis (Fig. 1).

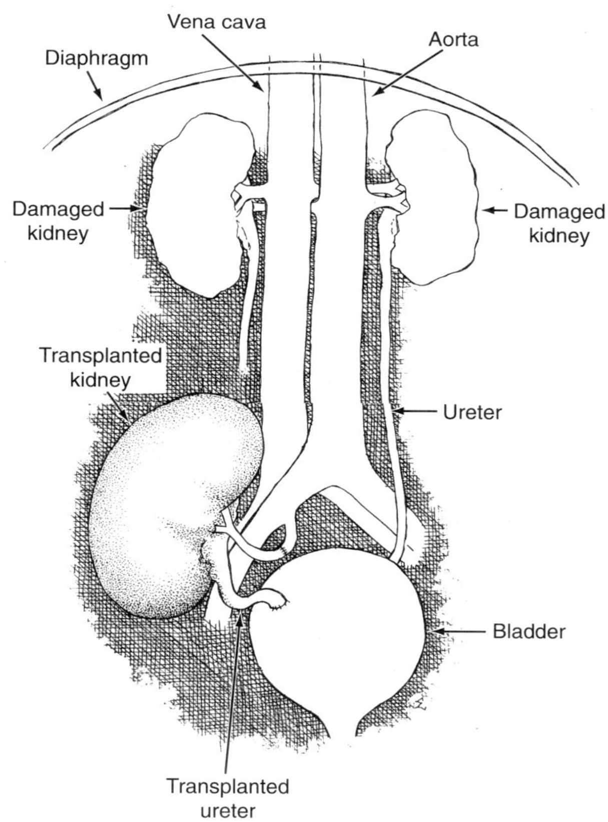

Figure 1. Usually the kidney is transplanted in the right lower part of the abdomen. Practically always, the patient's own kidneys are not disturbed at this time.

- Your own kidneys are not likely to be removed.
- The operation usually takes about 3 to 5 hours.
- You will be taken to a recovery room and observed. When your blood pressure, pulse, and breathing are stable you will be transferred to a hospital bed.
- Pain will be controlled with medicine.
- Your diet will be as you tolerate it.
- You should be able to go home in about 5 to 7 days.
- As with any operation, complications are always possible, some of them serious. With this type of operation, complications can include infection of the incision, poor healing, bleeding, blockage of the vessels of the new kidney, leakage or blockage of the ureter, and possibly others.
- Occasionally, the kidney does not work right away, and continued dialysis treatments are necessary for a period of time.
- Arrangements will be made for your medicine, follow-up office visit, and stitch removal.

HOME CARE

- You may walk about as you wish, even climb stairs, but don't overdo things.
- Take medicine as prescribed for your pain.
- You may eat as you did before the operation.
- It is very important that you understand the importance of your transplant medicines and that you never miss a dose.
- Do not drive a car until we first discuss it during your follow-up office visit.
- You may return to work when you feel up to it, but let's first talk about it.

CALL OUR OFFICE IF

- You develop any unusual signs or symptoms.
- The incision becomes red or swollen, or there is drainage from it.
- You develop a temperature higher than 100°F.
- You have any questions.

KNEE: Cartilage Tears

△ GENERAL INFORMATION

Cartilages of the knee joint are C-shaped, shock-absorbing cushions between the two bones, called the *femur* and the *tibia,* that make up the knee joint (Fig. 1). The majority of cartilage (meniscus) tears take place when a person is involved in a sport that requires sudden changes in direction, or "cutting." Arthritis of the knee can predispose a person to a different type of tear called a *degenerative cartilage tear.*

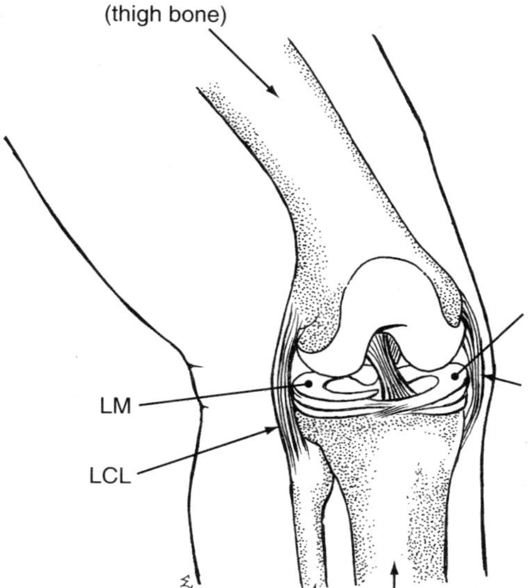

Figure 1. Knee joint. MM, Medial meniscus; LM, lateral meniscus; MCL, medial collateral ligament; LCL, lateral collateral ligament.

COMMON SIGNS AND SYMPTOMS

- Swelling of the knee joint.
- Possible "locking" or "catching" of the knee when attempting to straighten the knee.
- Pain localized to either side of the knee joint between the knee bones.
- Pain with twisting activity such as crossing the legs.

DIAGNOSIS

- Usually the diagnosis can be made by taking a detailed history and performing a thorough physical examination.
- The three characteristics of a cartilage tear are as follows:
  - Swelling of the knee.
  - Point tenderness at the joint space.
  - Pain with tests that compress the knee joint.
- MRI (magnetic resonance imaging): No x-rays are used with this technique. Instead, it is done with harmless magnetic fields and radio waves. A computer develops the pictures to show organs from several angles. It is especially valuable for examining bone and joint tissue and spaces.

○ TREATMENT

- Immediate treatment of a cartilage tear consists of rest, ice, compression, and elevation (RICE).
  - **Rest:** Avoid activities that can further aggravate the knee joint.
  - **Ice:** Apply a cloth over the knee joint and an ice bag over this for 30 minutes five times a day for the first 2 days after the injury.
  - **Compression:** Wear an elastic bandage or an elastic knee sleeve. This will help prevent or reduce swelling.
  - **Elevation:** Elevate the affected leg higher than the level of your heart to assist in reducing the swelling.
- Nonsteroidal anti-inflammatory medicine may be given for pain.
- An operation with an arthroscope may be recommended. The decision is influenced by the following:
  - The seriousness of the injury.
  - Whether this is a first or a repeat injury.
  - The degree of disability.
  - Your age, occupation, and health in general.
  - The need for you to be active as soon as possible.

After careful consideration of all factors, the recommendation is that you have an arthroscopy and correction of any cartilage problem found.

PREOPERATIVE PREPARATION

- You will have an examination of your blood, urine, and possibly your heart (EKG) and lungs (chest x-ray).
- Do not eat or drink anything for 8 hours before the operation.
- You may be given medicine that will make you feel drowsy before you are brought to the operating room.

□ OPERATION

The goal of surgery is to provide relief of pain and to restore range of motion, strength, and function of the knee joint.

- The operation is done on an outpatient basis, usually under general anesthesia.
- Three to four very small incisions will be made around the knee joint to insert the arthroscopes. The arthroscopes are as thick as your little finger and have lenses in them and a light at the tip.
- If the torn cartilage can be repaired, an accessory incision, approximately 1 inch long, may be made to accommodate suturing instead of removing the torn cartilage. If the torn cartilage cannot be repaired, the torn portion will be "trimmed out," leaving the remainder of the cartilage intact. The decision on whether to repair or remove a torn cartilage usually is made by the surgeon at the time of the operation.
- The operation usually takes about 30 to 60 minutes.

POSTOPERATIVE CARE

- You will be taken to a recovery room and observed until your blood pressure, pulse, and breathing are stable and you are completely alert. You should be able to go home that same day with a responsible adult.
- You will be given crutches to help you get around.
- A home program consisting of leg raising and range of motion exercises will be shown to you. You can begin these as soon as you are comfortable.
- Physical therapy to help restore function of the knee may be recommended.
- Arrangements will be made for your medicine, follow-up office visit, and stitch removal.
- As with any operation, complications are always possible. With this type of operation, complications can include infection, blood clots, and possibly others.

✣ HOME CARE

- Take it easy for the first day or two. When sitting or lying down, keep the knee above the level of your waist by resting your leg on one or two pillows. This will help reduce pain and any swelling.
- For the first 24 to 48 hours, place an ice bag over the knee for 20 minutes five times a day. This will help reduce any swelling.
- You may sponge bathe as you wish. If you choose to shower, however, the bandage must not get wet. Placing a plastic bag on the leg up to the thigh and sealing the bag with tape at the top is usually satisfactory.
- Perform your home exercises as instructed.
- Gradually get yourself off the crutches and pain medication as the discomfort decreases and knee function improves. Most individuals are off crutches 2 to 3 days after this type of an operation.
- There are a number of factors to consider before you can safely return to work. This will be discussed with you during your follow-up office visit.
- You may resume driving when you are off pain medication and crutches and you have regained function of the involved leg.

✆ CALL OUR OFFICE IF

- The incision becomes red or swollen, or there is drainage from it.
- The pain increases rather than decreases.
- You develop a temperature higher than 100°F.
- You have any questions.

△ GENERAL INFORMATION

Osteoarthritis of the knee is a breakdown of the smooth cartilage at the ends of bones that form the joint. Osteoarthritis of the knee may develop from the wear and tear of normal aging or from trauma such as a sports injury, a fall, or previous knee surgery. Quite often, knee arthritis involves the inner part of the knee joint. Also, this arthritis usually is associated with a *varus* (bowleg) deformity of the knee. This deformity doesn't have to be severe. It causes a shift in the weight from the center of the knee to the diseased portion of the inner knee.

COMMON SIGNS AND SYMPTOMS

- Pain localized to the inner part of the knee.
- Swelling or stiffness of the knee joint, or both.
- A mild, or quite obvious, "bowlegged" appearance of the leg.

DIAGNOSIS

- Usually the diagnosis can be made in an orthopedist's office by taking a detailed history and performing a thorough physical examination.
- X-rays are important to determine the location and degree of arthritis within your knee joint.
- A special x-ray of your entire leg (from hip to foot) will be performed with you standing so that the orthopedist can measure how much angulation there is at the knee joint. This information is important for the orthopedic surgeon to determine whether you would benefit from a surgical procedure called a *high tibial osteotomy*.
  - The goal of the osteotomy is to realign the mechanical axis of the leg to shift the weight bearing from the diseased inner side of the knee to a more normal alignment.
  - A high tibial osteotomy is performed by removing a predetermined wedge of the upper part of the shin bone, just below the knee joint.
  - A high tibial osteotomy is viewed as a pain-relieving procedure designed to provide several years of adequate knee function before a possible knee replacement surgery.
  - A high tibial osteotomy is not appropriate for significant arthritis of the knee cap, limited range of motion of the knee joint, excessive bowing, rheumatoid arthritis, or osteoporosis about the knee.

○ TREATMENT

- Taking a nonsteroidal anti-inflammatory medication.
- Applying an ice bag over the knee for 20 minutes, three to five times per day.
- Using a cane or crutches if needed for comfort.
- Seeing an orthopedic specialist for evaluation.
- A cortisone injection into the knee joint may be recommended for pain relief. This can be effective for a couple of days to many months. If conservative measures fail, a tibial osteotomy may be required.

After careful consideration of all factors, the recommendation is that you have a high tibial osteotomy.

PREOPERATIVE PREPARATION

- You will have an examination of your blood, urine, heart (EKG), and lungs (chest x-ray).
- Do not eat, drink, or smoke for 8 hours before the operation.
- You may be given medicine that will make you feel drowsy before you are brought to the operating room.

□ OPERATION

- The operation is done under general anesthesia.
- The incision will be just below the outer part of your knee joint.
- A small, triangular wedge of your shin bone will be removed, realigning the weight-bearing axis of the knee joint (Fig. 1).
- The operation usually takes 2 to 2½ hours.

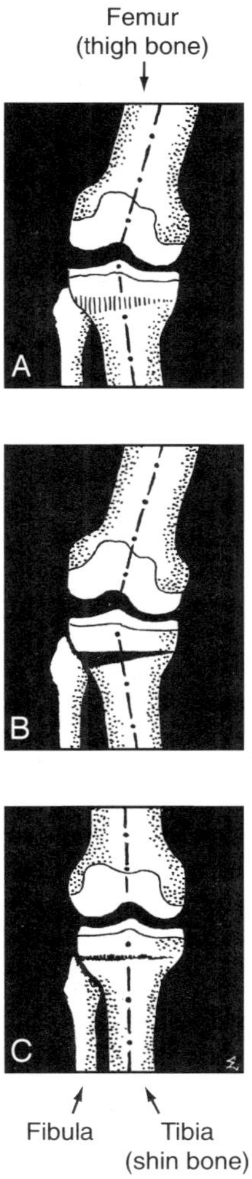

Figure 1. *A*, The knee is shown with a bowlegged angle. This angle places great pressure and does damage to the inner side of the knee joint. The wedge of bone that will be removed to make it possible to line up the bones properly is shown by the slanted lines. *B*, The wedge of bone has been removed. The knee is prepared for straightening. *C*, The knee joint is now in a straight line. A metal plate and screw are used to hold the bones in the correct position as they heal.

POSTOPERATIVE CARE

- You will be taken to a recovery room and observed. When your blood pressure, pulse, and breathing are stable, you will be taken to a regular hospital room.
- Pain will be controlled with medicine.
- A hinged knee brace or a long leg splint or cast will be applied to your knee, depending on your special requirements.
- You will receive crutches to help you get around.
- Gentle range of motion exercises to regain knee motion will begin several weeks after the operation and you will continue performing these exercises at home. Generally, patients readily recover their range of motion. Most patients can resume full weight bearing 6 to 8 weeks postoperatively.
- As with any operation, complications are always possible. With this type of operation, complications can include infection, blood clots, poor healing, heart problems, and possibly others.
- You should be able to go home in about 2 days.
- Arrangements will be made for your medicine, follow-up office visit, and stitch or clip removal.

HOME CARE

- You will be instructed on how much you may be up and about.
- Elevate the leg when sitting or sleeping by placing one to two pillows under it. This will help to reduce any swelling of the knee.
- You will be instructed on when you may bathe or shower and how to do this without getting the incision wet.
- Reduce the amount of pain medication you take as your discomfort decreases.

CALL OUR OFFICE IF

- The incision becomes red or swollen, or there is drainage from it.
- Postoperative pain increases rather than decreases.
- You develop a temperature higher than 100°F.
- You have any questions.

△ GENERAL INFORMATION

The *anterior cruciate ligament* (ACL) is one of the bands of tissue that connects the bones that make up the knee joint. Its main function is to maintain stability of the knee joint. Tears of the ACL are usually the result of sports such as downhill skiing, basketball, and volleyball, in which the foot is firmly planted on the ground and the knee is twisted. About 50% of people who tear their ACL sustain an associated tear of the *meniscus* (the cartilage of the knee).

COMMON SIGNS AND SYMPTOMS

- Often, a "pop" or "tearing" sensation inside the knee is heard or felt at the time of injury.
- Moderate to severe pain is felt at the time of injury, and the person can't continue to play the sport because of the pain.
- The knee joint swells usually within 24 hours, but frequently within 3 hours.
- The knee may become unstable or may feel as though it is "giving out."

DIAGNOSIS

- The diagnosis of an ACL tear can usually be made by taking a detailed history and performing a thorough physical examination of the knee.
- X-rays of the knee are essential to be certain there are no fractures or other related problems. An instrument called a knee ligament arthrometer can be used to measure looseness of the knee joint.
- MRI (magnetic resonance imaging): This technique uses no x-rays, only magnetic fields and radio waves. A computer develops pictures to show organs from several angles. It is especially valuable for examining bones, cartilage, ligaments, tendons, and muscles of the knee joint.

○ TREATMENT

- Immediate treatment consists of rest, ice, compression, and elevation (RICE)
  - **Rest:** Avoid activity that can further aggravate the knee joint.
  - **Ice:** Apply an ice bag to the knee for 20 minutes three to five times a day for the first 24 to 48 hours.
  - **Compression:** Wear an elastic bandage or Neoprene knee sleeve.
  - **Elevation:** Elevate the entire leg higher than the level of your heart to help reduce any swelling.
- Take a nonsteroidal, anti-inflammatory medication.
- Generally, ACL tears do not heal themselves. The torn ACL cannot be reattached or sewn back together; it simply does not work. It must be reconstructed to restore stability to the joint. This is usually done with a tendon graft, of which there are several choices available.
- People who choose to live with a torn ACL must alter their lifestyles significantly. Most likely, they will not be able to participate in activities that require pivoting, twisting, or turning of the affected leg.
- Custom braces are available for people with a deficient ACL. Their effectiveness can best be described by using the "rule of thirds." One-third of people with braces will be able to return to all of their preinjury activities, one-third will have to modify their activities significantly, and one-third will continue to have their knee "give out" on them. Many of these patients eventually go on to have their knee reconstructed.

After careful consideration of all factors, the recommendation is that you have an operation to try to correct your knee problem. The choice of operation will be discussed with you before anything is planned or done.

PREOPERATIVE PREPARATION

- You will have an examination of your blood, urine, and possibly your heart (EKG) and lungs (chest x-ray).
- Do not eat or drink anything for 8 hours before the operation.

□ OPERATION

The aim of the operation is to restore stability to the knee joint, give relief of pain, and provide normal function (Fig. 1). Generally, the operation is done on an outpatient basis.

- The choice of general or spinal anesthesia will be discussed with you beforehand.
- This operation is assisted by the use of an *arthroscope*, a smooth, metal instrument about as thick as a pencil with lenses and a light in it and the ability to cut various tissues. Two or three tiny incisions will be made to introduce the arthroscopic instruments and one longer one over the area from which the tendon graft will be obtained.
- If cartilage tears are found in the knee joint, they will be trimmed and removed if possible.
- The operation usually takes about 2 to 3 hours.

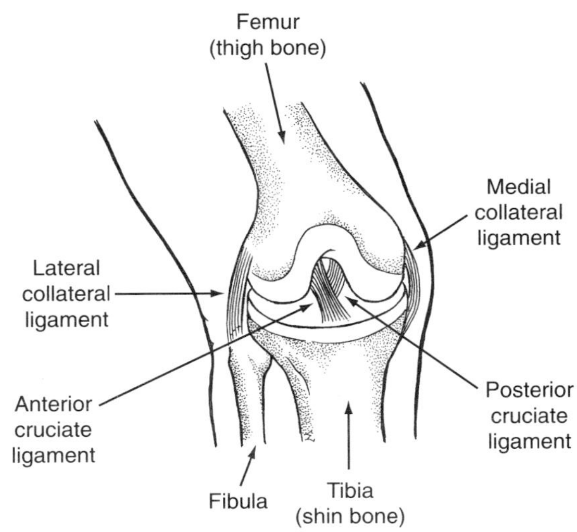

Figure 1. Knee: three-fourths view. The cruciate and collateral ligaments are shown. They can be injured in a variety of ways. The technique of repair is influenced by the ligament injured, the extent of the injury, the age and occupation of the person, and other clinical and technical considerations.

POSTOPERATIVE CARE

- You will be taken to a recovery room and observed until your blood pressure, pulse, and breathing are stable and you are completely alert. You should be able to go home that same day with a responsible adult. A knee immobilizer or hinged knee brace will be applied to your knee. The use of these appliances will be explained to you.
- Arrangements will be made for your medicine, follow-up office visit, and stitch removal.
- Home exercises consisting of leg raising and range of motion exercises will be shown to you. You will begin these as soon as you are comfortable.
- As with any operation, complications are always possible. With this operation, complications can include infection, blood clots, and possibly others.

✙ HOME CARE

- Take it easy for the first day or two. When sitting or lying down, rest your leg on one or two pillows to keep the knee above the level of your waist and reduce pain and swelling.
- For the first 24 to 48 hours, place an ice bag over the knee for 20 minutes five times a day.
- For the first 4 days, you may sponge bathe as you wish or shower with a shower bag properly secured over the knee to keep it dry.
- Perform the home exercises as instructed.
- Gradually wean yourself off the crutches and pain medication as the discomfort decreases and knee function improves, usually within 2 to 3 weeks.
- Do not resume driving or return to work before we discuss it during your follow-up office visit.

✆ CALL OUR OFFICE IF

- An incision becomes red or swollen, or there is drainage from it.
- The pain increases rather than decreases.
- You develop a temperature higher than 100°F.
- You have any questions.

△ GENERAL INFORMATION

Total knee replacement (or *arthroplasty*) is a method used to relieve the pain and disability caused by problems around the knee, most often arthritis.

Knee joint replacement involves replacing parts of the joint that actually move past one another. These surfaces are covered in cartilage, which makes it possible to have a smooth, pain-free movement of the knee. When this cartilage is damaged, movement of the joint is painful and the joint cannot move as much or work as well.

COMMON SIGNS AND SYMPTOMS

- Marked pain located about the knee and possibly radiating up and down the leg and limitation of motion are the most common.
- Difficulty in walking and putting on shoes and socks.
- The presence of a limp.
- A possible sense of instability.

DIAGNOSIS

The diagnosis can be made on the basis of the patient's complaints, findings on physical examination, and x-ray pictures of the knee. You may need some or all of the following tests:

- *Bone scan:* A fine needle is used to inject a solution with a tiny amount of a harmless radioactive material into your vein. The solution circulates throughout your entire body and attaches itself to any part of a bone that has something wrong with it. One hour after the injection, you will lie on a table, and a special machine will pass over your entire body taking a photograph (a *scan*) of all the bones from your skull to your toes. A specialist then examines the scan, looking for any abnormalities.
- *CT scan (computed tomography scan):* A machine shaped like a huge doughnut is used to take special x-rays. You will lie on a table inside the hole in the "doughnut." The x-rays are taken as very thin slices through the knee joint. This makes it possible to see the fine details in the knee joint.
- *MRI (magnetic resonance imaging):* No x-rays are used with this technique. Instead, it is done with harmless magnetic fields and radio waves. A computer develops the pictures to show organs from several angles. It is especially useful for examining your blood vessels, nerves, and bone tissue.

○ TREATMENT

- Anti-inflammatory and pain-relieving medicines.
- Modification of physical activity.
- Devices to help with walking.
- Physical therapy to strengthen muscles about the knee.
- Occasionally, cortisone injections may be very helpful in reducing pain and improving function.

If these methods do not bring sufficient pain relief or return of function, then replacement of the knee joint may be the most effective treatment.

After careful consideration of all factors, the recommendation is that you have an operation to replace your knee joint.

PREOPERATIVE PREPARATION

- Total knee replacement is a major operation. For this reason, it is necessary that you be in the best possible condition for it. This may require a separate visit with a medical doctor for a general examination to diagnose and treat any correctable problems.
- You will have an examination of your blood, urine, heart (EKG), and lungs (chest x-ray).
- Be certain your doctors are aware of medications you are now taking; any operations you have had; any history of blood clots, infections, or complications with prior operations; and any allergies you have.
- This operation may involve blood loss, making it necessary to give you a blood transfusion. Let's discuss donating some of your own blood before the operation so that it can be transfused back to you if needed during or after the operation.
- Stop taking aspirin and other anti-inflammatory medications at least 10 days before the operation if at all possible.
- Do not eat or drink anything for 8 hours before the operation.

□ OPERATION

- Most likely you will arrive at the hospital the morning of the operation.
- You may be given medicine that will make you feel drowsy before you are brought to the operating room.
- After you are asleep, wires from recording machines will be taped to your skin to keep track of your blood pressure, pulse, breathing, and level of oxygen in your blood.
- The operation consists of removing the diseased bone ends and implanting new joint ends (Fig. 1).
- The entire operation takes from 1 to 3 hours, depending on your special circumstances.

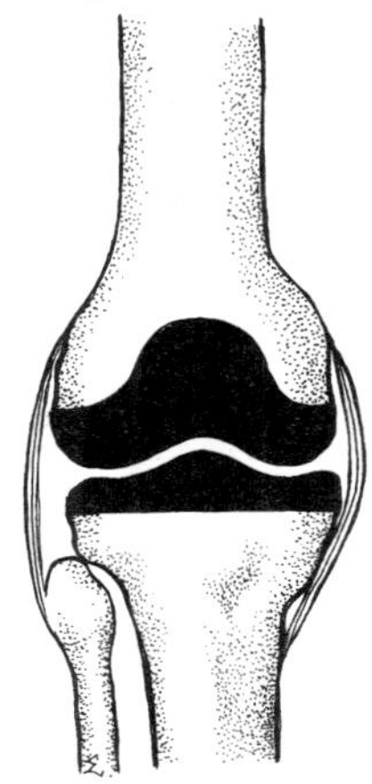

Figure 1. There are a number of ways to replace a knee. The technique used is greatly influenced by the specific needs of the patient. In the technique illustrated here, the replaced parts are in black.

POSTOPERATIVE CARE

- You will be taken to a recovery room and observed. When your blood pressure, pulse, and breathing are stable, you will be taken to a regular hospital room.
- Pain will be controlled with medicine.
- Your diet will be as you tolerate it.
- Rapid mobilization is the standard after knee replacement. Every individual responds somewhat differently, however, so you will have a customized therapy program.
- You will be discharged when you are eating and drinking well and your discomfort is well managed by oral pain medicines.
- As with any operation, complications are always possible. With this type of operation, complications can include infection of the operated area, blood clots in the legs or to the lungs, bleeding, pneumonia, heart problems, and possibly others.

✚ HOME CARE

- Continue with the program started while you were in the hospital.
- Very likely, arrangements will be made for a visiting nurse or therapist to assist you with the same exercises you did in the hospital.
- You will be advised about taking a shower or bath.
- Take medicine as prescribed for your pain.
- Include plenty of roughage and liquids in your diet.
- Do not engage in any stressful activity until we first discuss it.

✆ CALL OUR OFFICE IF

- The incision becomes red or swollen, or there is drainage from it.
- You have increasing pain, or your leg becomes swollen.
- You develop a temperature higher than 101°F.
- You have any questions.

△ GENERAL INFORMATION

The *larynx* (the "voice box," also referred to as "Adam's apple") is an important organ, not only because it makes it possible for us to speak but also because the air we breathe passes through it. Cancer of the larynx has a strong association with heavy smoking and alcohol use. It occurs most commonly in older men.

COMMON SIGNS AND SYMPTOMS

The signs and symptoms of cancer of the larynx depend on the location and size of the cancer and whether it has spread outside the larynx itself. The symptoms and signs may include the following:

- Hoarseness that persists.
- Difficulty breathing.
- The feeling of a lump in the throat.
- Painful or difficult swallowing.
- Enlarged lymph nodes in the neck.
- Recent but persistent cough.
- Ear pain.

DIAGNOSIS

A detailed history of your symptoms will be taken and a careful examination performed of your head and neck. Some or all of the following tests may be performed:

- *Indirect laryngoscopy:* Examination of your vocal cords done with a small, long-handled mirror.
- *Direct laryngoscopy:* This is done with a smooth, flexible instrument that is thinner than a pencil and has magnifying lenses and a light in it. The inside of your nose as well as your throat will be sprayed with an anesthetic to make it numb. The laryngoscope will be inserted gently into one side of your nose and then advanced down to the larynx. The throat can then be seen clearly. If anything suspicious is seen, a tiny piece of it can be taken (a *biopsy*) for microscopic examination.
- *CT scan (computed tomographic scan):* Special x-rays are taken as very thin slices through the area of the larynx. This makes it possible to see the fine details in the larynx and surrounding tissue.
- *MRI (magnetic resonance imaging):* No x-rays are used with this technique. Instead, it is done with harmless magnetic fields and radio waves. A computer develops the pictures to show organs from several angles. This technique is especially useful in determining the relationship of the tumor to the blood vessels, nerves, and bone tissue in this area.

○ TREATMENT

The treatment of cancer of the larynx depends on at least the following:

- The specific location of the cancer in the larynx.
- Its size.
- Involvement of any neighboring structures or the local lymph nodes.
- The age, occupation, and general medical condition of the patient.
- The patient's feelings about the various treatment options.

Based on the above, the treatment for cancer of the larynx can be as follows:

- Radiation treatment alone. This method preserves the speaking voice but is most effective for smaller cancers.
- Removal of superficial or localized cancer of the vocal cords with laser. There is no skin incision.
- Removal of part of the larynx. With this method, the person can breathe the normal way and can speak, but the voice is hoarse and somewhat weaker.
- Removal of the entire larynx. When the larynx is removed, it is necessary to breathe permanently through a stoma (the opening, *tracheostomy*) in the front of the neck. No air flows in and out of the mouth or nose. You will be taught how to speak, but by a different way (Figs. 1 and 2).

After the most careful consideration of all factors, especially the intent to give you the best chance for cure, the recommendation is that you have your entire larynx removed. Removal of the lymph nodes is sometimes necessary and can be done at the same time.

PREOPERATIVE PREPARATION

- You may have an examination of your blood, urine, heart (EKG), and lungs (chest x-ray).
- Do not eat or drink anything for 8 hours before the operation.
- You will have a specific meeting with the surgeon and the speech pathologist to discuss the several ways you can learn to speak after the operation.

□ OPERATION

- You will be asleep for the operation.
- You will not receive a blood transfusion unless it is absolutely necessary.
- The operation usually takes about 3 to 4 hours.

POSTOPERATIVE CARE

- You will be taken to a recovery room and observed. When your blood pressure, pulse, and breathing are stable, you will be taken to the intensive care unit to learn to take care of your tracheostomy properly.
- You will not be able to speak during this time. Pencil and paper will be provided for you so that you can communicate with the doctors and the nurses. Don't be concerned; someone will always be around to take care of your needs.
- Pain will be controlled with medicine.
- A very thin tube in your nose going down to your stomach will be used to give you all your nourishment for a week or so. As the tissue heals, little by little you will be able to eat food as usual.
- This operation causes the lungs and trachea (windpipe) to form a lot of mucus. The nurse will use a thin plastic tube to suck this mucus out through the tracheostomy. You will be taught to do this yourself without the nurse's help.

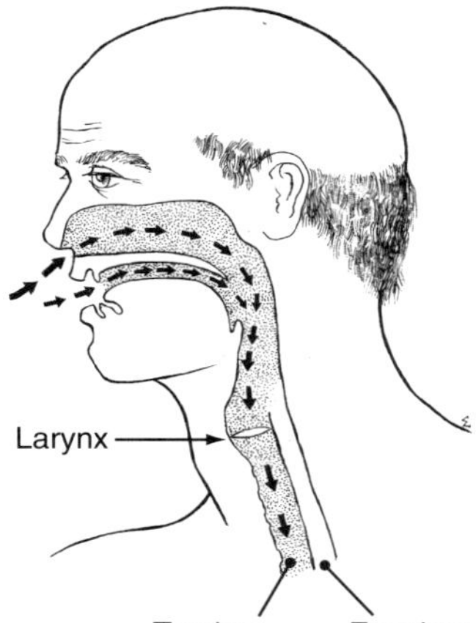

Figure 1. The air that a person breathes is humidified as it passes through the nose and the mouth on its way to the trachea and down into the lungs.

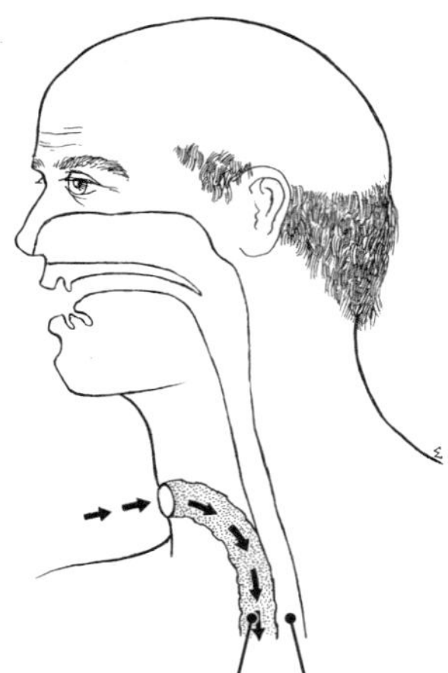

Figure 2. When the larynx is removed, the trachea (windpipe) comes through the skin directly to the outside. Now the air going into the lungs is much less humid than before. This state is not desirable and is the reason the air in the house must be kept humid.

- The air you normally breathe gets moistened as it passes through the nose on its way to the lungs. Now that you have a permanent tracheostomy, the air will be kept moist with a special humidifier.
- As with any operation, complications are always possible. With this type of operation, complications can include bleeding, infection, leakage of saliva through the incision, temporary difficulty swallowing, heart problems, and possibly others.
- You should be able to leave the hospital in about 1 week.
- Arrangements will be made for your medicine, follow-up office visit, and stitch removal.

HOME CARE

- Continue with the program started while you were in the hospital.
- You may walk about if you wish, even climb stairs, but don't overdo things.
- It is important to keep a high humidity level in the house, especially in the bedroom and wherever else you spend most of your time.
- Continue with suctioning of your trachea as you feel it to be necessary.
- Arrangements can be made for a home visiting nurse if one is needed. A suction machine will be ordered for you to have at home.
- You should *never* go swimming. Water would enter your stoma, and you would be at risk of drowning.
- You need special precautions if you feel that you should shower. In the beginning at least, bathing is preferable. A plastic bib-like cover can be purchased to protect your stoma.
- You may return to work when you feel up to it.
- Helpful information can be obtained through your local American Cancer Society or Laryngectomy Society.

CALL OUR OFFICE IF

- You have trouble breathing or swallowing.
- The incision becomes red or swollen, or there is drainage from it.
- Blood or blood clots come out of the stoma.
- You have any questions.

△ GENERAL INFORMATION

Laser is a relatively new method used to treat wrinkles and acne scars of the face. Laser is a specific, narrow, and sharp ray of light that "paints away" wrinkling and acne scars with light rather than burning them off. The laser helps prepare the skin's own collagen (the material that keeps the skin firm) and stimulates regrowth of new collagen. This rejuvenates, restores, and smoothes the skin.

CANDIDATES FOR LASER RESURFACING

- By far, most people have this procedure for cosmetic improvement.
- People with fair skin are more suitable for this procedure than those with darker skin.
- Small blood vessels on the skin of the face and body can be shrunk or eliminated by laser.
- Laser resurfacing is an excellent alternative for patients on blood-thinning medications (example: Coumadin) because the laser does not cause bleeding. This means that the person does not need to discontinue regular medication.

○ TREATMENT

Although laser technology offers some distinct advantages over conventional skin and resurfacing techniques, it is not intended to be a cure-all treatment. There are circumstances, such as deep scarring, deep wrinkles, and variations in skin pigmentation, in which conventional treatment, combined with laser surfacing, is indicated.

PREOPERATIVE PREPARATION

- The laser procedure will be carefully explained to you because it is important that you have realistic expectations and a full understanding of the healing process.
- A detailed history will be taken relative to your facial skin and any treatments or problems with it in the past.
- There will be a thorough physical examination as it pertains to the area to be treated.
- The surgeon will need to have assurance that you are not troubled with any significant illness or prone to keloids, scar formation, or cold sores.
- Please let the surgeon know if you have used Accutane medication for acne, especially within the last year. Also, be certain to let the surgeon and nurses know if you are allergic to any medications.
- Six weeks before the laser treatment:
  - Begin to use HQRA (a cream) on your face twice a day to prepare the skin for the laser.
  - Wear sunscreen daily with an SPF of at least 15 and both UVA and UVB protection.
  - Standard preoperative photographs will be taken of the area to be lasered.
  - Avoid tanning for 1 week before the laser procedure.
- You will be given prescriptions for the following:
  - Medication for preventing cold sore formation.
  - Medication for reducing any swelling of the face.
  - Prophylactic antibiotic.
  - A cream for use after your laser dressing is removed.
- The night before the procedure, use Dial soap to wash your face for 5 minutes. Rinse your face and do not put anything else on it. Repeat this the morning of the operation.
- On the morning of the procedure, start your medications as directed, taking small sips of water as necessary.
- Unless directed to do otherwise, do not eat or drink anything for 4 hours before the scheduled laser procedure.
- Wear comfortable clothing that will not need to be pulled over your head for removal. Remove your contact lenses.
- Arrange for someone to drive you home. You will be given medication to make you more comfortable after the operation, but this will reduce your alertness.

□ OPERATION

- You'll be given medicine that will make you feel drowsy before the procedure is begun.
- The procedure generally is done under local anesthesia. A short, fine needle is used to inject an anesthetic into the affected area to make it numb. Occasionally, the procedure is done under general anesthesia. In that case, you will have an examination of your blood, urine, heart (EKG), and lungs (chest x-ray). The choice of anesthetic will be discussed with you beforehand.
- During the procedure, you may feel some mild stinging.
- The procedure takes about 30 minutes to 1 hour, depending on how large an area is lasered.

POSTOPERATIVE CARE

- You will be taken to a recovery area and observed. When your blood pressure, pulse, and breathing are stable, you should be able to go home that very same day with a responsible adult.
- Arrangements will be made for your postoperative office visit.

✚ HOME CARE

- Restrict your activities the first 24 to 48 hours.
- Your face or lasered area may be swollen. At bedtime, sleep with your head elevated on two pillows.
- Use an ice bag (or a bag of frozen peas, which conforms well to the curves) for 20 minutes every hour for the first 24 hours during waking hours.
- During the first 24 to 48 hours, the lasered areas will weep a straw-colored fluid. This will be absorbed by the dressings on these areas.
- The skin will be quite pink: this will gradually fade during the next 4 to 6 weeks.
- The skin of your face will feel somewhat tense or tight. This is normal.

- Continue taking and complete your prescribed medications. If needed, you will be given medicine to help you sleep more comfortably.
- Avoid facial movement that will cause the lasered skin to move excessively.
- Avoid strenuous exercise for 2 to 3 weeks, both to avoid irritating the skin and also to avoid perspiring.
- Be alert that you do not become constipated. You may need some help with a laxative (example: milk of magnesia).
- Keep the dressings dry. After 1 week, gently wash your face with cold water. Ten days after the operation you may begin using light makeup.
- Do not pick at or rub away dead skin or crust.
- You will be given instructions on skin care.
- Avoid direct sunlight for 3 to 6 months. Use a sun cream as mentioned above.
- As with any procedure, complications are always possible. With this procedure, complications can include cold sores, which should immediately be treated with Zovirax, and blotching or dark pigmentation, which should be treated with the hydroquinone bleaching cream.

✆ CALL OUR OFFICE IF

- You develop any crust, cloudy drainage, increasing pain, unusual redness or swelling, cold sores or fever blisters, itchiness, or any blotching, lightening, or darkening of the skin.
- You develop a temperature higher than 100°F.
- You have any questions.

△ GENERAL INFORMATION

Leukoplakia means "white patch," which is what the affected area looks like. Leukoplakia usually involves the delicate lining of the mouth: the cheek, roof, and floor of the mouth and the side of the tongue. Leukoplakia in the mouth very often is associated with some type of chronic irritation. Examples are smoking or tobacco chewing, drinking hard liquor or hot coffee, eating spicy foods, and poor oral hygiene. Leukoplakia can become cancerous over time.

COMMON SIGNS AND SYMPTOMS

The appearance varies quite a bit:

- There may be a single area the size of a dime, but often there are several areas. They may be clustered together or spread around widely.
- The leukoplakia may look very filmy, as though you just drank some milk and didn't rinse your mouth.
- Ordinarily, leukoplakia is not abnormal to the feel, but an area may be firm or it may feel rough like sandpaper. There may be some raw areas in or around a lesion.

DIAGNOSIS

- The diagnosis can be made with certainty only by using a very fine short needle to inject an anesthetic in the involved area to make it numb. A small piece can then be taken (a *biopsy*) for laboratory examination.
- It is not reasonable for a doctor to biopsy *every* white lesion (most persons have more than one). Rather, considerable experience is needed to decide which lesions should be biopsied. It is advisable, however, to biopsy a *suspicious white lesion* that has the following characteristics:
  - It is firm to the touch.
  - It is raised from the surrounding flat, white tissue.
  - It has a raw area.
  - There is slight bleeding when the lesion is gently scraped.
  - It hurts.
  - It is enlarging in spite of treatment.

○ TREATMENT

- If seen early enough and the possible causes are stopped or reduced, leukoplakia can be reversed and the lining can become nearly normal. This is one of the few instances in which a precancerous lesion can be reversed.
- The first treatment, therefore, if there are no signs or symptoms of a cancer, is to *stop* what may be causing it.
- Certain forms of drug therapy can also reverse the progress of leukoplakia.

If a biopsy of a leukoplakia is done and it shows suspicious changes, then further treatment of the leukoplakia is necessary. If there are cancerous changes in the leukoplakia, this then becomes a more involved matter requiring more extensive surgery. If this becomes the case with you, we will have a detailed discussion about it.

PREOPERATIVE PREPARATION

- If a more extensive operation is to be done under general anesthetic, then you will have a general physical examination as well as testing of your blood, urine, heart (EKG), and lungs (chest x-ray).
- Do not eat or drink anything for 8 hours before the operation.
- You will be given medicine that will make you feel drowsy before you are brought to the operating room.

□ OPERATION

- Anesthesia:
  - If the operation is to be done under general anesthesia, the anesthetic will be given to you by vein. You will go to sleep promptly.
  - If the operation is going to be done under local anesthesia, a fine, short needle will be used to inject the area with an anesthetic and make it completely numb.
  - The decision on which anesthetic is to be used will be discussed with you beforehand.
  - Smaller, isolated lesions usually are removed under local anesthesia.
- If the lesion is large and suspicious, it will be removed under general anesthesia and the wound edges closed with dissolving sutures.
- If the leukoplakic lesions are not responding to medical treatment or are getting worse (but are not suspicious for cancer), they can be eliminated by being burned with electrocautery or laser therapy.
- As with any operation, complications are always possible. Although they are uncommon with your type of operation, complications can include separation of the wound, prolonged healing, and possibly others.
- You should be able to go home the same or the following day.

POSTOPERATIVE CARE

- Resume your usual activities.
- Rinse your mouth three times a day with room-temperature water in which you have dissolved 1/2 teaspoons of salt per quart of water. Do this for 3 to 5 days.
- Pain can be controlled with over-the-counter pain medicine.
- Soft, bland food is more comfortable to chew while the incision or raw areas are healing.

Note: Whatever treatment you have for your leukoplakia, you must be seen by your doctor at regular intervals. This is to detect any new lesions when they are in an early stage.

✆ CALL OUR OFFICE IF

- You notice any bleeding from the area.
- You have any unusual problems.
- You have any questions.

LIPOMA (FATTY TUMOR)

△ GENERAL INFORMATION

A lipoma is an abnormal collection of fat cells that is almost always under the skin but can sometimes be deeper, such as in the muscle. The mass usually is smooth and in the shape of a sphere or egg (Fig. 1). Lipomas can occur anytime after puberty in both females and males and can be found virtually anywhere in the body. Mostly, however, they are seen in the front and back of the chest and abdomen and in the arms and legs. The masses can be pea-size or the size of a grapefruit or even larger.

COMMON SIGNS AND SYMPTOMS

- Usually, a soft, painless, movable mass under the skin is discovered by chance.
- If it is large, it may interfere with function, especially of the arm or leg.

DIAGNOSIS

- Usually, the diagnosis can be made by taking a detailed history and doing a thorough physical examination. By far, most masses as described above are simple lipomas. Sometimes, however, additional tests may be necessary.
- *Ultrasound:* Harmless sound waves (ultrasound) are aimed at the area of the lipoma. The sound waves bouncing back (the echoes) from this area are seen as a picture on a screen. This is a painless and convenient way to examine such a mass and determine whether it is made of fat.
- *CT scan (computed tomography scan):* A machine that is shaped like a huge doughnut is used to take special x-rays. You will lie on the table inside the hole in the "doughnut." The x-rays are taken as very thin slices through the mass and surrounding tissue. This makes it possible to see inside the mass to estimate what it may be made of and whether it is benign or malignant. This technique is especially useful for examining deeper masses that cannot be felt well enough.
- *Biopsy:* If the mass is very large, stuck to the neighboring tissue, or more firm than the usual lipoma, the risk that it is a malignant lipoma (a *liposarcoma*) increases. If this is a concern, then just a small piece of it (a *biopsy*) needs to be taken for examination in the laboratory. The reason for taking a biopsy is that if the mass is malignant, the operation to remove it is entirely different from that for a benign lipoma. The biopsy can be performed in one of two ways as follows:
  - *Core needle biopsy:* The skin over the mass is swabbed with an antiseptic solution and injected with an anesthetic to make it numb. A special needle is placed through the skin and into the mass, and a core sample of the mass is obtained (about as thick as the lead in a pencil).
  - *Open biopsy:* The skin over the mass is swabbed with an antiseptic solution and surrounded with sterile towels. A thin, short needle is used to inject an anesthetic in the skin over the mass to make the area numb. An incision is made through the numb skin down to the mass, and a biopsy is taken for examination in the pathology laboratory.

○ TREATMENT

- Most lipomas do not need to be removed if they can be observed.
- An operation is advisable in the following circumstances:
  - The diagnosis of lipoma is not certain.
  - The lipoma is larger than 3 inches, because the chance of it being malignant increases when it is this size or larger.
  - The lipoma interferes with function.
  - The presumed lipoma is fixed to the surrounding tissue and so is not movable.
  - The lipoma is felt to be unsightly.

After careful consideration of all factors, the recommendation is that your fatty tumor be removed.

PREOPERATIVE PREPARATION

- Do not eat or drink anything for 8 hours before the operation.
- Shower or bathe as usual on the morning of the operation.

□ OPERATION

- You will lie on a comfortable table.
- The skin over the lipoma will be swabbed with antiseptic solution and surrounded with sterile towels.
- A thin, short needle will be used to inject an anesthetic in the skin over the mass to make the area numb.
- A cosmetic incision will be made, the lipoma removed, and the incision closed in a cosmetic fashion (Fig. 1).
- During the operation, you may feel some tugging but not pain.

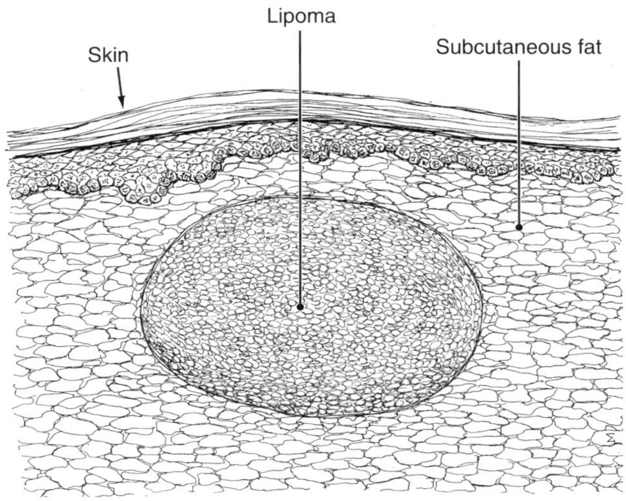

Figure 1. Once the lipoma is reached through the skin incision, it usually can be "shelled" out easily from the surrounding tissue, very much like removing the yolk in a hard-boiled egg.

POSTOPERATIVE CARE

- Your blood pressure, pulse, and breathing will be checked when they are stable. You then should be able to go home with a responsible adult.
- Arrangements will be made for any pain medicine and your follow-up office visit and suture removal.
- As with any operation, complications are always possible. Although they are uncommon with this type of operation, they can include bleeding, infection, and possibly others.

✚ HOME CARE

- You may resume your usual activities.
- You may shower if you wish and with any dressings on or off.
  - There may be narrow strips of tape across the incision. It's all right if they get wet; they will be removed in the doctor's office.
  - After you dry yourself, replace any dressings with clean, dry ones.

✆ CALL OUR OFFICE IF

- The wound becomes red or swollen, or there is any drainage from it.
- The wound becomes increasingly painful.
- You develop a temperature higher than 100°F.
- You have any questions.

△ GENERAL INFORMATION

Liposuction is a very effective and popular way of removing fat from certain areas of the body by sucking the fat away with special instruments. Liposuction is *not* meant to take off weight if you are overweight. The purpose of liposuction is to contour certain areas of your body so that they look better and are in proportion to the rest of your body.

Areas of the body that most commonly need to be contoured vary somewhat between women and men, as follows:

- *Women:* Cheeks, upper outer breasts, inner upper arms, upper hips ("saddle bags"), outer and inner thighs
- *Men:* Abdomen, upper waist ("love handles"), inner thighs
- *Both:* Jowls, neck, abdomen

Areas that seem to need contouring but are more difficult to do successfully include buttocks, calves, and ankles.

FAVORABLE CONDITIONS FOR LIPOSUCTION

- You have good skin tone. This means that when the fat is removed from under the skin, the skin will be able to spring back rather than remain loose and sagging. If the skin is loose and flabby to begin with, the results won't be as pleasing.
- You have tried to take off body fat with proper exercise and diet.
- You realize that liposuction is not for weight reduction and that the few pounds of fat that may be removed won't do anything for your weight.
- It is best if you have taken off as much weight as possible and then have the bulges contoured. The ideal then is not to put on weight again. Fortunately, even if you do put on weight, the contour (and proportions) frequently remain esthethically pleasing.
- Liposuction is not meant to improve on an unfavorable appearance caused by cellulite. Cellulite is not just a condition of too many or too large fat cells. Instead, it is caused by strands of fibrous tissue that pull down on the skin and give it an uneven appearance.

EXPECTATIONS OF LIPOSUCTION

- Liposuction is not a magic cure. It is not meant for quick and easy beauty. You should be realistic about what to expect.
- Liposuction (as with other cosmetic procedures) is something for you to decide that you want done for yourself. It should not be done primarily because you wish to please someone else.
- With most successful cosmetic procedures, a person's self-esteem improves. Be sure you understand this effect, because liposuction in itself in no way ensures that you will experience a dramatic change in your personal or professional life.

PREOPERATIVE PREPARATION

- Preoperative (and, later, postoperative) pictures will be taken.
- You will have an examination of your blood and urine. For persons older than 40 years of age there may also be an examination of the heart (EKG) and lungs (chest x-ray).
- Depending on the area of your body having the liposuction, you will be asked to wear a girdle-like garment (of your own) to firmly press down on the tissue that was worked on. This helps prevent bleeding; it presses down on the skin so that it can properly attach itself to the tissue deep to it; and it helps the injected fluid be absorbed in a better fashion. If your abdomen is to be done, bring such a garment with you.
- Do not eat or drink anything for 8 hours before the operation.
- Shower as usual on the morning of the operation.
- You may be given medicine that will make you feel drowsy before you are brought to the operating room.

□ OPERATION

- The nurse will thoroughly wash the area that will undergo liposuction with an antiseptic soap.
- While you are awake, areas on your body that are to have liposuction will be outlined by the surgeon with a special marker.
- The areas to be done will be draped with sterile towels.
- The surgeon will inject a large amount of fluid under your skin. This fluid will contain the anesthetic. Also, it will have in it a medicine that will make the capillaries close down some; this helps to reduce bleeding during the operation. Injecting this medicine may take 30 minutes or longer, depending on how wide an area is to be done. Because your tissue will swell with this fluid, this method of doing the procedure is called the *tumescent technique* of liposuction.
- You may be given some medicine to make you feel drowsy during the operation. Sometimes liposuction is done under general anesthesia.
- The liposuction needles *(cannulas)* range in size from a toothpick to a straw. They have openings on their sides so that as the cannula is advanced, tiny amounts of fat bulge into the needle. As the needle is moved back and forth, the tiny goblets of fat bulging into the needle are cut away and are sucked back up tubing that is connected to the needle and to a powerful suction machine (Figs. 1 and 2).
- The needles will be inserted through tiny incisions, which are usually made in a natural crease of the skin, where they will show the least.
- During the procedure, you will hear the machine and feel some tugging but you should not feel any pain.

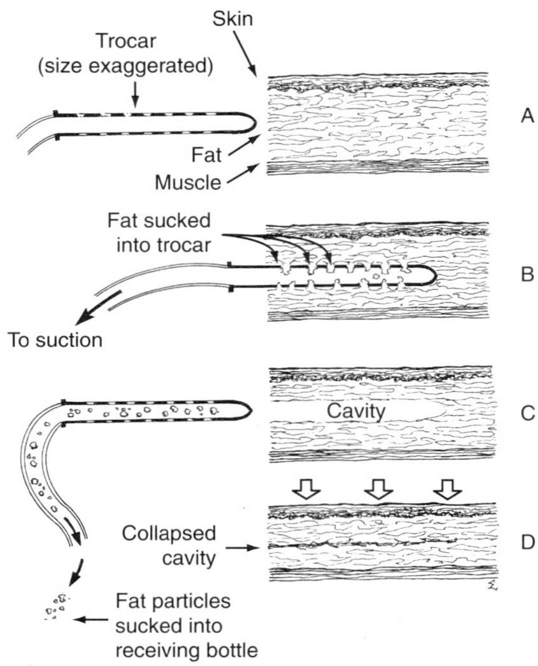

Figure 1. *A,* A section of the body surface showing skin, fat, and muscle. The trocar (the size is exaggerated) has multiple holes that have sharp cutting edges throughout its length. *B,* When the trocar is introduced into the fat, a small amount of fat bulges through each of the holes and into the trocar that has suction applied to it. *C,* As the trocar is withdrawn, it cuts off the small amounts of fat bulging inside it. They are sucked into a receiving bottle. This process is repeated as often as necessary. *D,* The created cavities collapse so that the entire area does not bulge as before.

- The operation can take from half an hour to several hours, depending on how large an area needs to be done.
- You will not need a blood transfusion.
- The short incisions used to insert the cannula will be closed in a cosmetic fashion.

POSTOPERATIVE CARE

- You will be taken to a recovery room. When your blood pressure, pulse, and breathing are stable and you are completely alert, you should be able to go home that same day with a responsible adult.
- Pain can be controlled with medicine.
- Arrangements will be made for your medicine, follow-up office visit, and stitch removal.

✣ HOME CARE

- Expect some straw-colored drainage from your incisions. Gauze pads over the incision can be changed as needed.
- You may walk about as you wish, even climb stairs.
- Your diet can be the same as before the liposuction.
- When you remove your girdle, do it slowly and carefully.
- You may shower as you wish, with any dressings on or off.
  - There may be narrow strips of tape across the incisions. It's all right if they get wet; they will be removed in the doctor's office.
  - After you dry yourself, replace any dressings with clean, dry ones.
- Take medicine as prescribed for your pain.
- Your tissue will look swollen and bruised for a few weeks. It may take 3 to 6 months for you to see the "final" result. However, in a month or so you will see about 75% of what will be the final appearance.
- You may drive if you are not stiff or in pain and are not taking pain medicines.
- You may resume sexual activity whenever you choose.
- You may return to work when you feel up to it.

✆ CALL OUR OFFICE IF

- You develop sudden swelling or a bruised area.
- The incision becomes red or swollen, or there is drainage from it.
- You develop a temperature higher than 100°F.
- You have any questions.

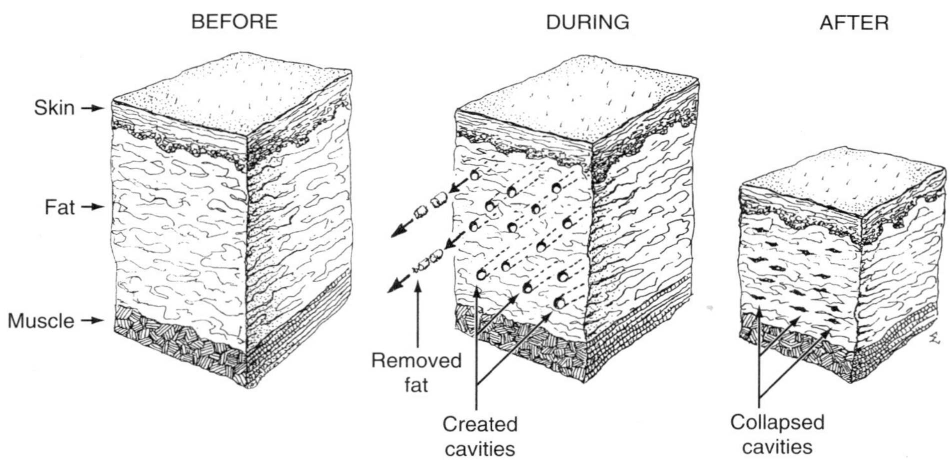

Figure 2. The liposuction process shown in a three-dimensional way.

△ GENERAL INFORMATION

Echinococcus granulosus is a tapeworm that lives in the intestines of dogs. Eggs of this tapeworm pass in the stool of the dog and can be found in the dust where dogs run loose. The eggs that are in the dust can be transferred to humans' hands and can be ingested at an early age. The eggs then travel to the liver, grow there, and can produce an echinococcal cyst.

This disease generally is found in middle-aged or older people from areas where humans and working dogs live in intimate proximity. It is rare in the United States, but immigration from countries where *Echinococcus* is common may increase the chances of seeing it in this country.

COMMON SIGNS AND SYMPTOMS

- Abdominal pain, especially in the right side of the upper abdomen.
- There may be fever, chills, hives, or jaundice.
- A mass in the right side of the upper abdomen.

DIAGNOSIS

- The diagnosis can be suspected in a person with the above signs and symptoms, especially if that person is from an area where *Echinococcus* is common.
- *X-ray of the abdomen:* This may show a calcified ring, something that occurs with ecchinococcal cyst.
- *Ultrasound*: Harmless sound waves are aimed at the liver. The sounds waves bouncing back (the echoes) from this area are seen as a picture on a screen. This is a convenient and painless way to examine the liver.
- *CT scan (computed tomography scan)*: A machine shaped like a huge doughnut is used to take special x-rays. You will lie on the table inside the hole in the "doughnut." The x-rays are taken as very thin slices through the liver. This makes it possible to see the fine details in the liver.

○ TREATMENT

The treatment usually is an operation both to relieve symptoms and to prevent complications.

PREOPERATIVE PREPARATION

- In addition to the liver, the heart (EKG) and lungs (chest x-ray) will be carefully examined for possible problems that might have an effect on the treatment.
- Do not eat or drink anything for 8 hours before the operation.
- You may be given medicine that will make you feel drowsy before you are brought to the operating room.

□ OPERATION

- The incision will be made over the liver in the right side of your upper abdomen.

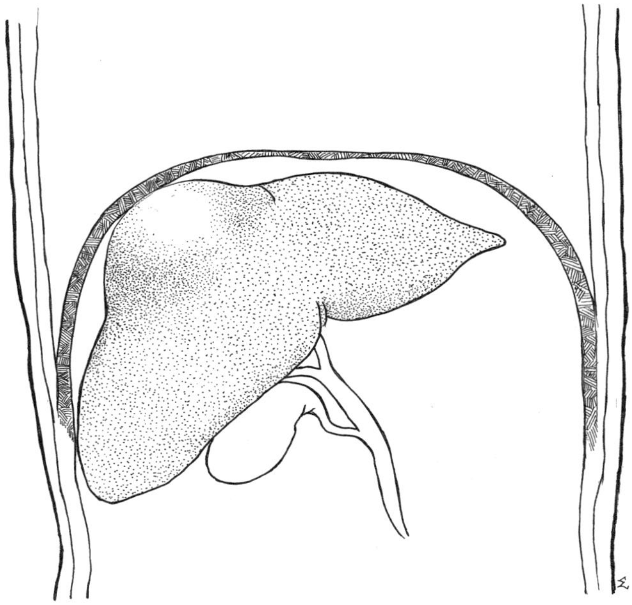

Figure 1. A typical appearance of the liver with an echinococcal cyst in it.

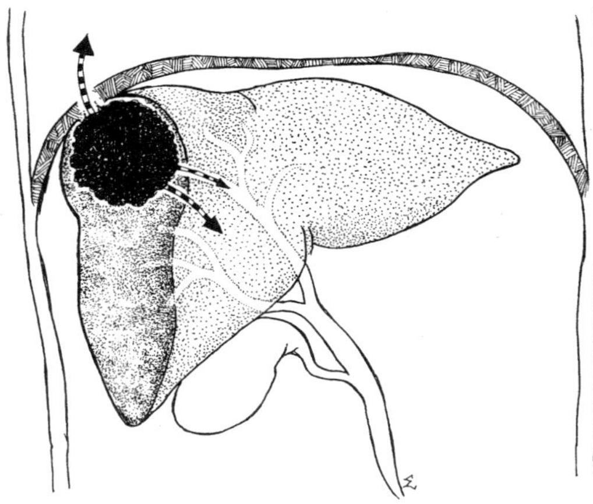

Figure 2. A cutaway of the liver in Figure 1. It shows some of the ways an echinococcal cyst may cause serious harm: upward extension through the diaphragm and into the chest cavity; rupture into the bile ducts or into the abdomen.

- The aims of the operation are as follows:
  - To remove the cyst *entirely*, if possible, because if any tissue is left behind it may cause another cyst to form (Figs. 1 and 2).
  - To remove "daughter" cysts from the bile ducts.
  - To remove the gallbladder.
  - To close the holes in the bile ducts.
- You will not receive a blood transfusion unless it is absolutely necessary.
- The operation usually takes 2 to 3 hours.

POSTOPERATIVE CARE

- You will wake up in a recovery room. When your blood pressure, pulse, and breathing are stable, you will be taken to a regular hospital room.
- The evening after the operation you will be helped to sit up in bed and on the next day to get out of bed.
- Pain can be controlled with medicine. The nurse will give it to you. Or, you can give yourself a preset amount of pain medicine when you feel the need for it. This is done with a device for patient-controlled analgesia (PCA) that is connected to the tubing giving you intravenous fluids.
- You may have a thin plastic tube in your nose. It goes down to your stomach to suck up the air you swallow. It will be removed when your bowels start working.
- Your diet will be increased as you tolerate it.
- As with any operation, complications are always possible. With your type of operation, complications can include bleeding, pneumonia, heart problems, jaundice, wound infection, and possibly others.
- Arrangements will be made for your medicine, follow-up office visit, and stitch removal.
- With early treatment, survival and cure are possible in nearly all patients with this condition.

✣ HOME CARE

- Resume your usual activities.
- You may walk about as you wish, even climb stairs, but don't overdo things.
- Take medicines as prescribed for your pain.
- You may eat as you did before the operation.
- Be careful that you do not become constipated.
  - Include enough roughage and liquid in your diet.
  - You may need a mild laxative (example: milk of magnesia).
- You may shower as you wish and with any dressings on or off.
  - There may be narrow strips of tape across the incision. It's all right if they get wet; they will be removed in the doctor's office.
  - After you dry yourself, replace any dressings with clean, dry ones.
- Driving a car with an automatic shift is not too demanding, but if you suddenly have to slam on the brakes or twist to turn the wheel, you may strain the sutures or tear something. During your follow-up visit, let's discuss when you can resume driving.
- You may resume sexual activity whenever you choose.
- You may return to work when you feel up to it but let's first talk about it during your follow-up office visit.

✆ CALL OUR OFFICE IF

- The incision becomes red or swollen, or there is drainage from it.
- You develop a temperature higher than 100°F.
- You have any questions.

△ GENERAL INFORMATION

An abscess of the liver can be difficult to diagnose and treat, but if it is not treated early and properly, there can be serious problems.

An amebic liver abscess can occur as follows:

- Transmitting amebas from hand to mouth with food.
- The amebas can come from an amebic dysentery, in which the amebas have caused an ulceration in the bowel. The amebas travel through the vein (portal vein) that drains all of the blood from the intestine into the liver.

COMMON SIGNS AND SYMPTOMS

- Pain in the right side of the upper abdomen.
- Sometimes there is pain in the right shoulder or neck.
- Fever, chills, and jaundice.
- Decreased breath sounds in the lower part of the right lung. The amebic abscess is located just under this part of the right lung.
- Nausea, vomiting, loss of appetite, or weight loss.
- Tenderness in the right side of the upper abdomen caused by the abscess there.

DIAGNOSIS

- A detailed history is taken and a thorough physical examination is done to search for a cause of the abscess.
- Serum blood tests.
- Stool is examined for the presence of amebas or salmonellae.
- *Chest x-ray*: The right lung can be affected up to 50% of the time.
- *Ultrasound*: Harmless sound waves are aimed at the abdomen, with special attention to the liver. The sound waves bouncing back (the echoes) from this area are seen as a picture on a screen. This is a convenient and painless way to examine the inside of the entire abdomen, and especially the liver, for any abnormality. Also, ultrasonography can tell whether the abnormality is a solid tumor or something with liquid in it.
- *CT scan (computed tomographic scan)*: These special x-rays are taken by a machine that is shaped like a huge doughnut. You will lie on the table inside the hole in the "doughnut." The x-rays are taken as very thin slices through the liver. This makes it possible to see fine details in the liver and to tell whether the abnormality is a solid tumor or something with fluid in it.
- *Colonoscopy*: This is done with a smooth, flexible optical instrument as big around as your little finger with a light at its tip. During the procedure you will be given medicine that will make you feel drowsy. The tip of the instrument will be lubricated and then gently inserted into your anus. The entire inside of your colon will be examined for evidence of infection with amebas.

○ TREATMENT

- The requirements for successful treatment are to make the correct diagnosis of amebiasis by means of a thorough history or serum tests, or by aspirating some of the abscess fluid with a needle for laboratory examination.
- If you now have, or in the recent past have had, amebic dysentery, or if there is strong evidence that amebic infection is the cause of the liver abscess, treatment with medicine against amebas is appropriate. The treatment consists of pills and drainage with a needle.
- In the rare case in which there is a poor response to medical therapy, then an operation is the recommended treatment.

After careful consideration of all factors, it is recommended that you have an operation for your liver abscess (Fig. 1). The reasons for this recommendation have already been explained to you.

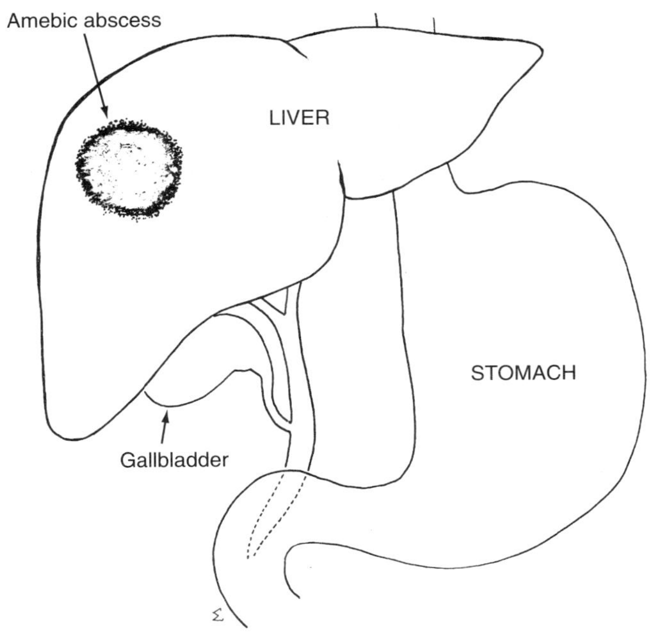

Figure 1. A single abscess is shown. There may be more than one, however, which is sometimes not discovered until the liver is exposed in the operating room. Such unexpected findings can change the planned therapy.

PREOPERATIVE PREPARATION

- You will have an examination of your heart (EKG), blood, and urine.
- Do not eat or drink anything for 8 hours before the operation.
- You may be given medicine that will make you feel drowsy before you are brought to the operating room.

☐ OPERATION

- You will be asleep for the operation.
- The exact procedure will depend on what is found and what needs to be done to correct the problem.

POSTOPERATIVE CARE

- You will wake up in a recovery room. When your blood pressure, pulse, and breathing are stable, you will be taken to a regular hospital room.
- Pain can be controlled with medicine. The nurse will give it to you, or you can give yourself a preset amount of pain medicine when you feel you need it. This is done with a device for patient-controlled analgesia (PCA) that is connected to the tubing giving you intravenous fluids.
- The evening after the operation you will be helped to sit up in bed and on the next day to get out of bed.
- You may have a thin plastic tube in your nose. It goes down to your stomach to suck up the air you swallow. When your bowels start working, it will be removed and you will be started on a liquid diet.
- Conditions that influence how well you do include the following:
  - Your age.
  - The number of abscess cavities in the liver.
  - The number of different bacteria in the abscess cavity.
  - Other medical problems you might have.
- As with any operation, complications are always possible. With this type of operation, complications can include pneumonia, wound infection, bleeding, heart problems, and possibly others.
- Arrangements will be made for your medicine, follow-up office visit, and stitch removal.

✚ HOME CARE

- You may walk about as you wish, even climb stairs.
- Take the medicine prescribed for your pain.
- Eat as you wish.
- Be careful that you do not become constipated.
  - Include enough roughage and liquid in your diet.
  - You may need a mild laxative (example: milk of magnesia).
- You may shower if you wish, with any dressings on or off.
  - There may be narrow strips of tape across the incision. It's all right if they get wet; they will be removed in the doctor's office.
  - After you dry yourself, replace the dressings with clean, dry ones.
- Driving a car with an automatic shift is not too demanding, but if you suddenly have to slam on the brakes or twist to turn the steering wheel, you may get into an accident. Or you may strain the sutures or tear something. During your follow-up visit let's discuss when you can resume driving.
- You may resume sexual activity whenever you choose.
- You may return to work when you feel up to it, but let's talk about it first during an office follow-up visit.

✆ CALL OUR OFFICE IF

- You develop any unusual signs or symptoms.
- The incision becomes red or swollen, or there is drainage from it.
- You develop a temperature higher than 100°F.
- You have any questions.

LIVER ABSCESS: Pyogenic (Bacterial)

△ GENERAL INFORMATION

An abscess of the liver can be difficult to diagnose and to treat, but if it is not treated early and properly, it can have serious consequences.

A liver abscess can develop in several ways:

- From an infected gallbladder and bile ducts (which are attached to the liver).
- Infections of the intestines or the appendix (all of the blood from the intestines drains into the liver).
- After abdominal surgery.

Liver abscess is seen in persons of both sexes and more often in older people.

COMMON SIGNS AND SYMPTOMS

- Signs and symptoms can come on suddenly or slowly and can be vague.
- The lower part of the right lung may not work well enough because of an abscess that is just beneath it.
- Fever and shaking chills.
- Pain or tenderness in the right side of the upper abdomen, or in the shoulder or the neck, especially on deep breathing.
- Nausea, loss of appetite, weight loss, and fatigue.

DIAGNOSIS

Making the diagnosis is not always easy because a number of diseases can act like a liver abscess. Any or all of the following tests may be done:

- Chest x-ray to see if the right lung is affected (up to 50% of the time).
- *Ultrasound*: Harmless sound waves are aimed at the abdomen, with special attention to the liver. The sound waves bouncing back (the echoes) from this area are seen as a picture on a screen. This is a painless and convenient way to examine the inside of the entire abdomen, and especially the liver, for any abnormality. Also, ultrasonography can tell whether the abnormality in the liver is a solid tumor or something with liquid in it.
- *CT scan (computed tomography scan)*: A machine shaped like a huge doughnut is used to take special x-rays. You will lie on the table inside the hole in the "doughnut." The x-rays are taken as very thin slices through the liver. This makes it possible to see fine details in the liver and to tell whether the abnormality is a solid tumor or something with fluid in it.
- Occasionally it is appropriate to place a needle in the suspected area to see if any pus is present (needle aspiration).

○ TREATMENT

- The important things for successful treatment are the following:
  - To find the cause of the abscess and to correct it (Fig. 1).
  - To vigorously give appropriate antibiotics.
  - To drain the abscess.
- If a liver abscess caused by bacteria is not treated at all, or does not respond to treatment that is only medical, it is almost always fatal.

After careful consideration of all factors, the recommendation is that you have an operation to drain your liver abscess.

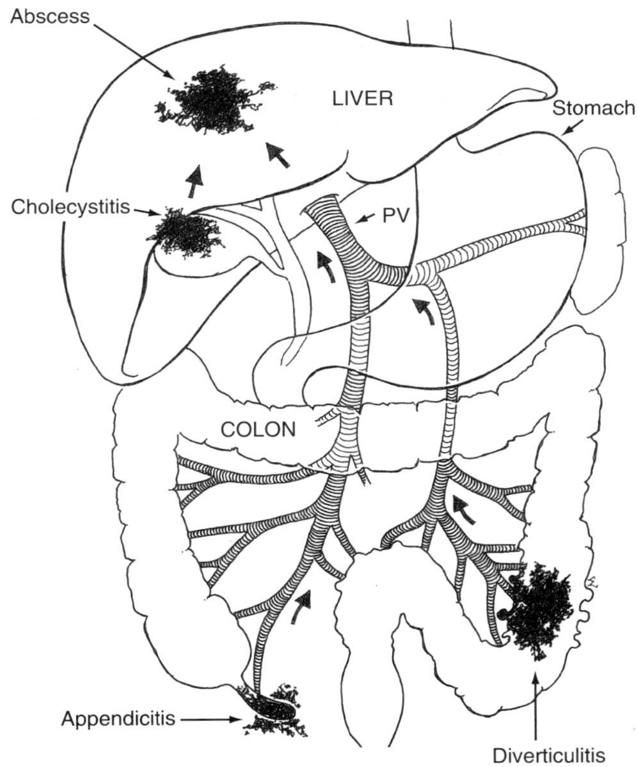

Figure 1. An abscess may form in the liver directly or may extend into it from an infected gallbladder that is attached to the liver. Also appendicitis or diverticulitis from which bacteria travel up the vein to the portal vein (PV) and into the liver.

PREOPERATIVE PREPARATION

- You will have an examination of your blood, urine, heart (EKG), and lungs (chest x-ray).
- Any associated problems you might have will be corrected as much as possible before the operation.
- Every effort will be made to find the cause of the abscess before the operation so that, if possible, it can be treated at the same time as the abscess.
- Do not eat or drink anything for 8 hours before the operation.
- Shower as usual on the morning of the operation.
- You may be given medicine that will make you feel drowsy before you are brought to the operating room.

☐ OPERATION

- You will be asleep for the operation.
- During the operation, there will be a careful search for other smaller abscesses that may not have been picked up by the tests.
- Sometimes the abscess can be safely emptied with a thin tube that is placed in the cavity and brought through to the outside.
- If the cause of the abscess is found before or even during the operation, this will be taken care of at the same time, if possible.

POSTOPERATIVE CARE

- You will be taken to a recovery room and observed. When your blood pressure, pulse, and breathing are stable, you will be taken to a regular hospital room.
- You will have a thin plastic tube in your nose. It goes down to your stomach to suck up the air you swallow. It will be removed when your bowels start working.
- There may be a drain coming to the outside from the abscess cavity to release any additional fluid present.
- Pain will be controlled with medicine.
- The evening after the operation you will be helped to sit up in bed and on the next day to get out of bed.
- You will be given an incentive spirometer. Breathing into this as you are instructed will help you expand your lungs and reduce the risk of developing pneumonia.
- After the tube in your nose is removed, your diet will start off with fluids and be increased as you tolerate it.
- Your recovery time will depend on how extensive the operation was and your condition in general.
- As with any operation, complications are always possible. With this type of operation, complications can include additional abscesses that are not found, pneumonia, blood clots, heart problems, wound infection, and possibly others.
- Arrangements will be made for your pain medicine, antibiotics, follow-up office visit, and stitch and drain removal.

✣ HOME CARE

- You may walk about as you wish, even climb stairs.
- You may eat as you did before the operation.
- Be careful that you do not become constipated.
  - Include enough roughage and plenty of liquids in your diet.
- You will be instructed on how to take care of your incision and when you may shower or bathe.
- Arrangements can be made for a visiting nurse if this is necessary.
- You may resume sexual activity whenever you choose.
- You may return to work when you feel up to it.

✆ CALL OUR OFFICE IF

- You develop any unusual signs or symptoms.
- The incision becomes red or swollen, or there is drainage from it.
- You develop a temperature higher than 100°F.
- You have any questions.

LIVER BIOPSY: Needle Aspiration

△ GENERAL INFORMATION

A *biopsy* is the removal and examination of tissue cells or fluid from the living body. This can be necessary for several purposes.

- To make or confirm a diagnosis.
- To examine for hormonal or other chemical clues on how to treat a disease.
- To determine whether there have been changes following treatment.
- To periodically gauge the course of a disease.

The liver is an organ that often needs to have a biopsy taken for some of the above reasons.

PREOPERATIVE PREPARATION

- Do not eat or drink anything for 8 hours before the operation.
- You will have an examination of your blood count and of the bleeding and clotting capabilities of your blood.
- Shower as usual on the morning of the operation.
- You may receive some medicine that will make you drowsy before the procedure.

□ OPERATION

- You will be positioned flat on a comfortable table.
- Ultrasound: Harmless sound waves will be aimed at the area of your liver. The sound waves bouncing back (the echoes) from this area are seen as a picture on a screen. Ultrasonography is a convenient and painless way to examine your liver and locate the area that needs to have the biopsy.
- The skin over this area will be painted with an antiseptic solution and draped.
- A very fine needle will be used to inject an anesthetic into the skin and deeper tissue. The area will become numb.
- A special needle will be inserted through the skin and into the liver and a biopsy sample taken. This part of the procedure usually takes less than 2 minutes. Many times, ultrasonography is used to watch the needle while the biopsy is being performed.
- The removed tissue will be sent to the pathology laboratory for examination.

POSTOPERATIVE CARE

- You will be asked to lie flat for several hours.
- When you are fully alert and your blood pressure, pulse, and breathing are stable, you should be able to go home directly with a responsible adult.
- As with any operation, complications are always possible. Although they are uncommon with this type of operation, complications can include bleeding at the level of the skin or inside the abdomen.

✣ HOME CARE

- Do not do anything strenuous that day.
- Do not lift anything that day.
- Lie down at every opportunity.
- You may eat as you did before the operation.
- You may shower as you wish, with any dressings on or off.
  - After you dry yourself, replace any dressing with a clean, dry one.

✆ CALL OUR OFFICE IF

- You develop any unusual signs or symptoms.
- You feel faint.
- You develop abdominal pain.
- The incision becomes red or swollen, or there is drainage from it.
- You develop a temperature higher than 100°F.
- You have any questions.

△ GENERAL INFORMATION

A *biopsy* is the removal and examination of tissue cells or fluid from the living body. This can be necessary for several purposes:

- To make or confirm a diagnosis.
- To examine for hormonal or other chemical clues on how to treat a disease.
- To determine whether there have been changes following treatment.
- To periodically gauge the course of a disease.

The liver is an organ that often needs to have a biopsy taken for some of the above reasons.

An *open* biopsy is done:

- If more tissue (the size of a sugar cube or larger) is needed.
- So as to place the ultrasound probe directly on the liver for greater accuracy in localizing the tissue that is being biopsied.
- If it would be too dangerous to stick a needle in the liver, as in the case of certain lesions like a blood vessel tumor; also to see if such a lesion can or should be removed.

PREOPERATIVE PREPARATION

- You will have an examination of your blood, urine, heart (EKG), and lungs (chest x-ray).
- Do not eat or drink anything for 8 hours before the operation.
- Shower as usual on the morning of the operation.
- You may be given medicine that will make you feel drowsy before you are brought to the operating room.

□ OPERATION

- The skin of your upper right abdomen will be swabbed with an antiseptic solution and draped with sterile towels.
- The operation will be done under local anesthesia. The skin over the liver will be made numb.
- You will be given medicine that will keep you drowsy.
- There will be a short incision under your right ribs.
- During the operation, you may feel some tugging, but no pain.
- The operation usually takes less than 1 hour.
- The removed tissue will be sent to the pathology laboratory for examination.

POSTOPERATIVE CARE

- When you are fully alert and your blood pressure, pulse, and breathing are stable, you should be able to go home directly with a responsible adult.
- As with any operation, complications are always possible. Although they are uncommon with your type of operation, complications can include bleeding inside the abdomen and wound infection.

✙ HOME CARE

- Do not do anything strenuous that day.
- Do not lift anything that day.
- Lie down at every opportunity.
- You may eat as you did before the operation.
- You may shower as you wish, with any dressings on or off.
  - There may be narrow strips of tape across the incision. It's all right if they get wet; they will be removed at the doctor's office.
  - After you dry yourself, replace any dressings with clean, dry ones across the incision.
- Take medicine as prescribed for your pain.

✆ CALL OUR OFFICE IF

- You develop any unusual signs or symptoms.
- You feel faint.
- You develop pain in your abdominal area.
- The incision becomes red or swollen, or there is drainage from it.
- You develop a temperature higher than 100°F.
- You have any questions.

LIVER CANCER: Cryosurgery (Cryoablation)

△ GENERAL INFORMATION

Until just a few years ago, if someone had a cancer in the liver that had started or traveled there *(metastasized)* from elsewhere in the body, the chances of cure were thought to be hopeless because it was too dangerous to remove the portion of the liver with the cancer in it. Now, this is no longer true. A number of new techniques have made it possible to remove with intent to cure up to three-fifths of the cancerous liver and to do it without too much risk.

COMMON PATIENT HISTORY

- There is a history of cancer elsewhere in the body (specifically the large bowel) that was removed but now has spread to the liver.
- There is a vague pain in the upper abdomen.
- A new cancer just developed in a normal liver or in a liver with cirrhosis.

COMMON SIGNS AND SYMPTOMS

- Pain in the right part of the upper abdomen.
- Some new abnormalities in the liver test results.
- Worsening or some additional abnormalities in a patient with chronic hepatitis.

DIAGNOSIS

A person who has the above history and symptoms should have some or all of the following tests done to see whether liver metastases are present.

- You will have an examination of your blood, urine, heart (EKG), and lungs (chest x-ray).
- *Ultrasound*: Harmless sound waves are aimed at the area of your liver. The sound waves bouncing back (the echoes) from this area are seen as a picture on a screen. This is a convenient and painless way to examine the liver.
- *CT scan (computed tomography scan)*: Special x-rays are taken as very thin slices through the area of the upper abdomen. This makes it possible to see the fine details in the liver.
- *MRI (magnetic resonance imaging)*: No x-rays are used with this technique. Instead, it is done with harmless magnetic fields and radio waves. A computer develops the pictures to show organs from several angles. It is especially valuable for examining blood vessels in relation to tissue.
- *Liver biopsy*: This can determine whether any abnormality seen with other studies is really cancer. The skin over the tumor area is made numb and a special fine needle is used to go through the numbed skin and into the suspected area in the liver. A tiny piece of the suspected tissue (a *biopsy*) is obtained for laboratory examination.
- *Bone scan*: A tiny amount of a harmless radioactive solution is injected into your vein, which then circulates throughout your entire body and attaches itself to any part of a bone that has something wrong with it. You will lie on a table as a special machine passes over your entire body taking a series of photographs (a *scan*) of all the bones from your skull to your toes. A specialist then examines the scan, looking for any abnormalities.

It has been determined that you have cancer in your liver. There is no evidence of cancer elsewhere in your body.

○ TREATMENT

The cancer in your liver is so close to important structures that it cannot be removed without very great risk or leaving you with too little healthy liver. It is possible, however, to kill the tumor where it sits by freezing it. The body can then slowly absorb this killed cancer tissue.

After taking all factors into consideration, it is recommended that you have an operation to freeze these cancers.

PREOPERATIVE PREPARATION

- In addition to your other tests, special attention will be given to your heart (EKG), lungs (chest x-ray), and kidneys.
- Do not eat or drink anything for 8 hours before the operation.

□ OPERATION

- Several patterns of cancer in the liver are shown that are suitable for treatment by freezing (Figs. 1–3).

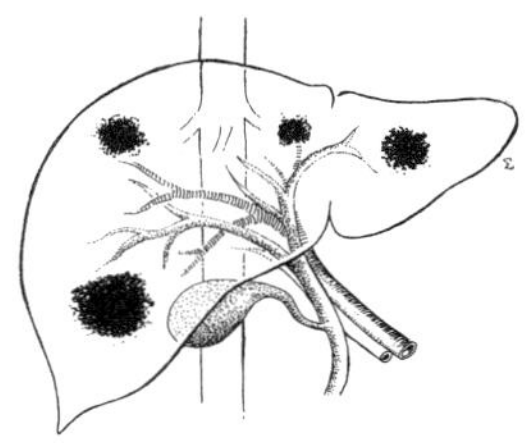

Figure 1. The metastatic lesions *(dark spots)* are spread too far apart, so too much surrounding normal tissue would be lost in removing them.

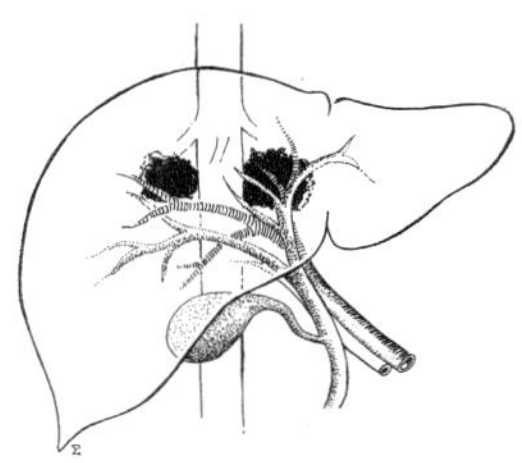

Figure 2. The location of these lesions tightly against each side of the big vein (vena cava) running through the center of the liver makes it too risky to try to remove them.

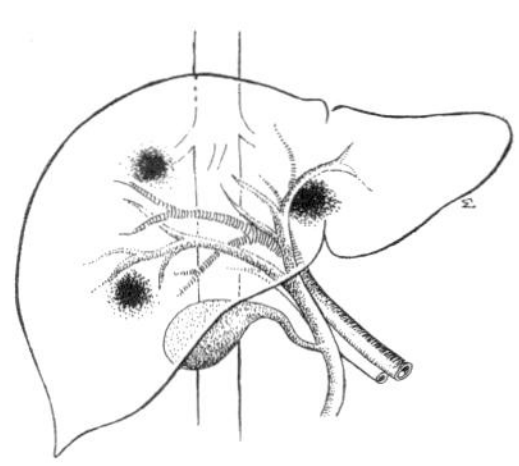

Figure 3. The lesions are not too large, but they are widely spread and are attached to blood vessels. If these blood vessels were removed, too much normal liver tissue would die.

- The abdomen will be opened, and the specially designed freezing needles will be guided to the metastases with the help of ultrasonography.
- The operation takes about 3 to 4 hours.

POSTOPERATIVE CARE

- You will be taken to a recovery room and observed. When your blood pressure, pulse, and breathing are stable, you will be taken to a regular hospital room.
- A thin plastic tube coming out of your nose goes down to the stomach to keep it empty until it starts working again.
- Pain will be controlled with medicine.
- You should be able to go home in several days.
- Arrangements will be made for your pain medicines, office visit, and stitch removal.
- As with any operation, complications are always possible, some of them serious. With your type of operation, complications can include bleeding, infection, pneumonia, heart problems, jaundice, bowel obstruction, wound infection, liver failure, and possibly others.

✚ HOME CARE

- You may walk about as you wish, even climb stairs, but don't overdo things.
- Take the medicines prescribed for you.
- Your diet can be as you tolerate it.
- Include plenty of roughage and liquids in your diet to help prevent constipation.
- You will be instructed on showering or bathing.
- Do not drive a car until we discuss it first during your follow-up office visit.

✆ CALL OUR OFFICE IF

- You develop any unusual signs or symptoms.
- The incision becomes red or swollen, or there is drainage from it.
- You develop a temperature higher than 100°F.
- You have any questions.

△ GENERAL INFORMATION

Whenever a person is receiving chemotherapy for cancer, the entire body is exposed to chemotherapy, even though in most areas of the body, there is no cancer. The reason all of the body tissue gets the chemotherapy is that once the medicine is swallowed or given into the vein, it travels throughout the entire body.

The thinking behind giving chemotherapy by an infusion pump is as follows: If anticancer medicine distributes itself all over the body when it is given by vein or by mouth, then why not find a way to give the chemotherapy so that it goes only to, or mostly to, the organ with the cancer in it. In this way, the areas of the body without cancer would not be exposed as much to the risks of chemotherapy.

○ TREATMENT

To be able to do this, several things are necessary:

- The anticancer medicine should be given through an artery feeding that organ or area of the body.
- The artery into which the medicine would be injected should be the only artery supplying blood to that organ.
- Because chemotherapy has to be given over a long period of time, the artery should be usable for a long period.
- Because this is the only artery supplying blood to the organ, the artery should not be damaged while it is being used for delivering chemotherapy.

Suitability of the Liver for Therapy by Infusion Pump

- The liver sometimes is the only organ in the body involved with metastatic cancer.
- The liver often has a main vessel that supplies all the areas of it.
  - Several methods have been used to get medicine into this single artery. The best way, however, is to do it by an operation.
  - As a bonus, the chemotherapy could be given in small amounts (a drop or two) at a time but over 24 hours throughout the day.

Before Treatment

- There needs to be a search for cancer at places in the body other than in the liver.
- The liver will be looked at carefully to see if the cancer in it can be destroyed by other, more effective ways, such as removing it or freezing it.

Some of the tests that may be done include the following:

- *CT scan (computed tomography scan)*: Special x-rays are taken as very thin slices through the liver and surrounding area. This makes it possible to see the fine details in the liver.
- *MRI (magnetic resonance imaging)*: No x-rays are used with this technique. Instead, it is done with harmless magnetic fields and radio waves. A computer develops the pictures to show organs from several angles. This technique is especially useful for examining your blood vessels in relation to the tumor.
- *Bone scan*: This is a way to take pictures (a *scan*) of all the bones in your body to see if cancer has spread to them.

After careful consideration of all factors, the recommendation is that you have an operation and have an infusion pump installed (Figs. 1 and 2).

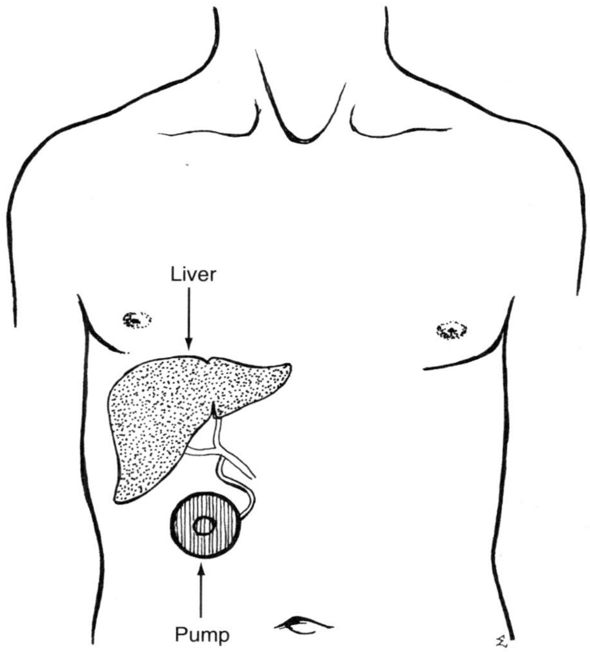

Figure 1. Infusion pump in position.

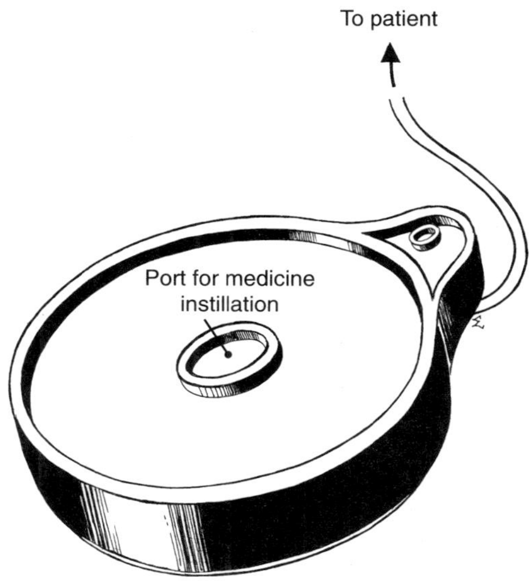

Figure 2. The liver infusion pump can be refilled with medicine as necessary by inserting a needle with the attached syringe containing the medicine straight down to the center of the pump and through a thick rubber cover into the medicine reservoir.

PREOPERATIVE PREPARATION

- There will be an examination of your blood, urine, heart (EKG), and lungs (chest x-ray).
- Do not eat or drink anything for 8 hours before the operation.
- You may be given medicine that will make you feel drowsy before you are brought to the operating room.

☐ OPERATION

- You will be asleep for the operation.
- The pump: This gadget is hollow and about the size of a pack of cigarettes. On one end of the pump there is a very small opening that is designed to let out a drop of fluid from inside the pump every few minutes. One end of a thin plastic tube is connected to this opening; the other end will be placed in the *hepatic* artery (the artery supplying the liver). One flat side of the pump has a special rubber wall. A needle can be inserted through this wall to refill the pump with medicine as necessary.
- The abdomen will be opened and the artery to the liver exposed. There is a small side branch of the hepatic artery that is not important. This side branch will be opened and used to place the tiny plastic tube (the size of angel hair spaghetti) into the hepatic artery.
- The infusion pump itself is placed in your abdominal wall just under the skin with the rubber side facing the skin. The abdomen is then closed.
- You now have a pump just under your skin that is connected to the blood supply to your liver by a small plastic tube.

POSTOPERATIVE CARE

- You will be taken to a recovery room and observed. When your blood pressure, pulse, and breathing are stable, you will be taken to a regular hospital room.
- You may have a thin plastic tube in your nose. It will be removed when your bowels start working and you start eating.
- The evening after the surgery you will be helped to sit up in bed and on the next day to get out of bed.
- Pain will be controlled with medicine.
- You should be able to go home in about 4 days.
- Arrangements will be made for your first follow-up office visit and preparation for filling the pump with anticancer medicine.
- As with any operation, complications are always possible. With this type of operation, complications can include infection, clotting in the pump tubing, bleeding, and possibly others.

✚ HOME CARE

- You may walk about as you wish, even climb stairs.
- You may eat as you did before the operation, but include plenty of roughage and liquids in your diet to help prevent constipation.
- Take medicine as prescribed for your pain.
- Unless instructed otherwise, you may shower as you wish, with any dressings on or off. After you dry yourself, replace any dressings with clean, dry ones.
- You will be informed of the schedule to have your pump refilled. Because a larger share of the medicine will be going to the liver, the side effects should be less than if you received the medicine by mouth or by vein. Also, because the medicine gets to the liver first and before it is diluted, it may be more effective against the tumor in the liver.

✆ CALL OUR OFFICE IF

- The incision becomes red or swollen, or there is drainage from it.
- You develop a temperature higher than 100°F.
- You have any questions.

△ GENERAL INFORMATION

Until just a few years ago, if someone had a cancer in the liver that had started or traveled there *(metastasized)* from elsewhere in the body, the chances of cure were thought to be hopeless because it was too dangerous to remove the portion of the liver with the cancer in it. Now, this is no longer true. A number of new techniques have made it possible to remove with intent to cure up to three-fifths of the cancerous liver and to do it without too much risk.

COMMON PATIENT HISTORY

- There is a history of cancer elsewhere in the body (specifically the large bowel) that was removed but now has spread to the liver.
- There is a vague pain in the upper abdomen.
- A new cancer just developed in a normal liver or in a liver with cirrhosis.

COMMON SIGNS AND SYMPTOMS

- Pain in the right part of the upper abdomen.
- Some new abnormalities in the liver test results.
- Worsening or some additional abnormalities in a patient with chronic hepatitis.

DIAGNOSIS

A person who has the above history and symptoms should have some or all of the following tests done to see if liver metastases are present.

- You will have an examination of your blood, urine, heart (EKG), and lungs (chest x-ray).
- *Ultrasound*: Harmless sound waves are aimed at the area of your liver. The sound waves bouncing back (the echoes) from this area are seen as a picture on a screen. This is a convenient and painless way to examine the liver.
- *CT scan (computed tomography scan)*: Special x-rays are taken as very thin slices through the area of the upper abdomen. This makes it possible to see the fine details in the liver.
- *MRI (magnetic resonance imaging)*: No x-rays are used with this technique. Instead, it is done with harmless magnetic fields and radio waves. A computer develops the pictures to show organs from several angles. This technique is especially valuable for examining blood vessels in relation to the tumor.
- *Liver biopsy*: This can determine whether any abnormality seen with other studies is really cancer. The skin over the tumor area is made numb and a special fine needle is used to go through the numbed skin and into the suspected area in the liver. A tiny piece of the suspected tissue (a *biopsy* specimen) is obtained for laboratory examination.
- *Bone scan*: A tiny amount of a harmless radioactive solution is injected into your vein, which then circulates throughout your entire body and attaches itself to any part of a bone that has something wrong with it. You will lie on a table as a special machine passes over your entire body taking a series of photographs (a *scan*) of all the bones from your skull to your toes. A specialist then examines the scan, looking for any abnormalities.

○ TREATMENT

It has been determined that you have cancer of the liver with no evidence that it is elsewhere in your body. The cancer is in a part of the liver that can be removed and still leave you with enough healthy liver.

Taking all factors into consideration, it is recommended that you have an operation to try to remove these tumors.

PREOPERATIVE PREPARATION

- In addition to your other tests, special attention will be given to your heart (EKG), lungs (chest x-ray), and kidneys.
- Do not eat or drink anything for 8 hours before the operation.

□ OPERATION

- Several types of resection are possible (Figs. 1–3).
- You will not receive a blood transfusion unless it is absolutely necessary.
- The operation takes about 3 to 5 hours.

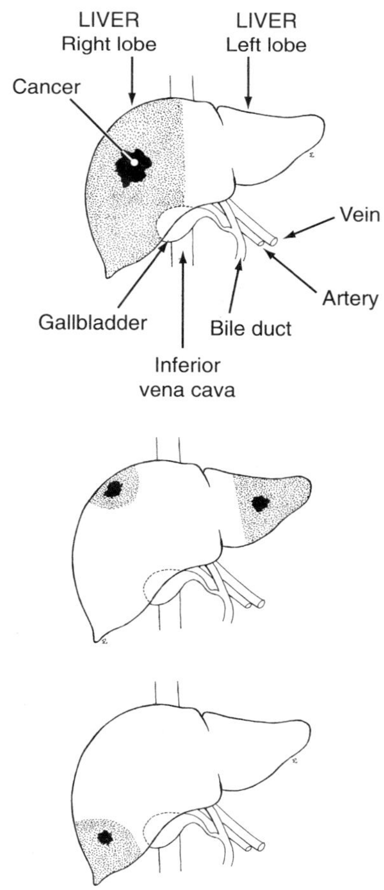

Figures 1–3. Some locations of metastatic cancer suitable for resection *(stippled area)*.

POSTOPERATIVE CARE

- You will be taken to the Surgical Care Unit, where the doctors and nurses are very experienced in taking care of patients with your condition. As soon as you are coming along well enough, you will be transferred to a regular hospital room.
- A thin plastic tube coming out of your nose goes down to the stomach to keep it empty until it starts working again.
- Pain will be controlled with medicine.
- You should be able to go home in about 7 to 10 days.
- Arrangements will be made for your pain medicine, office visit, stitch removal, and a home visiting nurse if this is necessary.
- Your condition can be cured. An estimate of your chances can be made only after all the test results are back.
- As with any operation, complications are always possible, some of them serious. With your type of operation, complications can include hemorrhage, infection, pneumonia, heart problems, jaundice, bowel obstruction, wound infection, liver failure, and possibly others.

✚ HOME CARE

- You may walk about as you wish, even climb stairs, but don't overdo things.
- Take medicine as prescribed for your pain.
- Your diet can be as you tolerate it, but include plenty of roughage and liquids to help prevent constipation.
- You will be instructed on showering or bathing.
- Do not drive a car until we discuss it first during your follow-up office visit.

✆ CALL OUR OFFICE IF

- You develop any unusual signs or symptoms.
- The incision becomes red or swollen, or there is drainage from it.
- You develop a temperature higher than 100°F.
- You have any questions.

LUNG CANCER (BRONCHOGENIC CANCER)

△ GENERAL INFORMATION

Cancer of the lung is the most common cancer of men in the United States. Smoking is considered the most important associated factor.

COMMON SIGNS AND SYMPTOMS

- Early cancer may not have any symptoms at all; it is found on a routine chest x-ray.
- When the cancer gets large enough to produce symptoms, these usually depend on the following:
  - Its location in the lung.
  - How deeply the cancer has penetrated.
- The most common signs and symptoms are as follows:
  - A persistent cough.
  - Occasional coughing up of bloody mucus.
  - "Heaviness" to severe constant pain in the chest.
  - Weight loss.

DIAGNOSIS

- Usually the diagnosis can be made by taking a detailed history, doing a thorough physical examination, and considering the laboratory reports carefully.
- *X-ray of the lungs*: This is the most common method by which the cancer is first seen. Even though the diagnosis is *suspected* on the basis of x-rays, it can be *confirmed* only by examining a piece of lung tissue under the microscope.
- *CT scan (computed tomography scan)*: A machine shaped like a huge doughnut is used to take special x-rays. You will lie on a table inside the hole in the "doughnut." The x-rays are taken as very thin slices through the area of the lung and the upper abdomen. This makes it possible to see the fine details in the lungs and liver.
- *Bronchoscopy*: The examination is done with a *bronchoscope*. This is an optical instrument about as big around as your little finger with a light at its tip. Your mouth and throat will be sprayed with anesthetic to make them numb. The bronchoscope will be carefully placed inside your bronchial tubes and both the right and left lungs carefully examined. If anything suspicious is seen, a small piece (a *biopsy* specimen) will be taken for examination in the laboratory.

○ TREATMENT

- An operation to remove the cancer provides the most favorable chance for cure.
- Sometimes it is advisable to give chemotherapy or x-ray therapy before the operation. If this is the case with you, there will be a detailed discussion with you before anything is planned or done.

PREOPERATIVE PREPARATION

- An examination of your blood, urine, and heart (EKG) will be done.
- Your heart will get special attention. In addition to the EKG, possibly other tests will be done, depending on your symptoms, because heart problems can give the most trouble after a lung operation.
- You will have a brain scan to be certain everything is clear there.
- You will have some breathing tests performed to see how well your lungs are functioning.
- Do not eat or drink anything for 8 hours before the operation.
- Shower as usual on the morning of the operation.
- You will be given medicine that will make you feel drowsy before you are brought to the operating room.

□ OPERATION

- You will be asleep for the operation.
- The incision will be on the side of your chest.
- The amount of lung removed will depend on what will give you the best chance for cure.
- You will not receive a blood transfusion unless it is absolutely necessary.
- The operation usually takes 2 to 4 hours.

POSTOPERATIVE CARE

- You will be taken to the Surgical Care Unit, where the doctors and nurses are very experienced in taking care of patients with your condition. As soon as you are coming along well enough, you will be transferred to a regular hospital room.
- Pain can be controlled with medicine. The nurse will give it to you, or you can give yourself a preset amount of pain medicine when you feel you need it. This is done with a device for patient-controlled analgesia (PCA) that is connected to the tubing giving you intravenous fluids.
- Two soft plastic tubes will be coming from your chest. They will drain fluids and help your lungs expand properly.
- The evening after the operation you will be helped to sit up in bed and on the next day to get out of bed.
- You will be given an incentive spirometer. Breathing into this as you are instructed will help you expand your lungs and reduce the risk of developing pneumonia.
- Your diet will be as you tolerate it.
- The tubes in your chest will be removed when there is no more drainage from them.
- You should be able to go home in about 1 week.
- As with any operation, complications are always possible. Although they are uncommon with this type of operation, complications can include pneumonia, infections, and heart problems, among others.
- Your condition can be cured. An estimate of your chances can be made only after all the test results are back.
- Arrangements will be made for your medicine, follow-up office visit, and stitch removal and discussion of possible additional therapy.

✚ HOME CARE

- Continue with the program started while you were in the hospital.
- You may walk about as you wish, even climb stairs. At first you may be short of breath after such activity, but as your body adjusts, your breathing capacity will improve.
- Your diet can be as before the operation, but include enough roughage and liquid to help prevent constipation.
- Take medicine as prescribed for your pain.
- Don't lift anything heavier than 5 pounds. Ask someone to do it for you.
- Walking and otherwise moving about—in moderation—is good for your circulation, your breathing, and your muscle tone. Remain active as long as it doesn't hurt you or tire you.
- You may shower as you wish, with any dressings on or off.
  - There may be narrow strips of tape across the incision. It's all right if they get wet; they will be removed in the doctor's office.
  - After you dry yourself, replace any dressings with clean, dry ones.
- Be careful that you do not become constipated.
  - You may need some help with a mild laxative (example: milk of magnesia).
- You can help "loosen" your shoulder by using your arm. Also, a good exercise is to stand next to a wall and "climb" up the wall with your hand.
- Driving a car with an automatic shift is not too demanding, but if you suddenly have to slam on the brakes or twist to turn the steering wheel, you may get into an accident or strain the sutures or tear something. During your follow-up visit, let's discuss when you can resume driving.
- You may resume sexual activity whenever you choose.
- You may return to work when you feel up to it, but let's talk about it first during one of your follow-up visits.

✆ CALL OUR OFFICE IF

- You develop any unusual signs or symptoms.
- You cough up any red sputum.
- You develop any difficulty with your breathing.
- You develop a temperature higher than 101°F.
- You have any questions.

LYMPH NODE BIOPSY

△ GENERAL INFORMATION

Just about every part of the body is outfitted with a huge number of microscopic channels that drain fluid (called *lymph*) from it. These channels pass through *lymph nodes,* whose function it is to filter out and trap bacteria, viruses, white blood cells, cancer cells, and other foreign particles in the lymph. When the lymph nodes trap a lot of material, they swell. Sometimes they swell simply as part of their job in helping the body fight off an infection. The lymph nodes are more concentrated in certain areas, for example, the neck, armpit *(axilla),* and groin.

It is sometimes difficult to know the cause of swelling in lymph nodes. In such situations, a portion or all of the lymph node needs to be removed. This is called a *lymph node biopsy.*

COMMON SIGNS AND SYMPTOMS

- The enlarged lymph node can be as small as a pea or as large as a walnut. Only one node may be felt, or there may be many. They may be separate or stuck together.
- Usually, they don't hurt, or they may just ache a bit.

The surest way to be certain of the nature of a lymph node is to remove a piece of it (a *biopsy* specimen) for examination in the laboratory. However, there are a number of considerations on whether a biopsy is necessary or advisable.

- The lymph nodes may not truly be enlarged. The person may be thin enough that normal, small lymph nodes can be felt.
- The cause of the enlargement is clear and not a serious one. The proper first step is to treat the cause (example: an infection), expecting the lymph node to get smaller.
- Sometimes the specific cause of the lymph node swelling is not clear to the doctor, but the possible causes are not alarming. In such cases, it may be reasonable to simply observe the patient for several weeks.
- The diagnosis may not be clear, but there may be serious harm in waiting and watching to see what happens. In such a case, a biopsy is warranted.
- The diagnosis is quite obvious (and serious). However, the treatment for the presumed disease is extensive and carries some risk. It would not be correct to start treatment without first knowing the *exact* diagnosis through a biopsy.

THE BIOPSY

If the decision is to perform a biopsy, the next decision is on what method of biopsy to use. The choices are as follows:

- *Fine needle aspiration biopsy:* A fine needle is inserted into the lymph node and some cells are sucked out for examination in the laboratory. This is an office procedure and takes just a few minutes to perform.
- *Core needle biopsy:* The skin over the swollen lymph node is swabbed with an antiseptic solution and surrounded with sterile towel drapes. A fine needle is used to inject an anesthetic into the skin to make it numb. A somewhat larger needle is then inserted in the lymph node and a core of lymph node tissue (about the thickness of the lead in a pencil) is removed and sent to the laboratory. This is an office procedure.
- *Open biopsy:* The area over the swelling is swabbed with an antiseptic solution and surrounded with sterile towel drapes. A fine short needle is used to inject an anesthetic in the skin and surrounding tissue to make the area numb. An incision is made and the enlarged lymph node exposed. Part or all of the node is removed. A small portion of the biopsy specimen may be sent to the laboratory to be examined for the presence of bacteria. The main portion will be sent to the pathology laboratory so that it can be examined for the presence of cancer.

After careful consideration of all factors, the recommendation is that you have an open biopsy of one of your enlarged lymph nodes.

PREOPERATIVE PREPARATION

- Don't drink or eat anything for 8 hours before the operation.
- You may shower (and shave) as usual that morning.
- You may be given medicine that will make you feel drowsy before you are brought into the operating room.

□ OPERATION

- The operation commonly is done in an outpatient surgical facility.
- During the operation, you may feel some tugging but no pain.
- The operation usually takes about 1 hour.

POSTOPERATIVE CARE

- You will be taken to a recovery room where you will stay until your blood pressure, pulse, and breathing are stable and you are completely alert. You should be able to go home that same day with a responsible adult.
- Arrangements will be made for your pain medicine, office visit, stitch removal (if necessary), a full discussion of your laboratory findings, and any further therapy.

✚ HOME CARE

- Resume your usual activities.
- Take medicine as prescribed for your pain.
- You may shower as you wish, with any dressings on or off.

- There may be narrow strips of tape across the incision. It's all right if they get wet; they will be removed in the doctor's office.
- After you dry yourself, replace any dressings with clean, dry ones.

✆ CALL OUR OFFICE IF

- The incision becomes red or swollen, or there is drainage from it.
- You develop a fever higher than 100°F.
- You have any questions.

△ GENERAL INFORMATION

Mammography is the best single test you can have to pick up potentially serious abnormalities in the breast that you *cannot* feel. Mammography also is extremely valuable in giving the doctor and you a very good idea of the nature of a lump that you *can* feel. So, regular mammography plus *regular* breast self-examination in addition to *regular* routine physical examination of your breasts by your physician—*all together*—is the best way to find, in its early stages, something that may be serious. Remember, *early* detection and treatment of a tumor has the best chance of being successful.

The American Cancer Society recommends that a baseline mammogram be done by age 40 years, and mammograms should be repeated every 1 or 2 years between the ages of 40 and 49 (depending on your particular risk factors). There should be an annual mammogram after age 50. However, there are exceptions to this:

- Your breast may be "lumpy," and while nothing in it appears ominous, it may be difficult for both you and your doctor to be certain without a mammogram.
- There may be a strong family history of breast cancer, making it wise for you to start having routine mammograms at an earlier age.

Discuss this issue with your doctor. The important point is to get mammograms and a physical examination on a *regular* basis.

WHAT IS A MAMMOGRAM?

A mammogram is a picture of the breast tissue that is done with a very low and safe dose of radiation. Some radiation does go through the breast, but if mammograms are properly ordered and performed, the information you get about your breasts is *far more* valuable than the virtually negligible risk of the very small dose of radiation passing through your breasts.

PREPARATION

Minimal preparation is necessary, but several suggestions are worth mentioning:

- Shower or bathe as usual on the day of your scheduled mammography, but do not use underarm deodorants, especially any dusting powders. Some of these have little particles in them that might cause very tiny shadows on the mammogram and possibly cause confusion.
- If you experience a lot of breast pain or tenderness before your menstrual periods, it may be wise to avoid scheduling your mammography at such a time. The breasts have to be compressed during the procedure, which would only aggravate your discomfort.
- If you are pregnant, or think you are pregnant, be certain to make this known to the technologist. Special arrangements may need to be made.
- You will be asked to disrobe from the waist up for the examination. Wearing a blouse or a two-piece outfit instead of a dress may make this easier for you.

THE MAMMOGRAM

- You will be standing or sitting for the mammogram, depending on the type of x-ray machine being used. Limited views can be taken of a patient in a wheelchair.
- Your breasts will be positioned and then compressed with a plastic shield or a plate sponge. This may cause some temporary discomfort.
- X-ray pictures of your breast will be taken as follows:
  - From top to bottom.
  - From an angle aimed toward your armpit (Fig. 1).

  These two views are routine and are necessary to take a picture of as much of the inside of your breast tissue as possible. Just one view simply is not enough. Even with three views, it sometimes is difficult to see 100% of the breast tissue. In some instances, a straight sideways view is also taken.
- On occasion, certain shadows may be seen on these routine mammograms that are not entirely clear. If so, additional pictures from a different angle may need to be taken. Sometimes a magnified view may need to be taken of a small area. This technique enlarges and sharpens any small abnormalities so that they can be seen more clearly.

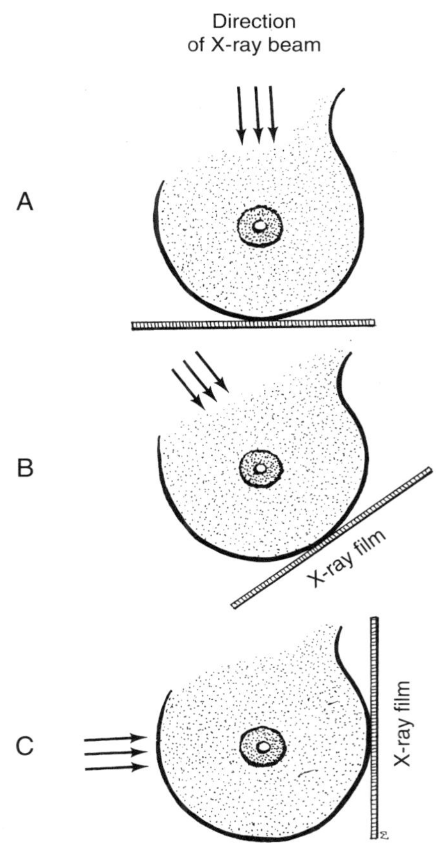

Figure 1. Typical views of the breast. *A*, Top to bottom (cephalocaudal); *B*, diagonal (oblique); *C*, side-to-side (lateral).

The Need to Compress Your Breast

For technical reasons, if the x-rays pass through the *same thickness* of tissue throughout the breast the pictures made are much clearer and sharper. To achieve uniform thickness in the average breast, it is necessary to flatten the breasts as much as possible (Fig. 2). This can be uncomfortable, but remember that the result a much clearer picture for the radiologist to look at, which is of benefit to you. Also, the thinner the breast is compressed, the less radiation dose is absorbed by the breast tissue.

Occasionally, this compression may produce some redness of the skin as well as discomfort. Neither of these is harmful, and both are temporary.

Your mammograms will be done by a highly trained technologist who does this all day long. Everyone's concern is to get the very best quality mammogram with the least number of films and the least discomfort for you. At the completion of the mammography, you'll be asked to wait a short while so that the technologist can make sure that the films are of good quality. After this, you are free to leave.

In some places, your mammograms will be carefully examined right away by a radiologist who is an expert in the field of mammography. You will then be told the results right away. In other places, the mammograms will be read later and the results will be reported to your personal physician.

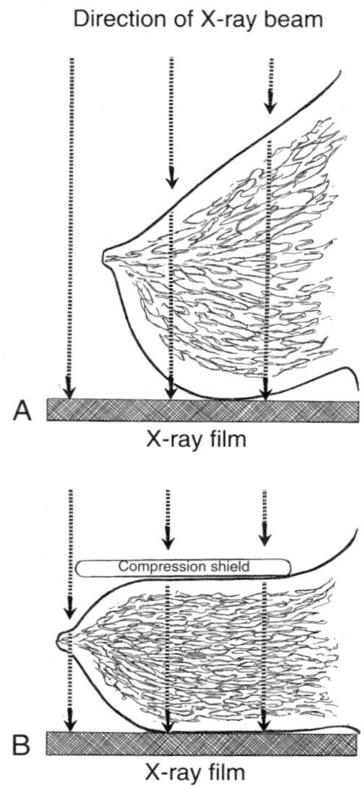

Figure 2. *A*, The breast as it normally lies on the x-ray films. *B*, The breast must be compressed so that it is uniform in thickness as much as possible. This produces more accurate detail on the x-ray films.

△ GENERAL INFORMATION

The small intestine starts at the stomach and ends in the right side of the lower abdomen, where it empties into the large bowel. About a foot and a half or so before the small intestine ends, it sometimes has a side pocket (called a *diverticulum,* and *Meckel's* after the person who first described it almost 200 years ago) (Fig. 1). The side pocket usually is about as big around as your thumb. It may not be much longer than the tip of your thumb, or it can be as long as your entire thumb.

About one or two out of 100 people is born with a diverticulum. About half of such diverticula have a lining in them that is just like the lining found in the stomach.

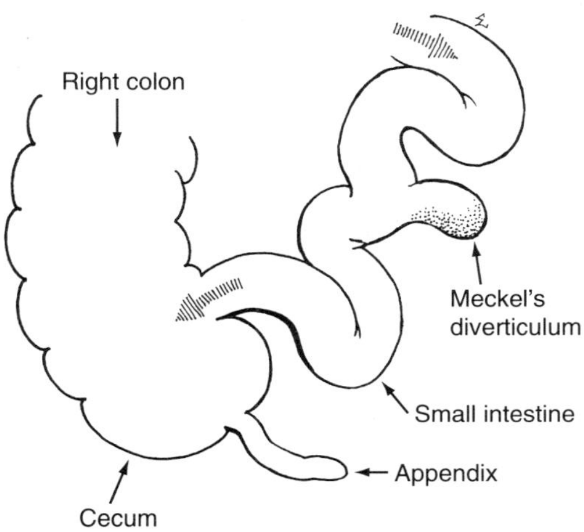

Figure 1. When a Meckel's diverticulum does not produce symptoms and is found incidentally, the indication to remove it is influenced by its length, the likelihood that it will cause a problem, the primary diagnosis causing the abdomen to be opened, and the local conditions present at the time.

COMMON SIGNS AND SYMPTOMS

Most of the time, Meckel's diverticulum does not produce any symptoms. Occasionally, however, it can cause trouble, as follows:

- The lining that is like the lining in the stomach can form an ulcer and bleed just as it can in the stomach. When this happens, blood is seen in the stool.
- Sometimes a diverticulum, especially a long one, can become twisted. This chokes off its blood supply and also blocks the intestine. The symptoms it produces can include the following:
  - Abdominal cramps.
  - Swelling of the abdomen.
  - Possible peritonitis if a twisted diverticulum develops gangrene.
- The diverticulum can cause the part of the small intestine in which it is located to slip into the small intestine just ahead of it. This causes blockage of the intestine and the following conditions:
  - There is abdominal cramping.
  - The abdomen becomes distended with gas that cannot pass.
- The diverticulum can become infected and irritate the tissue around it, with the following signs and symptoms:
  - There is pain in the right side of the lower abdomen.
  - There is distention of the abdomen.
  - There is fever and an elevated white blood cell count.

DIAGNOSIS

- The diagnosis can be suspected from the symptoms. However, making an exact diagnosis is not easy. Often, the diagnosis is made only when the abdomen is opened, because then it is obvious that something is happening inside the abdomen.
- Having you swallow barium and taking pictures of it as it travels through the small intestine sometimes will show the diverticulum.
- Other tests can be done with some success.

○ TREATMENT

- There is no need to open the abdomen to remove a Meckel's diverticulum that is not causing symptoms.
- A Meckel's diverticulum that produces symptoms however, should be removed. This requires an operation.

PREOPERATIVE PREPARATION

- You will have an examination of your blood, urine, heart (EKG), and lungs (chest x-ray).
- Do not eat or drink anything for 8 hours before the operation.
- Shower as usual on the morning of the operation.
- You may be given medicine that will make you feel drowsy before you are brought to the operating room.

□ OPERATION

- You will be asleep for the operation.
- The abdomen will be opened, the diverticulum removed, and the intestine put together again.
- You will not need a blood transfusion.
- The operation usually takes about 1 hour.

POSTOPERATIVE CARE

- You will be taken to a recovery room and observed. When your blood pressure, pulse, and breathing are stable, you will be taken to a regular hospital room.
- You may have a thin, plastic tube in your nose. The tube will be removed as soon as your bowels start working.
- The evening after the operation you will be helped to sit up in bed and on the next day to get out of bed.
- Pain will be controlled with medicine.
- You should be able to go home in 3 to 4 days.
- As with any operation, complications are always possible. With this type of operation, complications can include leakage where the opened intestine was

reconnected, bleeding, infection, bowel obstruction, and possibly others.

- Arrangements will be made for your medicine, follow-up office visit, and stitch removal.

✚ HOME CARE

- You may walk about as you wish, even climb stairs.
- Your diet can be as before the operation.
- You may shower as you wish, with any dressings on or off.
    - There may be narrow strips of tape across the incision. It's all right if they get wet; they will be removed in the doctor's office.
    - After you dry yourself, replace any dressings with clean, dry ones.
- Driving a car with an automatic shift is not too demanding, but if you suddenly have to slam on the brakes or twist to turn the steering wheel, you may strain the sutures or tear something. During your follow-up visit, let's discuss when you can resume driving.
- You may resume sexual activity whenever you choose.
- You may return to work when you feel up to it, but let's first talk about it during one of your follow-up visits.

✆ CALL OUR OFFICE IF

- The incision becomes red or swollen, or there is drainage from it.
- You develop a temperature higher than 100°F.
- You have any questions.

△ GENERAL INFORMATION

Melanoma is a malignancy of the cells in the skin that give the skin its color. Melanoma can be seen in people of any race but is more common in fair-skinned people.

COMMON SIGNS AND SYMPTOMS

- The lesion may start in clear skin, but the majority of lesions start in an already existing mole.
- The melanoma often starts as a dark mole and then begins to spread. The margins become irregular and many times can become fuzzy.
- The melanoma may be deep brown throughout or have some lighter tones in it.
- It can be quite smooth or have a rough surface. Some lesions have an ulcer in them.

DIAGNOSIS

- Anyone with the above signs should be suspected of having a melanoma.
- A detailed history and a thorough physical examination are often enough to make this diagnosis.
- The only way to be certain of the diagnosis is to remove a piece of the lesion (called a *biopsy*) for laboratory examination. The biopsy is performed as follows: The area containing the lesion is swabbed with an antiseptic solution and surrounded with sterile towels. A very fine, short needle is used to inject an anesthetic around the lesion to make the entire area numb. A small piece of tissue is taken and a bandage applied. This is an outpatient procedure.

○ TREATMENT

The best chance for cure is to remove, by an operation, the melanoma and any lymph nodes to which it has spread. The extent of the operation depends on several things:

- What type of melanoma it is.
- How deeply the melanoma has penetrated.
- Its location on the body.
- Whether or not the lymph nodes draining the area are involved.

After careful consideration of all factors, the recommendation is that you have an operation to remove your melanoma.

PREOPERATIVE PREPARATION

- You will have an examination of your blood, urine, heart (EKG), and lungs (chest x-ray). Melanoma can spread to almost any area of the body. This means that different special tests may need to be done to see if specific areas are involved. These may include the following:
  - *CT scan (computed tomography scan)*: A machine shaped like a huge doughnut is used to take special x-ray pictures. You will lie on the table inside the hole in the "doughnut." The x-rays are taken as very thin slices through the area in question (this can be the liver, brain, or region of the melanoma). This makes it possible to see the fine details in those organs as well as in the lymph node area near the melanoma.
  - *MRI (magnetic resonance imaging)*: No x-rays are used with this technique. Instead, it is done with harmless magnetic fields and radio waves. A computer develops the pictures to show organs from several angles. This technique is especially valuable for examining your blood vessels and nerve tissue.
  - *Bone scan*: A fine needle is used to inject a solution with a tiny amount of a harmless radioactive material into your vein. The solution circulates throughout your entire body and attaches itself to any bone that has anything wrong with it. One hour or so after the injection, you will lie on the table and a special machine will pass over your entire body taking a series of photographs (a *scan*) of all the bones from your skull to your toes. A specialist then examines the scan, looking for any abnormalities.
  - *PET scan (position emission tomography scan)*: With this technique, it is possible to see what activity is going on in a tumor. Radioactive forms of basic chemicals are used that are part of the body's chemical activity. They are injected into the blood stream and will become attached to the tumor (if there is activity present). The scanning machine measures how much activity is present and thus can determine how fast or slowly the tumor is growing.
- Do not eat or drink anything for 8 hours before the operation.
- Shower or bathe on the morning of the operation.
- You may be given medicine that will make you feel drowsy before you are brought to the operating room.

□ OPERATION

- The operation that is necessary can be very different for each patient.
- The aim is to remove the melanoma with a one-half inch margin of normal tissue around it.
- If the lymph nodes draining the area that contains the melanoma are enlarged, or otherwise are shown to contain melanoma, they will also be removed.
- Sometimes the area from which the melanoma is removed is large and the skin edges cannot be brought together. If so, skin may need to be taken from another area in your body to cover this open area. This is called a *skin graft*.
- The specific operation that applies to you will be discussed with you beforehand.
- You may be asleep for the operation, or it may be done with local anesthesia and sedation, depending on your special circumstances. This too will be explained to you beforehand.

POSTOPERATIVE CARE

- You will be taken to a recovery room and observed until your blood pressure, pulse, and breathing are stable. If this was a rather minor procedure done under local anesthesia, you should be able to go home that same day with a responsible adult. Otherwise, you will be transferred to a regular hospital room.
- If you are kept in the hospital, the evening after the surgery you will be helped to sit up in bed and on the next day to get out of bed.
- Pain will be controlled with medicine.
- Your condition can be cured. An estimate of your chances can be made only after all the test results are back.
- As with any operation, complications are always possible. With this type of operation, complications can include pneumonia, bleeding, infection, blood clots to the lung, and some others.
- Arrangements will be made for your medicine, follow-up office visit, and stitch removal.

✣ HOME CARE

- Resume your usual activities.
- You may walk about as you wish, even climb stairs.
- Eat as you wish.
- If you do not have a skin graft, you may shower as you wish, with any dressings on or off.
  - There may be narrow strips of tape across the incision. It's all right if they get wet; they will be removed in the doctor's office.
  - After you dry yourself, replace any dressings with clean, dry ones.
- If you have a skin graft, you will be instructed on showering or bathing and how to take care of your dressings.

✆ CALL OUR OFFICE IF

- Your incision becomes red or swollen, or there is drainage from it.
- You develop a temperature higher than 100°F.
- You have any questions.

MESENTERIC LYMPHADENITIS

△ GENERAL INFORMATION

Lymph nodes are found in practically all areas of the body. Normal lymph nodes can range in size from a poppy seed to an olive. Lymph channels carry lymph fluid in and out of these nodes.

Lymph fluid is present in all parts of the body. As the lymph passes through the lymph nodes, organisms or dead material in the lymph is filtered out. In other words, lymph nodes clean up fluid in the body. That's why when there's an infection, the lymph nodes in the area enlarge.

Lymph nodes are more common in some areas than others. A lot of them can be found in the neck, the armpits, and the groin. Inside the abdomen, however, one area that has a lot of lymph nodes is the *mesentery*. The mesentery is the structure that supports the intestine and carries the arteries and veins and which the lymph channels and lymph nodes follow.

Sometimes, when a person has a "cold"—a viral infection—the lymph nodes in the mesentery can enlarge from the size of a pea to five times bigger, or even more. This is called *mesenteric lymphadenitis*. This happens more in the mesenteric lymph nodes near the appendix. These large lymph nodes irritate the abdominal wall and cause pain in this area (Fig. 1).

This enlargement of the lymph nodes happens most often in younger people, especially children up to the age of 15 years.

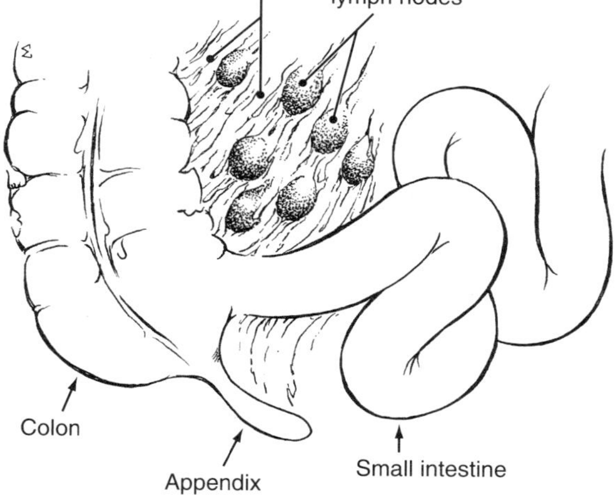

Figure 1. The enlarged lymph nodes *(stippled areas)* which can cause irritation and pain, can be seen near the area of the appendix.

COMMON SIGNS AND SYMPTOMS

- There is pain in the right side of the lower abdomen, the same area in which the pain of appendicitis is felt.
- Often, there is a history of a recent "cold," but this disorder can occur when someone has not been sick at all.

DIAGNOSIS

Usually the diagnosis can be made by taking a detailed history, doing a thorough physical examination, and considering the laboratory reports carefully. Unfortunately, often the diagnosis of mesenteric lymphadenitis cannot be made with certainty. This can present the surgeon with a problem.

- The biggest problem is to tell the difference between *mesenteric lymphadenitis* and *appendicitis*.
- Mesenteric lymphadenitis does not require an operation; it will go away by itself.
- Acute appendicitis requires an operation, and often very quickly.
- The surgeon must make the diagnosis as accurately as possible because the treatment is an operation or no operation, depending on the diagnosis. Unfortunately, sometimes it is not safe to wait to see whether the condition will go away; it might be something more serious like appendicitis.
- *Ultrasound*: Harmless sound waves are aimed at the area of the appendix. The sound waves bouncing back (the echoes) from this area are seen as pictures on a screen. This is a convenient, painless, and safe way to examine to see if the appendix is swollen.
- *CT scan (computed tomography scan)*: A machine shaped like a huge doughnut is used to take special x-rays. You will lie on a table inside the hole in the "doughnut." The x-rays are taken as very thin slices through the area of the lower abdomen. This makes it possible to see the fine details in this area, specifically in the appendix.
- If the decision is made to operate, the following will take place:

PREOPERATIVE PREPARATION

- Do not eat or drink anything for 8 hours before the operation.
- There will be an examination of your blood and possibly of your heart (EKG), and lungs (chest x-ray).
- Medicine will be given to you that will make you feel drowsy before you are brought to the operating room.

□ OPERATION

- You will be asleep for the operation.
- If the appendix is infected, it will be removed and the operation will be over. If the appendix is normal, then the area will be examined for another cause of the pain. If only mesenteric lymphadenitis is found, the appendix will be removed anyway to prevent possible future problems.
- The operation usually takes 1 hour.

POSTOPERATIVE CARE

- You will wake up in a recovery room. When your blood pressure, pulse, and breathing are stable, you will be taken to a regular hospital room.
- In a few hours you will be helped to get out of bed and the next day to go home.

- Pain will be controlled with medicine.
- Your diet will be as you tolerate it.
- Arrangements will be made for your medicine, follow-up office visit, and stitch removal.

✣ HOME CARE

- You may walk about as you wish, even climb stairs.
- You may eat as you did before the operation.
- You may shower as you wish, with any dressings on or off.
  - There may be narrow strips of tape across the incision. It's all right if they get wet; they will be removed in the doctor's office.
  - After you dry yourself, replace any dressings with clean, dry ones.
- Be careful that you do not become constipated.
  - Include enough roughage and liquid in your diet.
  - You may need a mild laxative (example: milk of magnesia).

✆ CALL OUR OFFICE IF

- You develop any unusual signs or symptoms.
- The incision becomes red or swollen, or there is drainage from it.
- You develop a temperature higher than 100°F.
- You have any questions.

△ GENERAL INFORMATION

People are considered morbidly obese if they are two times, or 100 pounds over, their ideal weight. Up to 3 million Americans may be morbidly obese.

There can be several reasons for morbid obesity:

- One eats more food than is needed.
- We have more food and more fattening food available in the United States.
- In some people, there may be a genetic factor.
- A number of emotional problems may lead a person to eat far beyond the daily requirements.
- A lifestyle of no exercise or a physical problem of not being able to move about leads to too few calories being burned off.
- There may be a lack of a support system for a person who is trying to take off excess weight.

EFFECTS OF MORBID OBESITY

Morbid obesity can do damage to almost every organ in the body.

- The bones and joints wear down early because of the great weight they carry.
- A large amount of fat in the chest and breasts prevents the heart and lungs from working as they should. The oxygen in the blood is not at the best level.
- The heart is overworked.
- High blood pressure is three times more common. Stroke is seen more frequently.
- Diabetes is five times more common.
- Gallbladder disease is seen more frequently.
- There are social consequences: the person cannot get or hold a job.
- Driving an automobile becomes increasingly difficult.
- There is a higher divorce rate.
- There is difficulty in engaging in sports activities.
- There is difficulty in finding or being able to dress in tasteful clothing.
- The risk of breast cancer increases.
- There is a greater risk with any illness or operation.

COMMON HISTORY

- The person has been obese—a lot or a little—for many years, often since childhood. All types of appetite medicines, diets, exercise programs, and psychologic therapies have been tried, often more than once. They didn't help, or the person didn't stick with the plan.
- Often, doctors and patients believe that morbid obesity is due to hormone problems, and many tests are done to see if this is the cause. Actually, it rarely is the cause because hormone problems lead to weakness and cause the patient to look for help early before they become morbidly obese.

○ TREATMENT

- Most experts agree that many morbidly obese persons cannot be helped to cut down their appetite very much or for very long by diet or medicines.
- Weight loss requires behavioral changes or exercise.
- An operation is considered as a last resort. It is considered when everyone—especially the morbidly obese person—feels that something should be done.

PREOPERATIVE PREPARATION

- A number of preparations are done, including a psychotherapy evaluation and conferences with dietitians and an endocrinologist.
- You will have a thorough physical examination with special emphasis on your heart and lungs. Any medical problem will be taken care of as much as possible.
- Do not eat or drink anything for 8 hours before the operation.
- You may be given medicine that will make you feel drowsy before you are brought to the operating room.

□ OPERATION

- You will be asleep for the operation.
- The operation planned for you will be to place staples across some of the stomach to make it smaller. Also, the opening for food leaving the stomach will be made smaller (Fig. 1). This will make you feel full after a much smaller meal.
- If other important conditions are found, they will be taken care of; for example, if gallstones are found, the gallbladder will be removed.
- You will not receive a blood transfusion unless it is absolutely necessary.
- The operation usually takes 2 to 3 hours.

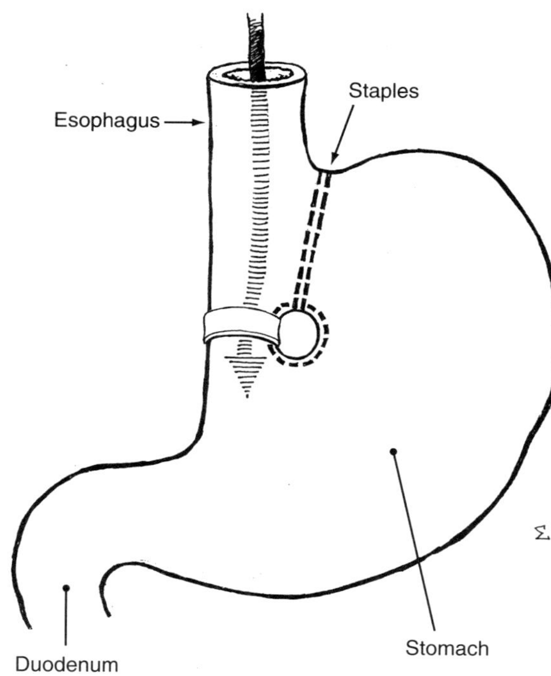

Figure 1. A common operation used in the surgical treatment of morbid obesity severely limits the amount of space available for food in the stomach and the speed at which the food can leave the stomach.

POSTOPERATIVE CARE

- You will be taken to the Surgical Care Unit, where the doctors and nurses are very experienced in taking care of patients with your condition. As soon as you are coming along well enough, you will be transferred to a regular hospital room.
- The evening after the surgery you will be helped to sit up in bed and on the next day to get out of bed.
- You will have a thin plastic tube in your nose. It goes down to your stomach to suck up the air you swallow. It will be removed within 2 to 3 days.
- You will be helped to arrange a diet schedule.
- As with any operation, complications are always possible. With your type of operation, complications can include wound infection; blood clots; infection inside the abdomen; swelling and blockage of the opening out of the stomach; the need to remove your spleen, which is right next to the stomach; and a hernia incision, among others. Rarely, the operation may not work because the staples across the stomach come loose, or the opening left may be too large and too much food can go into and out of the stomach. Possibly, the opening from the stomach is too small and the food cannot get out properly.
- You should be able to go home in 7 to 10 days.
- Arrangements will be made for your medicine, follow-up office visit, and stitch removal.

✚ HOME CARE

- Continue with the program started while you were in the hospital.
- You may walk about as you wish, even climb stairs. Walking and otherwise moving about—in moderation—are good for your circulation, your breathing, and your muscle tone. Remain active as long as it doesn't hurt you or tire you.
- You may shower as you wish, with any dressings on or off.
  - There may be narrow strips of tape across the incision. It's all right if they get wet; they will be removed in the doctor's office.
  - After you dry yourself, replace any dressings with clean, dry ones.
- Eat *slowly*. Chew each bite of food 30 times. If you eat beef, first slice it into tiny pieces. Do not eat raw vegetables. Do not swallow big pills.
- Weight loss will not occur if you often drink high-calorie liquid or soft foods, which easily pass through the small opening of your stomach.

✆ CALL OUR OFFICE IF

- You develop nausea or vomiting.
- You develop other new or unusual symptoms.
- The incision becomes red or swollen, or there is drainage from it.
- You develop a temperature higher than 100°F.
- You have any questions.

△ GENERAL INFORMATION

The tongue and the floor of the mouth are the main areas in the mouth cavity where cancers originate. The front two-thirds of the tongue is primarily responsible for forming words and also for maneuvering food to the back of the throat. The back one-third of the tongue is more responsible for starting the swallowing of foods toward the esophagus. The floor is under and to the sides of the tongue. Factors that are associated with cancer in this area are heavy use of tobacco, chronic alcoholism, and chronic irritation. Cancer in these areas occurs most commonly in older men.

COMMON SIGNS AND SYMPTOMS

Signs and symptoms of cancer of the tongue can vary, depending on the location and size of the cancer: An early cancer may appear as a small bump, ulcer, or white firm area on the tongue. There may be minor irritation. With larger tumors, there usually is persistent pain.

DIAGNOSIS

- Any new sore on the tongue or the floor of the mouth that persists for longer than 3 weeks should be investigated.
- Most cancers of the tongue are on the anterior two-thirds of the tongue and can be seen directly. Cancers on the back one-third of the tongue often need to be examined using a long-handled small mirror. This office examination takes just a few minutes.
- *CT scan (computed tomography scan)*: Special x-rays are taken as very thin slices through the area of the mouth. This makes it possible to see the fine details in the mouth tissue.
- *MRI (magnetic resonance imaging)*: No x-rays are used with this technique. Instead, it is done with harmless magnetic fields and radio waves. A computer develops the pictures to show organs and tissues in your mouth from several angles. This technique is especially useful to see the relationships of blood vessels, nerves, and bone tissue.
- Removing a small piece of any suspicious tissue (a *biopsy*) is the only sure way to make a diagnosis.

○ TREATMENT

Cancer of the tongue and the floor of the mouth can be treated by an operation or by radiation therapy or a combination of both (Fig. 1).

- Small lesions in either area of the tongue can be treated either with an operation or with radiation, with equal rates of cure.
- Generally, cancers in the front part of the tongue behave differently from those toward the back part. This must be taken into account when planning treatment.
- Cancer of the tongue can be like an iceberg; much of it can be under the surface.
- Roughly half the cancers of the tongue or floor of mouth already have spread to the lymph nodes in the neck, sometimes in microscopic fashion. For this reason, the lymph nodes in the neck often are removed, regardless of their appearance.

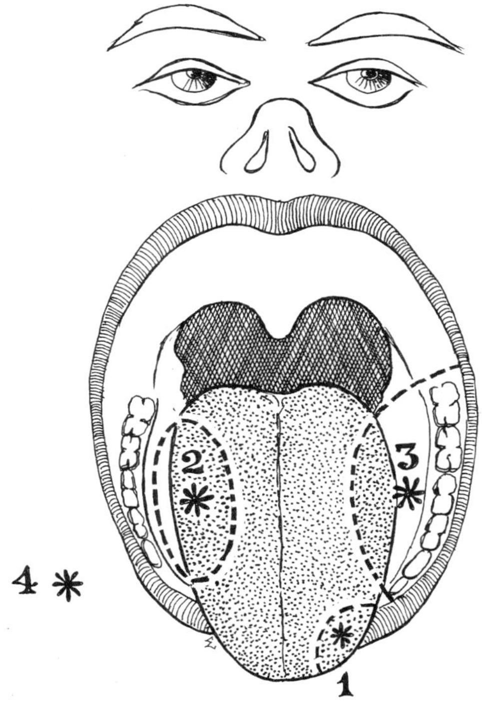

Figure 1. Four examples of cancer of the tongue or floor of the mouth and how they might be treated. *1*, Tip of tongue only: local resection. *2*, Tongue extending to floor of mouth with no evidence of lymph node involvement: excision of tongue and floor of mouth as shown. Possible x-ray treatment to the neck area. *3*, Tongue, floor of mouth, and jaw involved: resection of all areas involved as well as the lymph nodes in the neck (radical neck dissection) *4*, If lymph nodes are palpated, all of the lymph nodes in the neck are removed as well as the area from which the cancer originated.

- Some cancers of the tongue or the floor of the mouth involve some of the mandible (the jaw bone), so a portion of the bone also needs to be removed.
- Sometimes radiation therapy is given after an operation in an effort to kill any microscopic cells that may be left behind.
- An operation on the tongue and mandible can cause a lot of swelling of the tongue, making it difficult to bring up and spit out mucus, to eat, and even to breathe. For this reason, sometimes a temporary opening is made directly from the skin in the low part of the neck into the trachea (a *tracheostomy*) so that the mucus can be coughed up or sucked out this way. Also, a thin plastic tube is placed through the nose and down the stomach so that liquid food can be given this way for a few days. Both tubes will be removed when tissues in the mouth are properly healed.

After careful consideration of all factors, the recommendation is that you have an operation to remove the cancer in your mouth. The specific operation will be discussed with you in detail before anything is planned or done.

PREOPERATIVE PREPARATION

- You will have an examination of your blood, urine, heart (EKG), and lungs (chest x-ray).
- Do not eat or drink anything for 8 hours before the operation.

☐ OPERATION

- You will be asleep for the operation.
- The duration of the operation depends on what needs to be done.Generally, it is 2 to 4 hours.

POSTOPERATIVE CARE

- You will be taken to a recovery room and observed. When your blood pressure, pulse, and breathing are stable, you will be taken to a Surgical Care Unit, where the doctors and nurses have special experience in taking care of patients following this operation.
- You will not be able to speak well at this time because your tongue has sutures in it and will be swollen. Also, if you have a tracheostomy, your breathing will temporarily pass in and out of the neck and not through your mouth.
- Pain will be controlled with medicine.
- The evening after the operation you will be helped to sit up in bed and on the next day to get out of bed.
- As with any operation, complications are always possible, some of them serious. With this type of operation, complications can include infection, separation of the wound, heart problems, and possibly others.
- Depending on the extent of the operation performed, you should be able to go home in 2 to 7 days.
- Arrangements will be made for your medicine, follow-up office visit, and stitch or clip removal.

✣ HOME CARE

- Continue with the program started while you were in the hospital.
- You may walk about if you wish, even climb stairs, but don't overdo things.
- You may bathe as you wish. Don't shower if you had a tracheostomy.
- Arrangements can be made for a home visiting nurse if one is needed.
- Do not drive a car until we discuss this at your postoperative office visit.
- You may return to work when you feel up to it.

✆ CALL OUR OFFICE IF

- You have any breathing problems.
- The incision becomes red or swollen, or there is drainage from it.
- You have any bleeding from the mouth.
- You develop a temperature higher than 100°F.
- You have any questions.

MRI (MAGNETIC RESONANCE IMAGING)

Magnetic resonance imaging is a special way of looking inside your body. MRI can provide your doctor with important information that cannot be gotten in any other way.

HOW DOES MRI WORK?

An MRI machine does not use x-rays. Instead it uses a magnet, harmless radio waves, and a computer that converts all the information into photographs. MRI is one of the best ways to look at the brain, the spinal cord, muscles, and other soft tissues and is an excellent way of looking inside bones. It can also be very helpful in diagnosing abnormalities in the abdomen, pelvis, and chest. Finally, MRI can look at these structures from many angles.

One of the most important parts of an MRI machine is a very large, very strong magnet. MRI magnets come in various shapes. Many of the best machines have magnets that are shaped like long tubes or tunnels. Others, referred to as "open" magnets, are C-shaped or have large plates that go above and below the patient but are open on the sides. These are useful for very large patients or patients with claustrophobia.

PREPARATION

Although MRI is very safe for most patients, some people should not have MRI examinations, because the strong magnets of MRI machines can cause problems for them.

- You will be asked to remove anything with metal in it. This includes hairpins or clips, coins, watches, jewelry, keys, and clothing with metal hooks or zippers.
- Be sure to tell the technicians if you have any metals inside your body. This can include heart valves, clips on an aneurysm in your brain, bone plates, joint replacement, or implants in your middle ear.
- Do not wear eyeliner.
- It is very important that you tell the doctor and the technologist if you are pregnant.

THE PROCEDURE

- You will be placed on a padded table and made comfortable. The magnet will surround you (Fig. 1).
- You will be alone in the room, but the technologist will be just outside watching you constantly. You will be able to speak with each other at any time.
- The machine will examine a thin segment of your body, one segment every minute, until all of the desired area is examined.
- Every so often during the process, the machine makes some loud tapping noises. Don't be concerned; that's how it works.
- The scan takes 20 to 60 minutes, depending on how much of your body is examined.

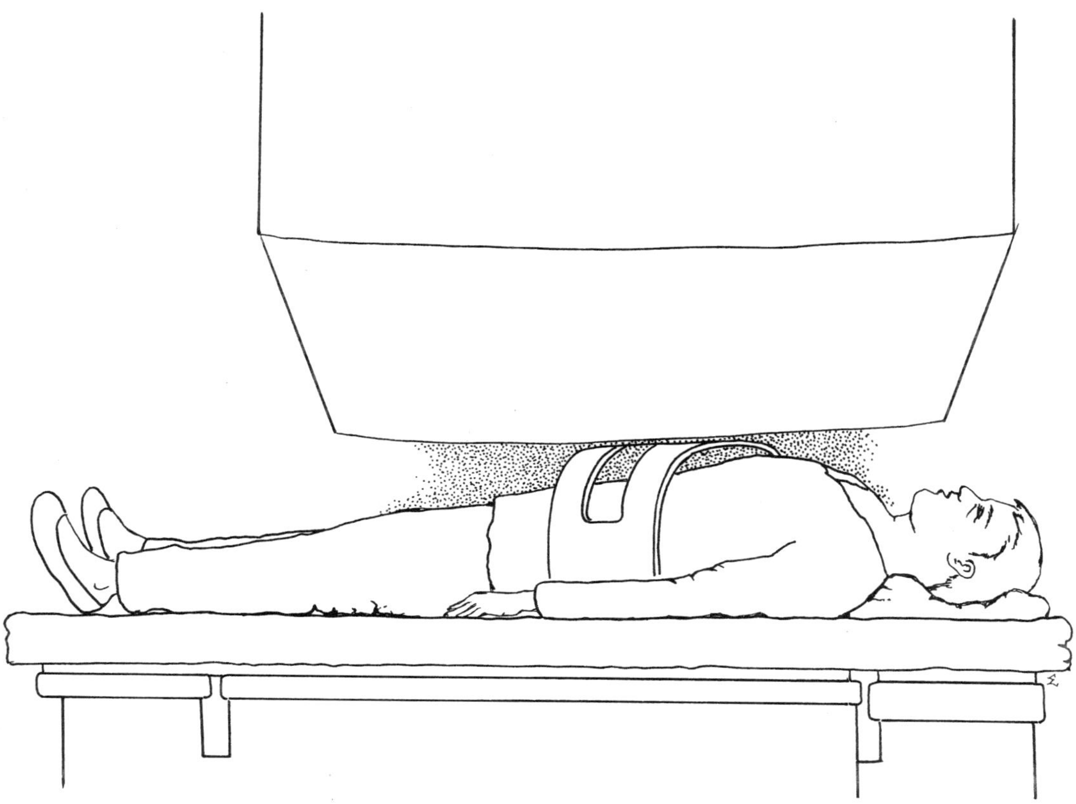

Figure 1.

- You will be free to leave after the examination. The examination will not have any aftereffects. You will be able to go about your business promptly.
- All the MRI pictures will be assembled and examined by MRI specialists. Their findings will be reported to your physician.

MYASTHENIA GRAVIS (THYMOMA)

△ GENERAL INFORMATION

Myasthenia gravis is a disease in which the body works against its nerves so that they do not properly stimulate the muscles to which they are connected. The result is that the muscles that are used to move the various parts of the body are weak and tire easily.

Myasthenia gravis is an autoimmune disease (meaning the body tries to reject some of its own tissue). The *thymus gland* is thought to be related to this disease process. The thymus gland is located beneath the upper part of the *sternum* (breast bone) (Fig. 1).

Myasthenia gravis most often affects younger women and older men.

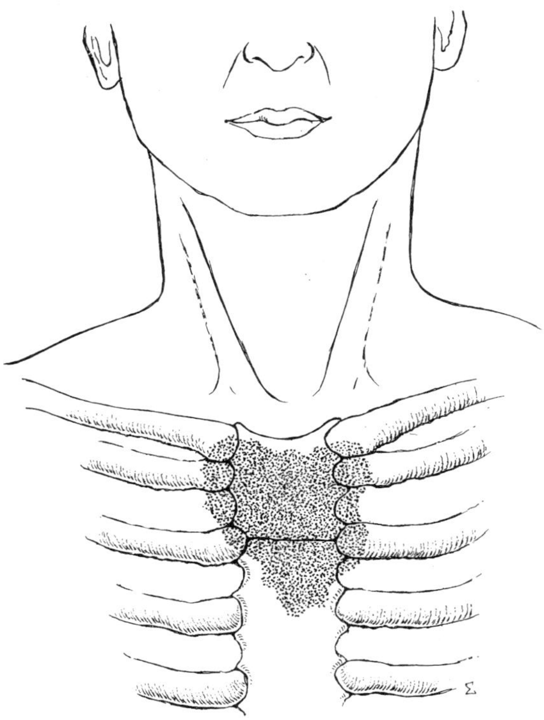

Figure 1. The diseased thymus gland *(stippled area)* is shown under the upper part of the sternum. Its size and shape can vary considerably.

COMMON SIGNS AND SYMPTOMS

- Early on, there is involvement only of the eye muscles. This produces drooping eyelids and double vision.
- Later, there may be difficulty with speaking, chewing, and swallowing. Breathing is not affected at this time.
- Later, the myasthenia may not respond well to medical therapy and there may be problems with breathing.
- At the beginning, about half of affected people have eye problems. Ultimately, about 90% develop eye problems.

DIAGNOSIS

- If anyone has the above history or symptoms, there should be concern about myasthenia gravis. Just the same, there are some other conditions that can produce some of the same symptoms.
- There are tests to determine how well the muscle receives a stimulus, and once it is stimulated, how well it responds.
- There is a test to measure how strongly the body is fighting to prevent the nerve signals from reaching the muscles.
- CT scan (computerized tomography scan): A machine shaped like a huge doughnut is used to take special x-rays. You will lie on the table inside the hole in the "doughnut." The x-rays are taken as very thin slices through the lower neck and upper part of the chest. This makes it possible to see if there's any abnormality in the thymus gland.

○ TREATMENT

- The initial treatment of myasthenia gravis should be medical.
- Operation is usually not recommended
  - For someone with only eye problems.
  - If the disease has been present for a long time and is not changing.
  - If the myasthenia develops late in life and is associated only with difficulty in chewing and swallowing.
- An operation is advisable
  - If medicines fail to control symptoms.
  - If muscle weakness develops.
  - If a tumor is seen in the thymus when the area is examined by CT scan.

After careful consideration of all factors, the recommendation is that you have your thymus removed by an operation.

PREOPERATIVE PREPARATION

- Improve the condition of the lungs as much as possible.
- Do not eat or drink anything for 8 hours before the operation unless you are specifically directed to do so by the doctor or nurse.
- Shower as usual on the morning of the operation.
- You may be given medicine that will make you feel drowsy before you are brought to the operating room.

□ OPERATION

- You will be asleep for the operation.
- The location of the incision varies; generally, however, it is over your sternum (breastbone).
- The aim of the operation is to totally remove the thymus gland.
- You will not receive a blood transfusion unless it is absolutely necessary.
- The operation takes 1 to 3 hours.

POSTOPERATIVE CARE

- You will be taken to the Surgical Care Unit, where the doctors and nurses are very experienced in taking care of patients who have undergone major surgery. As soon as you are coming along well enough, you will be transferred to a regular hospital room.
- There may be a small plastic drainage tube from your incision for several days.
- Pain will be controlled with medicine.
- You will be given an incentive spirometer. Breathing into this as you are instructed will help you expand your lungs and reduce the risk of developing pneumonia.
- You should be able to go home in a few days.
- As with any operation, complications are always possible. With this type of operation, complications can include wound infection, bleeding, heart problems, and pneumonia.
- Arrangements will be made for your medicines, follow-up office visit, and stitch removal.

✣ HOME CARE

- Continue with the program started while you were in the hospital.
- You may walk about as you wish and even climb stairs, but don't overdo things.
- Eat as you wish.
- Be certain to take your medicines exactly as prescribed.
- You may shower as you wish, with any dressings on or off.
    - There may be narrow strips of tape across the incision. It's all right if they get wet; they will be removed in the doctor's office.
    - After you dry yourself, replace any dressings with clean, dry ones.
- Driving your car may be important to you, but when you can do this safely depends on the operation you had, the medicines you are taking, and your condition in general. During your follow-up visit, talk with your doctor about when you can resume driving.
- You may resume sexual activity whenever you choose.
- You may return to work when you feel up to it, but let's talk about it first during a follow-up office visit.

✆ CALL OUR OFFICE IF

- You develop any unusual signs or symptoms.
- The incision becomes red or swollen, or there is drainage from it.
- You develop a temperature higher than 100°F.
- You have any questions.

NAVICULAR-SCAPHOID FRACTURE (WRIST FRACTURE)

△ GENERAL INFORMATION

The *navicular-scaphoid* (often just called scaphoid) is one of the small bones in your wrist. If it gets fractured (broken), this can be a real problem because it is the most important small bone in the wrist. Some breaks of the scaphoid produce a crack that is so faint an x-ray won't show it at the time of injury (Fig. 1). Often, the wrist must be put in a cast or splint and new x-rays taken weeks later when cracks in the bone become more visible. Unfortunately, the scaphoid has one of the most precarious blood supplies of any bone in the body. Even simple cracks in this bone can take months to heal in a cast.

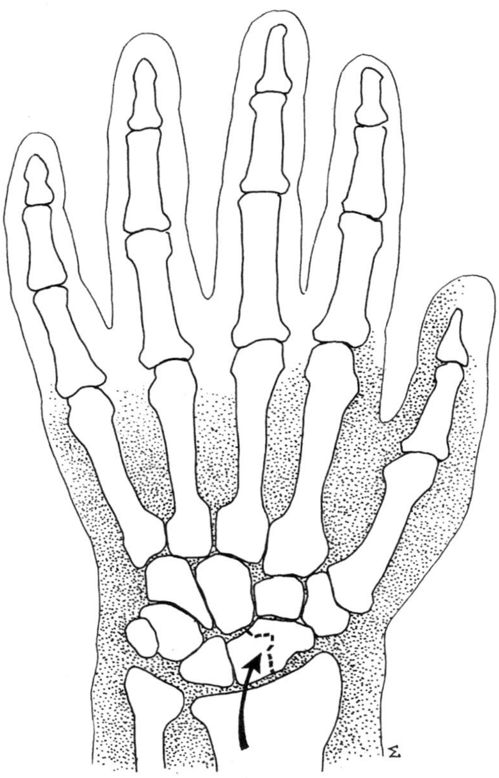

Figure 1. A typical location of a fracture is shown. However, it is not as obvious as shown; occasionally, when first seen, it can be not much wider than a human hair.

Owing to its poor blood supply, the bone occasionally does not heal properly. Sometimes it is necessary to operate if the bone does not heal. An operation may be needed if the fracture has caused the bone to be out of place and not fit in with the other bones.

DIAGNOSIS

- Every effort should be made to see that the correct diagnosis is made when a person with such a history and physical findings is seen.
- It is important to take a careful history and do a detailed physical examination, including discovering the following:
  - How the wrist was hurt and what position it was in during the accident.
  - Area of tenderness: the inside (thumbside) of the wrist hurts during movement with a scaphoid fracture.
  - Whether there is pain when pressure is applied over the proper position of the bone in the wrist.
- The wrist must be examined for areas that are swollen or bruised.
- Motion of the wrist must be tested and compared with that of the opposite (normal) wrist.

TESTS

- X-rays are taken with the wrist in several positions. If they show a fracture, then treatment can be started. If they are *negative* but the above symptoms are present, more tests are necessary.
- Magnified x-ray pictures sometimes can show very fine cracks.
- Tomography: this technique makes x-rays that look at the bone in thin slices, a layer at a time.
- CT scans or bone scans are also occasionally used in an effort to detect cracks not visualized on plain x-rays.

○ TREATMENT

- The proper treatment for this fracture is to have your arm and palm in a plaster cast if the fracture is a simple crack (not out of line). The healing time depends somewhat on where the crack is located.
- If you have pain specifically over the scaphoid bone after such an injury, you must be treated for a fracture even if the x-rays don't show a fracture.
- The wrist is immobilized, and several weeks later the cast is removed and new x-rays are taken. If originally there was a crack that could not be seen, it usually has become visible by x-ray by this point in the healing process.
- If the x-ray results are now positive for scaphoid fracture, that's bad news and good news: bad news because you have a fracture but good news because you had it treated correctly from the very beginning. This greatly improves the chances that the fracture will heal.
  - A cast will be reapplied. This will be repeated in about 4 weeks.
  - You will need a cast until the x-rays show adequate healing. Generally, this takes approximately 4 months, depending on many individual factors.
- Surgery is needed in two situations:
  - If, after all of the above guidelines are followed, the bone does not heal.

- If the initial fracture leads to bending or separation of the two halves of the scaphoid bone. In such a case, the wrist needs to be opened to get the bone back into place. Often, pins or a screw are needed to hold the bone in position during the healing phase.

△ GENERAL INFORMATION

Nephrostomy is a way to make it possible for urine to come straight to the outside through the skin instead of through the usual route.

The kidney makes urine that carries out waste products and extra water from your body. The urine passes from the kidneys down soft tubes (the *ureters*) that are the size and consistency of cooked macaroni and into the bladder. The urine stays in the bladder until you feel the urge to urinate. Sometimes the ureter is blocked for one reason or another, so urine cannot get to the bladder.

A procedure called a *percutaneous nephrostomy* (PCN) is necessary to let the urine come straight to the outside.

COMMON SIGNS AND SYMPTOMS

Even though the ureter is blocked and urine cannot get by, the kidney still keeps on making urine for a while.

- The ureter and the kidney become swollen from the backed-up urine.
- There is pain, mostly in the flank area.
- There is loss of appetite, nausea, and vomiting.
- If an infection develops in the ureter, there can be shaking chills and a high fever.

DIAGNOSIS

If the diagnosis is not known, some or all of the following tests will be necessary:

- *Ultrasound*: Harmless sound waves are aimed at the kidney, ureters, and bladder. The sound waves bouncing back (the echoes) from this area are seen as a picture on a screen. This is a convenient and painless way to see the condition of the kidneys and ureters.
- *CT scan (computed tomography scan)*: Special x-rays are taken as very thin slices through the area of the kidneys, ureters, and bladder. This makes it possible to see details in this area.
- *Cystoureteroscopy*: You will be put to sleep. This procedure involves placing a flexible tube (a *catheter*) that is about as big around as angel hair spaghetti into your bladder and up the ureters. Dye will be injected into the ureter and x-rays taken to show where the ureter is blocked, possibly by what it is blocked, and how serious the situation may be.

PURPOSE AND CONDITIONS FOR A KIDNEY PELVIS OR URETER TUBE

Placing a tube in the kidney pelvis or ureter is helpful for the following purposes:

- To be able to inject dye in the kidney pelvis to get pictures that may show what is causing the blockage and its location.
- To collect urine to see how well the kidney is working.
- To collect urine to determine the cause of the infection.
- To collect cells lining the kidney to see if cancer is present.
- To relieve back pressure caused by a stone, scar, or tumor, or to drain urine that is full of pus.
- To stretch a narrowed ureter.
- To break up and remove stones.

After careful consideration of all factors, the recommendation is that you have a nephrostomy soon. If the kidney remains blocked much longer, it may stop working. If it stops working too long, it dies and won't make urine, even if the blockage is removed at a later time.

PREPARATION FOR THE PROCEDURE

- You will have an examination of your blood, urine, heart (EKG), and lungs (chest x-ray).
- Do not eat or drink anything for 8 hours before the procedure.
- You will be given antibiotics.

□ OPERATION

- You may be given medicine that will make you feel drowsy.
- You will lie on your stomach.
- Your back in the area of your lower ribs will be painted with an antiseptic solution and surrounded with sterile towels. The skin will be made numb.
- A soft tube the size of spaghetti will be inserted through the numbed skin and into the kidney and possibly down into the ureter (Fig. 1).
- The procedure usually takes about 1 hour.

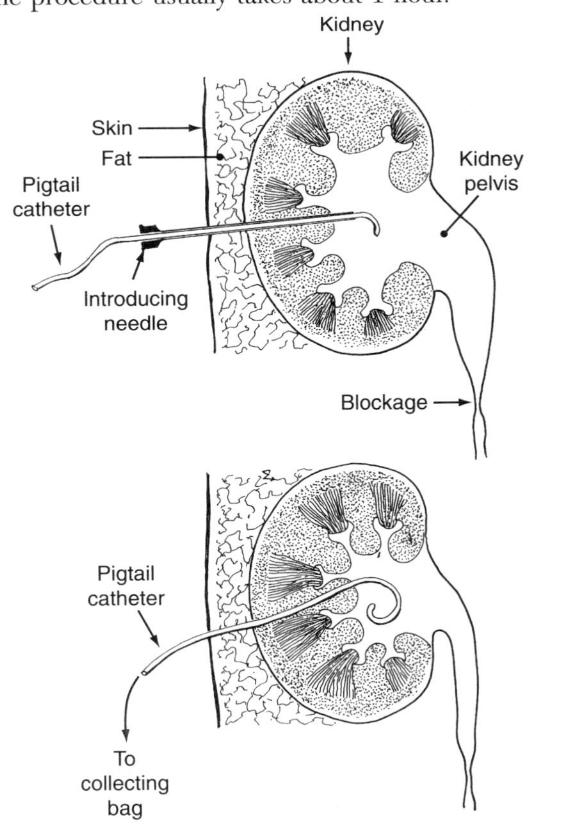

Figure 1. The nephrostomy tube is flexible and curled. This discourages it from accidentally falling out. When it is pulled for removal, it straightens out easily.

POSTOPERATIVE CARE

- You will be taken to a recovery room. When your blood pressure, pulse, and breathing are stable, you will be taken to a regular hospital room.
- There will be a tube coming out from your flank and connected to a special bag to collect the urine.
- Pain will be controlled with medicine.
- The evening after the surgery you will be helped to get out of bed and the next day to walk about.
- The hospital team of doctors and nurses will show you how to take care of the tube and how to empty the bag when it is full; it is not difficult.
- You should be able to go home the next day.
- As with any operation, complications are always possible. With this type of operation, complications can include infection, bleeding, blood clots, heart problems, and some others.
- Arrangements will be made for your medicine and follow-up office visit.

✚ HOME CARE

- You may walk about as you wish and even climb stairs, but don't overdo things.
- You may eat as you wish.
- Arrangements can be made for a home visiting nurse if one is needed.
- Take medicines as prescribed for you.
- You may drive a car if you wish, but only if you are not taking medicines that reduce your alertness.

✆ CALL OUR OFFICE IF

- The urine in the collecting bag becomes cloudy, red, or foul-smelling.
- There is very little urine in the bag.
- The area where the tube comes through the skin becomes red or swollen, or there is drainage from it.
- You develop a temperature higher than 100°F.
- The tube is accidentally pulled out, even part-way.
- You have any questions.

△ GENERAL INFORMATION

Neurolytic (or *neuroablative*) techniques are aimed at either damaging or destroying nerves. Neurolytic techniques can be useful in treating chronic pain; however, they must be used with extreme care, both in the selection of the patient and in the actual performance of the procedure.

THE NERVOUS SYSTEM

Nerves go to various parts of the body either directly from the brain or from the spinal cord. The spinal cord passes through a tunnel in the back part of the backbone (the spine) and goes from the underside of the brain down to the waist. At this point, it divides into many separate nerves. Along its length, the spinal cord gives off branches to the right and left every inch or so. These branches carry signals (including those of pain) to the brain from various parts of the body. Also, from the brain, signals go to various parts of the body to make things work.

NERVES SUITABLE FOR NEUROLYSIS

Some of the nerves from the spinal cord carry both types of signals—those for pain and those that make things move. Such nerves are not suitable for neurolysis. If an attempt is made to destroy the part of the nerve that carries the pain sensation to the brain, there is too much risk of injuring the portion of the nerve that makes things move. This, of course, is unacceptable.

For this reason, neurolytic procedures are performed for those nerves that carry only pain sensations to the brain and have nothing—or very little—to do with making things move. Some examples of nerves treated include the following:

- Nerve networks in the abdomen. The two important ones are the *celiac plexus* and the *hypogastric plexus*. Blocking these nerves can give relief from certain kinds of chronic abdominal pain.
- Nerves that travel under each rib (the *intercostal nerves*). Blocking these nerves can give relief of pain from certain types of chest trauma and of abdominal pain.
- Nerves that carry pain sensations from the joints of the spine.
- *Sympathetic nerves*. Blocking these nerves can help relieve pain caused by poor blood flow to the legs or by shingles.

HOW A NERVE BLOCK IS PERFORMED

Neurolytic procedures require considerable skill in several ways.

- Accurately determining whether a patient with pain is suitable for a nerve block.
- Having proper technical experience to be able to place the needle with the blocking agent in the correct spot.
- Avoiding complications.

Most neurolytic procedures are done on an outpatient basis.

- The position of the patient depends on the area being treated.
- The skin over the area is prepared in a sterile fashion.
- A spot on the skin over the target area is made numb with an anesthetic.
- A special needle is placed through the numbed skin and down to a nerve. Then a temporary anesthetic is injected in the desired spot of the nerve.
  - If there is no relief from this injection, it indicates that the person will not benefit from a neurolysis.
  - If there is relief, the patient can have an idea of how helpful the relief will be. If this is favorable, then preparations can be made to inject a longer-lasting neurolytic drug.

TYPES OF NEUROLYTIC PROCEDURES

The neurolysis can be performed in several ways.

- **Surgical:** This involves actually exposing the involved nerve or nerves by a surgical incision and then cutting the nerve, removing a portion of the nerve, or crushing the nerve with a surgical clamp. The first two procedures actually destroy the nerve, while crushing the nerve only damages it. This allows the nerve to recover at a later date.
- **Physical:** These neurolytic procedures involve applying controlled heat or cold to the nerve. This can be done under direct vision at the time of the operation or, more commonly, by reaching the nerve with a special type of needle inserted through the skin. Heat neurolysis is commonly called *thermocoagulation* and uses a radio-frequency electric current generation. Cold neurolysis is called *cryoablation* and utilizes a special freezing needle called a *cryoprobe.*
- **Chemical:** This technique involves injecting a caustic chemical into the nerve. Again, this can be done under direct vision at the time of the operation but is much more commonly done with a needle inserted through the skin *(percutaneously)*. The most commonly used agents for chemical neurolysis are either alcohol or phenol; however, there are several other chemicals that are occasionally used.

Percutaneous neurolytic procedures are usually done while using x-rays to see where the needle is going, except for those procedures that only require a very shallow insertion of the needle.

COMPLICATIONS

As with any procedure, complications are always possible. With neurolytic procedures, complications can include the following:

- The neurolytic agent may spread to block nerves one does not wish to be included in the block, particularly nerves that stimulate things to move.
- The neurolytic agent or cryoablation or thermocoagulation may cause a painful inflammation of the nerves and actually produce an increase in the pain (this is called reactive neuritis).

The use of ultra-long-lasting local anesthetics, which are now being developed, may one day eliminate most of the hazards of neurolytic blocking agents.

As you see, neurolytic nerve blocks require great skill to administer and carry appreciable risk. However, for the proper patient and with the procedure performed correctly and successfully, a neurolytic nerve block can give precious relief of pain and dramatically affect a person's quality of life.

NEUROSTIMULATION: Peripheral Nerve and Spinal Cord

△ GENERAL INFORMATION

The *spinal column* extends from the base of the skull to the waist. In the back part of the spine is a tunnel (the *spinal canal*). Down this canal runs the *spinal cord*, which is about as thick as the tip of your little finger. On its way down toward the waist, the spinal cord gives off nerve branches to the right and left every inch or so. They range in size from spaghetti to macaroni (Fig. 1).

These nerve branches look solid, but, in fact, they are made up of many small fibers. Each of these small fibers has a special job: Some fibers carry signals from the brain to the various parts of the body to make things move. Other fibers carry different kinds of sensation (smell, cold, warm, as well as the sensation of *pain*) back to the brain. It is only when these sensations reach the brain that a person actually *experiences* the feeling.

HOW NEUROSTIMULATION (NERVE STIMULATION) WORKS

It so happens that the fibers that carry the sensation of pain back to the brain work more slowly than the fibers that carry other sensations. So, if the nerves from an area can be stimulated artificially (by a very tiny electrical current), so many nonpain sensations will reach the spinal cord and brain right away that they will crowd out the sensations of pain that get there later. So, fewer sensations of pain will be felt. As an analogy, if there are 100 seats in a theater and when the doors open 125 people rush for those seats, the 25 slowest walkers will be less likely to find a seat.

The principle of nerve stimulation to relieve pain is to artificially stimulate a nerve coming from a painful area of the body so that the pain sensation traveling along these fibers can be crowded out by the nonpain sensation traveling faster along these fibers. Remember, it is only when the sensations of pain reach the brain that a person has a feeling of pain; if that nerve sensation cannot reach the brain, then there won't be a feeling of pain.

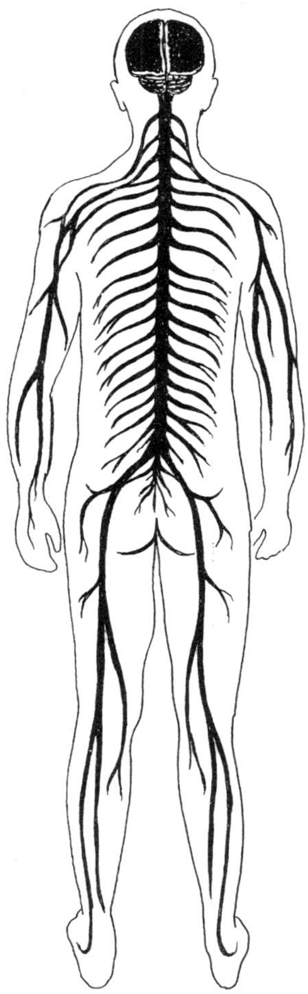

Figure 1.

HOW NEUROSTIMULATION IS USED

One simple use of electrostimulation is called transcutaneous electrical neurostimulation (TENS). This involves stimulation at the skin level with electrode pads that are placed on the skin *(transcutaneous)* to stimulate (by electrical means) certain nerves going to muscle *(neuromuscular)*. This is done to nerves traveling underneath the skin. The technique of spinal cord stimulation and peripheral nerve stimulation is more sophisticated and takes place deeper in the tissue. They are procedures generally done by anesthesiologists who have a special interest in pain management.

PEOPLE WHO CAN BENEFIT FROM NEUROSTIMULATION

Spinal cord stimulation is known to relieve chronic pain that has not responded to other treatment, for example, persistent pain following one or more spinal operations or chronic pain in the arms or legs due to nerve irritation and nerve damage.

HOW NEUROSTIMULATION IS DONE

With spinal cord stimulation, a series of tiny electrodes is placed within the spinal canal and will be used to stimulate the spinal cord. These electrodes are then connected to a battery unit that sends continuous impulses to the electrodes.

This stimulation of the spinal cord produces a tingling sensation in the area where the patient has pain, for example, in the arm, low back, or leg region. The stimulation of the painful part then crowds out the number of pain impulses that can reach the spinal cord and travel upward to the brain, where they would be interpreted as pain.

The practice of spinal cord stimulation is usually done as a two-stage event. The first stage is a temporary period of stimulation done with an electrode that is inserted into the spinal canal through the skin with a special needle. The fine electrode is left within the spinal canal to stimulate the spinal cord.

HOW DECISION IS MADE TO USE NEUROSTIMULATION

The patient is usually sent home and observed as an outpatient. The trial period of stimulation is continued over the next several days to see if there is relief of pain. Pain relief is usually judged to be successful if 50% or more of the pain goes away. If the patient has very little or no relief of pain, the fine electrode is withdrawn. If, however, the patient experiences 50% or greater relief of pain, that patient is considered to be suitable to receive a permanent implant.

After careful consideration of all factors, the recommendation is that you have an operation for permanent implantation of a nerve stimulator next to your spinal cord.

PREOPERATIVE PREPARATION

- You will have an examination of your blood, urine, heart (EKG), and lungs (chest x-ray).
- Do not eat or drink anything for 8 hours before the operation.

□ OPERATION

- You will be asleep for the operation.
- After you are asleep you will be turned so that you are lying on your stomach. A short incision will be made lengthwise over your spine.
- The stimulating electrode will be placed inside the spinal canal and passed up to the area through which the impulses start. The electrode will then be connected to a small pulse generator battery that is placed nearby, under the skin. When the operation is completed, everything will be under the skin.

POSTOPERATIVE CARE

- You will be taken to a recovery room and observed. When your blood pressure, pulse, and breathing are stable, you will be taken to a regular hospital room.
- Stimulation will be turned on within 24 hours.
- Doctors and technicians will work closely with you because you will need to be an active partner in knowing how this works and when and how you will need to make adjustments.
- As with any operation, complications are always possible, some of them serious. With this type of operation, complications can include electrode migration, which results in poor stimulation of the painful area. If such migration occurs, it may require the implanting surgeon to remove the old electrode and reinsert a new electrode. More serious possible complications are infection or bleeding in the spinal canal. These problems may require a spine surgeon to perform an operation. While extremely rare, the potential nerve injury associated with spinal surgery may leave the patient with numbness or weakness below the waist.

✣ HOME CARE

- There is no limitation on your activity if it does not interfere with your care.
- You will be advised on when you can start taking baths or showers and how to take care of the incision.
- Once the unit is in place, you will need to adjust it, usually on a daily basis. You are sent home with a portable programmer that allows you to do so.
- Remember, this device is not meant or expected to eliminate all of your pain; it almost never does. It is hoped that the device will decrease the severity of your pain and therefore the amount of pain medicine you need to take. The doctors and nurses will work closely with you on a proper schedule of pain medicines.
- You should not drive a car or otherwise use power tools if your medicines reduce your alertness.

✆ CALL OUR OFFICE IF

- You develop any unusual signs or symptoms.
- The incision becomes red or swollen, or there is drainage from it.
- You develop a temperature higher than 100°F.
- You have any questions.

△ GENERAL INFORMATION

Onycho (toe or finger*nail*) *mycosis* (a *fungus* infection), namely, a fungus infection of the toenail or fingernail, is very common.

COMMON SIGNS AND SYMPTOMS

The appearance is fairly typical. The end of the nail becomes thicker, and, with time, this thickening progresses up toward the base of the nail or across the entire front, or both.

- Soon it becomes difficult to trim the nail properly.
- Usually, the condition has been present for a long time.
- The toenail can become so thick and twisted that it is uncomfortable to walk. Also, it is unsightly.

DIAGNOSIS

Usually, the diagnosis can be made by taking a detailed history and doing a thorough physical examination.

THERAPY

- Most fungus infections of the toenail are ignored; some can be treated with medicines.
- Occasionally, however, the whole nail is so totally involved and twisted and bothersome that removing the toenail to give a new nail a fresh start is a reasonable thing to do.

PREOPERATIVE PREPARATION

- Shower or bathe as usual on the morning of the operation.
- Bring along an open-toed sandal. The bandage on your toe right after the operation will be bulky, which will prevent you from putting on a regular shoe.

□ OPERATION

- You will lie on a table. Your foot will be painted with an antiseptic solution and draped with sterile towels.
- A very fine, short needle will be used to inject an anesthetic into the nerves of the toe. This will make the toe entirely numb.
- The toenail with the fungus can then be removed.
- While this is being done, you will feel some tugging but no pain.
- This procedure removes the nail but it does not remove the cuticle, that part of the nail that can make a new nail.
- The area of your toenail will now be open but will not be painful because the toe will still be numb.
- A vaseline dressing will be applied over the raw area. A snug bandage will be wound around the toe.
- The operation usually takes 30 minutes.
- You should be able to go home directly after the operation. You will be able to walk on that foot.
- Arrangements will be made for pain medicine and a follow-up office visit.

✚ HOME CARE

- You may walk about for the first day, but only for essential things such as going to the bathroom. Mostly, lie on a couch with your leg elevated on a pillow. It will be more comfortable.
- Take medicine as prescribed for your pain.
- Some blood may seep through the bandage. This is common and should not alarm you.
- Do not get the bandage wet.
- You may return to work when you feel able to do so. If possible, try to rest the toe for 10 minutes several times during the day by sitting down and placing the leg on another chair.
- Do not drive your car. It is too dangerous. Let's discuss this during your follow-up office visit.
- On the morning of the first follow-up visit, take a shower and allow the foot to get wet. Dry and dress yourself as usual. This soaking of the toe will make it much easier and more comfortable for the first dressing to come off when you reach the doctor's office.
- Only a light dressing will be applied after the first dressing is removed.
- You'll be surprised at how soon the raw area will become dry (usually within 24 hours). A clean sock over this usually is enough.
- For a few days you will need to improvise, wearing shoes that are comfortable.
- A "new" toenail will start growing back soon. It usually takes about 2 months before it is fully grown. Also, the first new nail may be a little wavy. Usually, but not always, it becomes smooth like your opposite toenail.

✆ CALL OUR OFFICE IF

- Red blood continues to seep through the bandage wrapped around the toe.
- The toe continues to hurt and throb even after you lie down, elevate your foot, and take pain medicine.
- You develop a temperature higher than 100°F.
- You have any questions.

△ GENERAL INFORMATION

Bilateral orchiectomy is an operation in which the two testicles are removed. These are the two egg-shaped organs in the left and right side of the *scrotum*, which is the sac behind the penis. The testicles produce male hormones as well as sperm.

Often, a man with cancer of the prostate will receive hormone therapy for this condition, and this treatment works. After a while, however, the medicine may no longer be effective. A choice has to be made on how to cancel out the male hormones so they will not stimulate the cancer to grow.

○ TREATMENT

The options in treatment are as follows: Option 1: To give you female hormones, a medication which shuts down the male hormone system. Option 2: To remove your male hormones (they are made in your testicles).

- Removing both of your testicles will make you sterile permanently. You will not be able to father a child. Also, you likely will not be able to have an erection.
- Of course, the effects will be similar with female hormones.

After careful consideration of all factors, it is recommended that removing your testicles is the best treatment for you. The reasons for this have been explained to you.

On occasion, it is possible to place two egg-shaped plastic pieces in your scrotum so that it looks "full." This step, however, can create some problems with infection later. Nonetheless, if you think you would like this done, let's discuss it.

PREOPERATIVE PREPARATION

- You will have an examination of your blood, urine, heart (EKG), and lungs (chest x-ray).
- Do not eat or drink anything for 8 hours before the operation.
- Shower (and shave) as usual on the morning of the operation.
- You may be given medicine that will make you feel drowsy before you are brought to the operating room.

□ OPERATION

- You will be asleep for the operation.
- You will not need a blood transfusion.
- The operation usually takes about 1 hour.

POSTOPERATIVE CARE

- You will wake up in a recovery room. When your blood pressure, pulse, and breathing are stable, you should be able to go home with a responsible adult. Occasionally, one has to stay in the hospital overnight.
- There will be a snug dressing over the incisions. Jockey-type shorts will be placed over the dressings to keep the scrotum collapsed.
- Pain will be controlled with medicine.
- Arrangements will be made for your medicine and follow-up office visit. The stitches are absorbable.
- As with any operation, complications are always possible. With this type of operation, complications can include bleeding into the scrotum, infection, temporary problems with urination, and possibly others.

✙ HOME CARE

- You may walk about as you wish, even climb stairs, but don't overdo things.
- Lie down for 15 minutes three to four times a day. This will help keep down any swelling of your scrotum and make you more comfortable.
- You may eat as you did before the operation.
- Don't lift anything heavier than 5 pounds. Ask someone to do it for you.
- You may shower if you wish, with any dressings on or off. After you dry yourself, replace any dressings with clean, dry ones.
- Wear jockey-type shorts.
- Take medicine as prescribed for your pain.
- Driving a car with an automatic shift is not too demanding, but if you suddenly have to slam on the brakes or twist to turn the steering wheel, you may strain the sutures or tear something. During the follow-up visit, let's discuss when you can resume driving.
- You may return to work when you feel up to it.

✆ CALL OUR OFFICE IF

- The scrotum swells to a size larger than when you left the hospital.
- The incision becomes red or swollen, or there is drainage from it.
- You develop a temperature higher than 100°F.
- You have any questions.

OTITIS MEDIA: Myringotomy and Tube Placement

△ GENERAL INFORMATION

The ear has three parts to it (Fig. 1). The *outer* ear describes the part that is most visible as well as the canal (C) leading inward to the eardrum (ED). The eardrum is struck by sound waves, which cause it to vibrate. On its opposite surface, the eardrum is connected to three little bones that are in a small chamber about the size of a cranberry. This is the *middle* ear (ME). These three little bones pass the vibrations to the *inner* ear (IE), which sends them along the auditory nerve (AN) to the brain. The brain then interprets them as understandable sounds and words.

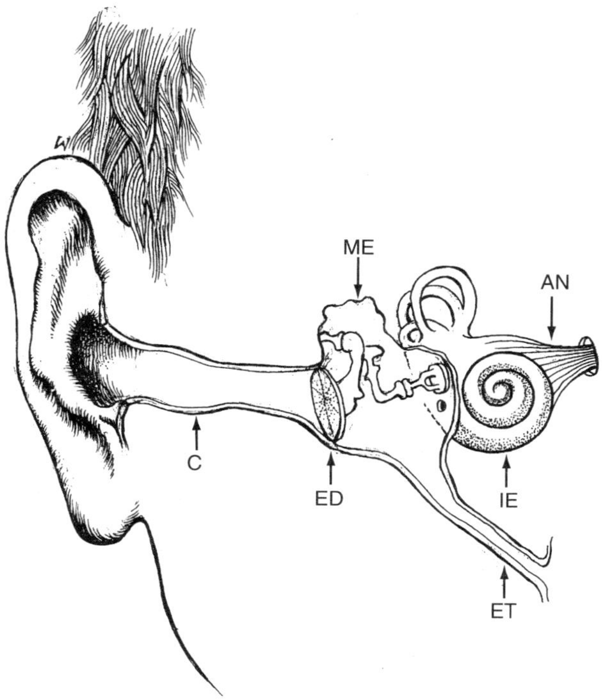

Figure 1.

The middle ear space normally is filled with air. The middle ear connects with the back of the nose through a collapsible tube called the *eustachian* tube (ET), which opens and closes with swallowing. Air in the throat can go in and out of the middle ear cavity through the eustachian tube. This allows air to enter and fluid to drain from the middle ear.

The eustachian tube is proportionally larger and at a different angle in infants and children than in adults. This makes it easier for bacteria to get from the throat to the middle ear cavity and cause an infection. Such an infection is called *otitis media*. A typical story is that of an infant or child with a "cold" who has developed otitis media. About 90% of children have such an attack by the age of 7 years. If the otitis media occurs suddenly, it is *acute* otitis media. If the infection comes and goes, or there is persistent infection, it is *chronic* otitis media.

COMMON SIGNS AND SYMPTOMS

- There is pain deep inside the affected ear. There may be a fever, but most often the temperature is normal.
- There may be evidence of a "cold," such as a cough or runny nose.
- The three little bones in the middle ear now are suspended in fluid so they and the eardrum don't move as well; hearing ability decreases. This may create speech delay and learning problems in school.
- Sometimes the pressure of fluid in the middle ear causes the eardrum to crack open, releasing liquid to the outer ear.
- In infants, irritability may be the only visible indication that an infection is present. Hearing probably is decreased, but this is not easily noticeable.

DIAGNOSIS

Anyone with the above history, symptoms, and findings, especially an infant or a young child, should be evaluated by a doctor for otitis media.

- Looking at the eardrum through the ear canal is a reliable (but not absolute) way to make the diagnosis.
- Hearing tests can help determine if fluid is present in the middle ear.
- A *tympanogram* is a measurement of the eardrum and its ability to move and is a good way to determine whether fluid is present.
- A hole in the eardrum with fluid coming out through it also establishes the diagnosis.

○ TREATMENT

- Most (90%) cases of acute otitis media treated with antibiotics get completely well, but sometimes this takes up to 3 months.
- If the fluid does not clear properly by 3 months despite antibiotics, a *myringotomy* may be suggested. This is a tiny cut made in the eardrum to drain out the fluid. At the same time, a tiny tube (the size of a grain of rice) is placed to keep the hole open and allow drainage.
- Medicated drops can be placed in the ear canal to flow through the tube into the middle ear to treat future infections.

After careful consideration of all factors, the recommendation is that your child have the fluid drained from the middle ear and at the same time a small, temporary tube placed in the eardrum.

PREOPERATIVE PREPARATION

- Do not let the child eat or drink anything for 8 hours before the operation.

□ OPERATION

- The operation will be done under quick-acting general anesthesia.
- The operation itself usually takes less than 10 minutes for both ears.

POSTOPERATIVE CARE

- Your child will be taken to a recovery room and observed. When the blood pressure, pulse, and breathing are stable and there is complete return of consciousness, your child can be taken home the same day.
- Arrangements will be made for medicines and the follow-up office visit.
- The tiny tube that was placed in the eardrum will fall out by itself in 6 to 12 months. Once in a while, it needs to be removed. All this will be explained to you in further detail.
- As with any operation, complications are always possible. They are uncommon with this type of operation and are related to being put to sleep. You should be clearly aware, however, that a number of acute and chronic problems can occur in the middle ear as a result of infection and *not* the operation. They can include acute or chronic infection of the mastoid bone, paralysis of the nerve to the face, permanent hearing loss, scarring of the eardrum, chronic perforation of the eardrum, brain abscess, and possibly others.

✚ HOME CARE

- Allow your child to engage in the usual activities.
- The diet can be as before the operation.
- Tylenol usually is sufficient for control of any pain.
- Be certain that any prescribed medicines are taken as instructed.
- When bathing your child, be certain that water does not get into the ear. You will be given suggestions on how to safeguard against this.

✆ CALL OUR OFFICE IF

- Your child develops a temperature higher than 101°F.
- Your child develops dizziness or staggering.
- The hearing is getting worse.

△ GENERAL INFORMATION

Otoplasty is derived from the Greek words *ota* (ears) and *plassein* (to mold or form). There are a variety of operations whose aim is to mold or form the ears so that they have a more "normal" and "natural" relationship to the head.

Techniques to correct ear deformity were first described more than 1,000 years ago. However, the operation to correct protruding ears was first performed just over a century ago.

About 5% of white people have some degree of abnormally protruding ears. A number of such individuals come to the plastic surgeon for consultation and treatment.

A typical history is one of merciless and relentless teasing by schoolmates with all types of unkind epithets such as Dumbo, Donkey-ears, Droopy, and others. Although this does not seriously affect many children, there are others in whom the psychosocial consequences can be very important. Further, such handicaps often persist in later social relationships as well as employment opportunities.

CANDIDATES FOR OTOPLASTY

Naturally, there can be differences of opinion among the patient, family, friends, and the consulting surgeon on what degree of deformity needs surgical correction. It is important to be aware, however, of how you yourself feel about matters rather than to be influenced by what others think.

CHOOSING A SURGEON

When deciding that something needs to be done to correct a cosmetic ear problem, there are a number of things to consider:

- Choose a plastic surgeon who has a continued interest, specific training, appropriate experience, and demonstrated technical skills in performing otoplasty. Equally important, the surgeon must have a full understanding of the psychosocial impact of what, to some, may appear an unimportant deformity.
- Getting opinions from two plastic surgeons is appropriate. Also, you should have your questions answered to your satisfaction.
- Be certain that the reasons you are seeking help are important to you and are not necessarily just to satisfy the opinions of others.
- Have realistic expectations.

○ TREATMENT

Each type of ear deformity requires some individualization of operative technique. The technique that will be used has been explained to you beforehand.

PREOPERATIVE PREPARATION

- There will be a careful examination of the head and neck, with special emphasis on the ears. A number of photographs will be taken. You may be shown a gallery of postoperative photographs of other patients to give you an idea of possible results.
- You may have an examination of your blood, urine, heart (EKG), and lungs (chest x-ray).
- Do not eat or drink anything for 8 hours before the operation.
- Shower or bathe on the morning of the operation.
- You may be given medicine that will make you feel drowsy before you are brought to the operating room.

□ OPERATION

- You will be asleep for the operation.
- You will not need a blood transfusion.
- Most often, both ears will need to be done.
- The operation usually takes about 2 hours.

POSTOPERATIVE CARE

- You will wake up in a recovery room. When your blood pressure, pulse, and breathing are stable, you will be taken to a regular hospital room.
- You will have a bandage encircling your head completely that will also snugly cover your ears.
- Pain is expected and sometimes is significant, but it can be controlled with medicine.
- Your diet will be as tolerated.
- As with any operation, complications are always possible. With this type of operation, complications can include bleeding, infection, loss of some skin around the incision, and possibly others.
- You should be able to go home the day after the operation.
- Arrangements will be made for your medicine, follow-up office visit, and stitch removal.

✣ HOME CARE

- You may walk about as you wish, even climb stairs.
- You may eat as you did before the operation.
- You may bathe as you wish. It is important not to get the dressing wet, so as a precaution, wear a shower cap.

✆ CALL OUR OFFICE IF

- You have pain under the dressings that is not letting up, even with the pain medicine prescribed for you, or you have pain that is more prominent on one side.
- You develop any unusual signs or symptoms.
- You develop a temperature higher than 100°F.
- You have any questions.

△ GENERAL INFORMATION

Otoplasty is derived from the Greek words *ota* (ears) and *plassein* (to mold or form). There are a variety of operations whose aim is to mold or form the ears so that they have a more "normal" and "natural" relationship to the head.

Techniques to correct ear deformity were first described more than 1,000 years ago. However, the operation to correct protruding ears was first performed just over a century ago.

About 5% of white people have some degree of abnormally protruding ears. A number of such individuals are brought to the plastic surgeon for consultation and treatment.

The person for whom surgical advice is sought most often is a young child. A typical history is one of merciless and relentless teasing by schoolmates with all types of unkind epithets such as Dumbo, Donkey-ears, Droopy, and others. The psychosomatic impact on a young child is not insignificant and should not be taken lightly.

CANDIDATES FOR OTOPLASTY

Naturally, there can be differing viewpoints among the patient, family, and surgeon on what degree of deformity needs surgical correction. It is important to respect how the *patient* feels about matters and not just what others think about it.

CHOOSING A SURGEON

When deciding that something needs to be done to correct a cosmetic ear problem for your child, there are a number of things to consider:

- Choose a plastic surgeon who has a continuing interest, specific training, appropriate experience, and demonstrated technical skills in performing plastic surgery procedures on ear abnormalities. Equally important, the surgeon must have a full understanding and sympathy with the psychosocial impact on a child being called names. It also should be realized that the social handicaps of a person with protruding ears are not necessarily confined to just the childhood years.
- Getting opinions from two plastic surgeons is appropriate. Also, you should have your questions answered to your satisfaction.
- Be certain that the reasons for seeking help for your child have to do with a legitimate deformity and any psychosocial consequences from it.
- Seek help on how to keep your child informed, without causing undue anxiety, about an operation.
- Have realistic expectations.
- Inform the relevant school personnel of any pending operation.

○ TREATMENT

Each type of ear deformity requires some individualization of operative technique. The technique that will be used with your child has been explained to you beforehand.

PREOPERATIVE PREPARATION

- There will be a careful examination of the head and neck, with special emphasis on the appearance and possible solution to the ear problem.
- A blood cell count may be ordered.
- A number of photographs will be taken. You may be shown a gallery of postoperative photographs of other patients to give you an idea of possible results.
- Do not let the child eat or drink anything for 8 hours before the operation.

□ OPERATION

- The operation will be done under general anesthesia.
- Often, both ears need to be done.
- Generally, the operation takes 2 hours.

POSTOPERATIVE CARE

- The child will wake up in a recovery room. When the blood pressure, pulse, and breathing are stable, the child will be taken to a regular hospital room.
- There will be a bandage going completely around the head, very much like a large sweatband. It will cover both ears.
- Pain is expected and sometimes is significant, but it can be controlled with medicine.
- The diet can be as tolerated.
- As with any operation, complications are always possible. With this type of operation, complications can include bleeding, infection, loss of some skin around the incision, and possibly others.
- You should be able to take your child home the day after the operation.
- Arrangements will be made for medicine, follow-up office visit, and stitch removal.

✣ HOME CARE

- The child may walk about as he or she wishes, even climb stairs.
- The child may eat as before the operation.
- The child may bathe as desired, but the dressing should not be allowed to become wet. Wearing a shower cap while bathing is a worthwhile precaution.

✆ CALL OUR OFFICE IF

- The child has pain under the dressing that is not letting up despite pain medication, or if the pain is more severe on one side.
- There is the development of any unusual signs or symptoms.
- The child develops a temperature higher than 100°F.
- You have any questions.

△ GENERAL INFORMATION

A very large number of operations are done on an outpatient basis or with a hospital stay of less than 24 hours. Some patients who are scheduled to have an operation performed in such a setting become anxious, but there is little reason for this. Advances have been made in so many ways and areas that, when properly selected and done, outpatient surgery is just as safe and effective as when you are admitted to a hospital. Very likely, you will be pleasantly surprised how well things will go. Much of this will go more smoothly if you read the following and if you participate as much and as well as you can.

Once the diagnosis is made and the recommendation is that you have your operation as an outpatient, there will be a full discussion with you on the reasons this is best for you. Some of these considerations and reasons may be as follows:

- There is a short recovery time.
- There can be less emotional strain on you; you will be able to return to familiar surroundings much sooner.
- The atmosphere of an outpatient facility (or the doctor's office) often is more relaxed than it is in a hospital.
- Often it is more convenient for you and your family.
- Because you will not stay in the hospital, the cost generally is lower.

TYPE OF FACILITY

The outpatient surgical facility can be one that is attached to a hospital, is free-standing, or simply is in the surgeon's office.

PREOPERATIVE EXAMINATION

The history of your problem will be carefully noted, as will any information that might influence the way to proceed with your operation. Such information can include allergies to any medicines, whether you take medicines that might change your blood clotting (example: aspirin, Coumadin), any unusual reactions to previous operations, and whether you take any illicit drugs (cocaine, marijuana, LSD) of any type and at any time.

PREOPERATIVE TESTS

What tests you have will again be influenced by your surgical problem and the planned operation.

- Often it is not necessary to have any laboratory tests at all.
- Sometimes the blood is examined to see whether it clots properly.
- A common routine is to have your blood and urine examined for any unexpected abnormality.
- If you are older than 50 years of age or your past medical history or the operation warrants it, you may have an examination of your heart (EKG) and your lungs (chest x-ray).
- If any other tests are needed, they will be explained to you beforehand.

PREOPERATIVE PREPARATION: Medical

- There may be diet restrictions preoperatively. You will be instructed on these. If there is any question about what you should do in this respect, ask the nurse/anesthesia service at the outpatient surgery facility about it.
- Some operations require you to have your bowel cleansed beforehand. You will be given instructions on how to do this.
- If you need to take medicines regularly, be certain to discuss with the surgeon or the anesthesiologist what you should do about this on the day of the operation.
- Shower or bathe (and shave) as usual on the day of the operation, unless instructed otherwise.
- Do not wear lipstick, fingernail polish, or mascara. If you are having surgery on your face or neck, take off all makeup as instructed.

PREOPERATIVE PREPARATION: Personal

- If anything prevents you from keeping your appointment (example: a cold, cough, or fever) inform the surgeon and the outpatient surgical facility promptly.
- Wear loose-fitting clothing.
- Leave all jewelry and valuables at home.
- You must have a responsible escort to accompany you home if you have sedation or general anesthesia. Often, it is advisable to also make arrangements for someone to be with you the first 24 hours after the operation.
- Don't forget to bring any regular medicines with you.

REGISTERING AT THE OUTPATIENT FACILITY

- Be certain to bring along the results of all the laboratory tests that were done in preparation for this operation. If, for some reason, the results are not available at all, the operation may need to be postponed.
- Bring along any insurance information.
- You will be asked to sign a routine consent for the operation.
- A band with your name on it will be applied around your wrist.
- You will be shown where to disrobe and put on an appropriate gown, cap, and slippers. You then will be helped onto a comfortable cart.
- You may be given medicine to make you feel drowsy before you are brought into the operating room.

□ OPERATION

- The operating room is brightly lit and on the cool side, and a lot of activity takes place in it.
- The nurse will introduce herself or himself and be at your side while you are prepared for the operation.
- Intravenous fluids may be started. The medicines to make you drowsy or keep you asleep are given through them.
- A tiny oxygen catheter may be placed at the opening of your nose.

- The anesthesiologist or nurse anesthetist or the surgeon will have discussed with you beforehand the type of anesthesia to be used. This can be any of the following:
  - Local anesthesia: A very fine needle is used to place the anesthetic around the area of the incision to make it numb.
  - Local anesthesia along with medicine to make you feel drowsy during the operation.
  - Putting you totally asleep.
  - A nerve block: The nerve to an area of your body is injected with an anesthetic to make it numb.
  - A spinal type of anesthesia.
- The area to be operated on will be prepared with an antiseptic solution and surrounded with sterile drapes.
- If the operation is done with the help of a video screen, the lights in the room will be very dim.
- Wires attached to recording machines will be taped to several places on your skin. They will keep track of your blood pressure, heartbeat, breathing, and level of oxygen in your blood.
- If local anesthesia is used, you may feel some tugging during the operation, but no pain. If, however, you do feel any twinge of pain, mention it to the surgeon because this can easily be taken care of.
- Many patients who have anesthesia along with sedation do not remember very much afterward about the operation itself.

POSTOPERATIVE CARE

- You will be taken to a recovery room and observed. When your blood pressure, pulse, and breathing are normal and you are completely alert, you will be offered some fluids to drink. At this point you can go home with a responsible adult.
- As appropriate, you will be given instructions on your diet, activity, wound care, medicines, and your follow-up visit.

✣ HOME CARE

- Follow the instructions given to you.
- For the first day or so eat soft foods in small amounts.
- Do not use any power equipment or drive if you are taking medicines that may decrease your alertness or if you cannot move freely and without pain.
- Do not take pain medications on an empty stomach. They might cause nausea.

✆ CALL OUR OFFICE IF

- You develop any unusual signs or symptoms.
- You have chest pains or breathing problems.
- You vomit for longer than 4 hours.
- The incision becomes red or swollen, or there is drainage from it.
- You have any questions.

△ GENERAL INFORMATION

The two ovaries are each located on either side of the uterus in the pelvis. There are several different kinds of cancers of the ovaries, and they occur most commonly in women between the ages of 40 and 75 years (Fig. 1).

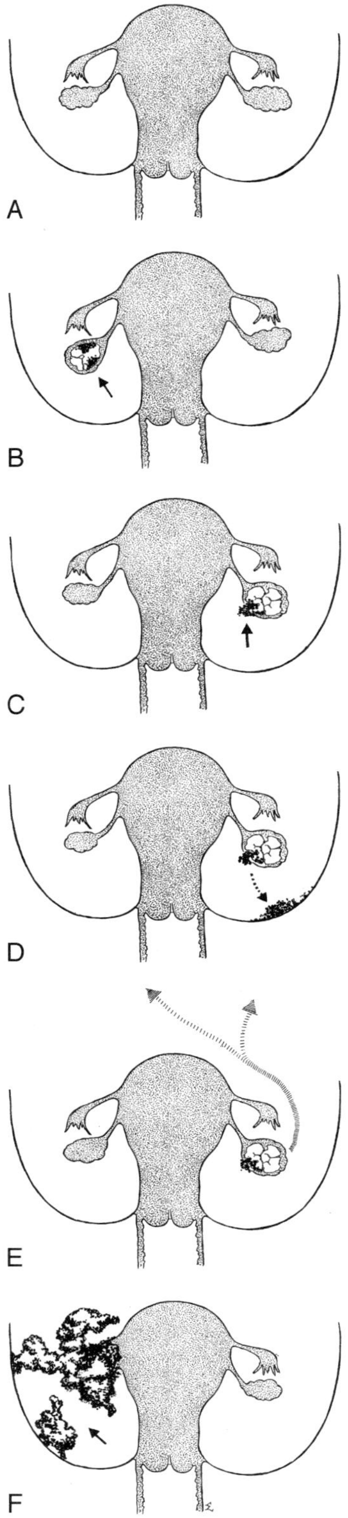

Figure 1. The treatment of ovarian cancer is influenced by the way the cancer manifests. *A*, Normal ovaries. *B*, Cancer of the ovary that appears to be confined to the inside of the ovary. *C*, Cancer that has broken to the outside surface of the ovary. *D*, Cancer cells have fallen from the ovary and implanted themselves on the lining of the abdominal cavity (called *drop* metastases). *E*, The ovarian cancer may appear confined, but microscopic cells have spread (metastasized) to distant areas. *F*, Bulky tumor may be present, and removing it for cure is not possible. Even so, removing as much of it as possible (called *debulking*) can relieve some present symptoms or prevent them from occurring in the future.

COMMON SIGNS AND SYMPTOMS

Cancer of the ovaries can produce a number of symptoms, but it does not often produce symptoms early in the disease. Some of these symptoms may be the following:

- Vague feelings of an upset stomach or intestines.
- Bloating and a sense of fullness.
- A swollen and painful abdomen.
- Vaginal bleeding or other fluid discharge.
- Fluid in the abdomen (called *ascites*).
- A mass in the pelvis.
- Pain during intercourse.
- Loss of weight (sometimes there is increase in weight from the accumulating ascites).

DIAGNOSIS

Some of the necessary tests include the following:

- An examination of your blood, urine, heart (EKG), and lungs (chest x-ray).
- *Ultrasound*: Harmless sound waves are aimed from outside your abdomen (and sometimes with a small instrument in your vagina) at the area of your pelvis. The sound waves bouncing back (the echoes) from this area are seen as a picture on a screen. Ultrasonography is a convenient and painless way to examine tissue inside your pelvis, especially the uterus and ovaries.
- *CT scan (computed tomography scan)*: A machine shaped like a huge doughnut is used to take special x-rays. You will lie on a table inside the hole in the "doughnut." The special x-rays are taken as very thin slices through the area of the pelvis. This makes it possible to see the fine details in your pelvic organs.
- *Stomach x-ray*: Barium is swallowed and x-rays are taken of it as it travels down to the stomach and beyond. This can be of value in determining whether there is a tumor of the stomach that has spread to the ovaries.
- *Barium enema (lower GI)*: Liquid barium is given as an enema (very much like a regular enema) and x-rays taken of it as it travels throughout the colon. This examination is of value in determining whether the symptoms are caused by a colon tumor that has involved the nearby ovary.

○ TREATMENT

The preferred treatment for cancer of the ovary is an operation to remove the uterus, tubes, ovaries, and the draining lymph nodes in the *omentum* (the fatty apron). This is called a *radical hysterectomy*.

Even if the tumor appears confined to just the ovary, the abdominal cavity is rinsed with a salt solution and the fluid collected for laboratory examination to see if any cancer cells are free in the abdominal cavity. In addition, tiny pieces of tissue (the size of a lentil) are removed from specified areas in the abdomen and examined for microscopic evidence of cancer. Even if all of the cancer cannot be removed, then removing most of it (this is called *debulking*) seems to improve the effectiveness of later chemotherapy or radiation therapy.

After the most careful consideration of all factors, the recommendation is that you have a radical hysterectomy.

PREOPERATIVE PREPARATION

- You will be instructed on how to cleanse your bowel before the operation.
- Do not eat or drink anything for 8 hours before the operation.
- Shower or bathe as usual on the morning of the operation.
- Do not douche or use a tampon on the day of the operation.
- You may be given medicine that will make you feel drowsy before you are brought to the operating room.

□ OPERATION

- You will be asleep for the operation, or be offered a spinal type of anesthesia.
- The operation usually takes about 3 hours.
- You will be taken to a recovery room and observed. When your blood pressure, pulse, and breathing are stable, you will be taken to a regular hospital room.
- You may have a thin plastic tube in your nose. It goes down to your stomach to suck up the air you swallow. It will be removed when your bowels start working.
- That evening you will be helped to sit up in bed and on the next day to get out of bed.
- There may be a catheter in your bladder. It will be removed as soon as it is felt you can comfortably pass urine on your own.
- Pain will be controlled with medicine.
- You should be able to go home in about 3 to 4 days.
- Arrangements will be made for your medicine, follow-up office visit, stitch or clip removal, and a discussion of possible additional therapy.
- As with any operation, complications are always possible. With this type of operation, they can include infection, bleeding, bowel obstruction, injury to the rectum, bladder, or ureter, and possibly others.

✚ HOME CARE

- You may walk about as you wish, even climb stairs, but don't overdo things.
- Take medicine as prescribed for your pain.
- Do not douche or use a tampon. A sanitary napkin is suitable for the usual vaginal discharge.
- Eat as you wish. Include plenty of roughage and liquids in your diet to help prevent constipation. You may need some help with a mild laxative (example: milk of magnesia).
- Unless otherwise instructed, you may shower if you wish, with any dressings on or off.
- Your incision and the muscles of the abdomen may ache, especially at the end of the day and after you have been standing for a long period. Your abdominal wall will feel more comfortable if you support it by wearing a somewhat loose-fitting girdle.
- If you are sent home with the elastic stockings you wore while in the hospital, keep using them for a week or so.
- Engaging in sexual intercourse too soon can be harmful to your recovery. If you wish, let's talk about this during your follow-up visit.
- Do not drive a car unless you can move freely and without pain and you are not taking medicines that decrease your alertness.
- You may return to work when you feel up to it.

✆ CALL OUR OFFICE IF

- The incision becomes red or swollen, or there is drainage from it.
- You develop a temperature higher than 100°F.
- There is a foul odor to any discharge from your vagina.
- You have any questions.

△ GENERAL INFORMATION

The two ovaries are located, one each, on either side of the uterus (Fig. 1). More types of tumors, benign and malignant, affect the ovaries than probably any other organ in the body.

COMMON SIGNS AND SYMPTOMS

- Few of these tumors produce symptoms early in their development unless they twist on themselves or a cyst ruptures or bleeds.
- There may be swelling of the abdomen.
- There may be symptoms in the colon or the bladder, if the tumor presses on either of these structures.

DIAGNOSIS

Tumors of the ovary may be solid, cystic (hollow and filled with fluid), or a mixture of solid and cystic. They may be "functional," that is, they produce hormones, or they may not be functioning at all.

It is estimated that in women younger than 30 years, 10% of ovarian tumors are malignant; this increases to 50% in women older than 50 years of age. The challenge, then, is to separate the benign from the malignant so that proper therapy can be given.

- Empty your bladder before coming to the doctor's office; the examination will be more comfortable for you.
- There will be a detailed record made of your symptoms and a thorough gynecologic and pelvic examination.

You will need some and possibly all of the following:

- Your blood will be examined in a routine manner as well as for "tumor markers," looking for any evidence that a cancer may be present.
- *Ultrasound*: Harmless sound waves are aimed from outside your abdomen, as well as with a small instrument in your vagina, at the area of your pelvis. The sound waves bouncing back (the echoes) from this area are seen as a picture on a screen. Ultrasonography is a convenient and painless way to examine organs and tissues inside your pelvis.
- *CT scan (computed tomography scan)*: A machine shaped like a huge doughnut is used to take special x-rays. You will lie on a table inside the hole in the "doughnut." The x-rays are taken as very thin slices through the area of the pelvis. This makes it possible to see the fine details in organs and tissues in the pelvis, especially the uterus and ovaries.
- *Barium enema*: Liquid barium (it looks and flows like buttermilk) will be introduced into your colon, which lies just next to the ovary, and x-ray pictures taken as the barium flows throughout the bowel. This can show if your problem is something in the colon rather than in the ovaries.

○ TREATMENT

The treatment of an ovarian tumor depends on the following:

- The size of the ovarian tumor.
- How long any symptoms have been present.
- How long the mass has been present.
- If the mass has been observed before, how long it has been there and whether there have been any changes during this time.
- The age of the person.

Other factors that influence treatment are as follows:

- Tumor characteristics: Is the tumor one cyst or more than one cyst? Or, is it both cystic and solid? Possibly it is all solid. These characteristics can be clues as to whether the tumor is benign or malignant.
- Are the various test results negative for the possible existence of cancer; worrisome for cancer but not conclusive; or indicating a high probability of cancer?
- Finally, it may not be possible to know the nature of the ovarian tumor without taking a look. A *laparoscopy* is advisable. This is done under general anesthesia with a long instrument as thick as your little finger with lenses in it and a light at its tip. The uterus and ovaries and surrounding tissue can be looked at directly. If it is clear that it is a benign tumor, then often nothing more need be done. However, plans can be made so that if something more serious is seen, it can be treated at that time. In this way, you won't have to be put to sleep a second time for the actual treatment.

Generally, an operation is recommended for an ovarian tumor whose exact nature is not known but

- Is larger than 6 cm (this is slightly smaller than a tennis ball).
- Persists (without getting smaller) for longer than 3 months.
- Twists on itself or bleeds significantly (this requires an immediate operation).

After careful consideration of all factors, it is recom-

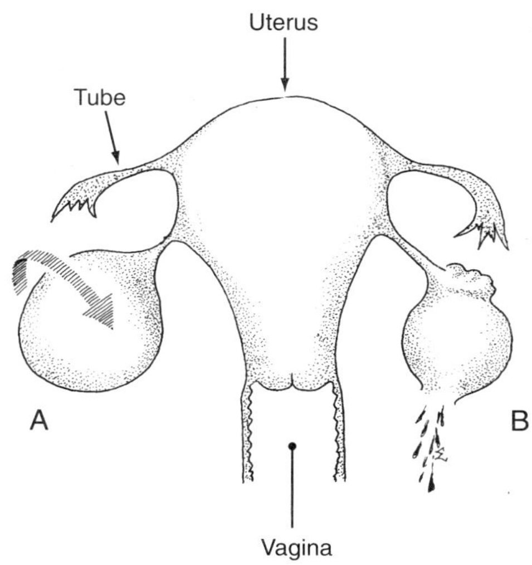

Figure 1. It cannot be known for sure whether a tumor of the ovary is benign unless the tissue is examined under the microscope. One of a number of reasons for removing an ovarian tumor is a large size or an increasing size. Other reasons to remove an ovarian tumor (usually on an urgent basis) are twisting *(torsion) (A)* and rupture with bleeding *(B)*.

mended that you have one operation to make a diagnosis and to treat your ovarian tumor at the same time (Fig. 1). If the tumor is found to be benign, the principles in treating it will be to remove all the tumor while conserving as much normal tissue as possible.

PREOPERATIVE PREPARATION

- In addition to any tests already done, you will have an examination of your blood, urine, heart (EKG), and lungs (chest x-ray).
- Do not eat or drink anything for 8 hours before the operation.
- You will be instructed on how to clean out your bowel before the operation.
- Do not douche or use a tampon on the day of the operation.
- Shower as usual on the morning of the operation.

☐ OPERATION

- You will be asleep for the operation.
- If possible and appropriate, the incision will be the "bikini" type.
- The operation usually takes about 2 hours, depending on what needs to be done.

POSTOPERATIVE CARE

- You will be taken to a recovery room and observed. When your blood pressure, pulse, and breathing are stable, you will be taken to a regular hospital room.
- The evening after the surgery you will be helped to sit up in bed and on the next day to get out of bed.
- Pain will be controlled with medicine.
- Your diet will be as you tolerate it.
- You should be able to go home in several days.
- Arrangements will be made for your medicine, follow-up office visit, and stitch or clip removal.

✚ HOME CARE

- You may walk about as you wish, even climb stairs, but don't overdo things.
- Take medicine as prescribed for your pain.
- Eat as you wish. Include plenty of roughage and liquids in your diet to help prevent constipation.
- Your abdominal incision may ache less if you can support your abdomen by wearing a girdle that is snug (but not too tight).
- Do not douche or use a tampon on the day of the operation.
- Do not drive a car unless you can move freely and without pain and you are not taking drugs that reduce your alertness.
- Engaging in sexual intercourse too soon can be harmful to your recovery. If you wish, talk about this with your doctor during your follow-up visit.
- You may return to work when you feel up to it.

✆ CALL OUR OFFICE IF

- The incision becomes red or swollen, or there is drainage from it.
- You develop a temperature higher than 100°F.
- You have any questions.

△ GENERAL INFORMATION

The pancreas is a gland that is located deep in the upper part of the abdomen. It is mostly behind the stomach (Fig. 1). It makes juices that help digest the meats and fats and other foods you eat. It also makes insulin that helps regulate the sugar level of the body.

Sometimes, the pancreas becomes inflamed; this is called *pancreatitis*. It can cause digestive fluids to leak out of the pancreas and collect in and around it. This fluid can digest tissue and cause serious problems. In many people, the fluid goes away as the pancreatitis gets better. Unfortunately, however, sometimes the fluid does not go away. This is a *pseudocyst* (Fig. 2).

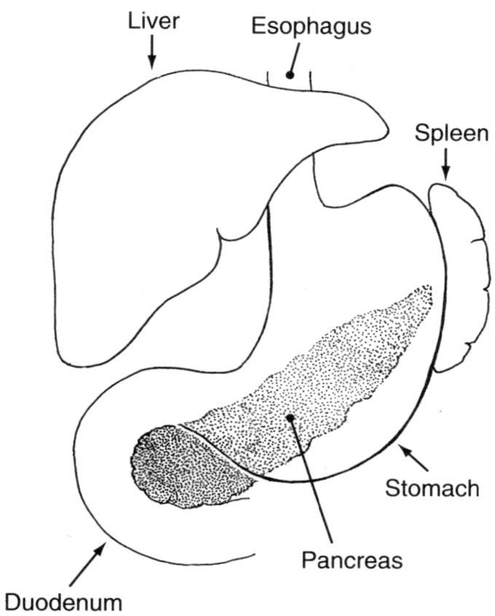

Figure 1. Normal pancreas.

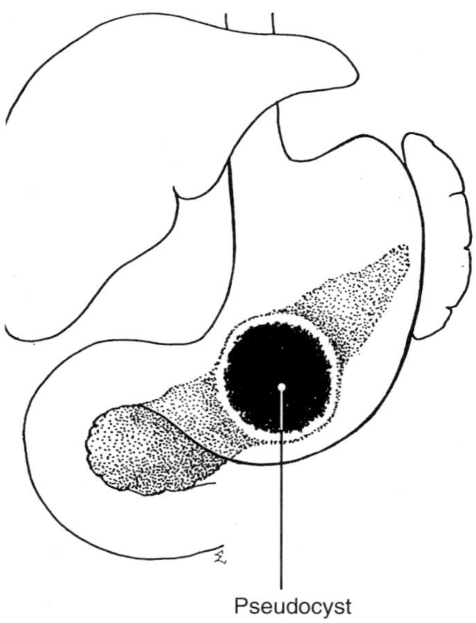

Figure 2. Pseudocyst of the pancreas.

COMMON SIGNS AND SYMPTOMS

- Pain or discomfort in the upper abdomen.
- Loss of appetite.
- Nausea and vomiting.
- Swelling of the upper abdomen.
- Weight loss.
- Fever and chills if the pseudocyst becomes infected.

DIAGNOSIS

Usually the diagnosis can be made by taking a detailed history, doing a thorough physical examination, and considering the laboratory reports carefully.

The pseudocyst can be seen by several methods:

- *Ultrasound*: Harmless sound waves are aimed at the pancreas. The sound waves bouncing back (the echoes) from this area are seen as a picture on a screen. This is a convenient and painless way to examine the pancreas.
- *CT scan (computed tomography scan)*: A machine shaped like a huge doughnut is used to take special x-rays. You will lie on the table inside the hole in the "doughnut." The x-rays are taken as thin slices through the area of the pancreas. This makes it possible to see a pseudocyst and the details inside it.

○ TREATMENT

- The pseudocyst should be treated in the following circumstances:
  - It is still there after 6 weeks and is still causing problems.
  - It is getting bigger.
  - The fluid in the pseudocyst becomes infected.
  - The cyst develops other complications (example: bleeding, blocking of the intestine).
  - There is a possibility of cancer in it.
- The treatment is to drain the pseudocyst by making a connection between it and the stomach, duodenum, or small intestine (Fig. 3).

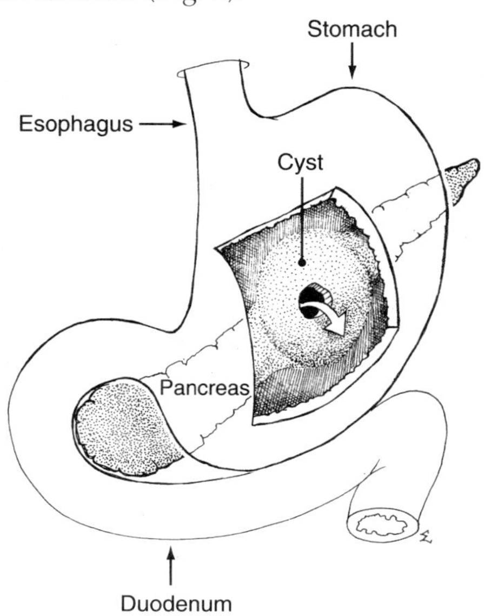

Figure 3. The pseudocyst is opened so that it drains directly into the stomach *(arrow)*.

After careful consideration of all factors, the recommendation is that you have an operation to correct the problem.

PREOPERATIVE PREPARATION

- You will have an examination of your blood, urine, heart (EKG), and lungs (chest x-ray).
- Do not eat or drink anything for 8 hours before the operation.
- You may be given medicine that will make you feel drowsy before you are brought to the operating room.

☐ OPERATION

- You will be asleep for the operation.
- The incision will be made at your upper abdomen.

POSTOPERATIVE CARE

- You will wake up in a recovery room. When your blood pressure, pulse, and breathing are stable, you will be taken to a regular hospital room.
- You will have a thin plastic tube in your nose. It goes down to your stomach to suck up the air you swallow. It will be removed when your bowels start working.
- The evening after the surgery you will be helped to sit up in bed and on the next day to get out of bed.
- Pain will be controlled with medicine.
- When you start eating, your diet will be liquid and then advanced as you tolerate it.
- You should be able to go home in about 3 to 5 days.
- As with any operation, complications are always possible. With this type of operation, complications can include bleeding, infection, leaking at a sutured area, blood clots, and possibly others.
- Arrangements will be made for your medicine, follow-up office visit, and stitch removal.

✚ HOME CARE

- Take medicine as prescribed for your pain.
- Unless otherwise instructed, you may eat as you wish.
- Do not drink alcohol.
- Unless otherwise instructed, you may shower as you wish, with any dressings on or off. After you dry yourself, replace any dressings with clean, dry ones.
- Do not drive a car unless you can move freely and without pain and you are not taking medicines that decrease your alertness.
- You may resume sexual activity whenever you choose.
- You may return to work when you feel up to it.

✆ CALL OUR OFFICE IF

- You have nausea, vomiting, or worsening abdominal pain.
- The incision becomes red or swollen, or there is drainage from it.
- You develop a temperature higher than 101°F.
- You have any questions.

△ GENERAL INFORMATION

The pancreas is located deep in your upper abdomen (Fig. 1). It makes insulin that controls your sugar levels and also makes juices that help digest the meats, fats, and other foods that you eat. Different types of tumors can grow in the pancreas. Most of them, whether they are benign or cancerous, need to be treated (Fig. 2).

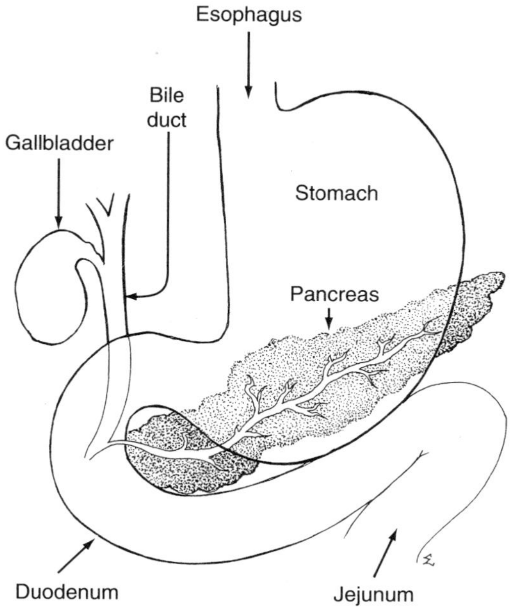

Figure 1.

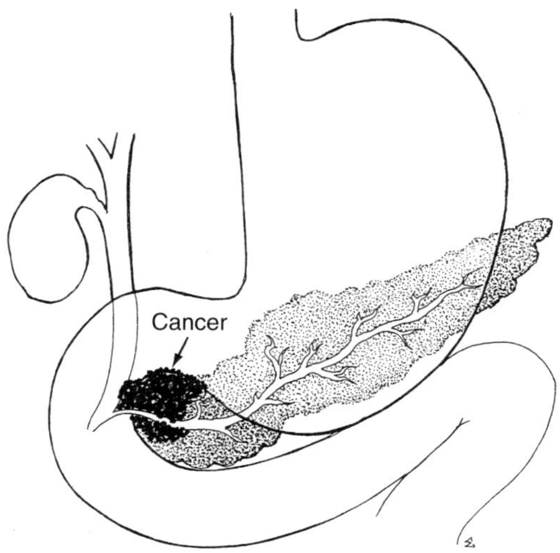

Figure 2. Cancer can affect any part of the pancreas. However, the head of the pancreas (the part closest to the duodenum) most often produces symptoms early enough that an operation for cure is possible. Such a cancer is shown here.

COMMON SIGNS AND SYMPTOMS

- Pain in the upper abdomen that sometimes is vague and other times is more severe and goes straight to the back.
- Jaundice (yellow eyes and skin).
- Loss of appetite and weight.

DIAGNOSIS

A detailed history and a thorough physical examination often lead to the diagnosis. You will have some and possibly all of these tests:

- *Ultrasound*: Harmless sound waves are aimed at the upper area of your abdomen. The sound waves bouncing back (the echoes) from this area are seen as a picture on a screen. Ultrasonography is a convenient and painless way to examine the pancreas and other organs and tissues in this area.
- *CT scan (computed tomography scan)*: A machine shaped like a huge doughnut is used to take special x-rays. You will lie on a table inside the hole in the "doughnut." The x-rays are taken as very thin slices through the area of the abdomen. This makes it possible to see the fine details in the pancreas and other organs in your abdomen.
- *ERCP (endoscopic retrograde cholangio-pancreatography)*: This test is done with an optical instrument (called an *endoscope*) that is soft, flexible, and about as thick as your little finger, with a light at its tip. Your mouth and throat will be sprayed with an anesthetic to make them numb. Also, you will be given medicine that will make you feel drowsy. The endoscope will be passed gently through your mouth and throat, down the stomach, and then out of it to just where the openings of the bile and pancreas ducts are. Dye is injected into the pancreas duct and x-ray pictures are taken to see where the problem might lie.
- *Needle aspiration biopsy*: Your upper abdomen will be painted with an antiseptic solution and surrounded with sterile drapes. The skin over the area of the pancreas will be made numb by being injected with an anesthetic. A special thin needle will then be inserted through the numbed skin and down to the tumor to take a small piece of it (a *biopsy*) for laboratory examination. The risk in making a diagnosis this way is that the needle could miss the tumor and a biopsy sent to the laboratory that would show up "negative" in the report. This "negative" result could lead to nothing more being done, which would be a serious mistake.

THERAPY

- An operation to possibly remove the cancer offers the best chance for cure.
- Because of the problems and risks in making the exact diagnosis *before* an operation, sometimes the diagnosis and the treatment are done at the same time in the operating room. Sometimes the cancer cannot be removed by an operation, but a number of things can be done to relieve symptoms that the cancer is causing.

After careful consideration of all factors, the recommendation is that you have an operation to try to remove the tumor.

PREOPERATIVE PREPARATION

- Your blood, urine, heart (EKG), and lungs (chest x-ray) will be carefully evaluated.
- Do not eat or drink anything for 8 hours before the operation.

☐ OPERATION

- You will be asleep for the operation.
- The incision will be in your upper abdomen.
- The operation involves removing the part of the pancreas with the cancer in it as well as surrounding tissue (Fig. 3).
- You will not receive a blood transfusion unless it is absolutely necessary.
- The length of the operation depends on what is found and what needs to be done.

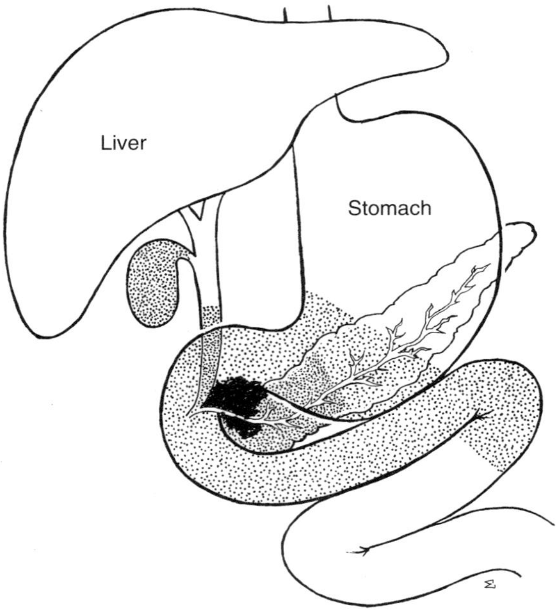

Figure 3. The tissue to be removed *(stippled area)* includes the distal part of the stomach, about half of the pancreas with the cancer in it, the duodenum, the gallbladder and most of the bile duct leading from the gallbladder, and the associated lymph nodes.

POSTOPERATIVE CARE

- You will be taken to the Surgical Care Unit, where the doctors and nurses are very experienced in taking care of patients with your condition.
- You will have a thin plastic tube in your nose for a few days.
- That evening you will be helped to sit up in bed and on the next day to get out of bed.
- There will be plastic tubes coming out of your abdomen to drain any fluids accumulating inside.
- Pain will be controlled with medicine.
- You will be given an incentive spirometer. Breathing into this as you are instructed will help you expand your lungs and reduce the risk of developing pneumonia.
- When you start to eat, your diet will first be liquids, and then advanced as you tolerate it.
- As with any operation, complications are always possible, some of them serious. With this type of operation, they can include bleeding, infection, heart problems, pneumonia, leakage from the sutured areas, and possibly others.
- You should be able to go home about 1 week after the operation.
- Arrangements will be made for your medicine, follow-up office visit, and stitch removal.

✚ HOME CARE

- You may walk about as you wish, even climb stairs, but don't overdo things.
- You will be given a suggested appropriate diet to follow during your convalescence.
- Take medicine as prescribed for your pain.
- Unless instructed otherwise, you may shower if you wish, with any dressings on or off. There may be narrow strips of tape across the incision. It's all right if they get wet; they will be removed in the doctor's office. After you dry yourself, replace any dressings with clean, dry ones.
- Arrangements can be made for a home visiting nurse if one is needed.
- During one of your follow-up office visits, let's discuss when you may drive, resume sexual activity, and return to work.

✆ CALL OUR OFFICE IF

- The incision becomes red or swollen, or there is drainage from it.
- You feel nauseated or vomit.
- You develop a temperature higher than 101°F.
- You have any questions.

△ GENERAL INFORMATION

The pancreas is located deep inside the upper part of your abdomen. It makes the strong juices that help digest the meats, fats, and other foods you eat. It also makes insulin, which helps regulate the sugar level in the body.

Sometimes, the pancreas becomes inflamed and the pancreas juices leak into the pancreas tissue itself as well as into the surrounding tissue. This is called *pancreatitis.* Most cases of pancreatitis are associated either with gallstones or with heavy drinking of alcohol.

COMMON SIGNS AND SYMPTOMS

When the pancreas juices leak into the tissue, what happens depends a lot on how much leakage takes place and how long the leakage lasts (Fig. 1).

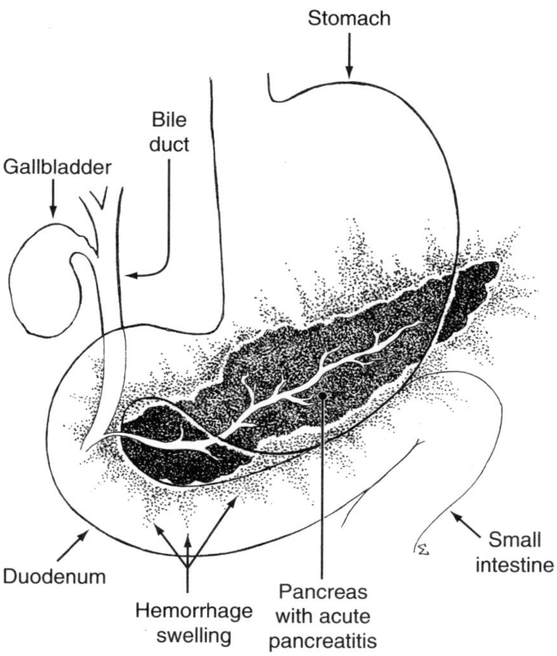

Figure 1. The severity and extent of inflammation seen with acute pancreatitis vary greatly. These can range from simple swelling and local accumulation of fluid to death of the entire pancreas and some surrounding tissue.

Mild Attack

- Pain in the upper abdomen and going to the sides or straight to the back.
- Nausea and vomiting.

Severe Attack

- Abdominal pain so severe that the person is unable to move.
- Shock: sweating, fast pulse, low blood pressure.
- Nausea and vomiting and even severe retching.
- Jaundice.

DIAGNOSIS

Tests that can help make the diagnosis include the following:

- X-ray of the abdomen.
- Examination of your blood, urine, heart (EKG), and lungs (chest x-ray).
- *Ultrasound*: Harmless sound waves are aimed at the abdomen, with special emphasis on the pancreas. The sound waves bouncing back (the echoes) from this area are seen as a picture on a screen. This is a convenient and painless way to examine the pancreas and other organs and tissues inside the abdomen.
- *CT scan (computed tomography scan)*: Special x-rays are taken as thin slices through the upper area of the abdomen. This makes it possible to see the fine details in the pancreas and surrounding tissue.

○ TREATMENT

The initial treatment includes the following:

- Giving fluids to make up for the loss by vomiting, not being able to take fluids by mouth, and the leaking of fluid around the inflamed pancreas.
- Giving oxygen to help with the breathing.
- Correcting any developing heart problems.
- Starting antibiotics to try to prevent an infection. The abdominal cavity may need to be rinsed out to remove the irritating pancreatic juices.

An operation is necessary for the following:

- A complication of the pancreatitis develops (for example: infection, which is almost always fatal if not treated by an operation).
- The diagnosis is not certain.
- Gallstones are also present.
- The pancreatitis is getting worse.
- To correct a condition that is not now causing a problem but that will surely make things worse if left alone.

PREOPERATIVE PREPARATION

The aim is to get you in the best possible shape for the operation. Associated problems will be taken care of as much as possible.

□ OPERATION

- You will be asleep for the operation.
- The exact operation cannot be decided on beforehand; the pancreas area may not require much dissection, or it may require extensive dissection and drainage.

POSTOPERATIVE CARE

- You will be taken to the Surgical Care Unit, where the doctors and nurses are very experienced in taking care of patients with your condition. As soon as you are coming along well enough, you will be transferred to a regular hospital room.
- You will have a thin plastic tube in your nose. It goes down to your stomach to suck up the air you swallow. It will be removed when your bowels start working again.
- There may be several soft rubber drains coming out from your abdomen.

- The evening after the operation you will be helped to sit up in bed and on the next day to get out of bed.
- Pain will be controlled with medicine.
- When the tube in your nose is removed you will be started on a liquid to soft diet.
- As with any operation, complications are always possible, some of them serious. With this type of operation, complications can include infection, bleeding, heart problems, blood clots, and possibly others.
- Arrangements will be made for your medicine, follow-up office visit, and stitch removal.

✙ HOME CARE

- You may walk about as you wish, even climb stairs, but take it easy. Take frequent rest periods.
- Follow the diet suggested for you.
- During one of your follow-up office visits, let's discuss when you may drive a car, resume sexual activity, and return to work.

✆ CALL OUR OFFICE IF

- You have nausea or vomiting.
- The incision becomes red or swollen, or there is drainage from it.
- You develop a temperature higher than 101°F.
- You have any questions.

△ GENERAL INFORMATION

The pancreas is located deep in your upper abdomen. It makes insulin, which controls the level of sugar in your blood. It also makes juices that help digest the meats, fats, and other foods you eat.

Sometimes the pancreas becomes inflamed, heals, but then becomes inflamed again. Often such attacks continue. Eventually, the attacks begin to destroy the pancreas so that it doesn't make digestive juices or even insulin as well. The pancreas becomes severely scarred, and the duct inside it through which the pancreas juices flow becomes blocked (Fig. 1). Chronic pancreatitis is often caused by heavy use of alcohol. There are other causes, and sometimes the cause is not known.

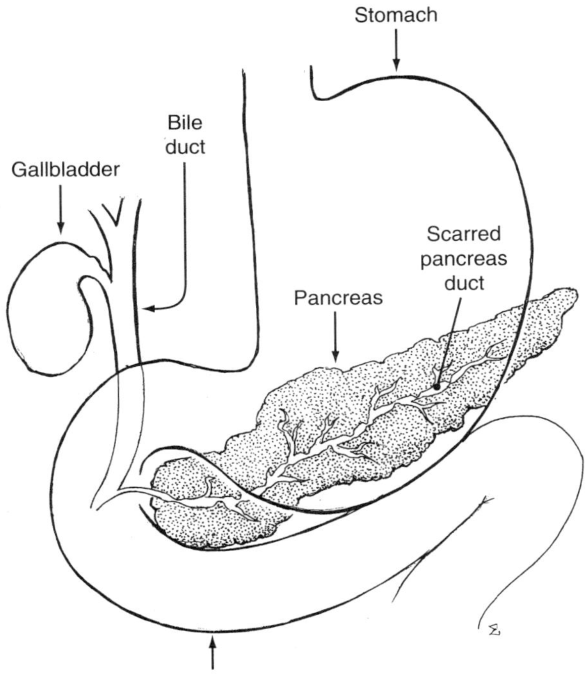

Figure 1. The extent of involvement of the pancreatic duct is an important factor in producing the symptoms that may make an operation necessary. This involvement can range from recurring local inflammation to extensive scarring, blockage of the duct, and destruction of some of the gland itself.

COMMON SIGNS AND SYMPTOMS

- Pain in the upper abdomen that may come and go or may be rather constant.
- The appetite is poor and there is weight loss. Eating may bring on pain.
- Diabetes can develop because insulin is not produced normally.
- Occasionally, the stools are loose and have a very foul odor.

DIAGNOSIS

Tests that can help establish the diagnosis include the following:

- An examination of your blood, urine, heart (EKG), and lungs (chest x-ray).
- X-ray of the abdomen may show deposits of calcium throughout the pancreas.
- CT scan (computed tomography scan): A machine shaped like a huge doughnut is used to take special x-rays. You will lie on the table inside the hole in the "doughnut." The x-rays are taken as very thin slices through the upper abdomen. This makes it possible to see the fine details in the pancreas.
- Showing the scarred pancreas ducts, by a special technique in which dye is placed in the pancreas duct, is very strong evidence of this condition.

○ TREATMENT

- The treatment is aimed at relieving pain.
- The treatment of chronic pancreatitis does not always require an operation.
- Drinking of alcohol must be stopped.
- An operation is reserved for patients who are suffering with pain every day and who have not been helped enough by all other forms of treatment.

After careful consideration of all factors, the recommendation is that you have an operation to try to improve your problem. It is important to understand that an operation does not make the damaged pancreas normal again. However, an operation can often substantially improve the symptoms.

PREOPERATIVE PREPARATION

- Do not eat or drink anything for 8 hours before the operation.
- Shower as usual on the morning of the operation.
- You may be given medicine that will make you feel drowsy before you are brought to the operating room.

□ OPERATION

Which one of the several possible operations is used to try to improve the problem depends on what is found. The following may be done:

- Removal of obstructions of your pancreas ducts.
- Removal of the pain nerve bundle in this area.
- Sometimes the only choice is to remove some of the pancreas.

POSTOPERATIVE CARE

- You will be taken to a recovery room and observed. When your blood pressure, pulse, and breathing are stable, you will be taken to a regular hospital room.
- You will have a thin plastic tube in your nose. It goes down to your stomach to suck up the air you swallow. It will be removed when it is safe to do so, usually in a few days.
- Pain will be controlled with medicine.
- The evening after the surgery you will be helped to sit up in bed and on the next day to get out of bed.
- You will be given an incentive spirometer. Breathing into this as you are instructed will help you expand your lungs and reduce the risk of developing pneumonia.
- You should be able to go home in about 1 week.

- Arrangements will be made for your medicine, follow-up office visit, and stitch removal.
- As with any operation, complications are always possible. With this type of operation, complications can include bleeding, infection, heart problems, pneumonia, leakage where tissue was stitched together, blood clots, and possibly others.
- Sometimes the operation goes perfectly well, yet the pain may not go away completely.
- Remember, when there is chronic pancreatitis, there is always some permanent damage to the pancreas.

✣ HOME CARE

- You may walk about as you wish, even climb stairs, but don't overdo things.
- Unless advised otherwise, you may eat as you wish.
- Do not drink any alcohol.
- Take medicine as prescribed for your pain.
- During your follow-up office visit, let's discuss when you may drive a car, resume sexual activity, and return to work.

✆ CALL OUR OFFICE IF

- You are nauseated, or you vomit.
- The incision becomes red and swollen, or there is drainage from it.
- You develop a temperature higher than 101°F.
- You have any questions.

PAP SMEAR AND PELVIC EXAMINATION

△ GENERAL INFORMATION

The Papanicolaou (Pap) smear studies, along with the pelvic examination, are the most common ways to pick up an early cancer of the sex organs in women. Don't forget that it is important to have a pelvic examination along with the Pap smear because there are a number of other problems of the female genital organs, beside those of the cervix, that can be seen or felt.

PREPARATION FOR EXAMINATION

- Do not douche or use a tampon for 24 hours before the examination.
- If you are pregnant, or think you are pregnant, let the doctor know beforehand.
- The examination should not be done if you are menstruating (unless you are seeing the doctor for abnormal or irregular menstrual flow).
- Empty your bladder before going into the doctor's office. It will make the examination more comfortable for you. If you are also having bladder or urine problems, mention this to the nurse before you see the doctor. You may be asked to supply a specimen of your urine.

HISTORY

There will be a detailed general history with special emphasis on any external or internal female genital problems.

EXAMINATION

The procedure is usually done as follows:

- The doctor's assistant will position and drape you as for a regular pelvic examination.
- With a strong light, the doctor will examine the outside of your pelvic area first for the following:
  - The general condition of the skin.
  - Any abnormal growths.
- A warm, slightly lubricated instrument (a speculum) of the correct size will be placed in your vagina to expose the *cervix* (the opening into the uterus), which is at the deep end of the vagina (Fig. 1).
- A specially shaped applicator (a spatula) will be used to gently scrape some cells from the surface of your cervix (Fig. 2). These will be sent to the laboratory and examined by a specialist (called a cytopathologist) for cancerous cells, precancerous cells, other types of abnormal cells, the cause of any infection you might have, and the hormone status of the cells lining your vagina. A sample may be taken from the vagina. This may be examined for the presence of any abnormal cells as well as for possible microorganisms if a vaginal infection is present.
- As the speculum is slowly removed, the lining of the vagina will be carefully inspected.
- Next, the doctor will place two gloved fingers in the vagina and the other hand over your lower abdomen. With the two hands, the inside of the abdomen is felt for any abnormalities. Occasionally, a rectal examination is done at the same time.

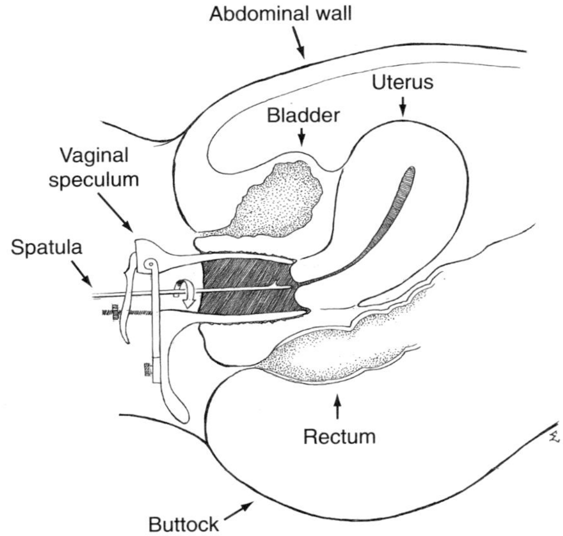

Figure 1. Side view of the female pelvis. The speculum is in the vagina, exposing the cervix. The spatula is moved in a rotary fashion, scraping cells off the cervix and vagina.

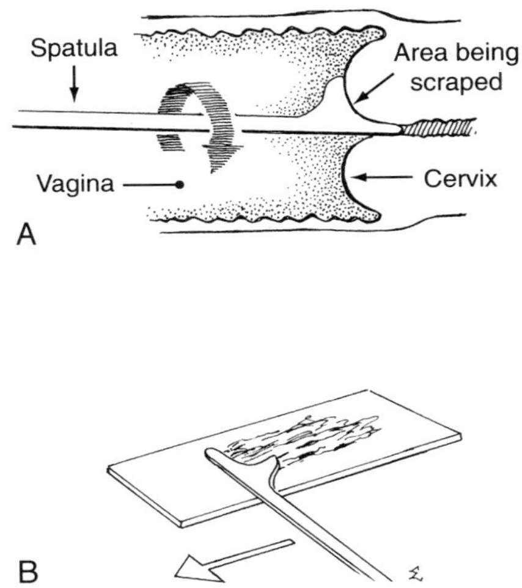

Figure 2. *A*, Enlarged view showing spatula scraping surface of cervix. *B*, The scraped material is spread on a glass slide and sent to the laboratory for testing.

- If for some reason the pelvic examination cannot be done properly, or if something suspicious is felt, other tests may be recommended.

THE EXAMINATION IS OVER

Arrangements will be made for you to be informed of the laboratory results.

You should know that, regardless of any positive findings of the Pap test, no treatment will be planned on these results alone, because the Pap test alone is not 100% accurate. If any serious abnormality is found, then additional tests that are somewhat more involved will need to be done. And, of course, if any of these tests are needed, they will be explained and discussed with you in detail.

△ GENERAL INFORMATION

Paracentesis is the removal of fluid (called *ascites*) from the abdominal cavity with a needle placed through the skin. There are a number of different causes of ascites. The cause of your ascites has been explained to you.

COMMON SIGNS AND SYMPTOMS

- The abdomen is swollen so much that it is uncomfortable.
- There may be difficulty with breathing, especially when lying down.
- Associated with this swelling of the abdomen, the ankles usually are quite swollen; walking is most difficult.

DIAGNOSIS

A number of tests can be done to find the specific cause of ascites. In your case, the cause of the ascites is known; the aim is to give you some relief.

○ TREATMENT

Some reasons for draining the fluid include the following:

- To relieve discomfort.
- To relieve the upward pressure on your diaphragm so that you can breathe more easily.
- To relieve pressure on your bladder, which in some people makes them have to urinate more frequently.
- Because medicines used to treat your condition are no longer working as well, or for other medical reasons, so treatment with medicines is now not recommended.
- To examine the fluid in the laboratory.

PREOPERATIVE PREPARATION

- Paracentesis can be done in the hospital, or in an outpatient surgical care unit, or even in the doctor's office.
- You will have a detailed history and careful physical examination. Also, there will be an examination of your blood, heart, and lungs.
- Do not eat or drink anything for 4 hours before the operation.
- Shower as usual on the morning of the operation.
- You will be asked to empty your bladder just before the paracentesis is done.

THE PARACENTESIS

- The paracentesis will most likely be done with your legs hanging over the examining table or bed.
- The skin of your abdomen will be painted with an antiseptic solution.
- A fine needle will be used to inject an anesthetic into the skin in the area just below your navel. This will make the entire area numb.
- A special needle that is attached to a tube connected to a bottle will be inserted through the numb skin and into the abdominal cavity.
- Your blood pressure and pulse will be checked carefully during the paracentesis.
- As the fluid is removed, you should feel more comfortable very soon.
- There is no pain associated with this procedure.
- Your abdomen will get smaller—sometimes much smaller.
- After the fluid has been removed, the needle will be withdrawn and the needle puncture site closed with several sutures and covered with a small bandage.
- You will be taken to a recovery room, where you will remain until your blood pressure, pulse, and breathing are stable and you are completely alert. You should be able to go home that same day with a responsible adult.
- Arrangements will be made for your medicine, follow-up office visit, and stitch removal.

✚ HOME CARE

- You may walk about as you wish, even climb stairs, but don't overdo things.
- You may eat as you did before the operation.
- You may shower if you wish, with any dressings on or off.
    - There may be narrow strips of tape across the incision. It's all right if they get wet; they will be removed in the doctor's office.
    - After you dry yourself, replace any dressings with clean, dry ones.

✆ CALL OUR OFFICE IF

- You develop any unusual signs or symptoms.
- You feel lightheaded or dizzy.
- Liquid starts or continues to leak out through the needle hole.
- You develop a temperature higher than 100°F.
- You have any questions.

△ GENERAL INFORMATION

A *paronychia* is an infection around the fold of the fingernail or toenail. It can be caused by aggressive manicuring in this area. Also, bacteria can more easily penetrate skin that is moist (and soapy) for long periods (example: moist soapy hands inside kitchen gloves) or hot and sweaty (example: feet inside tennis shoes in the summer). Many times the cause is not obvious.

COMMON SIGNS AND SYMPTOMS

- Tenderness and swelling around the nail fold (Fig. 1).
- There may be pus in this area as well as under the nail.
- The finger or toe can be moved without pain.
- There is no fever.

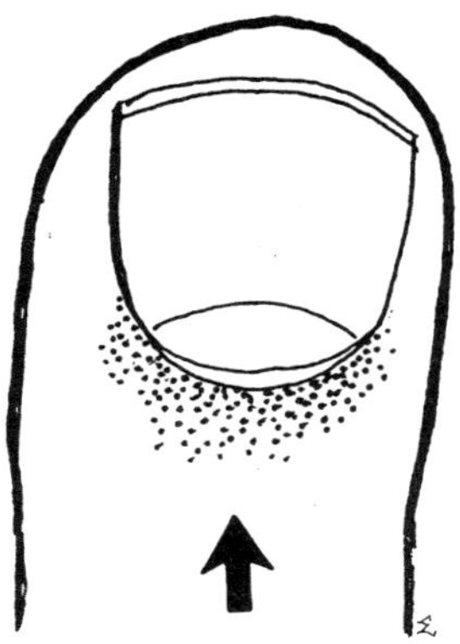

Figure 1.

DIAGNOSIS

The area of the nail fold is red, swollen, and very tender when touched.

○ TREATMENT

If it is caught early and no pus is present, it can be treated as follows:

- Antibiotics
- Warm, moist packs as follows:
  - Dissolve a teaspoon of ordinary salt in a quart of *warm* (not hot) tap water.
  - Place a clean washcloth in the solution, squeeze out most of the moisture, and then wrap the cloth around the finger or toe.
  - Cover the entire hand (or toe) with a piece of plastic (example: the plastic wrapper from the dry cleaner will do).
  - Cover all this with a dry face towel.
  - Rest the hand or toe with all the towels wrapped around it on a heating pad set on low.
  - Do this for 20 to 30 minutes three times per day.
  - As much as possible, keep the arm or leg elevated on pillows so that it is higher than the heart.

If pus has already collected, it will have to be drained.

□ OPERATION

- This minor operation is done as an outpatient procedure.
- The entire finger or toe will be painted with an antiseptic solution.
- A very thin, short needle will be used to inject an anesthetic into the nerve supplying the finger or toe. The finger or toe will become numb.
- An incision will be made to release the pus and a dressing applied.
- The operation takes less than 30 minutes.

POSTOPERATIVE CARE

- Arrangements will be made for your return office visit.
- You will be given a prescription for antibiotics.
- Over-the-counter pain medicine is adequate for any discomfort.

✚ HOME CARE

- Resume your usual activities.
- You will be shown how to change the dressing as necessary.
- You may be asked to soak the finger as described above to help with the healing.
- If you get the dressing wet, replace it with a clean, dry one.

✆ CALL OUR OFFICE IF

- Your finger swells and hurts as before.
- You develop a temperature higher than 100°F.
- You have any questions.

PAROTID TUMOR

△ GENERAL INFORMATION

A parotid tumor is an abnormal, uncontrolled growth in the *parotid gland,* one of the glands that makes saliva. The parotid gland is located low in front of the ear and at the angle of the jaw. (It is the gland that swells with mumps.) Most parotid tumors are benign. Fortunately, even the malignant ones do not often spread to distant parts of the body and usually are curable.

The cause of parotid tumors is not known.

COMMON SIGNS AND SYMPTOMS

- Usually, there is a painless, slow-growing mass at the angle of the jaw.

DIAGNOSIS

- Most often this is made by a detailed history and a thorough physical examination of your head and neck area.
- A specific diagnosis of whether the tumor is benign or malignant can be made by removing a tiny piece of it (a *biopsy*). This is done by making the skin over the mass numb with an anesthetic. Then a fine needle is pushed through the numbed skin and into the tumor to remove the piece for laboratory examination. Unfortunately, this method is not 100% accurate; the needle could miss the malignant area in the tumor. Biopsy is not always necessary, depending on the characteristics of a given tumor.
- CT scan (computed tomography scan): A machine shaped like a huge doughnut is used to take special x-rays. You will lie on a table inside the hole in the "doughnut." The x-rays are taken as very thin slices through the area of the parotid gland. This makes it possible to see the fine details in the parotid gland.

○ TREATMENT

An operation to remove the tumor is recommended for several reasons:

- The tumor may be malignant. An operation is the best way to cure this.
- Benign tumors can be cured only by an operation.
- In time, benign lesions can become malignant.
- Watching a benign nodule and removing it when it becomes larger increases the risk that a branch of the nerve will be injured in the operation.

After careful consideration of all factors, it is recommended that you have your parotid tumor removed.

PREOPERATIVE PREPARATION

- You will have an examination of your blood, urine, heart (EKG), and lungs (chest x-ray).
- Do not eat or drink anything for 8 hours before the operation.
- Shower (and shave) as usual on the morning of the operation.
- You may be given medicine that will make you feel drowsy before you are brought to the operating room.

□ OPERATION

- You will be asleep for the operation.
- A special feature of the parotid gland that influences the management of a parotid tumor is that the facial nerve (the one that controls smiling, puckering, blinking your eyes, etc.) runs through the middle of the gland. Because of its location, the nerve can be affected by tumors in the gland or injured during the operation (Fig. 1).
- The operation must be done with great skill so as to completely remove the tumor but not damage any of the nerve branches.
- The incision will be made in a cosmetic fashion in the crease immediately in front of the ear and behind the angle of the jaw.
- You will not need a blood transfusion.
- The operation usually takes about 2 hours.
- There will be a cosmetic closure.

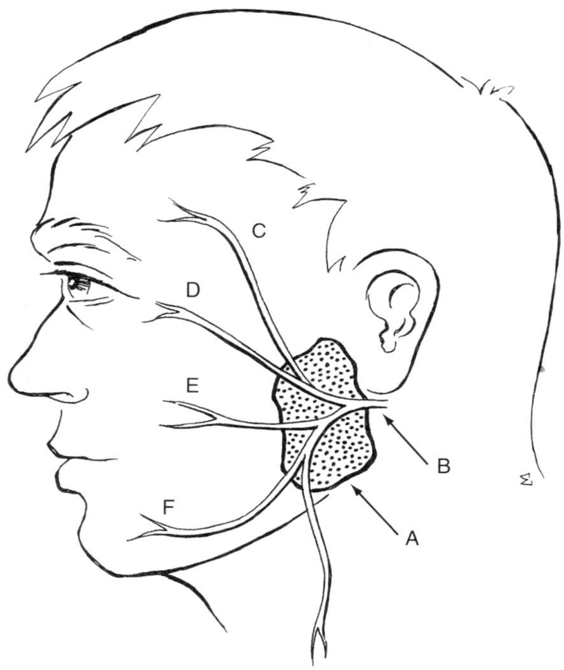

Figure 1. A, Parotid gland. B, Facial nerve. Branches of the facial nerve travel to the following muscles: forehead (C), eyelids (D), cheek (E), and lower lip (F).

POSTOPERATIVE COURSE

- You will wake up in a recovery room. When your blood pressure, pulse, and breathing are stable, you will be taken to a regular hospital room.
- There will be a bandage over the incision.
- There may be a small plastic tube coming from the incision, draining fluid from the area of the operation. It will be removed 1 to 2 days after the operation.
- The evening after the operation you will be helped to sit up in bed and on the next day to get out of bed.

- Pain is minimal and easily controlled with medicine.
- As with any operation, complications are always possible. With this type of operation, complications can include one or more branches of the facial nerve not working properly after the operation. Although most often this is temporary, in a very small percentage of patients it can be permanent. The result is weakness in the area of the face supplied by that branch of the nerve. Also, some numbness of the ear lobe is common and expected after this operation.
- You should be able to go home in a day or two.
- Arrangements will be made for your medicine, follow-up office visit, and stitch removal.
- Even if the tumor is malignant, your condition can be cured. An estimate of your chances can be made only after all the test results are back.

✚ HOME CARE

- Resume your usual activities.
- Eat as you wish.
- You will not notice any decrease in the amount of saliva you make.
- You may shower if you wish, with any dressing on or off.
  - There may be narrow strips of tape across the incision. It's all right if they get wet; they will be removed in the doctor's office.
  - After you dry yourself, replace any dressings with clean, dry ones.
- You can safely shave very close to the incision and the stitches. You may find it easier to do this with an electric shaver. Then you can cover the unshaved area with a narrow bandage if you wish.
- You may return to work when you feel up to it.

✆ CALL OUR OFFICE IF

- The area under the incision begins to bulge, or becomes red and warm, or there is drainage from it.
- You develop a temperature higher than 100°F.
- You have any questions.

PATENT DUCTUS ARTERIOSUS

△ GENERAL INFORMATION

In a normal person, the *right* side of the heart receives blood from the body and then pumps the blood under somewhat low pressure through the *pulmonary* (lung) artery to the lungs. There, the blood picks up oxygen and then goes to the *left* side of the heart. From there the blood is pumped under high pressure into the *aorta* (the large vessel from the heart) and out through all of the body.

Before a baby is born, it does not breathe. The baby's blood gets its oxygen from the mother through the placenta. Of course, during all this, the heart beats. The blood, however, instead of going out the pulmonary artery and to the lungs from the right side of the heart, is side-tracked and goes directly to the aorta. The side-tracking vessel is called a *ductus arteriosus*.

Soon after the baby is born, this ductus arteriosus scars down and closes and is called a *ligamentum arteriosum* (Fig. 1*A*). Now, all the blood in the pulmonary artery goes to the lungs and *not* directly to the aorta.

Rarely, however, the ductus arteriosus does not close after birth; it continues to remain *patent* (open) (Fig. 1*B*). So, blood goes from the high-pressure aorta to the low-pressure pulmonary artery that goes to the lungs (in the opposite direction to how it flows in the fetus). This high-pressure blood in the lungs can do serious damage to the lungs as well as to the heart.

COMMON SIGNS AND SYMPTOMS

- The symptoms can range from none at all to very severe, including difficulty with breathing and swelling of the tissue with water. This depends on the age of the child and the size of the patent ductus.
- Early, and if the condition is mild, there may be no symptoms.

DIAGNOSIS

- There is a very characteristic murmur in the heart area that can make the diagnosis 95% of the time.
- A chest x-ray may show some effect on the lungs.
- An electrocardiogram (EKG) may show a straining heart.
- **Echocardiogram:** Harmless sound waves are bounced off the heart and its vessels. The returning sound waves (the echoes) are seen as a picture on a screen. They can show the area involved.
- **Cardiac catheterization:** A tiny catheter is positioned in the heart so that the pressures can be measured in all its chambers and vessels. Also, dye can be injected and pictures of the dye taken as it flows through the heart and vessels. This study may be done to make certain of the diagnosis, although at times the echocardiogram should be all that is needed.

○ TREATMENT

- The condition can be corrected by an operation. This is best done at 1 to 2 years of age (Fig. 1*C*).
- The risk for the operation is virtually zero and the results very good.

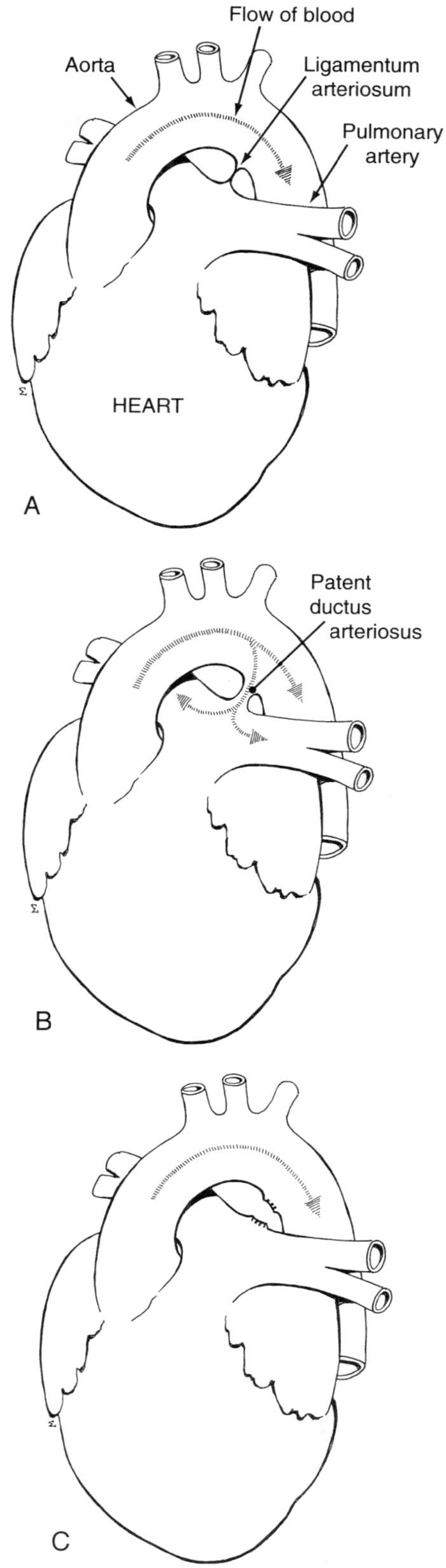

Figure 1. *A*, Normal heart. *B*, Patent ductus arteriosus. The blood is flowing both down the aorta and into the pulmonary arteries. *C*, The patent ductus is divided, and blood is flowing normally.

PREOPERATIVE PREPARATION

- All of the necessary studies will have been done while making the diagnosis.
- Do not give the child any food or liquids for 6 hours before the operation (the necessary fluids will be given by vein).

☐ OPERATION

- The operation is done under general anesthesia.
- The incision will be on the left side of the chest.
- The operation usually takes about 2 hours.

POSTOPERATIVE COURSE

- Your child will be taken to the Surgical Care Unit, where the doctors and nurses are very experienced in taking care of such patients. As soon as the child is coming along well enough, he or she will be transferred to a regular hospital room.
- Your child should be able to go home in about 4 days.
- Arrangements will be made for your child's medicine and follow-up office visit.

✣ HOME CARE

- Resume the usual activities.
- You may sponge bathe the child, with any dressings on or off. Do not let the child soak any longer than is necessary. After you dry the child, replace any dressings with clean, dry ones.

✆ CALL OUR OFFICE IF

- There are any unusual signs or symptoms.
- The incision becomes red or swollen, or there is drainage from it.
- The child develops a temperature higher than 100°F.
- You have any questions.

PEDIATRIC CAUDAL ANESTHESIA-ANALGESIA

△ GENERAL INFORMATION

Operating on infants and children requires special skills and techniques. Modern applications of anesthetic methods have made it possible to deliver better care to infants and children who are having simple or complicated operations. In addition, the operations can be done more safely, and a faster, more comfortable recovery can be expected.

One modern advance is *caudal anesthesia*, which can be combined with general anesthesia or with sedation. It is used to provide pain relief in infants and children who have operations in the lower abdomen, groin, legs, and feet. This type of anesthesia used alone or in combination with general anesthesia or sedation can be very effective in controlling pain during and after surgery.

ADVANTAGES OF CAUDAL ANESTHESIA

- Most children who have a caudal anesthetic do not require additional pain medicines during the first 6 to 12 hours following the operation. This reduces the need to treat pain with narcotics, given either by vein or in the muscle by injection. Narcotics often have undesirable side effects, such as nausea, vomiting, drowsiness, and suppression of breathing.
- Another advantage of caudal anesthesia before the operation is begun is that it blocks the nerves that carry pain signals before the painful incision is made. This results in less need for pain medicine after the operation.

WHO MIGHT BENEFIT FROM CAUDAL ANESTHESIA

In some infants and children who have diseases of the heart and lungs and in premature infants, there may be an increased risk to the child in giving a general anesthetic. In such children, having an operation in an area of the body below the navel, it may be safer to give caudal anesthesia alone. These children will additionally benefit from the pain relief that is experienced after the operation when using a caudal anesthetic.

HOW CAUDAL ANESTHESIA IS GIVEN

- In addition to examination by other doctors, the anesthesiologist will take a medical history and perform an examination to decide on the most appropriate anesthetic method.
- Medicine may be given to your child to bring on drowsiness.
- Thin wires from a recording machine will be placed on the skin to measure the oxygen supply in the blood, the pulse, and the blood pressure.
- An intravenous catheter will be placed to supply fluids and also will be used as a route to give medicines.
- The child will be positioned on his or her side with the hips and knees bent.
  - The skin over the lower back will be swabbed with an antiseptic solution and surrounded with sterile drapes.
  - A needle will be placed in a space in the lower part of the sacrum (the lowest portion of the backbone). The epidural space in which the needle is placed is an area of loose fatty tissue with blood vessels running through it. This epidural space surrounds the coverings of the spinal cord and the nerves coming from it. The spinal cord and its nerves carry signals (including those of pain) from the body to the brain.
  - A solution of the local anesthetic is injected *outside* the coverings of the spinal cord, especially outside the dura, the outermost membrane that surrounds the spinal cord. This is why it is called *epidural* anesthesia.

HOW IT WORKS

- The anesthetic is able to seep through the dura (and other coverings of the spinal cord) and mix with spinal fluid that surrounds the spinal cord and its nerve branches. The anesthetic binds to specific areas on these nerves and blocks painful sensations from the wound from reaching the brain.
- Caudal anesthesia can be given in one of two ways depending on the following:
  - The type of operation.
  - The length of time the operation will take.
  - Specific considerations for a particular patient.

TECHNIQUES

The anesthetic can be given as just a single injection into the epidural space. Or, a very thin plastic catheter is inserted into the epidural space and taped in position, which makes it possible for the anesthetic medication to be given continuously during the operation and even after the operation for relief of pain, if your child needs to remain in the hospital.

POSSIBLE COMPLICATIONS

As with any procedure, complications are always possible. Although they are uncommon (serious complications with caudal anesthesia occur once out of 40,000 anesthetics), they can include temporary breathing difficulty and disturbance of heart rhythm.

A more common problem is temporary difficulty passing urine. Temporary weakness in the legs can occur after caudal anesthesia. This usually resolves within 6 to 10 hours and normal movement and weight bearing can be done after this time, unless it is not permitted because of the type of operation that was performed.

SUMMARY

As you can see, caudal epidural anesthesia, along with sedation or general anesthesia, can provide a safe and effective method for providing pain relief for infants and children having an operation on the lower half of the body.

PELVIC INFLAMMATORY DISEASE (SALPINGO-OOPHORITIS)

△ GENERAL INFORMATION

Pelvic inflammatory disease (PID) is an infection of the internal female reproductive organs. This infection can spread to other organs in the abdominal cavity to cause peritonitis and the formation of abscesses. It is seen most commonly in younger women. It is caused by bacteria that enter the uterus through the cervix in the following ways:

- An infected sexual partner.
- The use of an intrauterine birth control device (IUD). Such a device makes it easier for bacteria in the vagina to enter the uterus.
- Douching. This may help bacteria enter the uterus and travel to the tubes.
- Infections of the cervix that can spread into the uterus and then to the tubes.

COMMON SIGNS AND SYMPTOMS

Early in the Disease

- There may be mild, vague pain on both sides of the lower abdomen, especially during the menstrual period.
- Heavier menstrual flow.
- Pain with intercourse.
- Foul-smelling vaginal discharge.
- Frequent urination or burning on urination.
- General ill feeling.
- Lower abdominal discomfort with walking.
- Pain over the liver area.

Later in the Disease

- Severe lower abdominal pain with tenderness in the abdomen, often requiring admission to the hospital.
- Fever.
- Generalized peritonitis if an abscess ruptures.

DIAGNOSIS

A high degree of awareness—always thinking of PID as a possible diagnosis—even with just a few symptoms, can help make the diagnosis, especially at an early stage (Fig. 1).

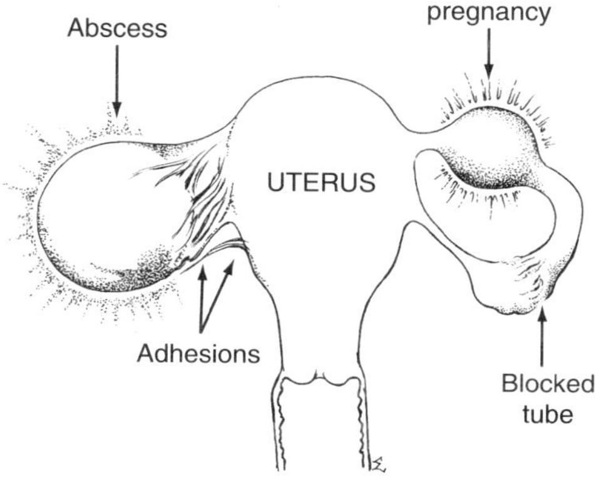

Figure 1. Pelvic inflammatory disease can manifest in a number of ways. Several of the more common ones are shown. They can occur singly or all together in a particular individual.

- A detailed history of symptoms and a thorough pelvic examination is essential.
- Obtaining any fluid in the vagina, especially if it is coming from the opening to the uterus (the cervix) for examination under the microscope for evidence of bacteria.
- *Ultrasound*: Harmless sound waves are aimed at the area of your pelvis. The sound waves bouncing back (the echoes) from this area are seen as a picture on a screen. Ultrasonography is a convenient and painless way to examine your uterus, tubes, and ovaries.
- *Colpocentesis*: A needle is placed through the tissue at the very uppermost part of the vagina. It will enter the area near the tubes and ovaries. If fluid is present, it is removed and examined under the microscope for evidence of bacteria.
- *Laparoscopy*: This is done when the symptoms are severe but the diagnosis not clear. A diagnosis needs to be made but if possible without opening the abdomen. The examination is done with a *laparoscope*, a smooth, flexible instrument about as thick as your finger, with lenses in it and a light at its tip. With the patient asleep, the laparoscope is placed in the abdominal cavity through a tiny incision in the navel. All the organs in the pelvis can be examined directly to provide the diagnosis as well as to indicate whether an open operation is necessary. If an operation is necessary, an incision can be made to carry it out at that time.

○ TREATMENT

Most patients with PID are treated medically and followed closely as necessary. The treatment can include the following:

- Antibiotics.
- Bedrest.
- Heating pad to the lower abdomen.
- Warm bath for 10 to 15 minutes three or four times a day.
- No douching.

An operation may be necessary for the following:

- Pelvic abscess.
- Ruptured pelvic abscess.
- Generalized peritonitis, the cause of which may be PID.
- Removal of the uterus and tubes for cases that are chronic or not responding to medical treatment, and in women past the childbearing age.

After careful consideration of all factors, the recommendation is that you have an operation to try to take care of your problem.

PREOPERATIVE PREPARATION

- You will have an examination of your blood, urine, heart (EKG), and lungs (chest x-ray).
- Do not eat or drink anything for 8 hours before the operation.

☐ OPERATION

- You will be asleep for the operation.
- The operation that is performed will depend on what is found. The possibilities will be explained to you as completely as possible before anything is planned or done.

POSTOPERATIVE CARE

- You will be taken to a recovery room and observed. When your blood pressure, pulse, and breathing are stable, you will be taken to a regular hospital room.
- There may be a catheter in your bladder for a day or so. This will be more comfortable for you.
- The evening after the operation you will be helped to sit up in bed and on the next day to get out of bed.
- Pain will be controlled with medicine.
- Your diet will be as you tolerate it.
- Arrangements will be made for your medicine, follow-up office visit, and stitch or clip removal.

✣ HOME CARE

- You may walk about as you wish, even climb stairs, but don't overdo things.
- You may eat as you wish, but include plenty of roughage and liquids in your diet to avoid constipation.
- Take medicine as prescribed for your pain.
- Do not douche or use a tampon. A sanitary pad can be used for the expected vaginal discharge.
- Unless instructed otherwise, you may shower if you wish, with any dressings on or off. After you dry yourself, replace any dressing with clean, dry ones.
- Do not drive a car unless you can move freely and without pain and are not taking drugs that reduce your alertness.
- Engaging in sexual intercourse too soon can be harmful to your recovery. Let's talk about this during your follow-up visit.
- You may return to work when you feel up to it.

✆ CALL OUR OFFICE IF

- The incision becomes red or swollen, or there is drainage from it.
- You develop a temperature higher than 100°F.
- You develop an increasing amount of foul-smelling discharge from your vagina.
- You have any questions.

PET (POSITRON-EMISSION TOMOGRAPHY) SCAN

△ GENERAL INFORMATION

PET scan stands for positron emission tomography scan. It is one of the latest and most sophisticated ways of looking at tumors.

There are a number of ways of looking at tumors:

- **X-rays:** With this technique, powerful electron beams are sent through the body and they strike a sensitive photographic film on the other side of the body. Some of the various organs and tissues of the part being x-rayed slow the x-rays down somewhat (for example, lung tissue), whereas others block x-rays almost completely (for example, bone). The result is the typical x-ray film. The drawback to x-rays is that if organs or tissues are located behind a bone, they cannot be seen at all or are seen poorly.
- **Ultrasound:** Harmless sound waves are aimed at an area of the body. The sound waves bouncing back (the echoes) from this area are seen as pictures on a screen. This is a convenient and painless way to examine organs and tissues inside your body. The details with this method are not quite as clear as with other methods.
- **CT scan (computed tomography scan):** This is a form of x-ray in which the machine takes pictures of the body as though it were in thin slices. This is something like being able to see all of the raisins and their exact location inside a loaf of bread without having to actually slice the bread.
- **MRI (magnetic resonance imaging):** This technique does not use x-rays. Instead, it uses harmless magnetic fields, radio waves, and computers. As the magnetic waves are sent back and forth through the area being examined, they are converted into pictures. Further, the organs being examined can be looked at from many different angles. With this technique, doctors can look around bones that might block other types of picture-taking. In addition, blood vessels and nerves can be seen more clearly.
- **PET scan:** With this technique, one can look at tumors, as with the other techniques, but it also is possible to tell what *activity* is going on in these tumors. This is possible for the following reasons: Radioactive forms of certain basic chemicals such as oxygen, nitrogen, carbon, and glucose have a very short life (a few minutes to 2 hours). These chemicals are chosen because they can become a part of the body's chemical activity. PET can record the activity of these chemicals with the body.

HOW IT IS DONE

A needle is used to inject the short-acting radioactive material (a *radiopharmaceutical*) into your vein. The radiopharmaceutical then circulates in the blood and becomes part of the body's chemical activities. Most important, it can become a part of the activity of any tumors that might be present.

THE MACHINE

- The PET scanner is shaped like a huge doughnut. You will lie on a table inside the hole in the "doughnut."
- The PET scanner will slowly pass over the part of the body being examined. As it does this, it records the radioactive signals from the radiopharmaceutical that has deposited itself in the various tissues (Fig. 1). These signals are converted into pictures that show the tumor in various colors: red for very active tumor, yellow for a less active tumor, green for even less, etc.

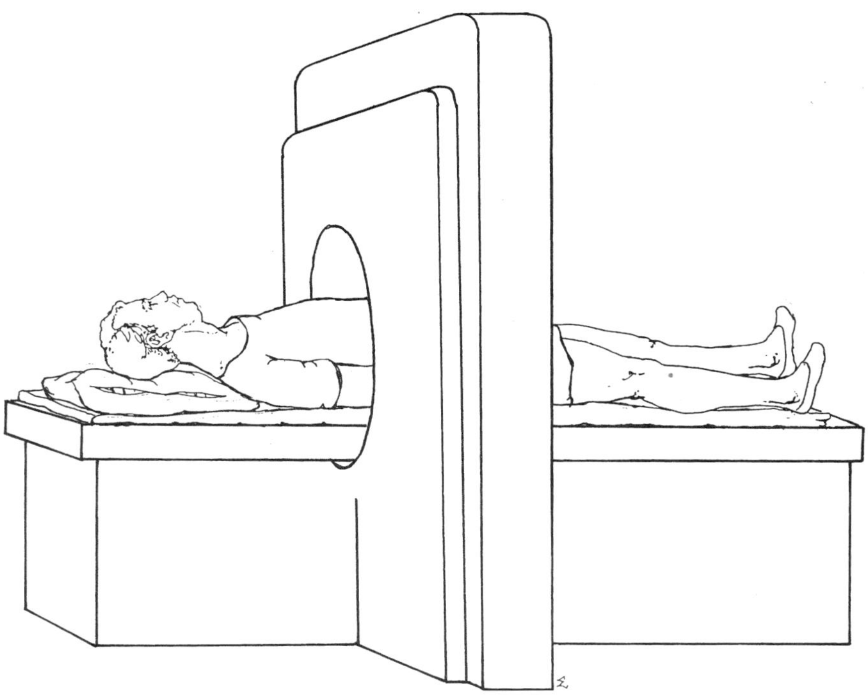

Figure 1.

THE RESULTS

Based on this color coding, the specialists who examine the pictures can determine several important things:

- Is a tumor present?
- If it is present, is it active or just not doing much, if anything?
- If it is active, how strong (or weak) is the activity?

COMMENTS

After the patient receives treatment for the tumor, the PET scan can be repeated to see what effect the treatment had on the chemical activity—the "life"—of the tumor.

In some instances, the information provided by a PET scan can be extremely important in making a diagnosis, guiding the therapy, and measuring the results of such therapy.

△ GENERAL INFORMATION

This is a disease of the penis. Scar tissue in the penis produces a deformity (usually a curvature) when the penis becomes erect (Fig. 1). It occurs in about 1% of the male population in this country. Trauma from sexual intercourse, constriction rings, self-injection therapy, and other injuries in susceptible patients may start the process of scar formation. However, the true cause of the disease is not definitely known.

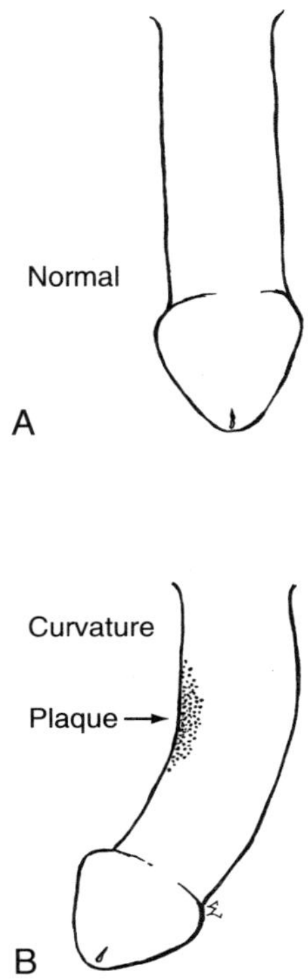

Figure 1.

COMMON SIGNS AND SYMPTOMS

- There is pain in the penis as it becomes erect.
- There is curvature of the penis as it becomes erect.
- Impotence: This may be caused by the curvature, or the curvature may exaggerate an already existing impotence.
- There is a *plaque* (localized scar) in the penis.

In some men, there may be associated conditions of excessive formation of scar tissue elsewhere in the body (example: keloid).

DIAGNOSIS

- Anyone with symptoms of pain in the penis followed by angulation or a plaque and with or without erection problems should be concerned about Peyronie's disease.
- The diagnosis can be made by taking a detailed history and doing a thorough physical examination of the genitalia.
- Penile injections, medicine by mouth, or vacuum devices may be used by the surgeon to cause penile erection so as to be able to examine the penis when it is erect.
- The individual may be asked to obtain photographs of the erect penis in the privacy of his home.
- An ultrasonogram may be done of the penis. Sound waves (they are like sonar) are aimed at the penis. The sound waves bouncing back (the echoes) are seen as pictures on a screen. This is a convenient, harmless, and painless way to examine the tissue inside the penis.
- An x-ray of the penis may be obtained to look for any calcium deposits.

○ TREATMENT

Surgical treatment of Peyronie's disease should be reserved for those individuals with severe deformity of the penis that prevents them from engaging in sexual activity.

There usually are three options available for treatment, depending on several factors:

- **Plication:** This is simply firming up the faulty tissue. It is most suitable for individuals with minimal curvature who are potent and sexually active.
- **Plaque excision and skin graft:** This involves removing the plaque and repairing the area with a skin graft. It is best for those persons with no pain who have significant curvature and who have a good response to injection of medicine into the penis to make it erect. It also is good for those who respond to a vacuum-constricting device. This is a method of preventing some of the blood from leaving the penis too early and so making the penis more erect.
- **Penile prosthesis:** One of several prostheses are placed in the penis. This is most suitable for those individuals who have no pain in the penis and who do not respond to medical therapy, self-injection, or a vacuum-constricting device. Finally, there are individuals who strongly desire some solution to their problem and this is the only available choice.

PREOPERATIVE PREPARATION

- You will have a thorough physical examination as well as an examination of your blood, urine, heart (EKG), and lungs (chest x-ray).
- Do not eat or drink anything for 8 hours before the operation.
- Shower as usual on the morning of the operation.
- Medicine may be given to you prior to the operation that will make you feel drowsy.

□ OPERATION

- Either you will be asleep for the operation, or the area of the penis will be anesthetized.
- An artificial erection of the penis will be created.
- An incision will be made behind the head of the penis.
- The curvature will be corrected by one of the procedures already mentioned.
- This operation usually takes 1 to 2 hours.

POSTOPERATIVE CARE

- You will wake up in the recovery room. When your blood pressure, pulse, and breathing are stable, you will be taken to a regular hospital room.
- The penis will have a bandage around it, but you should be able to urinate as usual.
- You will be given some medicine (probably for the next several weeks) to try to prevent your getting an erection.
- Pain will be controlled by medicine.
- You should be able to go home in 1 or 2 days.
- Arrangements will be made for your medicine, follow-up office visit, and stitch removal.
- As with any operation, complications are always possible. For this type of operation, complications can include bleeding, infection, and separation of the incision. Also, there may be some decrease in sensation over the penis for a few weeks. On occasion, the curvature may return.

✣ HOME CARE

- Lie down for 15 to 30 minutes every 2 hours; this helps reduce any swelling of the penis.
- You may walk about as you wish, even climb stairs.
- Be sure to take the medicines prescribed that will prevent your getting an erection. If your penis becomes erect, there is a risk that the stitches may tear.
- Do not place yourself in a situation of sexual arousal for 4 to 6 weeks. Do not engage in sexual intercourse for 6 weeks unless the surgeon agrees to a different timetable.
- You may eat as you did before the operation.
- You may shower as you wish, with any dressings on or off.
  - There may be narrow strips of tape across the incision. It's all right if they get wet; they will be removed in the doctor's office.
  - After you dry yourself, replace any dressings with clean, dry ones.
- Wearing boxer shorts may be more comfortable.

✆ CALL OUR OFFICE IF

- The penis begins to swell more than it did when you left the hospital.
- There is drainage of blood or other fluid through the incision.
- You develop a temperature higher than 101°F.
- You have any questions.

△ GENERAL INFORMATION

This is a condition in which some surface-type skin (the type that normally faces outward) gets trapped deep under the surface of the skin (Fig. 1). This happens in the area of the *sacrum* (tailbone).

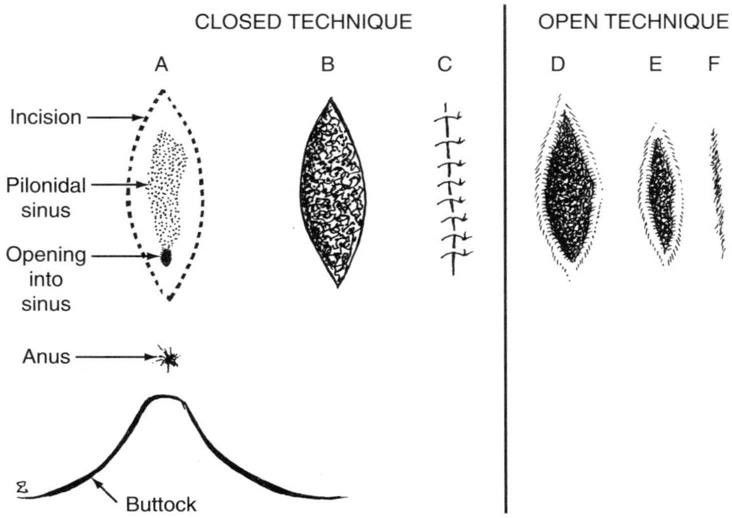

Figure 1. Generally, an infected pilonidal cyst that has developed into an abscess is treated initially by simple drainage to let the pus out and to permit the surrounding tissue to heal. Otherwise, the treatment of a cyst or sinus is the same, namely, excision. A, B, and C show the sequence of excision of the cyst with primary closure. D, E, and F show the healing process following the excision of the cyst when the wound is left open.

COMMON SIGNS AND SYMPTOMS

- The trapped skin grows hair, and the oil and sweat glands work, but this material has no place to empty. So, it forms what is called a pilonidal *cyst*.
- Most often, there is a small opening in the cyst through which the oil, and even hair, can find their way to the outside. This is a pilonidal *sinus*. Sometimes the cyst becomes infected, and an *abscess* forms.
- Pilonidal cyst and sinus occur most often in hairy young men.

DIAGNOSIS

Usually, the diagnosis can be made by taking a detailed history and doing a thorough physical examination.

○ TREATMENT

An operation is necessary to correct the problem if

- The condition repeatedly flares up and quiets down, but with no expectation that it will go away by itself.
- There is a foul-smelling, oily discharge from the sinus.
- An abscess forms.

After careful consideration of all factors, it is recommended that you have an operation to take care of your pilonidal problem.

PREOPERATIVE PREPARATION

- You will have an examination of your blood and urine. You may also have an examination of your heart (EKG) and lungs (chest x-ray).
- You will be given instructions on how to cleanse your bowel before the operation.
- Do not eat or drink anything for 8 hours before the operation.
- You may be given medicine that will make you feel drowsy before you are brought to the operating room.

□ OPERATION

- The operation is done either under local anesthesia along with some medicine to continue making you feel drowsy, or with you asleep. This will depend on how badly the area is infected and which one of several possible operations will be performed. This will be discussed with you beforehand.

The operation may be as follows:

- Simply opening the abscess (unroofing it) to let the pus out. This is to take care of an acute problem. The final operation is done at a later time when the infection quiets down.
- Removing all of the involved tissue but leaving the wound open to gradually close by itself over a period of 4 to 8 weeks.
- Removal of the involved tissue (cyst and sinus) with complete closure of the wound.
- The operation usually takes about 1 hour.

POSTOPERATIVE CARE

- You will be taken to a recovery room and observed until your blood pressure, pulse, and breathing are stable and you are completely alert. You should be able to go home that same day with a responsible adult. If the operation is more extensive, you will need to stay in the hospital for a day or two.
- Pain will be controlled with medicine.
- Arrangements will be made for your medicine, follow-up office visit, stitch removal, and instructions on wound care.

✚ HOME CARE

- You may walk about as you wish, even climb stairs, but don't overdo things.

- Take medicine as prescribed for your pain.
- Be certain to take any antibiotics prescribed for you.
- You will be instructed on taking sitz baths for 15 minutes twice a day if these are necessary. This involves sitting in a bathtub filled with enough warm (not hot) water to completely cover the operated area. It may be possible, and even more desirable, for you to take showers. If you wish, let's discuss this during your follow-up office visit.
- When you may return to work will depend on what operation you had. For example:
  - If the wound is closed completely, stitches will be removed in 10 or 14 days and you should be off work for about 2 weeks for proper healing.
  - If the wound is left open to gradually close by itself, it will drain and require change of dressings for 4 to 8 weeks. At the beginning, someone close to you can be taught how to do it; it's not difficult. After the first few days you should be able to do it yourself.
  - For some types of employment, a person with an open wound is not allowed to work.
- Be careful that you do not become constipated.
  - Include enough roughage and plenty of liquids in your diet.
  - You may need some help with a mild laxative (example: milk of magnesia).

✆ CALL OUR OFFICE IF

- A closed incision becomes red, swollen, or painful, or if there is drainage from it.
- There is bleeding from a wound that is left open.
- You develop a fever higher than 100°F.
- You have any questions.

△ GENERAL INFORMATION

Like a balloon, the lung is elastic and is filled with air. Also like a balloon, the lung cannot expand by itself; something needs to push it from the inside or pull it from the outside to make it get bigger.

When a person takes in a breath, the chest wall becomes bigger. This creates a vacuum between the inside of the chest wall and the lungs, so the lungs are pulled out, or expanded. The surface of the lungs is covered by a thin tissue membrane that keeps air in the lung. If a hole is made in this membrane, the lung collapses.

THE PNEUMOTHORAX

Things can happen that spoil the normal arrangement of the lung. Something makes a hole in the lung; for example, a bleb in the lung bursts, there is injury from a fractured rib, or there is a penetrating injury to the chest and lungs. As soon as the hole is made, the lung collapses.

Now every time the chest expands the lung does not go out with it; it remains collapsed. This is a *pneumothorax*. The air you breathe goes down your windpipe *(trachea)*, out through the hole in the lung, and into the chest cavity. So, there is air in the chest cavity that collapses the lung (Fig. 1).

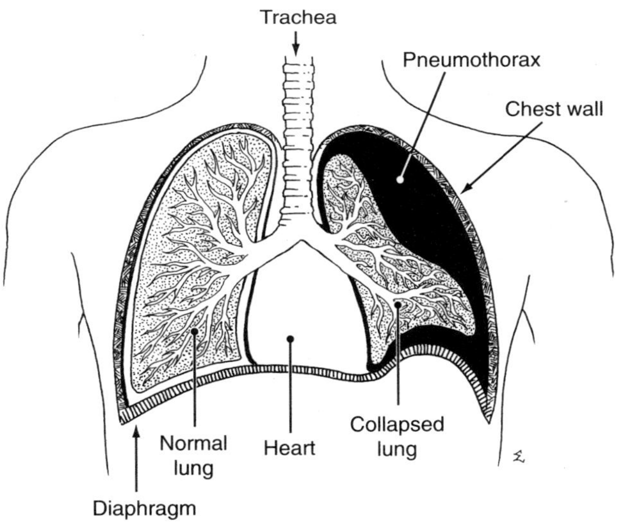

Figure 1. The extent of a pneumothorax varies considerably, ranging from a minimal amount that causes little difficulty to serious collapse of the lung that makes breathing very difficult. Also the heart and the vessels going in and out of it are shifted enough that the proper working of the heart is affected.

○ TREATMENT

- A procedure may be necessary to remove the air and expand the lung.
- This procedure involves placing a plastic tube about as big around as the tip of your little finger into the chest cavity. The purpose of this tube is to remove the air that is in the chest cavity and allow the lung to expand.
- If the hole is in the lung itself, the tube has to be left in because air will keep on leaking out of the lung and into the chest cavity.
  - Suction is applied on the tube so that the air is pulled out of the chest cavity faster than it leaks out of the lung. This brings back the vacuum between the chest wall and the lung, so the lung expands. This suction is kept up until the hole in the lung heals itself.
  - If the hole in the lung is too big and the above treatment does not work, an operation may be necessary to open the chest and repair the hole.

INSERTION OF CHEST TUBE

- The side of the chest with the pneumothorax is painted with an antiseptic solution and draped with sterile towels.
- A thin needle is used to inject an anesthetic into the skin to make it numb. A very short incision is made in the numbed skin and the plastic tube inserted.
- The plastic tube will be connected to a suction machine and the air that is *outside* of the lung itself removed. You will breathe much more easily very soon but you may cough quite a bit as the lung expands.
- An x-ray of your chest will be taken to be certain that the tube is in the right place and that the lung has expanded properly.

POSTOPERATIVE CARE

- You will be able to sit up as you wish.
- Pain can be controlled with medicine. The nurse will give it to you. Or, you can give yourself a preset amount of pain medicine when you feel you need it. This is done with a device called patient-controlled analgesia (PCA) that is connected to the tubing giving you intravenous fluids.
- You will be able to leave the hospital when your lung is expanded and healed.
- As with any operation, complications are always possible. With this type of operation, complications can include infection in the chest cavity, pneumonia, heart problems, and possibly others.
- Arrangements will be made for any medicine and follow-up office visit.

✚ HOME CARE

- Continue with the program started while you were in the hospital.
- You may eat as you did before the operation.
- Be careful that you do not become constipated.
  - Include enough roughage and liquid in your diet.
  - You may need some help with a mild laxative (example: mineral oil).
- Don't lift anything heavier than 5 pounds. Ask someone to do it for you.
- Inactivity is not good for you, but neither is overdoing it. Don't try to do too much too soon.

- Unless instructed otherwise, you may shower as you wish, with any dressings on or off.
  - There may be narrow strips of tape across the incision. It's all right if they get wet; they will be removed in the doctor's office.
  - After you dry yourself, replace any dressings with clean, dry ones.
- Driving a car with an automatic shift may not seem to be too demanding. However, if you suddenly have to slam on the brakes or twist to turn the steering wheel, you may strain the sutures or tear something. During your follow-up visit, let's discuss when you can resume driving.
- You may resume sexual activity whenever you choose.
- You may return to work when you feel up to it, but let's talk about it first during your follow-up office visit or by phone.

✆ CALL OUR OFFICE IF

- You develop any unusual signs or symptoms.
- You develop a temperature higher than 101°F.
- You have any questions.

POLYPOSIS COLI, FAMILIAL: Total Colectomy, Rectal Mucosectomy, and Ileal Pouch–Anal Anastomosis

△ GENERAL INFORMATION

A *colon polyp* is a growth that sticks out from the lining of the intestine. *Polyposis* ("many polyps") *coli* ("of the colon") is a condition in which many polyps, sometimes many hundreds of them, are in the colon and rectum. These polyps can be as small as a grain of rice or as large as a walnut. They sometimes cover the colon and rectum so completely that no normal lining of the colon can be seen. This condition is called *familial* because it can occur in families.

COMMON SIGNS AND SYMPTOMS

Often, these polyps don't produce any signs or symptoms. When there are symptoms, the most common is diarrhea or bleeding from the rectum.

DIAGNOSIS

- Taking a careful history of the symptoms can lead to the diagnosis.
- You will have a complete blood analysis.
- Colonoscopy: This is done with an optical instrument that is smooth, flexible, and as big around as your little finger, with a light at its tip. During the procedure, you will be given medicine that will make you feel drowsy. The instrument will be gently introduced through your anus, and the entire large bowel will be carefully examined. With colonoscopy, the doctor can see how much of the colon is involved. Also, if any suspicious areas are seen, a small piece (a *biopsy*) can be taken for laboratory examination. This examination will show what type of polyp it is. This is very important because there are some conditions that can look like polyposis coli but are not and so don't have the risk of developing cancer.

○ TREATMENT

In time, all patients with familial polyposis coli will develop cancer of the colon or rectum if the polyps are not removed. Removal of the polyps in polyposis coli requires removal of the colon. This can be done in several ways as follows:

Option 1. Removing the entire colon and rectum. A pouch is fashioned near the end of the small intestine (the ileum) to collect stool. The ileum is then brought directly to the outside (an *ileostomy*).

Advantages to This Method

- This is the simplest operation and eliminates the risk of cancer developing in the polyps.

Disadvantages to This Method

- There is the need to empty the pouch of stool several times each day or to wear a bag, or both.
- You have to wear a bag on the side to collect stool that may leak out the ileostomy.
- There is a very small chance that the operation may damage important nerves in the pelvis. For men, this means they would not be able to have an erection.

Option 2. Removing the colon **only.** A pouch is fashioned near the end of the small intestine (the ileum) and the end of the ileum is connected to the rectum.

Advantages to This Method

- The stool comes out through the anus.
- For men, the ability to have an erection is not changed.

Disadvantages to This Method

- There are 6 to 8 bowel movements per day.
- You will need to have proctoscopy at regular intervals for the rest of your life to be certain that cancer does not develop in the polyps that are left in the rectum.
- In spite of these precautions, the risk of developing cancer of the rectum is quite high.

Option 3. Removing the colon and then only the lining (the *mucosa*) of the rectum that grows the polyps. The small intestine is passed through the rectum (that no longer has mucosa) and is connected to the anus.

Advantages to This Method

- The end of the small intestine will be fashioned in such a way that it has a pouch in which stool can collect before it comes out the anus.
- It gets rid of all of the polyps.
- Bowel movements can come through the anus.
- This operation does not change the ability of a man to have an erection.

Disadvantages to This Method

- It is a more serious operation.
- You will have 6 to 8 bowel movements a day. However, you will be trained in exercises to learn how to squeeze your sphincter enough to keep the somewhat loose stool from soiling your underclothing. After 6 months, most individuals develop control of their stool during the waking hours. Once in a great while, there is leakage during sleep.

After the most careful consideration of all factors, it is recommended that you have the operation in Option 3. The reasons for this recommendation have been explained to you, but you should feel perfectly free to ask any questions you wish now or later.

PREOPERATIVE PREPARATION

- You will have an examination of your blood, urine, heart (EKG), and lungs (chest x-ray).
- Do not eat or drink anything for 8 hours before the operation.

□ OPERATION

- You will be asleep for the operation.
- This operation will be done both from above on the abdomen and from below in the anus area.
- The entire colon but only the lining of the rectum will be removed. The small intestine near its end (the ileum) will then be fashioned into a pouch to collect stool as it comes down into it. The end of the

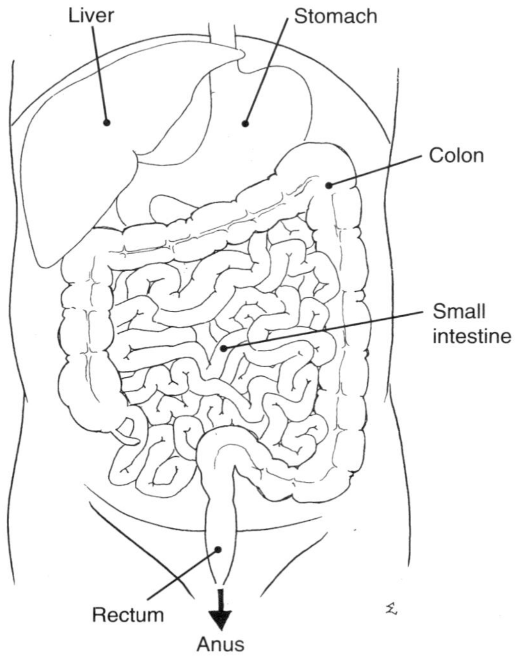

Figure 1. Normal relationships among the small intestine, colon, rectum, and anus.

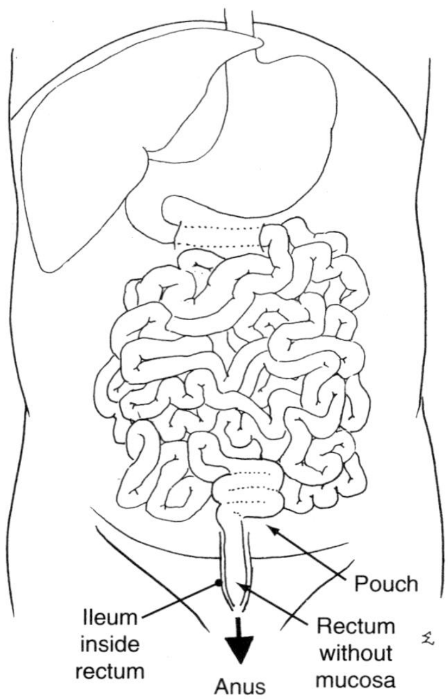

Figure 2. All of the colon is removed, and the small intestine (the ileum) is connected to the rectum.

ileum is passed through the rectum (without mucosa) and connected to the anus (Figs. 1 and 2).
- The operation usually takes about 4 or 5 hours.

POSTOPERATIVE CARE

- You will be taken to a recovery room and observed. When your blood pressure, pulse, and breathing are stable, you will be taken to a regular hospital room.
- You will have a thin plastic tube in your nose. It goes down to your stomach to suck up the air you swallow. It will be removed when your bowels start working.
- The evening after the operation you will be helped to sit up in bed and on the next day to get out of bed.
- Pain will be controlled with medicine.
- After your bowels start working, the tube in your nose will be removed and you will be started on a diet that you and the dietitian will arrange.
- The hospital support team of the doctors and nurses will work with you early and diligently to help you learn how to strengthen the sphincter of your anus.
- As with any operation, complications are always possible, some of them serious. With this type of operation, complications can include infections, leakage at one of the suture lines, bowel obstruction, blood clots, and possibly others.
- You should be able to go home in about 1 week.
- Arrangements will be made for your medicine, follow-up office visit, and stitch removal.

HOME CARE

- Continue with the program started while you were in the hospital.
- You may walk about as you wish, even climb stairs, but don't overdo things.
- You will be given a suggested appropriate diet to follow during your convalescence.
- Take the medicines prescribed for you.
- Arrangements can be made for a home visiting nurse if one is needed.
- You will be advised on how to go about taking a shower.

Remember that it will take a little time to become adjusted to this important change in your life. We will help you as much as we can so don't become discouraged during this period.

CALL OUR OFFICE IF

- The incision becomes red or swollen, or there is drainage from it.
- You develop a temperature higher than 100°F.
- You have any questions.

POLYPOSIS COLI, FAMILIAL: Total Colectomy with Ileal Pouch–Rectal Anastomosis

△ GENERAL INFORMATION

A *colon polyp* is a growth that sticks out from the lining of the intestine. *Polyposis* ("many polyps") *coli* ("of the colon") is a condition in which many polyps, sometimes many hundreds of them, are in the colon and rectum. These polyps can be as small as a grain of rice or as large as a walnut. They sometimes cover the colon and rectum so completely that no normal lining of the colon can be seen. The condition is called *familial* because it can occur in families.

COMMON SIGNS AND SYMPTOMS

Often, these polyps don't produce any signs or symptoms. When there are symptoms, the most common is diarrhea or bleeding from the rectum.

DIAGNOSIS

- Taking a careful history of the symptoms can lead to the diagnosis.
- You will have a complete blood analysis.
- Colonoscopy: This is done with an optical instrument that is smooth, flexible, and as big around as your little finger, with a light at its tip. During the procedure, you will be given medicine that will make you feel drowsy. The instrument will be gently introduced through your anus, and the entire large bowel will be carefully examined. With colonoscopy, the doctor can see how much of the colon is involved. Also, if any suspicious areas are seen, a small piece (a *biopsy*) can be taken for laboratory examination. This examination will show what type of polyp it is. This is very important because there are some conditions that can look like polyposis coli but are not and so don't have the risk of developing cancer.

○ TREATMENT

In time, all patients with familial polyposis coli will develop cancer of the colon or rectum if the polyps are not removed. Removal of the polyps requires removal of the colon. This can be done in several ways as follows.

Option 1. Removing the entire colon and rectum. A pouch is fashioned near the end of the small intestine (the ileum) to collect stool. The ileum is then brought directly to the outside (an *ileostomy*).

Advantages to This Method
- This is the simplest operation and eliminates the risk of cancer developing in the polyps.

Disadvantages to This Method
- There is the need to empty the pouch of stool several times each day, or to wear a bag, or both.
- You have to wear a bag on the side to collect stool that may leak out the ileostomy.
- There is a very small chance that the operation may damage important nerves in the pelvis. For men, this means they would not be able to have an erection.

Option 2. Removing the colon **only.** A pouch is fashioned near the end of the small intestine (the *ileum*) and the end of the ileum is connected to the rectum.

Advantages to This Method
- The stool comes out through the anus.
- For men, the ability to have an erection is not changed.

Disadvantages to This Method
- There are 6 to 8 bowel movements per day.
- You will need to have proctoscopy at regular intervals for the rest of your life to be certain that cancer does not develop in the polyps that are left in the rectum.
- In spite of these precautions, the risk of developing cancer of the rectum is quite high.

Option 3. Removing the colon and then only the lining (the *mucosa*) of the rectum that grows the polyps. The small intestine is passed through the rectum (that no longer has mucosa) and is connected to the anus.

Advantages to This Method
- The end of the small intestine will be fashioned in such a way that it has a pouch in which stool can collect before it comes out the anus.
- It gets rid of all of the polyps.
- Bowel movements can come through the anus.
- This operation does not change the ability of a man to have an erection.

Disadvantages to This Method
- It is a more serious operation.
- You will have 6 to 8 bowel movements a day. However, you will be trained in exercises to learn how to squeeze your sphincter enough to keep the somewhat loose stool from soiling your underclothing. After 6 months, most individuals develop control of their stool during the waking hours. Very rarely, there is leakage during sleep.

After the most careful consideration of all factors, it is recommended that you have the operation in Option 2. The reasons for this recommendation have been explained to you, but you should feel perfectly free to ask any questions you wish now or later.

PREOPERATIVE PREPARATION

- You will have an examination of your blood, urine, heart (EKG), and lungs (chest x-ray).
- Do not eat or drink anything for 8 hours before the operation.

□ OPERATION

- You will be asleep for the operation.
- This operation will be done through the abdomen.
- The colon will be removed, and the small intestine near its end (the ileum) will be fashioned into a pouch to collect stool as it comes down into it.

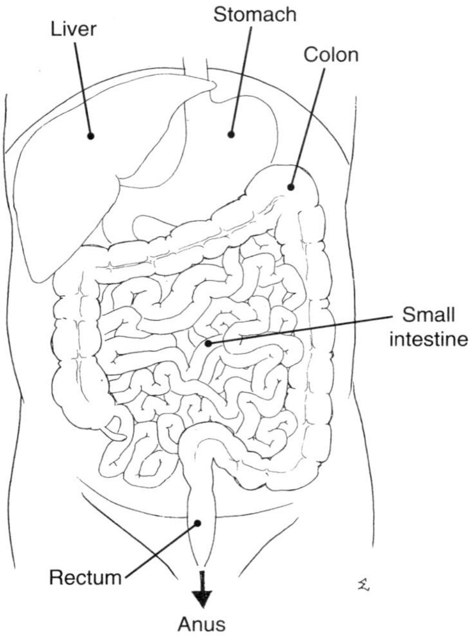

Figure 1. Normal relationships among the small intestine, colon, rectum, and anus.

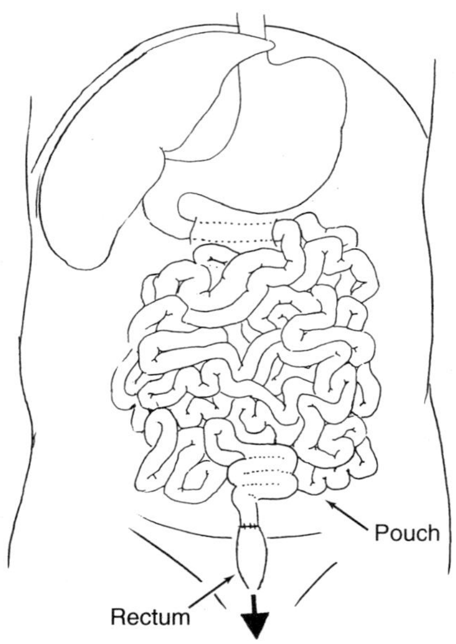

Figure 2. The entire colon is removed. A pouch will be fashioned near the end of the ileum, and the end of the ileum will be connected to the rectum.

The end of the ileum will then be connected to the rectum (Figs. 1 and 2).
- The operation usually takes about 3 hours.

POSTOPERATIVE CARE

- You will be taken to a recovery room and observed. When your blood pressure, pulse, and breathing are stable, you will be taken to a regular hospital room.
- You will have a thin plastic tube in your nose. It goes down to your stomach to suck up the air you swallow. It will be removed when your bowels start working.
- The evening after the surgery you will be helped to sit up in bed and on the next day to get out of bed.
- Pain will be controlled with medicine.
- After your bowels start working, the tube in your nose will be removed and you will be started on a diet that you and the dietitian will arrange.
- The hospital support team of the doctors and nurses will work with you early and diligently to help you adjust to your new condition.
- As with any operation, complications are always possible, some of them serious. With this type of operation, complications can include infections, leakage at one of the suture lines, bowel obstruction, blood clots, and possibly others.
- You should be able to go home in about 1 week.
- Arrangements will be made for your medicine, follow-up office visit, and stitch removal.

✣ HOME CARE

- Continue with the program started while you were in the hospital.
- You may walk about as you wish, even climb stairs, but don't overdo things.
- You will be given a suggested appropriate diet to follow during your convalescence.
- Take the medicines prescribed for you.
- Arrangements can be made for a home visiting nurse if one is needed.
- You will be advised on how to go about taking a shower.

Remember that it will take a little time to become adjusted to this important change in your life. We will help you as much as we can, so don't become discouraged during this period.

✆ CALL OUR OFFICE IF

- The incision becomes red or swollen, or there is drainage from it.
- You develop a temperature higher than 100°F.
- You have any questions.

POLYPOSIS COLI, FAMILIAL: Total Proctocolectomy with Ileostomy (Koch Pouch)

△ GENERAL INFORMATION

A *colon polyp* is a growth that sticks out from the lining of the intestine. *Polyposis* ("many polyps") *coli* ("of the colon") is a condition in which many polyps, sometimes many hundreds of them, are in the colon and rectum. These polyps can be as small as a grain of rice or as large as a walnut. They sometimes cover the colon and rectum so completely that no normal lining of the colon can be seen. This condition is called *familial* because it can occur in families.

COMMON SIGNS AND SYMPTOMS

Often, these polyps don't produce any signs or symptoms. When there are symptoms, the most common is diarrhea or bleeding from the rectum.

DIAGNOSIS

- Taking a careful history of the symptoms can lead to the diagnosis.
- You will have a complete blood analysis.
- Colonoscopy: This is done with an optical instrument that is smooth, flexible, and as big around as your little finger, with a light at its tip. During the procedure, you will be given medicine that will make you feel drowsy. The instrument will be gently introduced through your anus, and the entire large bowel will be carefully examined. With colonoscopy, the doctor can see how much of the colon is involved. Also, if any suspicious areas are seen, a small piece (a *biopsy*) can be taken for laboratory examination. This examination will show what type of polyp it is. This is very important because there are some conditions that can look like polyposis coli but are not and so don't have the risk of developing cancer.

○ TREATMENT

In time, all patients with familial polyposis coli will develop cancer of the colon or rectum if the polyps are not removed. Removal of the polyps in polyposis coli requires removal of the colon. This can be done in several ways as follows:

Option 1. Removing the entire colon and rectum. A pouch is fashioned near the end of the small intestine (the ileum) to collect the stool. The ileum is then brought directly to the outside (an *ileostomy*).

Advantages to This Method
- This is the simplest operation and eliminates the risk of cancer developing in the polyps.

Disadvantages to This Method
- There is the need to empty the pouch of stool several times each day, or to wear a bag, or both.
- You have to wear a bag on the side to collect stool that may leak out the ileostomy.
- There is a very small chance that the operation may damage important nerves in the pelvis. For men, this means they would not be able to have an erection.

Option 2. Removing the colon **only.** A pouch is fashioned near the end of the small intestine (the ileum) and the end of the ileum connected to the rectum.

Advantages to This Method
- The stool comes out through the anus.
- For men, the ability to have an erection is not changed.

Disadvantages to This Method
- There are 6 to 8 bowel movements per day.
- You will need to have proctoscopy at regular intervals for the rest of your life to be certain that cancer does not develop in the polyps that are left in the rectum.
- In spite of these precautions, the risk of developing cancer of the rectum is quite high.

Option 3. Removing the colon and then only the lining (the *mucosa*) of the rectum that grows the polyps. The small intestine is passed through the rectum (that no longer has mucosa) and is connected to the anus.

Advantages to This Method
- The end of the small intestine will be fashioned in such a way that it has a pouch in which stool can collect before it comes out the anus.
- It gets rid of all of the polyps.
- Bowel movements can come through the anus.
- This operation does not change the ability of a man to have an erection.

Disadvantages to This Method
- It is a more serious operation.
- You will have 6 to 8 bowel movements a day. However, you will be trained in exercises to learn how to squeeze your sphincter enough to keep the somewhat loose stool from soiling your underclothing. After 6 months, most individuals develop control of their stool during the waking hours. Very rarely, there is leakage during sleep.

After the most careful consideration of all factors, it is recommended that you have the operation in Option 1. The reasons for this recommendation have been explained to you, but you should feel perfectly free to ask any questions you wish now or later.

PREOPERATIVE PREPARATION

- You will have an examination of your blood, urine, heart (EKG), and lungs (chest x-ray).
- Do not eat or drink anything for 8 hours before the operation.

□ OPERATION

- You will be asleep for the operation.
- This operation will be done both from above on the abdomen and from below in the anus area.
- After the colon and rectum are removed, the small intestine near its end (the ileum) will be fashioned into a pouch to collect stool as it comes down into it.

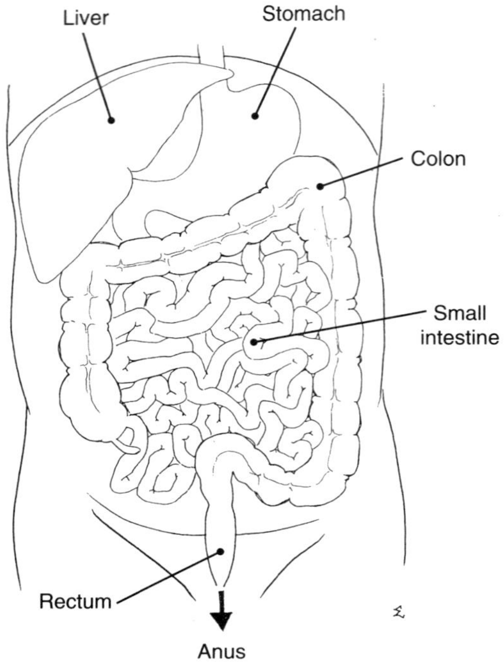

Figure 1. Normal relationships among the small intestine, colon, rectum, and anus.

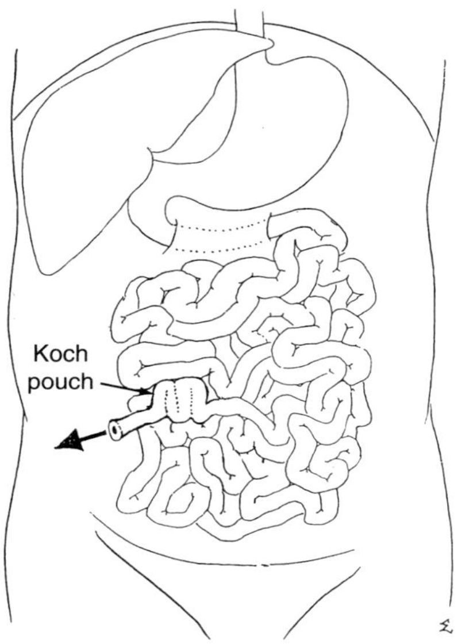

Figure 2. Entire colon, rectum, and anus are removed. A pouch (Koch pouch) for temporary collection of stool is fashioned almost at the end of the small intestine (ileum). The end of the small intestine is brought to the outside of the rectum (as an ileostomy).

This pouch will then be brought directly out through the abdominal wall as an *ileostomy* (Figs. 1 and 2).
- The operation usually takes about 3 hours.

POSTOPERATIVE CARE

- You will be taken to a recovery room and observed. When your blood pressure, pulse, and breathing are stable, you will be taken to a regular hospital room.
- You will have a thin plastic tube in your nose. It goes down to your stomach to suck up the air you swallow. It will be removed when your ileostomy starts working.
- The evening after the surgery you will be helped to sit up in bed and on the next day to get out of bed.
- Pain will be controlled with medicine.
- After the ileostomy starts working, the tube in your nose will be removed and you will be started on a diet that you and the dietitian will arrange.
- The hospital support team of the doctors and nurses will work with you early and diligently to help you learn how to take care of the ileostomy.
- As with any operation, complications are always possible, some of them serious. With this type of operation, complications can include infections, leakage at one of the suture lines, bowel obstruction, blood clots, and possibly others.
- You should be able to go home in about 1 week.
- Arrangements will be made for your medicine, follow-up office visit, and stitch removal.

✥ HOME CARE

- Continue with the program started while you were in the hospital.
- You may walk about as you wish, even climb stairs, but don't overdo things.
- You will be given a suggested appropriate diet to follow during your convalescence.
- Take the medicines prescribed for you.
- Arrangements can be made for a home visiting nurse if one is needed.
- You will be advised on how to go about taking a shower.

Remember that it will take a little time to become adjusted to this important change in your life. We will help you as much as we can, so don't become discouraged during this period.

✆ CALL OUR OFFICE IF

- The incision becomes red or swollen, or there is drainage from it.
- You develop a temperature higher than 100°F.
- You have any questions.

△ GENERAL INFORMATION

The *popliteal* artery runs behind the knee joint. An *aneurysm* is a ballooning out of a blood vessel.

An aneurysm of the popliteal artery is usually caused by weakening of the artery wall as the result of cholesterol deposits *(atherosclerosis)*. Popliteal aneurysms occur most frequently in older men. About half the time, the popliteal aneurysm can be present in both legs. Also, about 75% of such individuals have an aneurysm elsewhere in their body, mostly in the abdominal aorta.

COMMON SIGNS AND SYMPTOMS

- Rarely, it may cause pain and tenderness behind the knee.
- Sometimes there may be decreased blood flow to the leg because tiny clots forming in the aneurysm flow downward to block small vessels in the foot.

DIAGNOSIS

- Anyone with a pulsating mass behind the knee should be considered to have a popliteal artery aneurysm.
- *CT scan (computed tomography scan):* A machine shaped like a huge doughnut is used to take special x-rays. You will lie on the table inside the hole in the "doughnut." The x-rays are taken as very thin slices through the area of the knee. This makes it possible to see the size and other fine details of the arteries and surrounding tissues.
- *Arteriogram*: Dye is injected into the aorta and pictures taken as the dye travels down into the popliteal artery to show the aneurysm.

○ TREATMENT

- There is a real risk that the aneurysm could form a clot and block the popliteal artery completely, causing gangrene of the leg.
- There may be small clots breaking off a larger one in the aneurysm. These small clots block small arteries further down until enough of the small arteries get blocked that the leg cannot survive.
- Many times the above happens without any warning.
- The treatment is an operation as soon as possible, even though the aneurysm is not producing any symptoms or is small. There is too great a risk of what may happen if the problem is not corrected (Fig. 1).

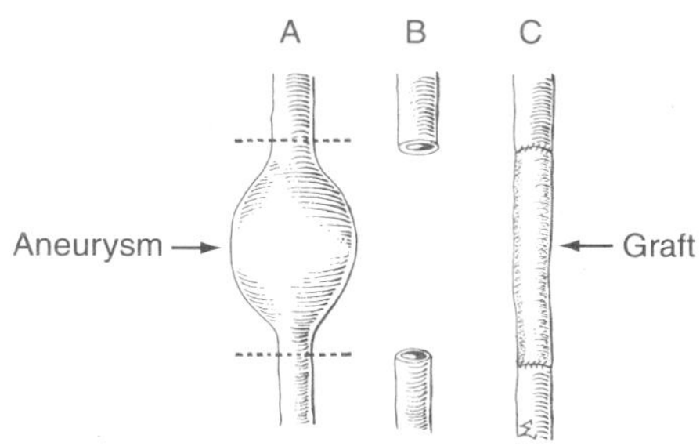

Figure 1. An aneurysm of the popliteal artery needs to be repaired expertly and with great care. A failure of the operation can risk the life of the affected leg.

PREOPERATIVE PREPARATION

- You will have a thorough physical examination with special attention to your aorta, the other leg vessels, and the arteries to your brain.
- You will have an examination of your blood, urine, heart (EKG), and lungs (chest x-ray).
- Do not eat or drink anything for 8 hours before the operation.
- Shower (and shave) as usual on the morning of the operation.
- You may be given medicine that will make you feel drowsy before you are brought to the operating room.

□ OPERATION

- You will be asleep for the operation, or epidural or spinal anesthesia will be given.
- Usually, a piece of vein from your leg is used to reconnect the vessels across the back of your knee after the aneurysm is removed.
- You will not receive a blood transfusion unless it is absolutely necessary.
- The operation usually takes 2 hours.

POSTOPERATIVE CARE

- You will be taken to a recovery room where the doctors and nurses are very experienced in taking care of patients with your condition. As soon as you are coming along well enough, you will be transferred to a regular hospital room.
- That day you will be helped to stand next to the bed.
- Bending your knees can be harmful during this healing period. A program will be worked out in which you either stand, walk, or you lie on a couch with your knees straight.
- As with any operation, complications are always possible, some of them serious. With this type of operation, complications can include clotting of the graft vein, which requires immediate reoperation; bleeding; gangrene of the foot or leg; heart problems; and possibly others.
- You should be able to go home in about 5 days.
- Arrangements will be made for your medicine, follow-up office visit, and stitch removal.

✚ HOME CARE

- Continue with the program started while you were in the hospital.
- You may walk about as you wish, and even climb stairs, but don't overdo it. Take frequent rest periods and don't forget: Do not bend your knees severely.
- You may eat as you did before the operation.
- Unless instructed otherwise, you may shower as you wish, with any dressings on or off.
  - There may be narrow strips of tape across the incision. It's all right if they get wet; they will be removed in the doctor's office.
  - After you dry yourself, replace any dressings with clean, dry ones.
- Take medicine as prescribed for your pain.

- Driving a car with an automatic shift may not seem too demanding. However, if you suddenly have to slam on the brakes or twist to turn the steering wheel, you may strain the sutures or tear something. During your follow-up visit, let's discuss when you can resume driving.
- You may resume sexual activity whenever you choose.
- You may return to work when you feel up to it, but let's talk about it first during an office follow-up visit.

✆ CALL OUR OFFICE IF

- Your foot or leg becomes pale or develops new pain that won't let up. If you cannot reach the surgeon right away, go to the hospital emergency room.
- You develop any unusual signs or symptoms.
- The incision becomes red or swollen, or there is drainage from it.
- You develop a temperature higher than 100°F.
- You have any questions.

AFTER CARE

The nature of your problem is such that you must be examined at regular intervals for the rest of your life to keep track of the other vessels in your body. For this reason, it is very important that you faithfully keep your doctors' appointments even if you are feeling perfectly well.

PORTAL HYPERTENSION: Esophageal Vein Sclerotherapy

△ GENERAL INFORMATION

Nearly the entire intestine drains its blood, with all the nourishment in it from the digested food, into the *portal vein.* The blood in the portal vein passes through the liver, which processes all this nourishment. The blood then leaves the liver to continue on to the heart.

If the liver is chronically diseased (most commonly with cirrhosis), scar tissue forms in the liver and blocks the flow of the portal vein. This causes the portal vein to back up (and swell) so that the veins draining the intestine find detours to reach the heart. Some of these detour veins are just under the lining of the esophagus. These detour veins can become swollen and cause serious problems. This is especially true of the veins in the esophagus.

COMMON SIGNS AND SYMPTOMS

- These exposed large veins in the esophagus can bleed. Blood may be found in the stool during a routine examination but sometimes the veins can hemorrhage in an alarming manner.
- The spleen, which is an important organ in the left part of your upper abdomen, becomes enlarged because the blood from it also is blocked. This prevents the spleen from functioning properly.
- There is poor nutrition because a lot of the blood with all its nourishment from the small bowel detours around the liver. The result is that the nourishment in this blood is not used properly.
- Mental confusion: The bowel blood with some of its waste products detours around the liver where it normally is cleansed. Instead, it goes directly to the brain, which causes mental confusion.
- Fluid (called *ascites*) can accumulate in the abdomen.

DIAGNOSIS

- You will have a detailed history taken and a thorough physical examination.
- You will undergo a number of tests of your blood to evaluate the condition of the liver. The ways to establish the diagnosis are not always the same for each person, even though the same disease is suspected. A test is done, and if the results don't make the diagnosis clear enough, then the next test is done. That's why the necessary tests on you will include at least some, and possibly all, of the following:
  - *Esophagogram*: You will be given barium to swallow (it looks and flows like buttermilk). X-rays will be taken as the barium goes down the esophagus. Often, these x-rays can show the dilated veins.
  - *Esophagoscopy*: This is done with an optical instrument that is smooth, flexible, and as big around as your little finger, with a light at its tip. Your mouth and throat will be sprayed with an anesthetic to make them numb. Also, you will be given some medicine to relax you and make you feel very drowsy. The instrument will be placed gently down your esophagus so that the esophagus can be examined thoroughly to determine the presence and condition of any swollen veins. Dilated veins can be seen just under the lining of the esophagus carrying the detoured blood.
  - Sometimes a tiny piece of the liver is taken (a *biopsy*) with a special needle made for this purpose. It will show, under the microscope, the state of the cirrhosis.

○ TREATMENT

- The treatment depends on a number of factors:
  - The size of the dilated veins in the lining of the esophagus.
  - The location of these dilated veins.
  - The condition of the liver (cirrhosis).
  - Whether these dilated veins have bled before, how seriously, and whether this is continuing.
  - Any associated illness and your general condition.
  - Whether the problem is caused by a diseased liver or something entirely separate from any liver disease.
- Because the distended veins can present in different ways, different treatments usually are necessary for each type of case. These can include the following:
  - Observation only.
  - Medicine only.
  - Clotting the veins in the esophagus (so they cannot bleed).
  - Making a small incision in the neck and inserting a small surgical gadget in the vein there that can be advanced down to the liver to make a new connection to improve the flow of blood in the portal veins.
  - Performing an open operation and making a large new connection to relieve the pressure in the portal vein as well as the veins in the esophagus.
  - Transplanting a new, healthy liver.

After very careful consideration of all factors, the recommendation is that the veins in the lining of your esophagus be treated directly. This can be done by clotting these veins in one of three ways:

Sclerotherapy is done with the help of an instrument very much like the one used for esophagoscopy. A fine needle can be brought out of the tip of this esophagoscope to inject the veins with the scarring solution.

In *electrocoagulation* a very thin electric wire can be brought out at the tip of the esophagoscope and used to burn the dilated veins.

In *banding*, special rubberbands can be applied around the vein to squeeze it shut and cause it to clot with an attachment to the esophagoscope designed specifically for this purpose. Which of the three methods is used will depend on the conditions found when examining the veins in your esophagus.

- You will be asleep for this procedure.
- Generally, it takes 1 to 2 hours.
- There may be additional sessions later.

POSTOPERATIVE CARE

- You will be taken to a recovery room where the nurses have experience in taking care of patients with your condition.
- Your general condition will be watched carefully, with special attention to any return of bleeding.
- That afternoon you will be helped to get out of bed and walk about as tolerated.
- At first, your diet will be liquids, and later soft foods will be added.
- You will need to stay in the hospital until the risk of your re-bleeding is reduced to an acceptable level.

✚ HOME CARE

- Continue with the program started while you were in the hospital.
- You may walk about as you wish, even climb stairs.
- Follow the diet outlined for you.
- Be careful that you do not become constipated.
  - Include plenty of roughage and liquid in your diet.
  - You may need some help with a mild laxative (example: milk of magnesia).
- Drive the car as you wish, provided you are not on medicines that might reduce your alertness.
- You may resume sexual activity whenever you choose.
- You may return to work when you feel up to it.

✆ CALL OUR OFFICE IF

- You develop any unusual signs or symptoms.
- You vomit blood or see that your bowel movement is very dark to black.
- You develop a temperature higher than 101°F.
- You have any questions.

△ GENERAL INFORMATION

Nearly the entire intestine drains its blood, with all the nourishment in it from the digested food, into the *portal vein*. The blood in the portal vein passes through the liver, which processes all this nourishment. The blood then leaves the liver to continue into the vena cava and on to the heart.

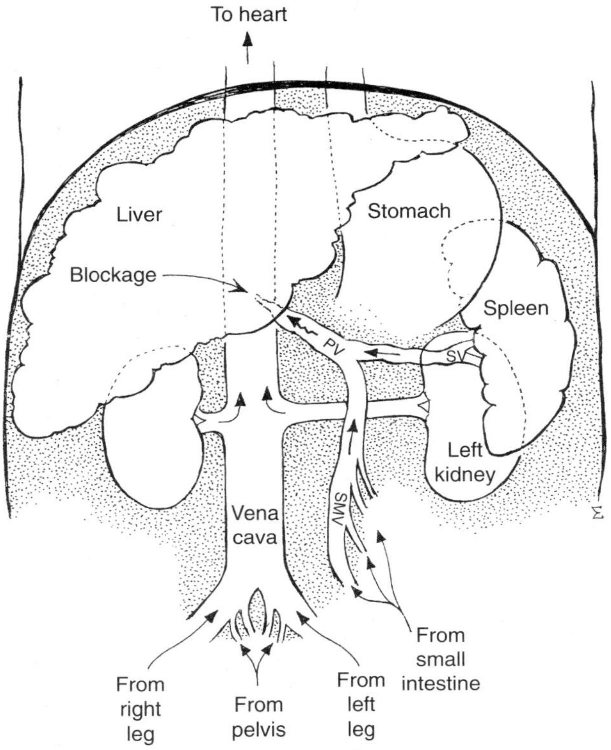

Figure 1. Blockage of flow of blood in the portal vein (PV). SV, splenic vein; SMV, superior mesenteric vein.

If the liver is chronically diseased (most commonly with cirrhosis), scar tissue forms in the liver and blocks the flow of the portal vein (Fig. 1). This causes the pressure in the portal vein to increase *(portal hypertension)* and all the veins to swell. The veins draining the intestine find detour veins to reach the heart. Some of these detour veins are just under the lining of the esophagus. These swollen detour veins in the esophagus can hemorrhage, causing serious problems.

COMMON SIGNS AND SYMPTOMS

- The swollen veins in the esophagus can rupture and hemorrhage.
- The spleen, which is an important organ in the left part of your upper abdomen, cannot work properly because it is swollen with backed-up blood.
- Nutrition suffers because a lot of the blood with all its nourishment from the small bowel detours around the liver.
- Mental confusion: The bowel blood with some of its waste products detours around the liver, where it normally is cleansed, and instead goes directly to the brain, which causes mental confusion.
- Fluid (called *ascites*) can accumulate in the abdomen.

DIAGNOSIS

- The diagnosis can be suspected by taking a detailed history and doing a thorough physical examination.
- Extensive examinations of the blood and of liver function are essential.
- *Esophagogram*: You will be given barium to swallow (it looks and flows like buttermilk). X-rays will be taken as the barium goes down the esophagus. Often, these x-rays can show the dilated veins.
- *Esophagoscopy*: This is done with an optical instrument that is smooth, flexible, and as big around as your little finger, with a light at its tip. Your mouth and throat will be sprayed with an anesthetic to make them numb. Also, you will be given medicine to make you feel very drowsy. The instrument will be placed gently down your esophagus so that the esophagus can be examined thoroughly to determine the presence and condition of any swollen veins carrying the detoured blood.
- Sometimes a tiny piece of the liver is taken (a *biopsy*) with a special needle and examined under the microscope to show the state of the cirrhosis.

○ TREATMENT

- The treatment of portal hypertension depends on the following:
  - The size of the dilated veins in the lining of the esophagus.
  - The location of these dilated veins.
  - The condition of the liver (cirrhosis).
  - Whether these dilated veins have bled before, how seriously, and whether this is continuing.
  - Any associated illness and the general condition of the individual.
  - Whether the problem is caused by a diseased liver or something entirely separate from any liver disease.
- Because the distended veins can manifest in different ways, different treatments usually are appropriate. These can include the following:
  - Observation only.
  - Medical therapy only.
  - Clotting the veins in the esophagus (so they cannot bleed).
  - Making a small incision in the neck and inserting a small surgical gadget in the neck vein that can be advanced down to the liver to make a new connection to improve the flow of blood in the portal vein.
  - Performing an open operation and making a large new connection for the portal vein to relieve the pressure in it as well as in the veins in the esophagus.

- Possibly performing a transplant and replacing the diseased liver.

After very careful consideration of all factors, the recommendation is that you have an operation to make the biggest new connection possible. In this operation, a short length of synthetic tubing that is roughly as big as the tip of your little finger will be used to make a connection between your mesenteric vein and your vena cava, which is wide open. This is called a *mesocaval shunt* (Fig. 2).

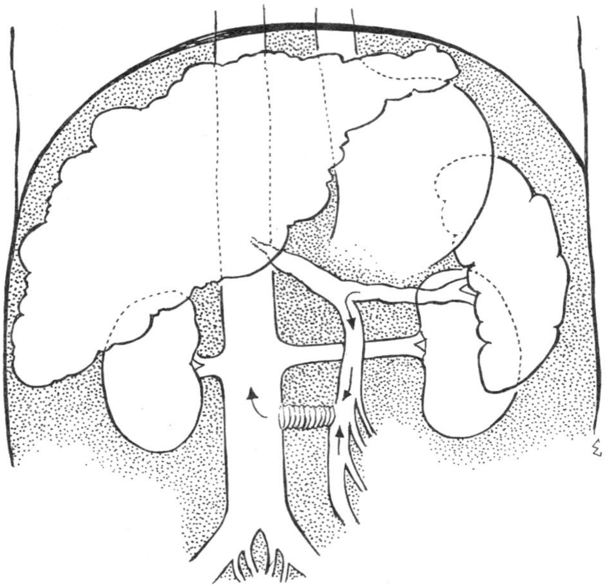

Figure 2. The flow of blood in the portal vein is blocked. A synthetic tube is used to connect the superior mesenteric vein with the inferior vena cava, which is wide open. Now the blood can flow freely (see arrows).

PREOPERATIVE PREPARATION

- Your blood, heart (EKG), kidneys, and lungs (chest x-ray) will be examined with great care. Any problems found in these areas will be corrected as much as possible.
- Do not eat or drink anything for 8 hours before the operation.

□ OPERATION

- You will be asleep for the operation.
- Occasionally, during the operation it is not possible to make the new connection as planned. If this is the case, then one of the alternate methods will be used.
- You will receive a blood transfusion if it is necessary.
- The operation usually takes about 5 hours.

POSTOPERATIVE CARE

- You will be taken to the Surgical Care Unit, where the doctors and nurses are very experienced in taking care of patients with your condition. As soon as you are coming along well enough, you will be transferred to a regular hospital room.
- You will have a thin plastic tube in your nose. It goes down to your stomach to suck up the air you swallow. It will be removed when your bowels start working.
- Pain will be controlled with medicine.
- The next day you will be helped to get out of bed.
- You will be given an incentive spirometer. Breathing into this as you are instructed will help you expand your lungs and reduce the risk of developing pneumonia.
- After the tube in your nose is removed, your diet will be as you tolerate it.
- You should be able to go home in about 10 days.
- Arrangements will be made for your medicine, follow-up office visit, and stitch or clip removal.

✚ HOME CARE

- You may walk about as you wish, even climb stairs, but don't overdo things.
- Take the medicines prescribed for you.
- Unless instructed otherwise, you may shower as you wish, with any dressings on or off. After you dry yourself, replace any dressings with clean, dry ones.
- Do not drive a car until we first talk about it.

✆ CALL OUR OFFICE IF

- You develop any unusual signs or symptoms, especially any type of vomiting.
- Your bowel movements are very dark.
- The incision becomes swollen or there is drainage from it.
- You develop a temperature higher than 101°F.
- You have any questions.

△ GENERAL INFORMATION

Nearly the entire intestine drains its blood, with all the nourishment in it from the digested food, into the *portal vein*. The blood in the portal vein passes through the liver, which processes all this nourishment. The blood then leaves the liver to continue into the vena cava and on to the heart.

If the liver is chronically diseased (most commonly with cirrhosis), scar tissue forms in the liver and blocks the flow of the portal vein (Fig. 1). This causes the portal vein to back up (and swell) so that the veins draining the intestine find detours to reach the heart. Some of these detour veins are just under the lining of the esophagus. These detour veins can become swollen and cause serious problems. This is especially true of the veins in the esophagus.

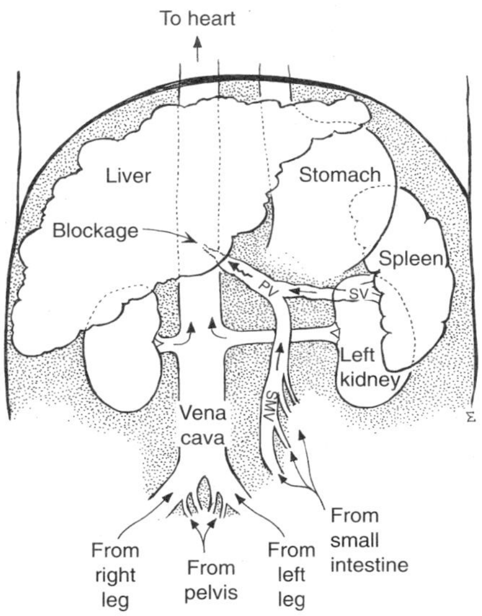

Figure 1. Blockage of flow of blood in the portal vein (PV). SV, splenic vein; SMV, superior mesenteric vein.

COMMON SIGNS AND SYMPTOMS

- As food passes these exposed large veins in the esophagus, it can scratch them, causing them to bleed. Blood may be found in the stool during a routine examination. Sometimes, they can hemorrhage in an alarming manner.
- The spleen, which is an important organ in the left part of your upper abdomen, becomes enlarged because the blood from it also is blocked. This prevents the spleen from functioning properly.
- There is poor nutrition because a lot of the blood with all its nourishment from the small bowel detours around the liver. The result is that the nourishment in this blood is not used properly.
- Mental confusion: The bowel blood with some of its waste products detours around the liver, where it normally is cleansed, and instead goes directly to the brain, which causes mental confusion.
- Fluid (called *ascites*) can accumulate in the abdomen.

DIAGNOSIS

- You will have a detailed history taken and a thorough physical examination.
- You will have a number of tests of your blood to evaluate the condition of the liver. The ways to establish the diagnosis are not always the same for each person, even though the same disease is suspected. A test is done, and if the results don't make the diagnosis clear enough, then the next test is done. That's why the necessary tests on you will include at least some, and possibly all, of the following:
  - *Esophagogram*: You will be given barium to swallow. X-rays will be taken as the barium goes down the esophagus. Often, these x-rays can show the dilated veins.
  - *Esophagoscopy*: This is done with an optical instrument that is smooth, flexible, and as big around as your little finger, with a light at its tip. Your mouth and throat will be sprayed with an anesthetic to make them numb. Also, you will be given some medicine to relax you and make you very drowsy. The instrument will be placed gently down your esophagus so that it can be examined thoroughly to determine the presence and condition of any swollen veins. Dilated veins can be seen just under the lining of the esophagus carrying the detoured blood.
  - Sometimes a tiny piece of liver is taken (a *biopsy*) with a special needle made for this purpose. It will show the state of the cirrhosis under the microscope.

○ TREATMENT

- The treatment depends on a number of factors:
  - The size of the dilated veins in the lining of the esophagus.
  - The location of these dilated veins.
  - The condition of the liver (cirrhosis).
  - Whether these dilated veins have bled before, how seriously, and whether this is continuing.
  - Any associated illness and your general condition.
  - Whether the problem is caused by a diseased liver or something entirely separate from any liver disease.
- Because the distended veins can present in different ways, different treatments usually are necessary for each type of case. These can include the following:
  - Observation only.
  - Medicine only.
  - Clotting the veins in the esophagus (so they cannot bleed).
  - Making a small incision in the neck and inserting a small surgical gadget in the vein that can be advanced down to the liver to make a new connection to improve the flow of blood in the portal veins.
  - Performing a formal operation and making a large new connection to relieve the pressure in the portal vein as well as in the veins in the esophagus.
  - Performing a transplant of a new, healthy liver.

After very careful consideration of all factors, the recommendation is that you have an operation to make the biggest new connection possible. This connection will make a new passage for blood from the portal vein into your vena cava, which is wide open. This is called a *portacaval shunt* (Fig. 2).

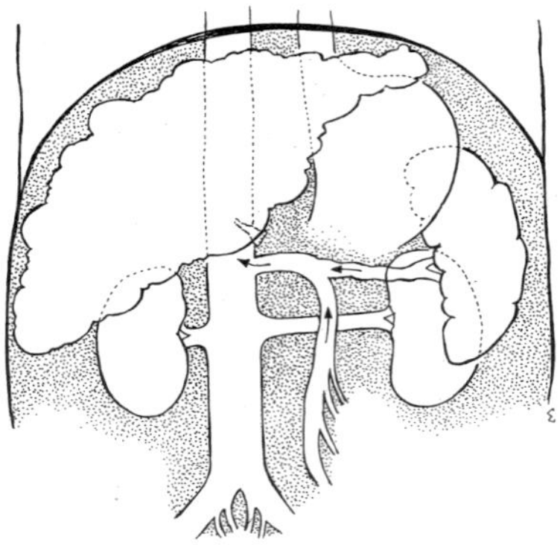

Figure 2. The flow of blood in the blocked portal vein is re-routed so that it flows into the vena cava, which is wide open.

PREOPERATIVE PREPARATION

- Your heart (EKG), kidneys, and lungs (chest x-ray) will be examined with great care. Any problems found in these areas will be corrected as much as possible.
- Do not eat or drink anything for 8 hours before the operation.
- Shower the morning of the operation.
- You will be given medicine that will make you feel drowsy before you are brought to the operating room.

☐ OPERATION

- The aim of the portacaval shunt is to connect the portal vein with the general *(systemic)* circulation because the normal way for the blood to get to the systemic circulation is blocked. Occasionally, during the operation it is not possible to make the new connection as planned. If this is the case, then one of the alternate methods will be used.
- You will receive a blood transfusion if it is necessary.
- The operation usually takes about 5 hours.

POSTOPERATIVE CARE

- You will be taken to the Surgical Care Unit, where the doctors and nurses are very experienced in taking care of patients with your condition. As soon as you are coming along well enough, you will be transferred to a regular hospital room.
- You will have a thin plastic tube in your nose. It goes down to your stomach to suck up the air you swallow. It will be removed when your bowels start working.
- Pain can be controlled with medicine. The nurse will give it to you, or you can give yourself a pre-set amount of pain medicine when you feel you need it. This is done with a device called patient-controlled analgesia (PCA) that is connected to the tubing giving you intravenous fluids.
- The evening after the operation you will be helped to sit up in bed and on the next day to get out of bed.
- You will be given an incentive spirometer. Breathing into this as you are instructed will help you expand your lungs and reduce the risk of developing pneumonia.
- After the tube in your nose is removed, your diet will be as you tolerate it.
- You should be able to go home in about 10 days.
- You will be given a suggested appropriate diet to follow during your convalescence.
- Arrangements will be made for your medicine, follow-up office visit, and stitch or clip removal.
- Arrangements can be made for a home visiting nurse if one is needed.

✜ HOME CARE

- Continue with the care and program as begun in the hospital.
- You may walk about as you wish, even climb stairs, but don't overdo things.
- Take medicine as prescribed for your pain.
- Be careful that you do not become constipated.
  - Include enough roughage and plenty of liquids in your diet.
  - You may need some help with a mild laxative (example: milk of magnesia).
- Don't lift anything over 5 pounds. Ask someone to do it for you.
- Unless instructed otherwise, you may shower as you wish, with any dressings on or off.
  - There may be narrow strips of tape across the incision. It's all right if they get wet; they will be removed in the doctor's office.
  - After you dry yourself, replace any dressings with clean, dry ones.
- Your incision and the muscles of the abdomen may ache, especially at the end of the day and after you have been standing for a long period. You can support them by wearing a girdle or similar garment that is snug (but not too tight). Wearing it over a cotton undergarment is easier on your incision and the stitches.
- Driving your car may be important to you, but when you can do this safely depends on the operation you had, the medicines you are taking, and your condition in general. During your follow-up visit, let's talk about when you can resume driving.
- You may resume sexual activity whenever you choose.
- You may return to work when you feel up to it, but first talk about it with your doctor during a follow-up office visit.

✆ CALL OUR OFFICE IF

- You develop any unusual signs or symptoms, especially any type of vomiting.
- Your bowel movements are very dark.
- The incision becomes swollen, or there is drainage from it.
- You develop a temperature higher than 101°F.
- You have any questions.

△ GENERAL INFORMATION

Nearly the entire intestine drains its blood, with all the nourishment in it from the digested food, into the *portal vein.* The blood in the portal vein passes through the liver, which processes all this nourishment. The blood then leaves the liver to continue into the vena cava and on to the heart.

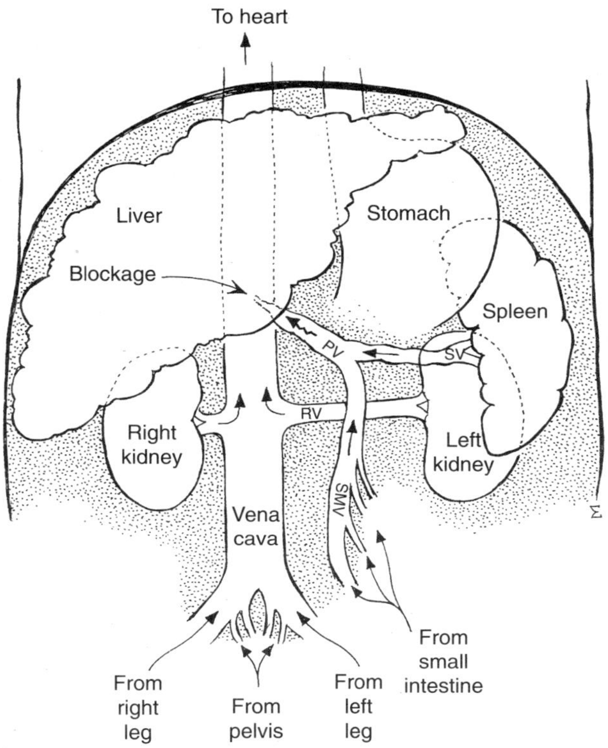

Figure 1. Blockage of flow of blood in the portal vein (PV). SV, Splenic vein; RV, renal vein; SMV, superior mesenteric vein.

If the liver is chronically diseased (most commonly with cirrhosis), scar tissue forms in the liver and blocks the flow of the portal vein (Fig. 1). This causes the pressure in the portal vein to increase *(portal hypertension)* and all the veins to swell. The veins draining the intestine find detour veins to reach the heart. Some of these detour veins are just under the lining of the esophagus. These swollen detour veins in the esophagus can hemorrhage, causing serious problems.

COMMON SIGNS AND SYMPTOMS

- The swollen veins in the esophagus can rupture and hemorrhage.
- The spleen, which is an important organ in the left part of your upper abdomen, cannot work properly because it is swollen with backed-up blood.
- Nutrition suffers because a lot of the blood with all its nourishment from the small bowel detours around the liver.
- Mental confusion: The bowel blood with some of its waste products detours around the liver, where it normally is cleansed, and instead goes directly to the brain, which causes mental confusion.
- Fluid (called *ascites*) can accumulate in the abdomen.

DIAGNOSIS

- The diagnosis can be suspected by taking a detailed history and doing a thorough physical examination.
- Extensive examinations of the blood and of liver function are essential.
- *Esophagogram*: You will be given barium to swallow (it looks and flows like buttermilk). X-rays will be taken as the barium goes down the esophagus. Often, these x-rays can show the dilated veins.
- *Esophagoscopy*: This is done with an optical instrument that is smooth, flexible, and as big around as your little finger, with a light at its tip. Your mouth and throat will be sprayed with an anesthetic to make them numb. Also, you will be given medicine to make you feel very drowsy. The instrument will be placed gently down your esophagus so that the esophagus can be examined thoroughly to determine the presence and condition of any swollen veins carrying the detoured blood.
- Sometimes a tiny piece of liver is taken (a *biopsy*) with a special needle and examined under the microscope to show the state of the cirrhosis under the microscope.

○ TREATMENT

- The treatment of portal hypertension depends on the following:
  - The size of the dilated veins in the lining of the esophagus.
  - The location of these dilated veins.
  - The condition of the liver (cirrhosis).
  - Whether these dilated veins have bled before, how seriously, and whether this is continuing.
  - Any associated illness and the general condition of the individual.
  - Whether the problem is caused by a diseased liver or something entirely separate from any liver disease.
- Because the distended veins can present in different ways, different treatments usually are appropriate. These can include the following:
  - Observation only.
  - Medical therapy only.
  - Clotting the veins in the esophagus (so they cannot bleed).
  - Making a small incision in the neck and inserting a small surgical gadget in the neck vein that can be advanced down to the liver to make a new connection to improve the flow of blood in the portal vein.
  - Performing an open operation and making a large new connection for the portal vein to relieve the pressure in it as well as in the veins in the esophagus.

- Possibly performing a transplant and replacing the diseased liver.

After very careful consideration of all factors, the recommendation is that you have an operation to make the biggest new connection possible. This connection will make a new passage for blood from the splenic vein into the renal vein (Fig. 2).

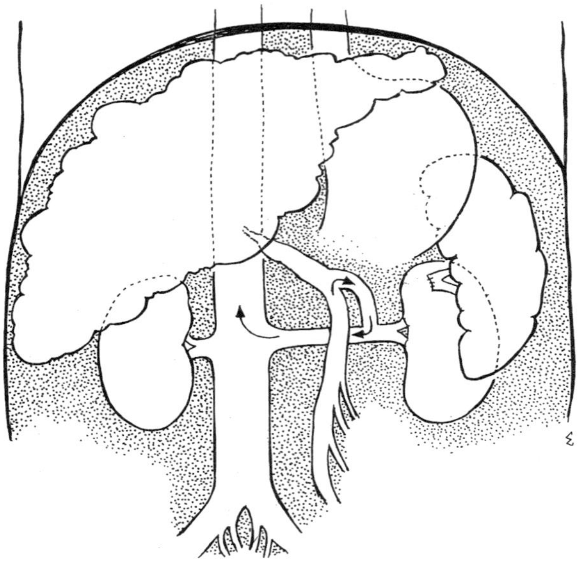

Figure 2. The flow of blood in the blocked portal vein is rerouted so that it now flows from the splenic vein (which is connected to the portal vein) into the renal vein, which empties into the vena cava. The arrows show the new direction of blood flow.

PREOPERATIVE PREPARATION

- Your blood, heart (EKG), kidneys, and lungs (chest x-ray) will be examined with great care. Any problems found in these areas will be corrected as much as possible.
- Do not eat or drink anything for 8 hours before the operation.

□ OPERATION

- You will be asleep for the operation.
- Occasionally, during the operation it is not possible to make the new connection as planned. If this is the case, then one of the alternate methods will be used.
- You will receive a blood transfusion if it is necessary.
- The operation usually takes about 5 hours.

POSTOPERATIVE CARE

- You will be taken to the Surgical Care Unit, where the doctors and nurses are very experienced in taking care of patients with your condition. As soon as you are coming along well enough, you will be transferred to a regular hospital room.
- You will have a thin plastic tube in your nose. It goes down to your stomach to suck up the air you swallow. It will be removed when your bowels start working.
- Pain will be controlled with medicine.
- The next day you will be helped to get out of bed.
- You will be given an incentive spirometer. Breathing into this as you are instructed will help you expand your lungs and reduce the risk of developing pneumonia.
- After the tube in your nose is removed, your diet will be as you tolerate it.
- You should be able to go home in about 10 days.
- Arrangements will be made for your medicine, follow-up office visit, and stitch or clip removal.

✣ HOME CARE

- You may walk about as you wish, even climb stairs, but don't overdo things.
- Take the medicines prescribed for you.
- Unless instructed otherwise, you may shower as you wish, with any dressings on or off. After you dry yourself, replace any dressings with clean, dry ones.
- Do not drive a car until we first talk about it.

✆ CALL OUR OFFICE IF

- You develop any unusual signs or symptoms, especially any type of vomiting.
- Your bowel movements are very dark.
- The incision becomes swollen or there is drainage from it.
- You develop a temperature higher than 101°F.
- You have any questions.

PORTAL HYPERTENSION: TIPS

△ GENERAL INFORMATION

Nearly the entire intestine drains its blood, with all the nourishment in it from the digested food, into the *portal vein*. The blood in the portal vein passes through the liver, which processes all this nourishment. The blood then leaves the liver to continue into the vena cava and on to the heart.

If the liver is chronically diseased (most commonly with cirrhosis), scar tissue forms in the liver and blocks the flow of the portal vein. This causes the pressure in the portal vein to increase *(portal hypertension)* and all the veins to swell. The veins draining the intestine find detour veins to reach the heart. Some of these detour veins are just under the lining of the esophagus. These swollen detour veins in the esophagus can hemorrhage, causing serious problems.

COMMON SIGNS AND SYMPTOMS

- The swollen veins in the esophagus can rupture and hemorrhage.
- The spleen, which is an important organ in the left part of your upper abdomen, cannot work properly because it is swollen with backed-up blood.
- Nutrition suffers because a lot of the blood with all its nourishment from the small bowel detours around the liver.
- Mental confusion: The bowel blood with some of its waste products detours around the liver, where it normally is cleansed, and instead goes directly to the brain, which causes mental confusion.
- Fluid (called *ascites*) can accumulate in the abdomen.

DIAGNOSIS

- The diagnosis can be suspected by taking a detailed history and doing a thorough physical examination.
- Extensive examinations of the blood and of liver function are essential.
- *Esophagogram*: You will be given barium to swallow (it looks and flows like buttermilk). X-rays will be taken as the barium goes down the esophagus. Often, these x-rays can show the dilated veins.
- *Esophagoscopy*: This is done with an optical instrument that is smooth, flexible, and as big around as your little finger, with a light at its tip. Your mouth and throat will be sprayed with an anesthetic to make them numb. Also, you will be given medicine to make you feel very drowsy. The instrument will be placed gently down your esophagus so that the esophagus can be examined thoroughly to determine the presence and condition of any swollen veins carrying the detoured blood.
- Sometimes a tiny piece of liver is taken (a *biopsy*) with a special needle and examined under the microscope to show the state of the cirrhosis.

○ TREATMENT

- The treatment of portal hypertension depends on the following:
  - The size of the dilated veins in the lining of the esophagus.
  - The location of these dilated veins.
  - The condition of the liver (cirrhosis).
  - Whether these dilated veins have bled before, how seriously, and whether this is continuing.
  - Any associated illness and the general condition of the individual.
  - Whether the problem is caused by a diseased liver or something entirely separate from any liver disease.
- Because the distended veins can present in different ways, different treatments usually are appropriate. These can include the following:
  - Observation only.
  - Medical therapy only.
  - Clotting the veins in the esophagus (so they cannot bleed).
  - Making a small incision in the neck and inserting a small surgical gadget in the neck vein that can be advanced down to the liver to make a new connection to improve the flow of blood in the portal vein.
  - Performing an open operation and making a large new connection for the portal vein to relieve the pressure in it as well as the veins in the esophagus.
  - Possibly performing a transplant and replacing the diseased liver.

After very careful consideration of all factors, the recommendation is that you have a new connection made to reduce the pressure in the veins in the esophagus. The operation is done by inserting a small surgical device through a vein in your neck. The procedure is called TIPS (transjugular intrahepatic portosystemic shunt).

PREOPERATIVE PREPARATION

- Your blood, heart (EKG), kidneys, and lungs (chest x-ray) will be examined with great care. Any problems found in these areas will be corrected as much as possible.
- Do not eat or drink anything for 8 hours before the operation.

□ OPERATION

This procedure will be done by a radiologist as follows:

- You will be lying on an x-ray table.
- The right side of your neck will be painted with an antiseptic solution. The skin over a vein (the *jugular* vein) in the neck will be made numb. A thin wire that has a very special cutting tool at its tip will be placed into your jugular vein. The wire is then advanced down the jugular vein and into the large vein below it (the *vena cava*) and to the area of the liver. This is next to the blocked portal vein.
- The special cutting tool at the end of the wire is then used to make a new connection between the blocked portal vein and the vena cava (which is wide open).
- Now that the portal vein can empty its blood more easily into the vena cava, the pressure in the portal vein and in the veins in the esophagus drops. The risk of bleeding is now markedly reduced.
- The procedure takes about 3 hours.

- *Note:* Occasionally, for technical reasons, this connection cannot be made. If that happens in your case, you will be returned to your room and alternate methods for correcting your problem will be discussed.

POSTOPERATIVE CARE

- You will be kept in the Radiology Department for a while and observed. When your blood pressure, pulse, and breathing are stable, you will be transferred to your regular hospital room.
- You will be able to sit up that day and eat a soft diet.
- You should be able to go home in 3 to 5 days.
- Arrangements will be made for your diet, medicines, and follow-up office visit.
- As with any operation, complications are always possible. With this type of operation, complications can include infection, bleeding, heart problems, injury to the veins, clotting of the new connection, and possibly others.

✣ HOME CARE

- You may walk about as you wish, even climb stairs.
- Follow the diet recommended for you.
- You may shower or bathe as you wish.
- Don't lift anything heavier than 5 pounds. Ask someone to do it for you.
- Inactivity is not good for you, but neither is overdoing it. Don't try to do too much too soon.
- You may drive a car and return to work when you feel up to it.

✆ CALL OUR OFFICE IF

- You have more than one very dark bowel movement.
- You vomit or cough up any blood.
- You develop a temperature higher than 101°F.
- You have any questions.

PRESSURE ULCERS (BED SORES)

△ GENERAL INFORMATION

A pressure sore *(decubitus ulcer)* is an area in which tissue over a hard surface (usually bone) has died because of pressure on it that was severe enough or lasted long enough. Such pressure blocks blood vessels, cutting off blood supply and oxygen to the tissue and causing it to die. It is surprising how quickly the tissue can suffer when enough and continuous pressure is applied to it. Four hours of enough and continuous pressure will temporarily damage the tissue. Eight hours of such pressure can produce permanent changes that develop into an ulcer.

Conditions under which pressure ulcers are commonly seen include the following:

- Older patients who are weakened and have to lie in bed because of a number of medical problems. Also, in such patients the skin is weak and unable to tolerate such blockage of its blood vessels.
- People with paraplegia: Often, such individuals have difficulty moving frequently enough. Also, they don't properly feel the pressure against their flesh.
- People with nerve conditions (example: multiple sclerosis) that keep them from moving properly.

COMMON SIGNS AND SYMPTOMS

The signs and symptoms depend on a number of factors, including the following:

- The location of the pressure.
- How long the pressure was present.
- The size of the ulcer.
- Whether or not the dead tissue has become infected.
- The general condition of the person with the ulcer.

Generally, there is a progression of events in the development of a pressure ulcer, as follows:

- At the beginning, there is a redness of the area that appears after the pressure is removed.
- With longer pressure, the redness does not go away soon.
- With even more prolonged pressure, redness and blisters may develop.
- In the next stage, tissue dies, forming a shallow ulcer.
- In the more advanced stage, the ulcer is deeper.
- Finally, the skin and tissue under it develop gangrene and become black.
- In later stages, the ulcer as well as the bone deep to it can be infected.

DIAGNOSIS

The diagnosis can be made when seeing someone with the above history and findings.

- Sometimes the skin has what appears to be an innocent-looking small hole over a raw area. This, however, can be misleading. Once the skin with the small hole is opened, a large amount of dead tissue may be found underneath.
- X-rays may be necessary to look for infection or dead bone at the bottom of the ulcer.
- A sample of any drainage from the ulcer can be taken to the laboratory to see what type of bacteria may be present and which antibiotic is the most effective against them.

○ TREATMENT

- Any underlying problems will be corrected as much as possible.
- Generally, if an ulcer has already developed infection and is producing symptoms, the person needs to be in a hospital for care.

The care given an ulcer when a person needs to be hospitalized varies considerably, depending on the special conditions of a patient, but it can include the following:

- Shallow ulcers can be treated with a variety of ointments.
- Antibiotics are given as necessary.
- Deeper ulcers need to have dead tissue trimmed—a little every day—and the area covered with appropriate dressings. Such ulcers can gradually heal without any further treatment.
- Gangrenous tissue also needs to be removed, either in stages or all in one setting.
- Larger or deeper ulcers (whether they first present that way or are what results when the gangrenous tissue is removed) frequently require an operation. Several types of operations can be used as follows:
  - All of the dead tissue is removed and the edges of the ulcer brought together, all at one time.
  - All of the dead tissue in a larger ulcer is trimmed down to where healthy tissue is available.
  - The skin with its attached fat and muscle from the area next to the ulcer is slipped sideways to cover the ulcer itself. This is called a *sliding pedicle graft*. Such a graft provides healthy, thick tissue and has the best chance for success in these situations.

After careful consideration of all factors, the recommendation is that you have an operation to clean up your ulcer. If simple closure is not possible, then the ulcer will be covered with a pedicle graft.

PREOPERATIVE PREPARATION

- You will be helped to achieve the best condition possible for the operation. This may include blood transfusions, improving your nutrition, and attention to problems of your lungs, heart, and kidneys, as well as other problems.
- Do not eat or drink anything for 8 hours before the operation.

□ OPERATION

- You will be asleep for the operation.

POSTOPERATIVE CARE

- You will be taken to a recovery room and observed. When your blood pressure, pulse, and breathing are stable, you will be taken to a regular hospital room.
- Pain will be controlled with medicine.
- Your diet will be as tolerated.

- Arrangements will be made for your wound care when you leave the hospital.
- As with any operation, complications are always possible. With this type of operation, complications can include breakdown of the repair, heart attack, stroke, pneumonia, blood clots, and possibly others.

AFTER CARE

- You will either go home or return to the nursing facility from where you came.
- Continue with the program started while you were in the hospital.

△ GENERAL INFORMATION

The prostate gland is part of the reproductive system in men. The average prostate gland is about the size of a walnut and is located in front of the rectum and at the bottom part of the bladder (Fig. 1). The prostate surrounds the urethra, the tube that carries urine from the bladder out through the penis. The primary role of the prostate is to produce fluid for semen. Prostate fluid mixes with sperm from the testicles to become semen and then both are transported out through the urethra with ejaculation during sexual intercourse.

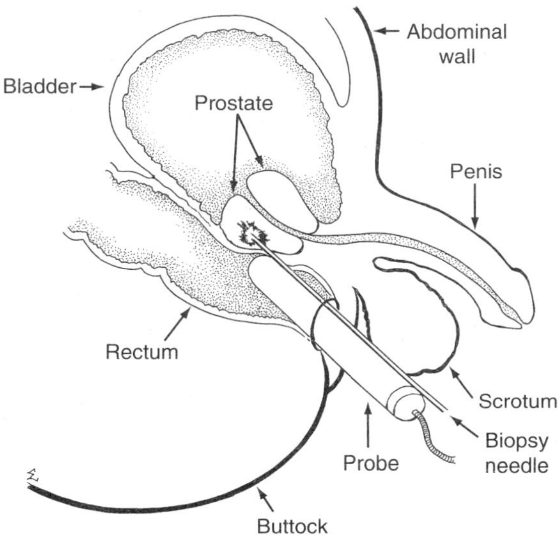

Figure 1. Side view of male pelvis.

The prostate gland can be felt by the doctor with an examining finger in the rectum. Sometimes, a suspicious lump can be felt in the prostate or a test of the blood shows an elevation of prostate-specific antigen (PSA). Either of these findings may—but only possibly—indicate that cancer of the prostate is present. However, the only certain way to know is to remove a small piece of abnormal prostate tissue (a *biopsy* specimen) so that it can be carefully examined in the laboratory. This is the situation with you.

Ultrasonography is used to look inside the prostate. Harmless, painless sound waves are aimed at your prostate and the sound waves bouncing back (the echoes) are seen as pictures on a screen. In this way the prostate gland itself and any abnormalities inside or around it can be seen.

PREPARATIONS FOR BIOPSY

You will have a general physical examination as well as a finger examination of your prostate before the biopsy is done.

- Be certain to tell the urologist and the nurse before the procedure of any medicines you may be taking that thin the blood (example: aspirin, Coumadin).
- You may have a light breakfast or lunch before the procedure.
- You may be given antibiotics to take by mouth before the biopsy.
- You will be instructed on what type of enema to take before the biopsy, if this is thought to be necessary.

THE PROCEDURE

The gadget that sends out the sound waves (it is called a probe or a transducer) is about the size of your finger. It will be lubricated and then gently placed through your anus (just as with an examining finger) and positioned right next to the prostate.

- You will feel some discomfort and the urge to have a bowel movement.
- Measurements of the prostate will be taken (from the pictures of the prostate on the screen) and of any suspicious areas in the prostate.
- If a biopsy is indicated, the urologist will place a small, thin needle into the suspicious area and perform the biopsies (usually six). The rectum in this area does not have any pain nerves, so the biopsy usually is not painful.
- The biopsy specimens will be sent to the laboratory for careful examination.
- You will be given antibiotics to take after the biopsy.
- You may have an urge to urinate or to have a bowel movement for the first several hours after this procedure. For this reason, you may wish to rest for an hour or two after the procedure and then go about your usual business.
- As with any procedure, complications are always possible. With this procedure, complications can include infection, excessive bleeding, and possibly others.
- Arrangements will be made for you to know the results of the biopsy when they are available and to have a discussion with the doctors about any further therapy.

✚ HOME CARE

- Continue with your usual activities.
- You may have blood in your urine, stool, and ejaculate. The blood in your urine and stool should clear up in a day or two. However, you may notice a brown or reddish color in your ejaculate for up to 1 month after the biopsy.

✆ CALL OUR OFFICE IF

- You develop any unusual signs or symptoms.
- You develop a temperature higher than 101.5°F.
- You have any questions.

PROSTATE CANCER: Suprapubic Prostatectomy

△ GENERAL INFORMATION

Prostate cancer is the most frequently diagnosed cancer (except for skin cancer) in men in the United States. The risk of having prostate cancer increases as a man gets older. In the past several years, earlier diagnosis and more aggressive treatment have enhanced the opportunities for cure.

COMMON SIGNS AND SYMPTOMS

- Prostate cancer can cause enlargement of the prostate, which in turn can result in the following:
  - Weak urinary stream.
  - Increased frequency of urination.
  - Imcomplete emptying of the bladder.
  - Blood in the urine or semen.
- These same symptoms can also be caused by benign, noncancerous enlargement of the prostate gland or other benign conditions such as infections of the urinary tract or stones.

Diagnosis

This is commonly done by the physician inserting a finger in the rectum to feel the prostate gland. A blood test, prostate-specific antigen (PSA), makes it possible to detect prostate cancer even before it can be felt by rectal examination.

Diagnostic Tests

If cancer is *suspected*, one or more of the following tests will need to be done:

- *Transrectal ultrasonography*: An instrument (a probe) slightly thicker than an examining finger is used. The probe is lubricated and inserted so that its tip lies over the prostate gland. From the tip of the probe, harmless, painless sound waves are beamed in the direction of the prostate. The waves bouncing back (the echoes) are seen on a television screen. This is a reliable way to see abnormalities within the prostate gland.
- *Prostate biopsy*: The skin just below the scrotum (the sac) is made numb with an anesthetic solution. With the help of the ultrasonography, a needle is guided through the numbed skin and to the abnormal area of the prostate and a tiny piece taken (a *biopsy*) for examination in the laboratory.

The following tests are commonly performed when a diagnosis of cancer has actually been *confirmed*.

- *Bone scan*: A fine needle is used to inject a solution with a tiny amount of a harmless radioactive material into your vein. The solution circulates throughout your entire body and attaches itself to any part of a bone that has something wrong with it. One hour after the injection, you will lie on a table, and a special machine will pass over your entire body taking a photograph (a *scan*) of all the bones from your skull to your toes. A specialist then examines the scan, looking for any abnormalities.
- *CT scan (computed tomography scan)*: A machine shaped like a huge doughnut is used to take special x-rays. You will lie on a table inside the hole in the "doughnut." The x-rays are taken as very thin slices through the area of the kidneys and pelvis. This makes it possible to see fine details in this area.
- *MRI (magnetic resonance imaging)*: No x-rays are used with this technique. Instead, it is done with harmless magnetic fields and radio waves. A computer develops the pictures to show organs from several angles. This technique is especially useful for examining your blood vessels, nerves, and bone tissue.

○ TREATMENT

If the cancer is limited to just the prostate gland, then treatment of the entire prostate gland by radiation or complete removal of the gland by an operation can be curative.

Radiation Treatment

The *advantages* are as follows:

- No major operation is necessary.
- As with an operation, there is a small (5%) risk of not being able to hold urine as well as you did before.
- A risk of impotence (but not as great as with an operation).

The *disadvantages* are as follows:

- The entire prostate gland is left in place and so is not available for detailed study to know more certainly that the cancer was localized.
- Determining the success of local treatment is more difficult.
- If radiation treatment fails, performing an operation later to remove the prostate has greater risk than if this area had not received radiation treatment.
- Scarring in the area in and around the prostate can occur later and continue to affect how you are able to hold and pass your urine.

An Operation

The *advantages* of an operation are as follows:

- The entire gland is actually removed and can be studied to determine whether the cancer is confined to the gland. This information can help plan any further treatment as well as more accurately determine the prognosis.
- Once the tissue is removed, very few side effects appear in later years.

The *disadvantages* are as follows:

- There is the need of an operation.
- A small (5%) risk of not being able to hold your urine as well as you did before the operation.
- A significant risk of impotence (loss of erection).
- In addition, there is the possibility of bleeding, infection, blood clots, and possibly other complications.

After careful consideration of all factors, the recommendation is that you have a radical prostatectomy to attempt to cure your prostate cancer.

PREOPERATIVE PREPARATION

To cure prostate cancer by an operation, the entire prostate must be removed.

The prostate can be removed through a small incision in the lower abdomen (the *suprapubic* or the *retropubic* approach) or through a small incision between the scrotum (the sac) and the anus (the *perineal* approach) (Fig. 1). One advantage of the suprapubic approach is that the lymph nodes in the abdomen (which can be the site of early spread of cancer) can be evaluated before the prostate is removed. If the removed lymph nodes show cancer (while you are still in the operating room), then the prostate usually is not removed. Instead, radiation or hormone therapy is planned. Which technique is chosen will be discussed with you beforehand.

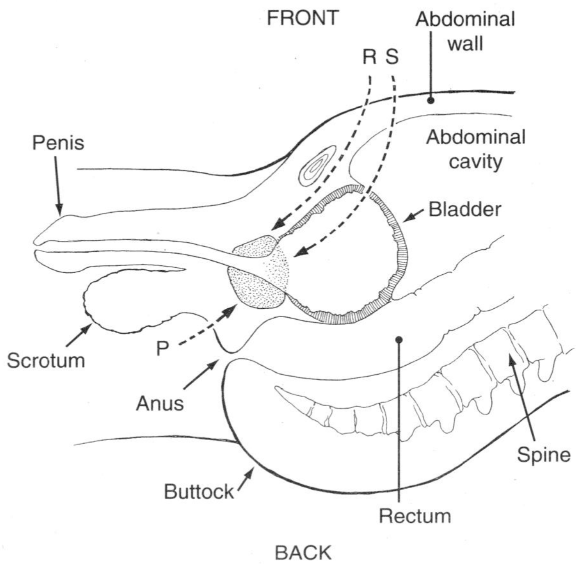

Figure 1. All of the prostate gland must be removed even when only part of it is cancerous. Several approaches are possible—suprapubic (S), retropubic (R), and perineal (P)—and each has its advantages and disadvantages. The choice of approach is influenced by the specific circumstances of a patient.

After careful consideration of all factors, the recommendation is that your prostate be removed through an incision in your abdomen (suprapubic).

- You will have an examination of your blood, urine, heart (EKG), and lungs (chest x-ray).
- Do not take aspirin or aspirin-containing medicines for 1 week before the operation.
- You will be instructed on how to clean out your bowels.
- Do not eat or drink anything for 8 hours before the operation.
- Shower and shave as usual on the morning of the operation.
- You may be given medicine that will make you feel drowsy before you are brought to the operating room.

☐ OPERATION

- You will be asleep for the operation.
- The operation generally takes about 2 hours.
- You will not receive a blood transfusion unless it is absolutely necessary.

POSTOPERATIVE CARE

- You will be taken to a recovery room and observed. When your blood pressure, pulse, and breathing are stable, you will be taken to a regular hospital room.
- You will have a catheter (a small tube coming from the penis) which drains the bladder until the area can heal completely. This takes approximately 2 to 3 weeks. You'll be given instructions on caring for the catheter at home (it is not difficult) until it can be removed in the doctor's office.
- Pain can be controlled with medicine. The nurse will give it to you, or you can give yourself a preset amount of pain medicine when you feel you need it. This is done with a device called patient-controlled analgesia (PCA) that is connected to the tubing giving you intravenous fluids.
- That evening after the operation you will be helped to sit up in bed and on the next day to get out of bed.
- You will be given an incentive spirometer. Breathing into this as you are instructed will help you expand your lungs and reduce the risk of developing pneumonia.
- A liquid diet will be started one day after the operation and will be advanced as you tolerate it.
- You should be able to go home in about 1 week.
- Arrangements will be made for your medicine, follow-up office visits, and stitch or clip removal.

✣ HOME CARE

- Continue with the program started while you were in the hospital.
- Inactivity is not good for you but neither is overdoing it. Don't try to do too much too soon.
- Eat as you wish, but include plenty of roughage and liquids in your diet to help prevent constipation.
- Take medicine as prescribed for your pain.
- You will be given a night drainage bag for draining the catheter during your first 2 weeks at home. This hangs off the side of the bed and gives better drainage through the night. During the day, you may wish to have the catheter directly connected to your leg bag. Before you leave the hospital, the nurse will instruct you on how to change from one bag to the other.
- During your office visit, let's discuss when you can resume driving.

✆ CALL OUR OFFICE IF

- The catheter stops draining properly or falls out.
- You develop any unusual signs or symptoms.
- The incision becomes red or swollen, or there is drainage from it.
- You develop a temperature higher than 100°F.
- You have any questions.

△ GENERAL INFORMATION

Prostate enlargement *(hyperplasia)* is benign overgrowth of the prostate gland. The prostate gland surrounds the outlet of the bladder (the *urethra*), and when the gland enlarges, it squeezes the urethra, preventing the urine from easily leaving the bladder.

COMMON SIGNS AND SYMPTOMS

Early: The flow of urine is not as fast or as strong as it used to be. The person has to urinate more frequently. When there is the urge to urinate it needs to be done without delay. Many men have to get up more often at night to urinate.

Later: The bladder does not empty completely. The flow of urine weakens and slows to a dribble. Other problems include blood in the urine and infection of the bladder or kidney.

DIAGNOSIS

- Usually, the diagnosis can be made by taking a detailed history, doing a physical examination, and performing several office and laboratory tests.
- *Uriflow*: This test measures how fast your urine is passed.
- Measuring *residual urine*: Residual urine is the amount of urine that is left in the bladder after you are finished urinating.
- *Cystoscopy*: The doctor looks directly inside of the urethra and the bladder and can examine the blocking prostate tissue with a telescope (called a *cystoscope*) that is about the size of a pencil with a light at its tip. This procedure can be performed in the office.
- *Ultrasound*: Harmless sound waves are aimed at your prostate. The sound waves bouncing back (the echoes) from this area are seen as a picture on a screen. Ultrasound is a convenient and harmless way to examine the prostate gland.
- *IVP (Intravenous pyelogram)*: A special liquid is injected into your veins, and x-rays are taken as it flows through your kidneys and bladder.

○ TREATMENT

The specific treatment depends on the following:
- How severe your symptoms are.
- Whether the prostate enlargement is causing other problems.
- The size, shape, and consistency of the prostate gland.
- Your age, sexual activity, and general health.

Less severe symptoms can often be controlled by making some adjustment in what you eat and when you drink fluids. There are medications that can help improve the flow of urine.

An operation usually is advisable if any of the following conditions are present:
- Severe obstruction.
- Early signs of kidney damage.
- Repeated urinary tract infections.
- Retention of urine.
- Repeated bleeding with urination.

Operations that are used to treat prostate hyperplasia include the following:

Transurethral Resection of the Prostate (TURP): This operation is performed through the urethra with a special cystoscope. No incision is made and the recovery period is shorter. Generally, this operation is not used to remove a very large prostate.

Suprapubic or Retropubic Prostatectomy: This operation is performed through an incision in the abdomen and is suitable when the prostate gland is too large to be safely removed with a cystoscope through the urethra.

Perineal Prostatectomy: This operation is performed through an incision just below the scrotum (the sac containing the testes).

Laser Hyperthermia: This is done by using a special instrument in the urethra that causes the portion of the prostate causing the obstruction to shrink.

After careful consideration of all factors, the recommendation is that the obstructive portion of your prostate gland be removed through the perineal route (Fig. 1).

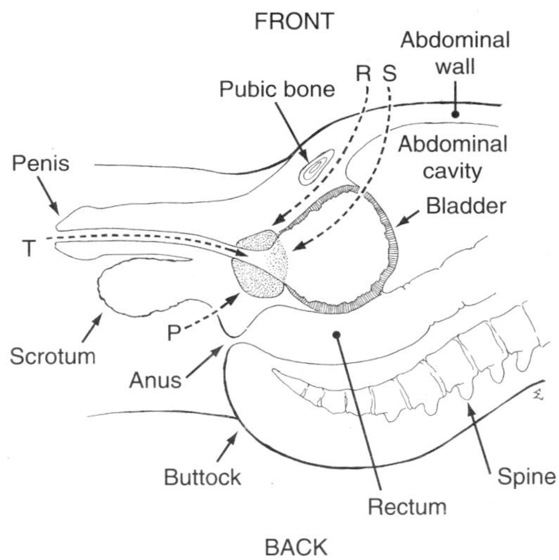

Figure 1. The prostate gland can be physically resected through several approaches—suprapubic (S), retropubic (R), transurethral (T), and perineal (P)—and each has its advantages and disadvantages. The choice of approach is influenced by the specific circumstances of a patient.

PREOPERATIVE PREPARATION

- You will have a general physical examination and an evaluation of your blood, heart (EKG), and lungs (chest x-ray).
- Do not eat or drink anything for 8 hours before the operation.

☐ OPERATION

- The choice of a general or a spinal anesthetic will be discussed with you beforehand.
- The incision will be made between the anus and the scrotum, and the obstructing part of the prostate will be removed.
- The operation usually takes about 2 hours.

POSTOPERATIVE CARE

- You will be taken to a recovery room and observed. When your blood pressure, pulse, and breathing are stable, you will be taken to a regular hospital room.
- There will be a catheter in your bladder for several days.
- You may have a strong urge to urinate right away. This is normal.
- Pain will be controlled with medicine.
- That evening you may sit up in bed and eat a soft diet.
- You will be given all the fluids your body needs directly into a vein in your arm for a day or two.
- When the catheter is removed, the flow of urine will be very full and strong. You will have to quickly go to the bathroom the minute you feel the urge to urinate because the sphincter muscle will not yet be strong enough to hold back the flow of urine. You will feel a burning sensation when you urinate.
- As with any operation, complications are always possible. With this type of operation, they can include bleeding and infection, and possibly others.
- This operation will not affect the sensation and strength of an orgasm (climax). It may, however, alter your ability to father children. If this is a concern, we should speak about it before any operation.
- You should be able to go home in about 3 days.
- Arrangements will be made for your medicine and follow-up office visit.

✚ HOME CARE

- You may walk about as you wish, even climb stairs, but don't overdo things.
- Unless instructed otherwise, you may shower if you wish.
- Include plenty of roughage and liquids in your diet to help prevent constipation.
- Do not drive a car or return to work before your follow-up office visit.

✆ CALL OUR OFFICE IF

- You experience heavy bleeding or pass clots with urination.
- The incision becomes red or swollen, or there is drainage from it.
- You develop a temperature higher than 100°F.
- You have any questions.

PROSTATE ENLARGEMENT (BPH): Suprapubic Prostatectomy

△ GENERAL INFORMATION

Prostate enlargement *(hyperplasia)* is benign overgrowth of the prostate gland. The prostate gland surrounds the outlet of the bladder (the *urethra*) and when the gland enlarges, it squeezes the urethra, preventing the urine from easily leaving the bladder.

COMMON SIGNS AND SYMPTOMS

Early: The flow of urine is not as fast or as strong as it used to be. The person has to urinate more frequently. When there is the urge to urinate it needs to be done without delay. Many men have to get up more often at night to urinate.

Later: The bladder does not empty completely. The flow of urine weakens and slows to a dribble. Other problems include blood in the urine and infection of the bladder or kidney.

DIAGNOSIS

- Usually, the diagnosis can be made by taking a detailed history, doing a physical examination, and performing several office and laboratory tests.
- *Uriflow*: This test measures how fast your urine is passed.
- Measuring *residual urine*: Residual urine is the amount of urine that is left in the bladder after you are finished urinating.
- *Cystoscopy*: The doctor looks directly inside of the urethra and the bladder and can examine the blocking prostate tissue with a telescope (called a *cystoscope*) that is about the size of a pencil with a light at its tip. This procedure can be performed in the office.
- *Ultrasound*: Harmless sound waves are aimed at your prostate. The sound waves bouncing back (the echoes) from this area are seen as a picture on a screen. Ultrasound is a convenient and harmless way to examine the prostate gland.
- *IVP (Intravenous pyelogram)*: A special liquid is injected into your veins and x-rays are taken as it flows through your kidneys and bladder. This provides valuable information about the kidneys and bladder.

○ TREATMENT

The specific treatment depends on the following:
- How severe your symptoms are.
- Whether the prostate enlargement is causing other problems.
- The size, shape, and consistency of the prostate gland.
- Your age, sexual activity, and general health.

Less severe symptoms can often be controlled by making some adjustment in what you eat and when you drink fluids. There are medications that can help improve the flow of your urine.

An operation usually is advisable if any of the following conditions are present:
- Severe obstruction.
- Early signs of damage to the kidneys.
- Repeated urinary tract infections.
- Retention of urine.
- Repeated bleeding with urination.

Operations that are used to treat prostate hyperplasia include the following:

Transurethral Resection of the Prostate (TURP): This operation is performed through the urethra with a special cystoscope. No incision is made and the recovery period is shorter. Generally, this operation is not used to remove a very large prostate.

Suprapubic or Retropubic Prostatectomy: This operation is performed through an incision in the abdomen and is suitable when the prostate gland is too large to be safely removed with a cystoscope through the urethra.

Perineal Prostatectomy: This operation is performed through an incision just below the scrotum (the sac containing the testes).

Laser Hyperthermia: This is done by using a special instrument in the urethra that causes the portion of the prostate causing the obstruction to shrink.

After careful consideration of all factors, the recommendation is that the obstructive portion of your prostate gland be removed through an abdominal incision (Fig. 1).

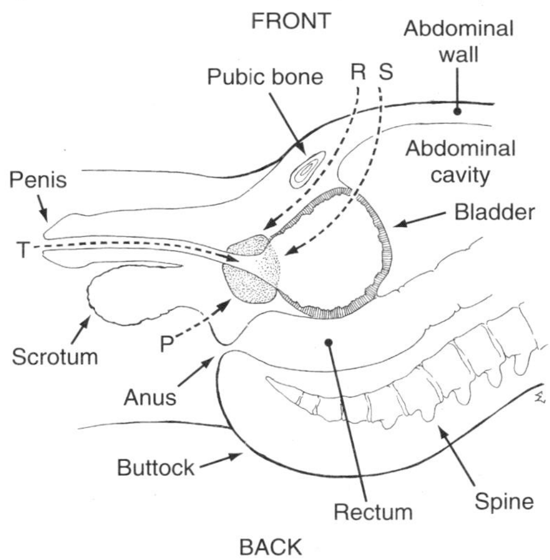

Figure 1. The prostate gland can be physically resected through several approaches—suprapubic (S), retropubic (R), transurethral (T), and perineal (P)—and each has its advantages and disadvantages. The choice of approach is influenced by the specific circumstances cf a patient.

PREOPERATIVE PREPARATION

- You will have a general physical examination and an evaluation of your blood, heart (EKG), and lungs (chest x-ray).
- Do not eat or drink anything for 8 hours before the operation.

☐ OPERATION

- The choice of a general or a spinal anesthetic will be discussed with you beforehand.
- The operation usually takes about 2 hours.

POSTOPERATIVE CARE

- You will be taken to a recovery room and observed. When your blood pressure, pulse, and breathing are stable, you will be taken to a regular hospital room.
- There will be a catheter in your bladder for several days.
- You may have a strong urge to pass your urine right away. This is normal.
- Pain will be controlled with medicine.
- That evening you will be helped to sit up in bed and the next day to get out of bed.
- You will be given all the fluids your body needs directly into a vein in your arm for a day or two.
- When the catheter is removed, the flow of urine will be very full and very strong. You will have to quickly go to the bathroom the minute you feel the urge to urinate because the sphincter muscle will not yet be strong enough to hold back the flow of urine. You will feel a burning sensation when you urinate.
- As with any operation, complications are always possible. With this type of operation, they can include bleeding and infection, and possibly others. The likelihood of not being able to control your urine or not being able to maintain an erection after this operation is very small.
- This operation will not affect the sensation and strength of an orgasm (climax). It may, however, alter your ability to father children. If this is a concern, we should speak about it before any operation.
- You should be able to go home in about 3 to 5 days.
- Arrangements will be made for your medicine, follow-up office visit, and stitch removal.

✣ HOME CARE

- You may walk about as you wish, even climb stairs, but don't overdo things.
- Take the medicines prescribed for you.
- Include plenty of roughage and liquids in your diet to help prevent constipation.
- Do not drive a car or return to work before your follow-up office visit.

✆ CALL OUR OFFICE IF

- You develop a temperature higher than 100°F.
- You are not able to easily eliminate the urine.
- There is drainage from the incision.
- You have any questions.

PROSTATE ENLARGEMENT (BPH):
Transurethral Microwave Thermotherapy

△ GENERAL INFORMATION

Prostate hyperplasia is benign overgrowth of the prostate gland. The prostate gland surrounds the *urethra*, which is the outlet of the bladder. When the prostate gland enlarges, it squeezes the urethra, making it difficult for urine to easily leave the bladder (Fig. 1).

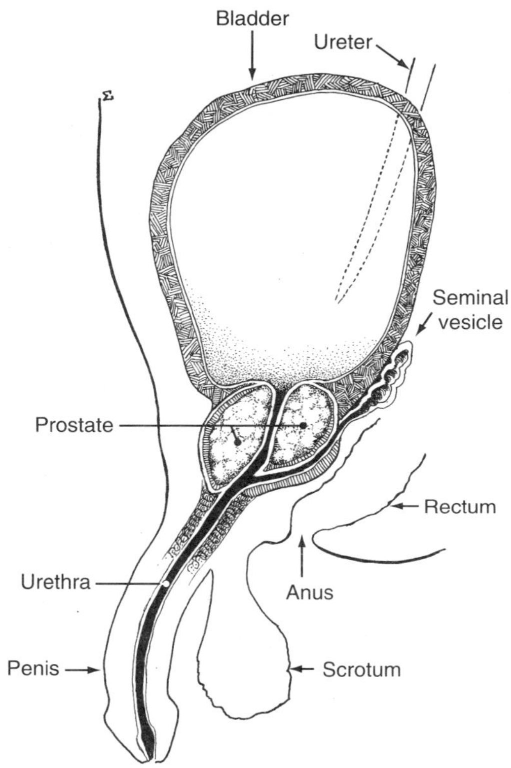

Figure 1. Side view of anatomy of prostate. Enlarged prostate causes narrowing of urethra.

COMMON SIGNS AND SYMPTOMS

Early: The flow of urine is not as fast or as strong as it used to be. There is a need to urinate more frequently. When there is an urge to urinate, it needs to be done without delay.

Later: The bladder may not be able to empty completely. The flow of urine slows to a dribble. There is blood in the urine. The bladder or kidney may become infected.

DIAGNOSIS

- Usually, the diagnosis can be made by taking a detailed history, doing a thorough physical examination, and performing several office and laboratory tests.
- *Uriflow*: You urinate into a collecting device that measures how fast the urine is passed.
- Measuring *residual urine*: Residual urine is the amount of urine left in the bladder after you are finished urinating.
- *Cystoscopy*: In this procedure, the urologist looks directly at the inside of the urethra and the bladder using a small telescope (called a *cystoscope*) that is about the size of a pencil with a light at its tip. Cystoscopy can be performed in the office and can help determine the size and shape of the obstruction that is caused by the enlarging prostate.
- *IVP (Intravenous pyelogram)*: A special liquid is injected into your veins, and x-rays are taken as it travels through the kidneys and draining tubes (the *ureters*). This provides valuable information about the kidneys and the bladder and the degree of obstruction caused by the enlarging prostate.

○ TREATMENT

There are a number of available treatments. Which treatment is best depends on a number of factors.

- How severe your symptoms are.
- Whether the prostate enlargement is causing other problems in the urinary tract, such as infection, bleeding, or kidney failure.
- The size, shape, and consistency of the prostate gland.
- Your age, sexual activity, and general health.

For less severe symptoms, it may be reasonable to just watch the problem carefully and to have regular examinations. With medications and with some adjustment in your diet and when you drink fluids, you may be able to reduce some of the bothersome symptoms.

An operation usually is advisable if any of the following conditions are present:

- More severe obstruction.
- Early signs of damage to the kidneys.
- Recurrent infections of the urinary tract.
- Retention of urine.
- Repeated bleeding in the urinary tract.

The operations used to treat prostate hyperplasia include the following:

Transurethral Resection of the Prostate (TURP): This operation is performed through the urethra using a special type of *cystoscope* that is the size of a pencil. No incision is made and the recovery period is shorter. This operation usually is not used to remove a very large prostate.

Suprapubic Prostatectomy or Retropubic Prostatectomy: This operation is performed through an incision in the abdomen and is more suitable for a larger prostate or when there are other conditions that need to be corrected at the same time.

Perineal Prostatectomy: The prostate is removed through an incision just below the scrotum (the sac holding the testicles).

Transurethral Microwave Thermotherapy (TMT): This is done by using a special instrument in the urethra that causes the portion of the prostate causing the obstruction to shrink. This technique is not used in the following circumstances:

- Enlargement of certain parts of the prostate.
- Prostate cancer.
- Prostate infection.
- Scarring and narrowing of the urethra.
- Urinary tract infection.
- Bladder cancer.
- Bladder stones.

After careful consideration of all factors, the recommendation is that you have your prostate hyperplasia treated through the urethra with TMT.

The advantages to this method are as follows:

- It is virtually as effective as a prostatectomy with other techniques.
- No anesthesia is necessary.
- Only one session treatment is needed and it takes a relatively short time.
- It is an outpatient procedure.
- The benefits last an average of at least 4 years.
- There is no significant bleeding after the operation.
- There is a 75% chance that your sexual performance will remain the same or get better.

PREOPERATIVE PREPARATION

- You will have a general physical examination and an evaluation of your blood, heart (EKG), and lungs (chest x-ray).
- Do not eat or drink anything for 8 hours before the operation.
- You may be given medicine that will make you feel drowsy before you are brought to the operating room.

☐ OPERATION

- You will be placed on a comfortable table.
- An anesthetic will be squirted into your urethra to make it completely numb.
- The flexible, smooth laser probe (about the size of a pencil) will be inserted into your urethra. That portion of the probe that sends out the microwaves will be positioned just inside the enlarged prostate. The urologist and the technician will be in constant attendance as the treatment is being administered. You should feel no significant discomfort. The procedure usually lasts about 30 minutes (Figs. 2–4).

POSTOPERATIVE CARE

- Your blood pressure, pulse, and breathing will be observed to make certain they are stable. When you are completely alert, you should be able to go home with a responsible adult.
- Arrangements will be made for your medicine and your postoperative follow-up visit.

✚ HOME CARE

- You may walk about as you wish, even climb stairs, but don't overdo things.
- Drink plenty of fluids for the next few days, especially water and juices.
- The catheter that is in your penis will be removed in the office during your postoperative visit.
- You may notice lightly blood-tinged urine in the catheter bag for 24 to 48 hours after the procedure. This is to be expected; don't be alarmed.
- There will be no significant change in the preoperative symptoms for about 1 month.
- Take any medicines as directed.
- Do not drive for 48 hours.
- Do not take any alcoholic beverages or caffeine for 1 week after the procedure.

✆ CALL OUR OFFICE IF

- You develop any unusual signs or symptoms.
- You develop a temperature higher than 100°F.
- You have any questions.

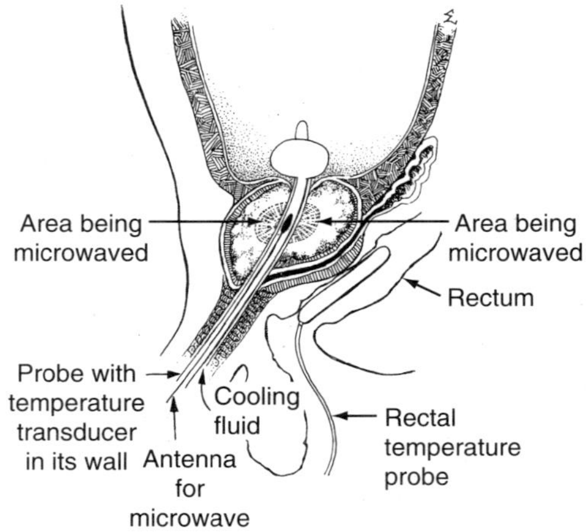

Figure 2. Same view as in Figure 1. Antenna from microwave is positioned next to enlarged obstructing portion of prostate gland. Treatment is in progress.

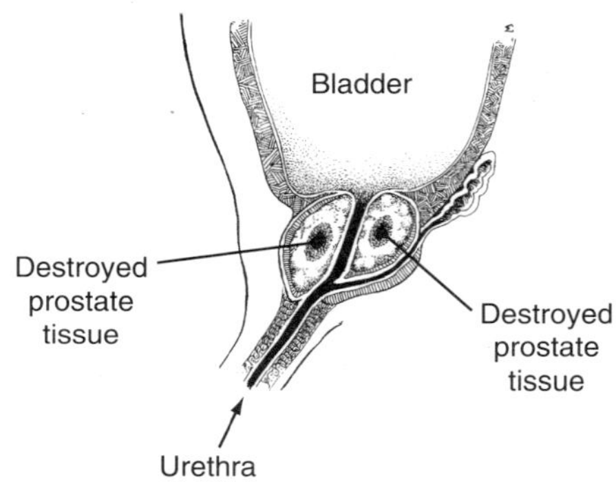

Figure 3. Same view as in Figures 1 and 2. Treatment completed and antenna withdrawn. This demonstrates areas of destroyed prostate.

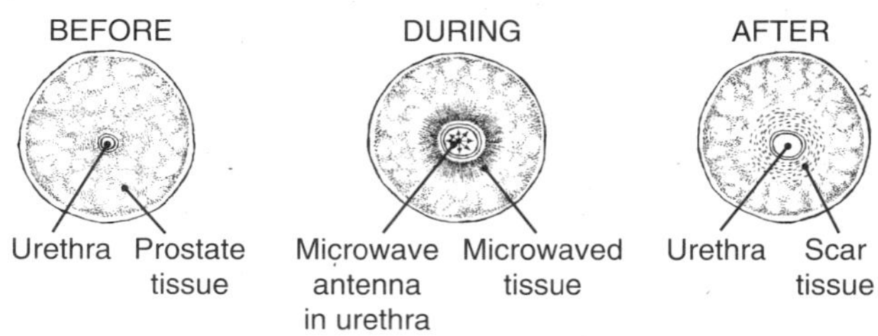

Figure 4. Cross-section of urethra at level of obstructing prostate demonstrates the area of the prostate destroyed and subsequent shrinkage of the destroyed tissue, which enlarges the narrowed urethra in this area.

PROSTATE ENLARGEMENT (BPH): Transurethral Resection

△ GENERAL INFORMATION

Prostate enlargement *(hyperplasia)* is benign (noncancerous) overgrowth of the prostate gland. The prostate gland surrounds the outlet of the bladder (the *urethra*) and when the gland enlarges, it squeezes the urethra, preventing the urine from easily leaving the bladder.

COMMON SIGNS AND SYMPTOMS

Early: The urine does not flow as fast or as strong as it used to. The person has to urinate more frequently. When there is the urge to urinate, it needs to be done without delay. Many men have to get up more often at night to urinate.

Later: The bladder does not empty completely. The flow of urine weakens and slows to a dribble. Other problems may include blood in the urine and infection of the bladder or kidney.

DIAGNOSIS

- Usually, the diagnosis can be made by taking a detailed history, doing a physical examination, and performing several office and laboratory tests.
- *Uriflow*: This test measures how fast your urine is passed.
- Measuring *residual urine*: Residual urine is the amount of urine that is left in the bladder after you are finished urinating.
- *Cystoscopy*: The doctor looks directly inside of the urethra and the bladder and can examine the blocking prostate tissue with a telescope (called a *cystoscope*) that is about the size of a pencil with a light at its tip. This can be done in the office.
- *Ultrasound*: Harmless sound waves are aimed at your prostate. The sound waves bouncing back (the echoes) from this area are seen as a picture on a screen. Ultrasound is a convenient and harmless way to examine the prostate gland.
- *IVP (Intravenous pyelogram)*: A special liquid is injected into your veins, and x-rays are taken as it flows through your kidneys and bladder.

○ TREATMENT

The specific treatment depends on the following:
- How severe your symptoms are.
- Whether the prostate enlargement is causing other problems.
- The size, shape, and consistency of the prostate gland.
- Your age, sexual activity, and general health.

Less severe symptoms can often be controlled by making some adjustment in what you eat and when you drink fluids. There are medications that can help improve the flow of your urine.

An operation usually is advisable if any of the following conditions are present:
- Severe obstruction.
- Early signs of kidney damage.
- Repeated urinary tract infections.
- Retention of urine.
- Repeated bleeding with urination.

Operations that are used to treat prostate hyperplasia include the following (Fig. 1):

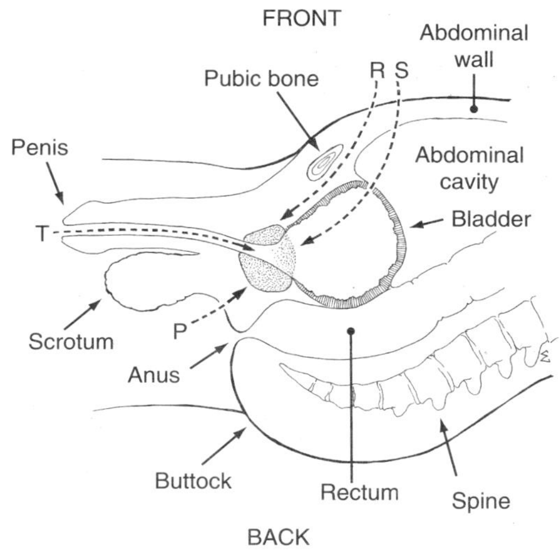

Figure 1. The prostate gland can be physically resected through several approaches—suprapubic (S), retropubic (R), transurethral (T), and perineal (P)—and each has its advantages and disadvantages. The choice of approach is influenced by the specific circumstances of a patient.

Transurethral Resection of the Prostate (TURP): This operation is performed through the urethra with a special cystoscope. No incision is made and the recovery period is shorter. Generally, this operation is not used to remove a very large prostate.

Suprapubic or Retropubic Prostatectomy: This operation is performed through an incision in the abdomen and is suitable when the prostate gland is too large to be safely removed with a cystoscope through the urethra.

Perineal Prostatectomy: This operation is performed through an incision just below the scrotum (the sac containing the testicles).

Laser Hyperthermia: This is done by using a special instrument in the urethra that causes the portion of the prostate causing the obstruction to shrink.

After careful consideration of all factors, the recommendation is that the obstructive portion of your prostate gland be removed through the urethra (TURP).

PREOPERATIVE PREPARATION

- You will have a general physical examination and an evaluation of your blood, heart (EKG), and lungs (chest x-ray).
- Do not eat or drink anything for 8 hours before the operation.

☐ OPERATION

- The choice of a general or a spinal anesthetic will be discussed with you beforehand.
- A cystoscope with an electrical cutting device is used to shave down and remove the obstructing part of the prostate gland.
- The operation usually takes about 1 hour.

POSTOPERATIVE CARE

- You will be taken to a recovery room and observed. When your blood pressure, pulse, and breathing are stable, you will be taken to a regular hospital room.
- There will be a catheter in your penis for several days to drain your bladder.
- You may have a strong urge to pass your urine right away. This is normal after the operation.
- Pain will be controlled with medicine.
- That evening you may sit up in bed and eat a soft diet.
- After the catheter is removed, you may have a strong urge to urinate, you may urinate more frequently, and you may note a burning sensation in your urethra when you pass your urine. This will get better every day, but it may take up to 4 to 6 weeks before things are normal.
- As with any operation, complications are always possible. With this type of operation, they can include bleeding and infection, and possibly others. The likelihood of not being able to control your urine or not being able to maintain an erection after this operation is very small.
- This operation will not affect the sensation and strength of an orgasm (climax). It may, however, alter your ability to father children. If this is a concern, we should speak about it before any operation.
- You should be able to go home in about 3 days.
- Arrangements will be made for your medicine and follow-up office visit.

✚ HOME CARE

- You may walk about as you wish, even climb stairs, but don't overdo things.
- Include plenty of roughage and liquids in your diet to help prevent constipation.
- Do not drive a car or return to work until your follow-up office visit.

✆ CALL OUR OFFICE IF

- You develop a temperature higher than 101°F.
- You are not able to easily eliminate the urine.
- The urine becomes very red or there are blood clots associated with passing urine.
- You have any questions.

△ GENERAL INFORMATION

The heart has a number of large vessels that bring blood from the lungs and all other parts of the body as well as taking blood back to the same areas.

The amount of blood coming in and going out of the heart has to be the same. If this is out of balance, the heart or lungs can develop problems. A pulmonary artery catheter (commonly called a PAC) is a special, small tube passed inside your heart to measure the pressures in your heart. This helps the doctors estimate how well your heart is working during complicated operations, when you are in the intensive care unit (ICU), or when you have heart problems. The surgical team uses the information obtained from these measurements to help make decisions on the amount of fluids you require during your operation and whether you need special medications to support the functions of your heart.

INDICATIONS FOR A PAC

- Most commonly, a PAC is used in open-heart surgery, such as coronary artery bypass of heart valve replacement.
- A PAC may also be required during other operations when you have an underlying problem with your heart.
- Even if the heart is healthy, certain complicated operations, such as liver transplantation or aneurysm repair, frequently require the use of a PAC because of the amount of fluid or blood that is required during the operation.
- A PAC may also be required in the ICU after the operation if your blood pressure becomes unstable.

THE PROCEDURE

- If the catheter is inserted under local anesthesia while you are awake, you will be given medicine to make you feel drowsy.
- You will lie flat on the operating room table or the hospital bed.
- You will be given some oxygen through a small tube in your nose.
- The skin on the side of your neck or below your clavicle (collarbone) will be swabbed with an antiseptic solution and surrounded with sterile towels.
- The operating table or bed will be tilted head down to enlarge the veins in the neck.
- A thin, short needle will be used to inject an anesthetic in the skin over the vein to make it numb.
- The PAC is as thin as spaghetti. It will be placed in the vein in your neck or below your clavicle. Its tip is then advanced along the vein until it reaches the pulmonary artery and from there into one of the chambers of the heart. The drapes and oxygen are removed and the PAC is ready for use.

USING THE PAC

- During the operation, the anesthesiologist uses the information supplied by the PAC in several ways:
  - To determine how much fluid you should be given.
  - During open-heart surgery, the PAC is especially important to help the cardiac surgeon determine how effectively the heart is working.
  - The information is used after the operation in the ICU to further guide the physicians in monitoring and treating your heart function. The PAC is used only while you are in the ICU and is always removed before you are sent to your regular room on the hospital floor, typically 1 to 2 days after your operation.
- As with any procedure, complications are always possible. With this operation, they can include infection. This usually happens only when the PAC needs to be kept in your heart for 5 to 7 days, at which time it must be removed.

Pulmonary artery catheterization is valuable in making certain operations safer and more successful.

△ GENERAL INFORMATION

All the veins draining blood from below the chest empty into a big vein about the size of your thumb, called the *inferior vena cava*, that takes the blood to the right side of the heart. The heart pumps it out through the *pulmonary artery*—also as big as your thumb—which takes it to the lungs. In the lungs, the pulmonary artery divides into smaller and smaller vessels until there are hundreds of them no bigger than the lead in a pencil. Here in the lungs, the blood picks up fresh oxygen and then flows to the left side of the heart, which pumps it throughout the body.

WHAT HAPPENS

Once in a while, a clot forms in one of the veins from the lower half of the body draining into the inferior vena cava. (A blood clot looks like grape Jell-O.) When some or all of the clot breaks off, it travels with the rest of the blood into the heart, then into the pulmonary artery, and then to the lung. But when it reaches the smaller branches in the lung, it can't get through: It blocks the artery and not enough blood can get through it to the lungs. This blood clot now is called a *pulmonary embolus* (Fig. 1).

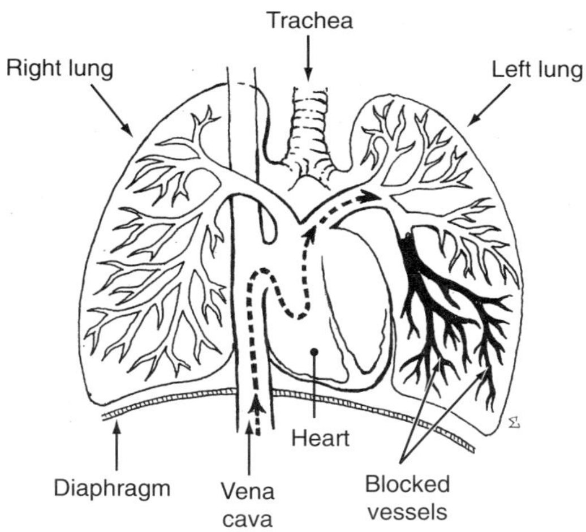

Figure 1. A "typical" pulmonary embolism is shown. Emboli, however, can be larger or smaller and in one or both lungs. These factors can influence the treatment and the outcome.

If the clot causes a complete blockage, many persons die within an hour. If some blood can get through, the condition is still serious, but the patient has a chance if treated promptly and correctly.

HOW A CLOT FORMS

A blood clot is likely to form when:

- **The blood stands still too long:** This can happen when patients are unable to move around because they have some chronic illness, are undergoing an operation, are in a plaster cast, are unconscious, or are simply old and weak.
- **Something irritates the inside of the vein:** The inside of the vein normally is as smooth as glass. If there is a rough area present, it encourages a clot to form there. This can happen when there is surgery around large veins, for example, an operation in the pelvis.
- **The blood just clots faster than normal:** This can happen with certain diseases, including cancer; in pregnant women; and in women taking contraceptive medicines.

CLOT PREVENTION

- **The blood stands still too long:**
  - Before the operation starts, the legs are positioned so that nothing blocks the flow of blood back to the heart.
  - Special air cushion stockings are placed on the legs and connected to a machine. During the operation, the stockings squeeze the legs every few minutes to keep the blood flowing.
  - Soon after the operation, the patient gets out of bed. While in bed, the patient wears elastic stockings to prevent the veins from filling up with blood that does not move well enough and is urged to move the legs at least every hour.
- **Something is irritating the inside of the vein:**
  - The surgeon is as gentle as possible during the operation, because rough handling of tissue increases the risk of clotting within adjacent veins.
- **Blood just clots faster than normal:**
  - Blood tests are taken before the operation to see how fast the blood clots and possibly to correct any problems.
  - Even if clotting is normal, certain types of patients are given a small dose of blood thinner to discourage clotting from occurring faster than normal.

COMMON SIGNS AND SYMPTOMS

- Shortness of breath, chest pain, spitting up frothy blood, and fast pulse.
- Unfortunately, many of the above symptoms are also seen with other diseases.

DIAGNOSIS

- The doctor considers the clinical setting, takes a detailed history, and does a thorough physical examination.
- A chest x-ray is taken to see the part of the lung affected by the blockage.
- An electrocardiogram (EKG) is done to see if the heart is struggling to pump blood past the blockage.
- Dye is injected into the pulmonary artery, and x-rays are taken of the dye to try to actually see the blockage.

○ TREATMENT

- If the clot does not block the vessels completely, treatment can include the following:
  - Treatment to help the heart that is struggling to pump blood past the blockage.

- Having the person breathe pure oxygen so that the part of the lung that is still working receives the maximum amount of oxygen.
- Aggressive treatment with blood thinners *(anticoagulants)* to prevent other clots from forming as well as to prevent the clot already present from getting even bigger.
- Fortunately, the body itself quickly makes chemicals that slowly dissolve the clot. So, if the patient can be helped for a time, the vessels can open up again.
- Special intravenous medications are available to dissolve clots when necessary.

- If the blockage is serious and the patient is not doing well, an operation may need to be done to remove the clot. This is a major, serious operation, but it can be successful.
- The patient usually needs to be on long-term anticoagulants, which are carefully regulated.
- If long-term blood thinners don't seem to work, and there's evidence that more small clots are forming, there is an operation to put a filter across the vena cava. Blood in the vena cava can get by this filter but the clots cannot.

This explanation may help you better understand why some things are done to you and for you before, during, and after your operation.

△ GENERAL INFORMATION

Pyogenic granuloma is a lesion found in older children and pregnant women. It can grow just about anywhere in the body but is most often found in the mouth area or on the shoulder. When it first appears, it is no larger than a poppy seed, but it quickly gets larger, sometimes growing to the size of a cranberry.

This lesion contains a lot of blood vessels, giving it a red to dark brown color. It does not come from an infection. It is not malignant and never becomes malignant.

The cause is unknown, but some think it is tied in with hormones, because pyogenic granulomas go away when the pregnancy is over. They often come back again with the next pregnancy, however.

COMMON SIGNS AND SYMPTOMS

- A raised or flat lesion on the lip, cheek, tongue, gum, or skin.
- It does not hurt. It bleeds easily when scratched or picked.

DIAGNOSIS

- Usually, the diagnosis can be made by taking a detailed history and doing a thorough examination of the lesion.

○ TREATMENT

- Most of the time, removal of the lesion is the best treatment.
- Observation usually is best in pregnant women, unless the lesion bleeds too often and is a real nuisance.

□ OPERATION

- This is an outpatient procedure.
- A very fine, short needle is used to inject a local anesthetic around the granuloma. This will make the area completely numb.
- The granuloma is simply cut off. The base of it (still numb) is burned slightly with the fine tip of an electrical instrument to prevent bleeding.
- In some patients, it is better to remove the granuloma through a cosmetic incision.
- A small bandage is applied.

POSTOPERATIVE CARE

- You will be instructed on how to take care of the treated area and how to apply the bandage.
- Pain is minimal and can be controlled with over-the-counter medicine.

✆ CALL OUR OFFICE IF

- There is bleeding from the operated area that doesn't stop after 15 minutes of firm pressure with a piece of gauze.
- The wound becomes red or swollen or is draining any pus.
- You develop a temperature higher than 100°F.
- You have any questions.

△ GENERAL INFORMATION

Rabies has been feared for many centuries because of the dreadful way in which a person dies once the disease takes hold. Fortunately, today human rabies in the United States is rare, mostly because of the practice of vaccinating dogs and cats.

It is estimated that each year about 2 million people are bitten by animals in the United States; about 25% of these are dog bites. There are roughly 5,000 laboratory-confirmed cases of rabies in animals each year.

Cats and dogs account for fewer than 5% of rabies cases. At least 90% of cases are caused by wild animals, with skunks and raccoons making up the majority (70%). Other animals frequently infected are bats, foxes, coyotes, and bobcats. Rats, mice, chipmunks, squirrels, rabbits, hamsters, guinea pigs, and gerbils are almost never a rabies threat to humans.

Rabies is caused by a virus found in the saliva of the sick animal. It gets into humans through an opening in the skin, almost always a bite. The virus grows in tissue along the nerve, causing the nerve to die.

COMMON SIGNS AND SYMPTOMS

- Early on, symptoms are not really specific. There may be fever, headache, tiredness, loss of appetite, and sore throat. The sore throat then progresses to painful spasms of the swallowing muscles.
- Later, there is increasing nervousness, loss of sleep, and anxiety.
- Finally, as the nerves die, breathing becomes ineffective and oxygen is low; the heartbeat becomes irregular; stroke occurs frequently; and finally, the patient lapses into a coma. Practically all persons die if they reach this stage.

DIAGNOSIS

- If anyone has the above history or symptoms, there should be concern about infection with rabies.
- The specific diagnosis can be made only after the biting animal is killed, an autopsy performed, and the brain examined for the telltale signs of rabies.
- How the biting took place can often help with the diagnosis. For example, was the biting animal:
  - A healthy, vaccinated, family pet that was provoked?
  - A strange dog or cat that was provoked, bit the person, and then escaped? Or, was it an unprovoked attack and escape?
  - A wild animal (raccoon, skunk, fox, bobcat, coyote, bat)?
  - One that is available for study, or did it escape?
  - A rat, mouse, chipmunk, squirrel, hamster, or gerbil?

○ TREATMENT

The Bite Wound

- The wound should be rinsed thoroughly with a salt solution. (It is helpful if some of the virus is washed away.)
- The wound should be rinsed with an antiseptic solution to reduce the chance of infection by ordinary bacteria. (The customary antiseptic solutions used on open wounds do not kill the rabies virus.)
- Antibiotics for protection against infection by bacteria should be strongly considered, depending on the biting circumstances and the condition of the wound itself. (Antibiotics do not kill the rabies virus.)
- Treatment against tetanus (lockjaw) should be strongly considered, depending on the biting circumstances and the wound itself.

The Bitten Person

The following are some principles of treatment for persons bitten by animals that might have rabies:

- Animals that have rabies almost always die within 10 days.
- It usually takes 3 to 6 weeks for rabies to develop in humans.
- Once a human actually shows symptoms, especially in the advanced stage, the condition almost always is fatal.
- For these reasons, it is necessary to start preventive treatment promptly. One cannot wait to see whether rabies develops; by then it would be too late.
- The treatment has two parts:
  - One part is medicine that gives temporary protection (called *passive immunization*). The medicine can give only temporary protection, but at least it works right away.
  - The other part of the treatment is to give a vaccine to help the body build up its own resistance (called *active immunization*). However, it takes some weeks before it starts taking effect.
- The vaccination to produce active immunity can have side effects, some of them very serious. For this reason, the vaccine should not be given without some serious thought.

Guidelines for treatment are listed below.

- All the circumstances related to the biting animal and to the bite wound itself have to be considered when deciding on whether to begin treatment for possible rabies.
- **It is important to have the biting animal, if at all possible.** If the biting animal is available, it is easier to decide whether rabies treatment should be started.
- No prophylactic treatment is necessary if the biting animal is a family pet that is healthy and vaccinated, the animal was provoked, the bite is superficial, and the animal can be isolated and observed.
- Prophylactic treatment is almost never necessary for bites by a rat, mouse, chipmunk, squirrel, rabbit, hamster, or gerbil. It is extremely rare for rabies to develop from bites by these animals.
- Prophylactic treatment should be started for the following:
  - Bites from a wild animal. This includes raccoons, skunks, foxes, coyotes, bobcats, and bats.
  - Bites from a domestic dog or cat that is suspected of having rabies and is isolated and available for study.

- Bites from a domestic dog or cat that has escaped.
- Multiple deep bites in the head and neck or hands.

All wild biting animals and all domestic animals suspected of having rabies should be killed (without too much damage to the head) and kept refrigerated if possible. Health authorities should be called promptly to start the process of performing an autopsy on the brain of these animals.

- The prophylactic and vaccination treatment is continued if
  - The wild animal escaped.
  - The brain autopsy of the wild animal or of the domestic dog or cat showed rabies.
  - The domestic dog or cat escaped.
  - The domestic dog or cat that was isolated and observed dies of rabies.
- The prophylactic and vaccination treatment can be stopped if
  - The brain autopsy of the wild or domestic animal fails to show rabies.
  - The isolated, observed domestic animal is well after 2 weeks of observation.
- There may be other special circumstances; treatment in these instances should be done on an individual basis, following the principles described.

All in all, approximately 25,000 persons in the United States each year need to have the complete therapy for rabies.

RADICAL NECK DISSECTION

△ GENERAL INFORMATION

Radical neck dissection involves removing the lymph nodes on one side of the neck along with a large muscle there, some rather unimportant nerves, and often an important nerve that helps lift the shoulder.

Most often, the operation is done for cancer that has spread to the neck from the mouth or throat cavity or sometimes the face or even from a cancer starting in an organ in the neck. An operation in which less tissue is removed is called a *modified radical neck dissection*.

Sometimes part of the jaw and tongue is removed during the radical neck dissection. This operation is called a *monobloc, tongue and jaw.*

COMMON SIGNS AND SYMPTOMS

- There is no set number of lymph nodes in the neck (or in any location), just as there is no set number of hairs in the scalp.
- Most of the time, lymph nodes are small; occasionally, a few can be felt even though there is nothing wrong with them.
- At other times they can get larger and be felt easily. This may occur for no apparent reason, or it may be because the nodes are reacting to an infection or are involved with cancer. These enlarged lymph nodes can get to be the size of an olive or larger. There can be only one or many of them.

DIAGNOSIS

If a person has, or has had, cancer in an area that drains into these neck lymph nodes and they later become enlarged, there should be concern about the possibility that cancer has spread to these lymph nodes. Obtaining a piece of this tissue (a *biopsy*) is recommended and can be done as follows:

- *Needle aspiration biopsy* is performed by inserting a needle through the skin and into the lymph node to obtain the tissue for laboratory examination.
- *Open biopsy*: The skin over the suspicious lymph node is painted with an antiseptic solution and surrounded with sterile towels. A thin needle is used to inject an anesthetic solution into the skin and surrounding tissue to make the entire area numb. A short incision is made through the numb skin, and the lymph node is removed for examination in the laboratory.

○ TREATMENT

- If the biopsy shows the presence of cancer in your nodes and if tests show that the cancer has not spread to any other part of your body, then a radical neck dissection is appropriate.
- After careful consideration of all the factors in your case, the recommendation is that you have a radical neck dissection.

PREOPERATIVE PREPARATION

- You will have an examination of your blood, urine, heart (EKG), and lungs (chest x-ray).
- A thorough examination will be done of your mouth and throat as well as the outside of your neck.
- *CT scan (computed tomography scan)*: These special x-rays are taken by a machine that is shaped like a huge doughnut. You will lie on a table inside the hole in the "doughnut." The x-rays are taken as very thin slices through the area of the neck. This makes it possible to see the fine details in the neck.
- It is possible you may need chemotherapy or radiation (x-ray) therapy before the operation. If this is so, it will be explained to you.
- Do not eat or drink anything for 8 hours before the operation.
- Bathe or shower as usual on the morning of the operation.
- You may be given medicine that will make you feel drowsy before you are brought to the operating room.

□ OPERATION

- You will be asleep for the operation.
- A curved or T-shaped incision will be made on the side of your neck. The lymph nodes and other tissue in this area will be removed (Fig. 1).
- The operation usually takes about 2 to 3 hours.

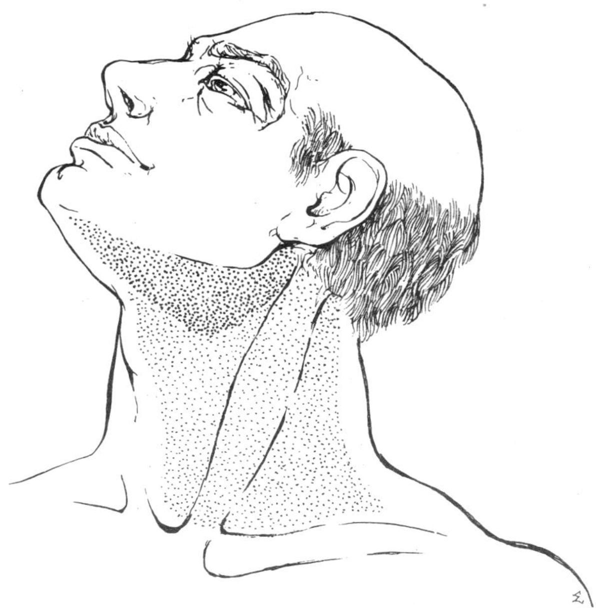

Figure 1. The tissue removed during a radical neck dissection includes that in the stippled areas. Sometimes less than a "radical" dissection is performed; most often this is limited to the upper neck *(heavier stippling)*. Such an operation is often referred to as an *upper neck* or *supraomohyoid* dissection.

POSTOPERATIVE CARE

- You will be taken to a recovery room and observed. When your blood pressure, pulse, and breathing are stable, you will be taken to a regular hospital room.
- There will be a small plastic tube from your wound connected to a plastic bag to collect any extra fluid in

the area. It usually is removed 3 to 5 days after the operation.

- That evening you will be helped to sit up in bed and on the next day to get out of bed.
- Pain will be controlled with medicine.
- You should be able to eat soft to solid food within a day.
- As with any operation, complications are always possible. With this type of operation, they can include bleeding, infection, loss of skin in the area of the incision, temporary and possibly permanent weakness of the lower lip on the side of the operation, heart problems, and possibly others.
- You should be able to go home in 3 to 4 days.
- Your condition can be cured. An estimate of your chances can be made only after all the laboratory results are back.

✣ HOME CARE

- You may walk about as you wish, even climb stairs, but don't overdo things.
- Take medicine as prescribed for your pain.
- You will be given a suggested diet to follow during your convalescence, if necessary. Include plenty of roughage and liquids in your diet to help prevent constipation. You may need a mild laxative (example: milk of magnesia).
- Unless instructed otherwise, you may shower with any dressings on or off. After you dry yourself, replace any dressings with clean, dry ones.
- Do not drive until your first follow-up visit. After that, do not drive unless you can move freely and without pain and you are not taking any medicine that decreases your alertness.
- You may resume sexual activity whenever you choose.
- You may return to work when you feel up to it.

✆ CALL OUR OFFICE IF

- The incision becomes red or swollen, or there is drainage from it.
- You develop a temperature higher than 100°F.
- You have any questions.

△ GENERAL INFORMATION

The rectum is that part of the large bowel that starts at the *anus* (the opening to the outside) and extends upward for about 10 inches. The rest of the large bowel is called the *colon*. Cancer of the rectum is common in older adults. The cause of cancer in a case such as yours is not truly known.

COMMON SIGNS AND SYMPTOMS

- In the early stages there often are no symptoms.
- Blood may be found in the stool by the patient or by the doctor when doing a routine physical examination.
- The stool may be thinner because it has to squeeze past the cancer.
- Sometimes the cancer produces the urge to have a bowel movement but nothing comes out.

DIAGNOSIS

- Often the diagnosis can be made by taking a detailed history, doing a thorough physical examination, and considering the laboratory report.
- *Flexible sigmoidoscopy*: This is a valuable, often routine procedure. A smooth, flexible optical instrument that is as thick as your little finger and has a light at its tip is used to examine the lower 25 or so inches of your bowel.
- *Colonoscopy*: This is done with an instrument that has lenses in it and a light at its tip, is smooth and flexible, and is as big around as your little finger. During the procedure you will be given medicine that will make you feel drowsy. The tip of the instrument will be introduced through the anus and carefully advanced up your entire large bowel, which is thoroughly examined. If any suspicious tissue is seen, a small piece of it can be taken (a *biopsy*) for laboratory examination.
- *Ultrasound*: A thin instrument very much like an enema tip (a *probe*) is placed in the rectum, and the tip is positioned over the tumor. Harmless sound waves coming from the tip of the probe are aimed at the tumor in your rectum. The sound waves bouncing back (the echoes) from this area are seen as a picture on a screen. Ultrasound is a convenient and painless way to examine the tumor to see how deeply it is penetrating the rectum. This helps determine the type of operation that will be needed.
- *CT scan (computed tomography scan)*: These x-rays are taken as very thin slices through the area of the rectum. This makes it possible to see details in the rectum and any growths outside it.
- *Cystoscopy*: This procedure involves looking into your bladder if it is felt the cancer is close by.
- In women, the vagina also is examined carefully.

○ TREATMENT

The best chance to cure a cancer of the rectum that has not spread to distant areas is by an operation.

- The type of operation required is influenced by the following:
  - The size of the cancer.
  - The exact location of the cancer.
  - How deeply it penetrates the wall of the rectum.
  - Whether the lymph nodes in the area are involved or are likely to be involved.
  - Your general condition.

The two operations most commonly used to treat cancer of the rectum are as follows:

- Removal of most of the rectum and the cancer in it through an abdominal incision. The cut ends of the rectum are reconnected. There is no colostomy. This operation is more suitable for a cancer that is not too close to the anus. This operation may affect your sex life.
- Removal of the rectum and the anus and creation of a permanent colostomy (Figs. 1 and 2). This operation will almost surely affect your sex life. This operation is best when the cancer involves some of the anus or when the entire rectum and anus need to be removed.

After the most careful consideration of all factors, including the best chance for cure, the recommendation is that you have an operation that involves removing your rectum and anus and establishing a permanent colostomy.

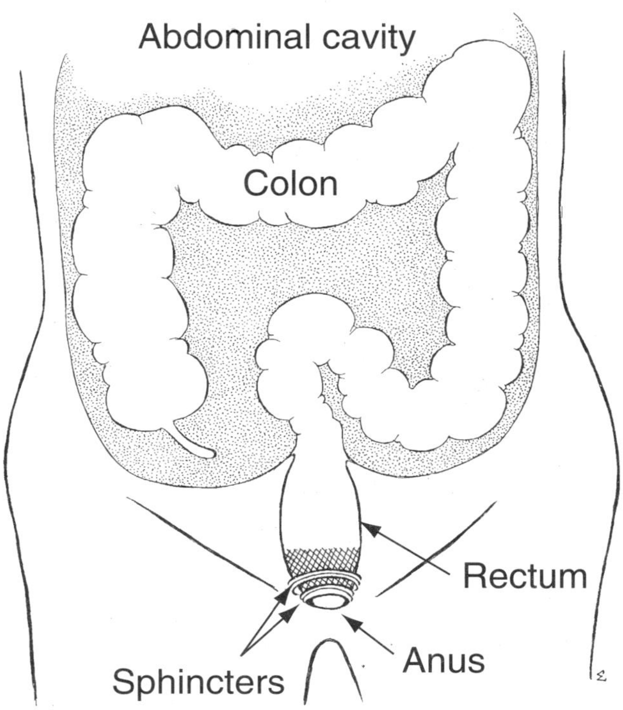

Figure 1. The type of cancer commonly found low in the rectum *(cross-hatched area)* very often affects the sphincters of the anus or is too close to them for the cancer to be removed properly and for the best chance for cure.

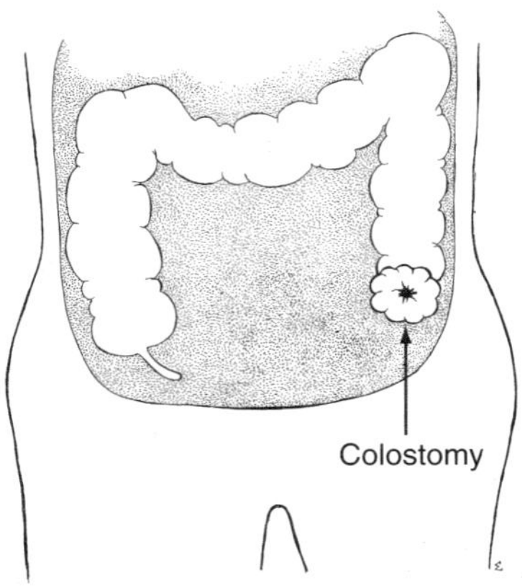

Figure 2. In the conditions illustrated in Figure 1, the anus and sphincter must also be removed and a permanent colostomy established.

PREOPERATIVE PREPARATION

- There will be an extensive discussion with you about the particulars of a colostomy.
- You will be given instructions on how to clean out your bowel.
- Do not eat or drink anything for 8 hours before the operation.

☐ OPERATION

- You will be asleep for the operation.
- The incision will run up and down your lower abdomen as well as around your anal area.
- The colostomy bag will be fitted and placed in position in the operating room.
- The operation usually takes about 3 hours.

POSTOPERATIVE CARE

- You will be taken to a recovery room and observed. After your blood pressure, pulse, and breathing are stable, you will be taken to a regular hospital room.
- You will have a thin plastic tube in your nose for a few days.
- A catheter will be in your bladder for several days.
- Pain will be controlled with medicine.
- After the tube in your nose is removed, you will be started on a liquid diet and advanced to solid food as you tolerate it.
- As with any operation, complications are always possible. With this type of operation, they can include bleeding, infection, pneumonia, blood clots, and possibly others.
- You should be able to go home in about 1 week.
- Arrangements will be made for your medicine, follow-up office visit, and stitch or clip removal.
- Arrangements will also be made for a home visiting nurse.

✚ HOME CARE

- Continue with the program started while you were in the hospital.
- You may walk about as you wish, even climb stairs, but don't overdo things.
- You will be given a suggested diet to follow during your convalescence.
- Take medicine as prescribed for your pain.
- While you are in the hospital, the nurse will teach you how to take care of your colostomy. Even so, in the beginning a visiting nurse will help you at home. Soon, you will be able to easily take care of things by yourself.
- You may return to work when you feel up to it.

✆ CALL OUR OFFICE IF

- The wound becomes swollen and red, or there is drainage from it.
- You develop a temperature higher than 100°F.
- Your bowels don't move for 48 hours.
- You have any questions.

△ GENERAL INFORMATION

The *rectum* is that part of the large bowel that starts at the *anus* (the opening to the outside) and extends up for about 10 inches. The rest of the large bowel is called the *colon*. Cancer of the rectum is common in older adults. The cause of cancer in a case such as yours is not truly known.

COMMON SIGNS AND SYMPTOMS

- In the early stages there often are no symptoms.
- Blood may be found in the stool by the patient or by the doctor when doing a routine physical examination.
- The stool may be thinner because it has to squeeze past the cancer.
- Sometimes the cancer produces the urge to have a bowel movement but nothing comes out.

DIAGNOSIS

- Often the diagnosis can be made by taking a detailed history, doing a thorough physical examination, and considering the laboratory report.
- *Flexible sigmoidoscopy*: This is a valuable, often routine procedure. A smooth, flexible optical instrument that is as thick as your little finger and has a light at its tip is used to examine the lower 25 or so inches of your bowel.
- *Colonoscopy*: This is done with an instrument that has lenses in it and a light at its tip, is smooth and flexible, and is as big around as your little finger. During the procedure you will be given medicine that will make you feel drowsy. The tip of the instrument will be introduced through the anus and carefully advanced up your entire large bowel, which is thoroughly examined. If any suspicious tissue is seen, a small piece of it can be taken *(biopsy)* for laboratory examination.
- *Ultrasound*: A thin instrument very much like an enema tip (a *probe*) is placed in the rectum, and the tip is positioned over the tumor. Harmless sound waves coming from the tip of the probe are aimed at the tumor in your rectum. The sound waves bouncing back (the echoes) from this area are seen as a picture on a screen. Ultrasound is a convenient and painless way to examine the tumor to see how deeply it is penetrating the rectum. This helps determine the type of operation that will be needed.
- *CT scan (computed tomography scan)*: These x-rays are taken as very thin slices through the area of the rectum. This makes it possible to see details in the rectum and any growths outside it.
- *Cystoscopy*: This procedure involves looking into your bladder if it is felt the cancer is close by.
- In women, the vagina also is examined carefully.

○ TREATMENT

The best chance to cure a cancer of the rectum that has not spread to distant areas is by an operation.

- The type of operation required is influenced by the following:
  - The size of the cancer.
  - The exact location of the cancer.
  - How deeply it penetrates the wall of the rectum.
  - Whether the lymph nodes in the area are involved or are likely to be involved.
  - Your general condition.

The two operations most commonly used to treat cancer of the rectum are as follows:

- Removal of most of the rectum and the cancer in it through an abdominal incision. The cut ends of the rectum are reconnected. There is no colostomy. This operation is more suitable for a cancer that is not too close to the anus. This operation may affect your sex life.
- Removal of the rectum and anus and creation of a permanent colostomy. This operation will almost surely affect your sex life. This operation is best when the cancer involves some of the anus or when the entire rectum and anus need to be removed.

After the most careful consideration of all factors, the recommendation is that you have an operation that involves removing most of your rectum and then reconnecting the cut ends. The anus is left in place and you can have bowel movements as before (Figs. 1 and 2).

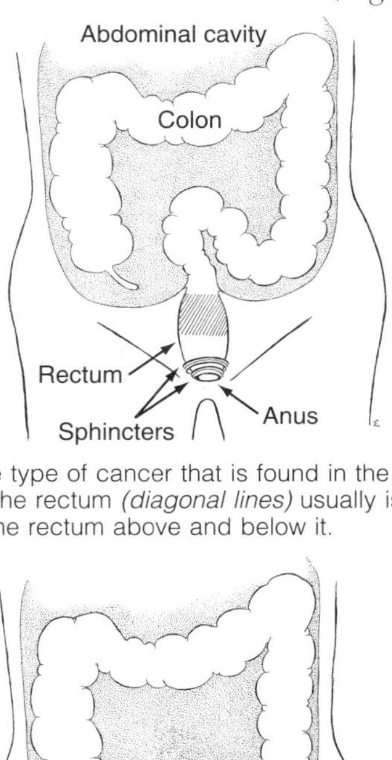

Figure 1. The type of cancer that is found in the middle and upper part of the rectum *(diagonal lines)* usually is removed along with some rectum above and below it.

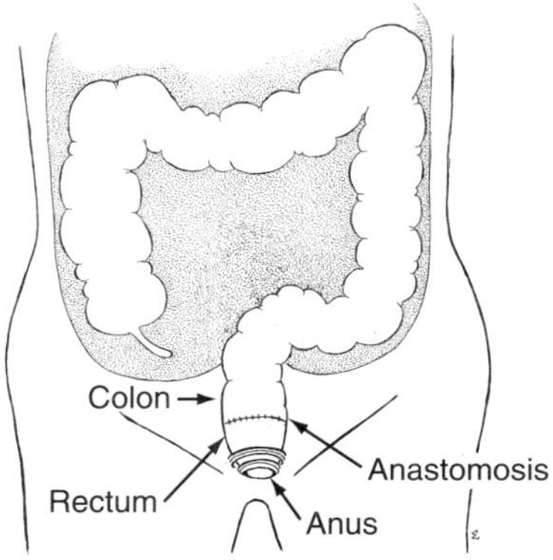

Figure 2. The divided ends of the rectum are reconnected. This makes it possible to continue having bowel movements the usual way. This operation is done through the abdomen.

PREOPERATIVE PREPARATION

- You will be given instructions on how to clean out your bowel.
- Do not eat or drink anything for 8 hours before the operation.

☐ OPERATION

- You will be asleep for the operation.
- The incision will run up and down your lower abdomen.
- The operation usually takes about 3 hours.

POSTOPERATIVE CARE

- You will be taken to a recovery room and observed. After your blood pressure, pulse, and breathing are stable, you will be taken to a regular hospital room.
- You will have a thin plastic tube in your nose for a few days.
- A catheter will be in your bladder for several days.
- Pain will be controlled with medicine.
- After the tube in your nose is removed, you will be started on a liquid diet and advanced to solid food as you tolerate it.
- As with any operation, complications are always possible. With this type of operation, they can include bleeding, infection, pneumonia, blood clots, and possibly others.
- You should be able to go home in about 1 week.
- Arrangements will be made for your medicine, follow-up office visit, and stitch or clip removal.

✚ HOME CARE

- Continue with the program started while you were in the hospital.
- You may walk about as you wish, even climb stairs, but don't overdo things.
- You will be given a suggested diet to follow during your convalescence. Include plenty of roughage and liquids in your diet to help prevent constipation.
- Take the medicines prescribed for you.
- Unless instructed otherwise, you may shower as you wish.
- You may return to work when you feel up to it.

✆ CALL OUR OFFICE IF

- The wound becomes swollen and red, or there is drainage from it.
- You develop a temperature higher than 100°F.
- Your bowels don't move for 48 hours.
- You have any questions.

△ GENERAL INFORMATION

The *rectum* is that part of the large bowel that starts at the *anus* (the opening to the outside) and extends up for about 10 inches. The rest of the large bowel is called the *colon*. Cancer of the rectum is common in older adults. The cause of cancer in a case such as yours is not truly known.

COMMON SIGNS AND SYMPTOMS

- In the early stages there often are no symptoms.
- Blood may be found in the stool by the patient or by the doctor when doing a routine physical examination.
- The stool may be thinner because it has to squeeze past the cancer.
- Sometimes the cancer produces the urge to have a bowel movement but nothing comes out.

DIAGNOSIS

- Often the diagnosis can be made by taking a detailed history, doing a thorough physical examination, and considering the laboratory report.
- *Flexible sigmoidoscopy:* This is a valuable, often routine procedure. A smooth, flexible optical instrument that is as thick as your little finger and has a light at its tip is used to examine the lower 25 or so inches of your bowel.
- *Colonoscopy:* This is done with an instrument that has lenses in it and a light at its tip, is smooth and flexible, and is as big around as your little finger. During the procedure you will be given medicine that will make you feel drowsy. The tip of the instrument will be introduced through the anus and carefully advanced up your entire large bowel, which is thoroughly examined. If any suspicious tissue is seen, a small piece of it can be taken (a *biopsy*) for laboratory examination.
- *Ultrasound:* A thin instrument very much like an enema tip (a *probe*) is placed in the rectum and the tip positioned over the tumor. Harmless sound waves coming from the tip of the probe are aimed at the tumor. The sound waves bouncing back (the echoes) from this area are seen as a picture on a screen. Ultrasound is a convenient and painless way to examine the tumor to see how deeply it is penetrating the rectum. This helps determine the type of operation that will be needed.
- *CT scan (computed tomography scan):* These x-rays are taken as very thin slices through the area of the rectum. This makes it possible to see details in the rectum and any growths outside it.
- *Cystoscopy:* This procedure involves looking into your bladder if it is felt the cancer is close by.
- In women, the vagina also is examined carefully.

○ TREATMENT

The best chance to cure a cancer of the rectum that has not spread to distant areas is by an operation.

- The type of operation required is influenced by the following:
  - The size of the cancer.
  - The exact location of the cancer.
  - How deeply it penetrates the wall of the rectum.
  - Whether the lymph nodes in the area are involved or are likely to be involved.
  - Your general condition.

There are several operations to treat cancer of the rectum:

- Removal of most of the rectum and the cancer in it through an abdominal incision. The cut ends of the rectum are reconnected. There is no colostomy. This operation is more suitable for a cancer that is not too close to the anus. This operation may affect your sex life.
- Removal of the rectum as well as the anus and creation of a permanent colostomy. This operation will almost surely affect your sex life.
- Another operation involves removing the cancer entirely through the anus without cutting the anus or making an abdominal incision (or a colostomy). This operation requires special instruments and techniques and is called transanal endoscopic microsurgical resection (TEM). This is a suitable operation for a cancer that is small, does not penetrate deeply into the wall of the rectum, is located away from the anus, and has not spread to the lymph nodes nearby. Few patients are suitable candidates for this type of operation.

After the most careful consideration of all factors, the recommendation is that you have an operation that involves removing your cancer entirely through the anus and without an abdominal incision (Fig. 1).

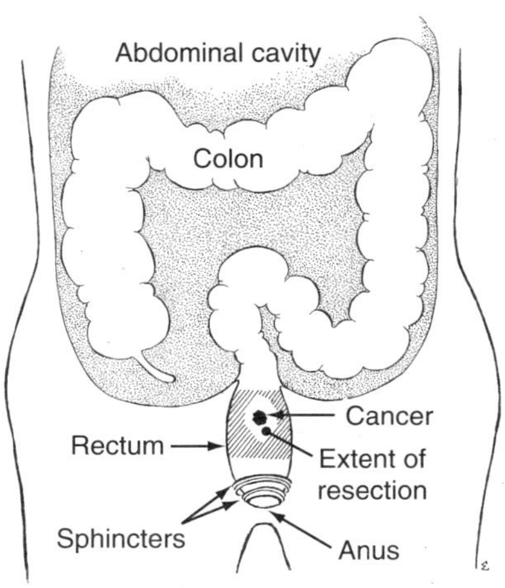

Figure 1. Cancer that is located in the middle and upper third of the rectum most often is removed along with normal rectum above and below it *(diagonal lines)* and the cut ends reconnected. Usually this operation is done through the abdomen. On occasion, small cancers *(dark area)* in this location that are superficial (they do not penetrate deeply) can be removed entirely through the anus with no abdominal incision. (Resection margins indicated by the white area around the cancer.) This technique requires special instruments and techniques.

PREOPERATIVE PREPARATION

- You will be given instructions on how to clean out your bowel.
- Do not eat or drink anything for 8 hours before the operation.

□ OPERATION

- You will be asleep for the operation.
- The operation usually takes about 3 hours.

POSTOPERATIVE CARE

- You will be taken to a recovery room and observed. After your blood pressure, pulse, and breathing are stable, you will be taken to a regular hospital room.
- A catheter will be in your bladder for several days.
- Your anus will be quite sore for several days. Pain will be controlled with medicine.
- You will be started on a liquid diet and then advanced to more solid foods.
- As with any operation, complications are always possible. With this type of operation, they can include bleeding, infection, blood clots, and possibly others.
- You should be able to go home in about 3 to 5 days.
- Arrangements will be made for your medicine and follow-up office visit.

✚ HOME CARE

- You may walk about as you wish, even climb stairs, but don't overdo things.
- You will be given a suggested diet to follow during your convalescence.
- Take medicines as prescribed for you.
- You may return to work when you feel up to it.

✆ CALL OUR OFFICE IF

- You develop a temperature higher than 100°F.
- Your bowels don't move for 48 hours.
- You have any questions.

RECTAL PROLAPSE: Perineal Repair

△ GENERAL INFORMATION

Rectal prolapse is a condition in which part of the rectum starts to come out through the anus or actually does come out (Fig. 1). It occurs most often in children younger than 3 years of age and in older women.

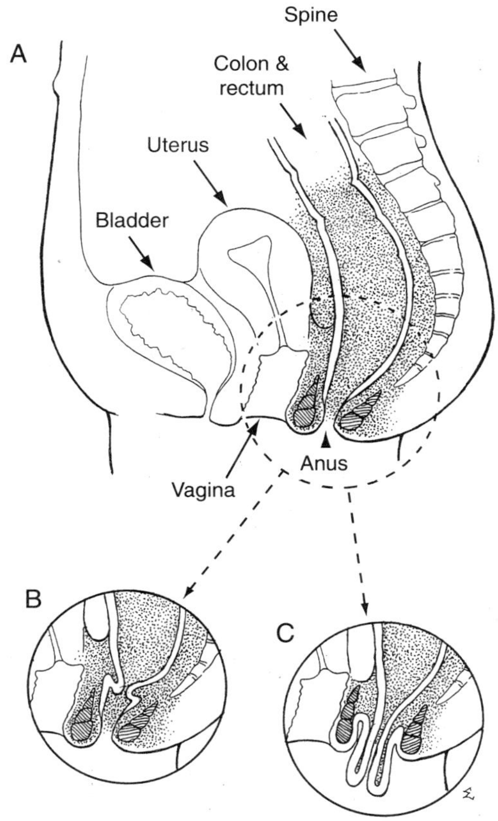

Figure 1. *A*, Normal anatomy of the female pelvis. *B*, Close-up view of the anus. *C*, Close-up view showing the lining *(mucosa)* of the rectum prolapsing through the anus and coming to the outside.

COMMON SIGNS AND SYMPTOMS

The symptoms depend a lot on the seriousness of the condition and can include the following:

- A little of the lining of the rectum (the *mucosa*) hangs out, giving the appearance of hemorrhoids.
- Mucus is discharged from the prolapsed mucosa.
- There is fecal soiling of the anal area or the underclothing.
- There is bleeding.
- A few inches of rectum hang out, especially after a bowel movement, and need to be pushed back in.
- Sometimes there is severe constipation.

DIAGNOSIS

- A meticulous history is taken, including, in females, the number of births and their difficulty and details of a hysterectomy if one has been done. You will be asked about any urinary or fecal incontinence, constipation, use of enemas, injuries to your back, nerve problems, and prior operations on the anus.

At least some, and possibly all, of the following will be done:

- An examination of your blood, urine, heart (EKG), and lungs (chest x-ray).
- *Barium enema:* Liquid barium (it has the consistency of buttermilk) will be given somewhat like a regular enema and x-rays taken of it as it flows throughout the colon. This can reveal unsuspected problems in the colon.
- *Colonoscopy:* This is done with an instrument that has lenses in it and a light at its tip, is smooth and flexible, and is as big around as your little finger. During the colonoscopy, you will be given medicine to make you feel drowsy. The tip of the instrument will be gently introduced into your anus and then advanced until your entire large bowel is examined.
- If you suffer from constipation, a detailed discussion will take place about your diet and eating habits. If you have done all the right things and they have not helped, special x-ray studies will be done to see how well your colon and rectum move.
- The strength of your sphincters will be measured.
- *Ultrasonography*: Harmless, painless ultrasound waves will be used to study your anal sphincter to see if it is scarred or torn, even though on the surface everything may appear normal.

○ TREATMENT

- There are a number of operations for rectal prolapse. Which one is best for you depends on the following:
  - The degree of prolapse.
  - Associated problems in the area.
  - The presence of fecal or urinary incontinence or constipation.
  - Other general conditions that may add to the problem.
  - The reasons for your wanting care.
- The goals of any operation are to improve the symptoms by anchoring the colon and the rectum inside your pelvis so that they are not able to slide down.
- The repair of rectal prolapse can be done either entirely from the bottom (perineal) area or entirely from the abdomen. From the abdomen, the operation can be done with the abdomen open, or it can be done without a regular incision by using long tubes called laparoscopes that are the size of your little finger. They are inserted into your abdomen through tiny incisions.

After careful consideration of all factors, the recommendation is that you have an operation to repair your prolapse and that this be done through the bottom, the perineal route.

PREOPERATIVE PREPARATION

- You will have an examination of your blood, urine, heart (EKG), and lungs (chest x-ray).
- Do not eat or drink anything for 8 hours before the operation.
- You will be instructed on how to clean out your bowel.

□ OPERATION

- You will be asleep for the operation.
- The incision will be entirely in your anal area; there will not be an abdominal incision.
- The length of the operation depends on what is found and what needs to be done.

POSTOPERATIVE CARE

- You will be taken to a recovery room and observed. When your blood pressure, pulse, and breathing are stable, you will be taken to a regular hospital room.
- There will be a catheter in your bladder to drain the urine for a short period.
- That evening you will be helped to sit up in bed and on the next day to get out of bed.
- When you are able to take food by mouth, your diet will be regulated so that you will have a soft, formed stool.
- You should be able to go home in about 3 days.
- Arrangements will be made for your medicine, follow-up office visit, and stitch removal.

✚ HOME CARE

- You may walk about as you wish, even climb stairs, but don't overdo things.
- An appropriate diet will be outlined for you.
- Include plenty of roughage and liquids in your diet to help prevent constipation.
- You may shower if you wish.
- Engaging in sexual intercourse too soon can be harmful to your recovery. If you wish, we can talk about this during your follow-up visit.
- You may return to work when you feel up to it.

✆ CALL OUR OFFICE IF

- The incision becomes red or swollen, or there is drainage from it.
- You develop a temperature higher than 100°F.
- You do not have a bowel movement for 2 days.
- You have any questions.

△ GENERAL INFORMATION

Rectal prolapse is a condition in which part of the rectum starts to come out through the anus or actually does come out (Fig. 1). It occurs most often in children younger than 3 years of age and in older women.

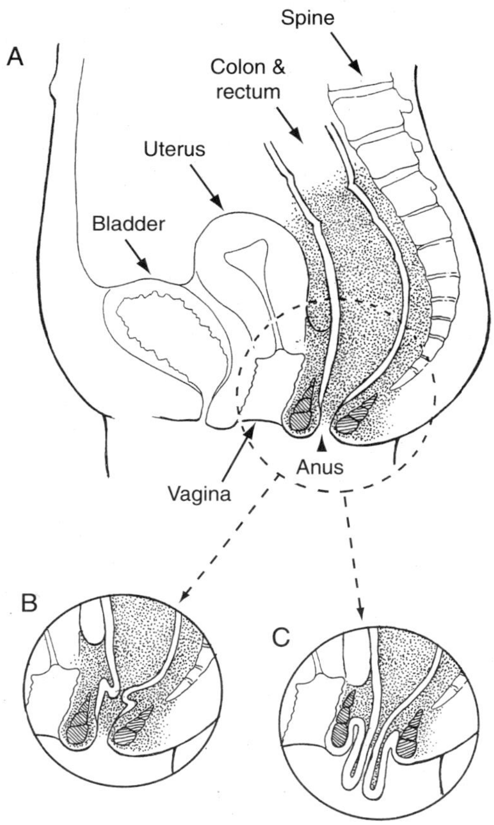

Figure 1. *A*, Normal anatomy of the female pelvis. *B*, Close-up view of the anus. *C*, Close-up view showing the lining (mucosa) of the rectum prolapsing through the anus and coming to the outside.

COMMON SIGNS AND SYMPTOMS

The symptoms depend a lot on the seriousness of the condition and can include the following:

- Some of the lining of the rectum (the *mucosa*) hangs out, giving the appearance of hemorrhoids.
- Mucus is discharged from the prolapsed mucosa.
- There is fecal soiling of the anal area or the underclothing.
- There is bleeding.
- A few inches of rectum hang out, especially after a bowel movement, and need to be pushed back in.
- Sometimes there is severe constipation.

DIAGNOSIS

- A meticulous history will be taken including, in females, the number of births and their difficulty and details of a hysterectomy if one has been done. You will be asked about any urinary or fecal incontinence, constipation, use of enemas, injuries to your back, nerve problems, and prior operations on the anus.

At least some, and possibly all, of the following will be done:

- An examination of your blood, urine, heart (EKG), and lungs (chest x-ray).
- *Barium enema:* Liquid barium (it has the consistency of buttermilk) will be given somewhat like a regular enema and x-rays taken of it as it flows throughout the colon. This can reveal unsuspected problems in the colon.
- *Colonoscopy:* This is done with an instrument that has lenses in it and a light at its tip, is smooth and flexible, and is as big around as your little finger. During the colonoscopy, you will be given medicine to make you feel drowsy. The tip of the instrument will be gently introduced into your anus and then advanced until your entire large bowel is examined.
- If you suffer from constipation, a detailed discussion will take place about your diet and eating habits. If you have done all the right things and they have not helped, special x-ray studies will be done to see how well your colon and rectum move.
- The strength of your sphincters will be measured.
- *Ultrasonography:* Harmless, painless ultrasound waves will be used to study your anal sphincter to see if it is scarred or torn, even though on the surface everything may appear normal.

○ TREATMENT

- There are a number of operations for rectal prolapse. Which one is best for you depends on the following:
  - The degree of prolapse.
  - Associated problems in the area.
  - The presence of fecal or urinary incontinence or constipation.
  - Other general conditions that may add to the problem.
  - The reasons for your wanting care.
- The goals of any operation are to improve the symptoms by anchoring the colon and the rectum inside your pelvis so that they are not able to slide down.
- The repair of rectal prolapse can be done either entirely from the bottom (perineal) area or entirely from the abdomen. From the abdomen the operation can be done with the abdomen open, or it can be done without a regular incision using long tubes called laparoscopes that are the size of your little finger. They are inserted into your abdomen through tiny incisions.

After careful consideration of all factors, the recommendation is that you have your rectal prolapse corrected through an abdominal incision.

PREOPERATIVE PREPARATION

- You will have an examination of your blood, urine, heart (EKG), and lungs (chest x-ray).

- Do not eat or drink anything for 8 hours before the operation.
- You will be instructed on how to clean out your bowel.

☐ OPERATION

- You will be asleep for the operation.
- The incision will run downwards from your umbilicus (belly button).
- The length of the operation depends on what is found and what needs to be done.

POSTOPERATIVE CARE

- You will be taken to a recovery room and observed. When your blood pressure, pulse, and breathing are stable, you will be taken to a regular hospital room.
- There will be a catheter in your bladder to drain the urine for a short period.
- That evening you will be helped to sit up in bed and on the next day to get out of bed.
- When you are able to take food by mouth, your diet will be regulated so that you will have a soft, formed stool.
- You should be able to go home in about 3 days.
- Arrangements will be made for your medicine, follow-up office visit, and stitch removal.

✚ HOME CARE

- You may walk about as you wish, even climb stairs, but don't overdo things.
- An appropriate diet will be outlined for you.
- Include plenty of roughage and liquids in your diet to help prevent constipation.
- You will be instructed on when you can bathe or shower.
- You may return to work when you feel up to it.

✆ CALL OUR OFFICE IF

- The incision becomes red or swollen, or there is drainage from it.
- You develop a temperature higher than 100°F.
- You do not have a bowel movement for 2 days.
- You have any questions.

△ GENERAL INFORMATION

Tumors that appear low in the rectum almost always are new growths that start in the lining (the *rectal mucosa*). Treatment usually depends on how deeply the tumor penetrates the mucosa and the tissue under the mucosa. This is especially important for tumors that are cancerous, for the following reasons:

- Tumors that are *superficial*, that is, shallow and not deeply penetrating, can sometimes be treated with a local operation and x-ray treatment without having to remove the rectum.
- On the other hand, tumors that are *penetrating* need wide and deep excision. Because such tumors are so close to the anus, it means that the anus also must be removed. Such a patient would end up with a permanent colostomy. In a colostomy, the stool empties into bag attached to the side of the abdomen.

Because of these important differences in treatment for two different conditions that on the surface can appear the same, it is necessary to find out how deeply the tumor penetrates into the wall of the rectum. This can help the surgeon to avoid giving a colostomy to a patient who could be treated just as well with a more limited operation. This is where ultrasound comes in.

ULTRASOUND

- Ultrasound involves the use of harmless and painless sound waves that are aimed at an area of your body. The sound waves bouncing back (the echoes) from the area are seen as pictures on a screen. This is a convenient, painless, and harmless way to examine organs and other tissue inside your body.

RECTAL ULTRASOUND

Preparation

- You will be given an enema an hour or so before the procedure.

Equipment

- The part of the ultrasound apparatus that sends out and receives the sound waves needs to be as close to the tumor as possible to produce the clearest and most accurate pictures.
- In rectal ultrasound a probe as big around as your little finger that is shaped like an enema nozzle is inserted into your rectum. The sound waves come out of its tip and go in all directions. The sound waves cannot be heard and they produce no sensation at all, so you won't feel any discomfort (Fig. 1).

Procedure

- You will lie on your side on a comfortable table.
- If you have not had a proctoscopy very recently, one will be done now. This is to double-check the placement of the probe so that it lies on top of the tumor during the next step of this procedure.
- The ultrasound probe will be lubricated and gently inserted inside your rectum.
- The tip of the probe will be passed back and forth across the tumor growth and the sound waves bouncing back will be observed on a screen. Permanent pictures will be taken of any important views.
- At the conclusion of the examination, the probe will be slipped out of the rectum, and you will be free to go about your business. In the meantime, all the pictures will be assembled and carefully examined.
- Arrangements will be made for an office visit to discuss the findings with you and how they will influence your care.

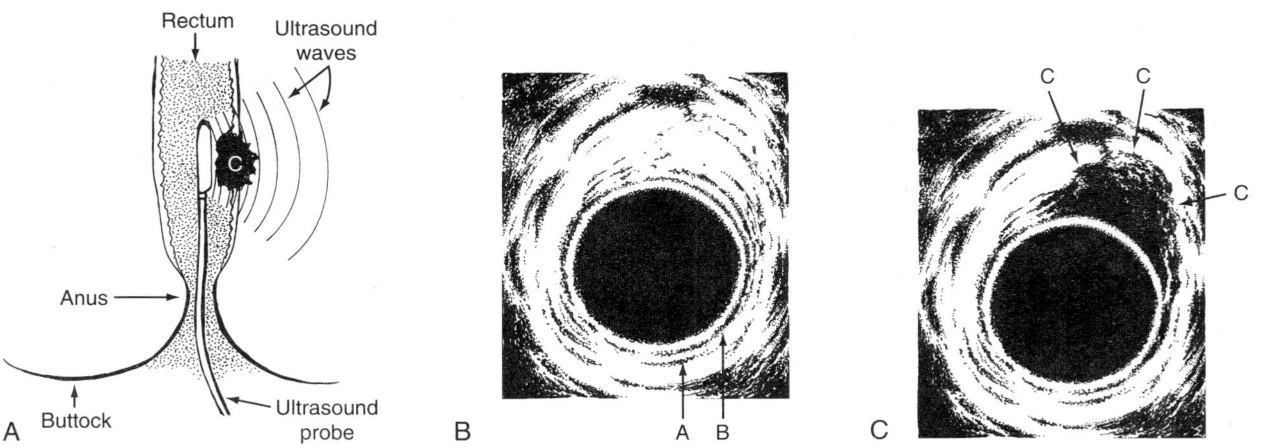

Figure 1. *A,* Side view of the rectum, showing the ultrasound probe positioned over a cancer. *B,* Ultrasound view of a normal rectum. The dark central area is the inside of the rectum. The circles marked A and B are the muscles around the rectum. *C,* A rectum with cancer in it. The arrows (C) indicate where the cancer has penetrated deeply into the muscle layers surrounding the rectum.

△ GENERAL INFORMATION

The vagina is located immediately in front of the rectum and behind the bladder (Fig. 1). The rectum is separated from the vagina by a thick sheet of muscle and tissue that can stretch remarkably. During childbirth, the vaginal tissue stretches and never completely regains its strength and tone. This happens with each delivery. As a woman ages, the tissue relaxes even more. If this weak tissue bulges into the vagina, it is called a *rectocele* (Fig. 2).

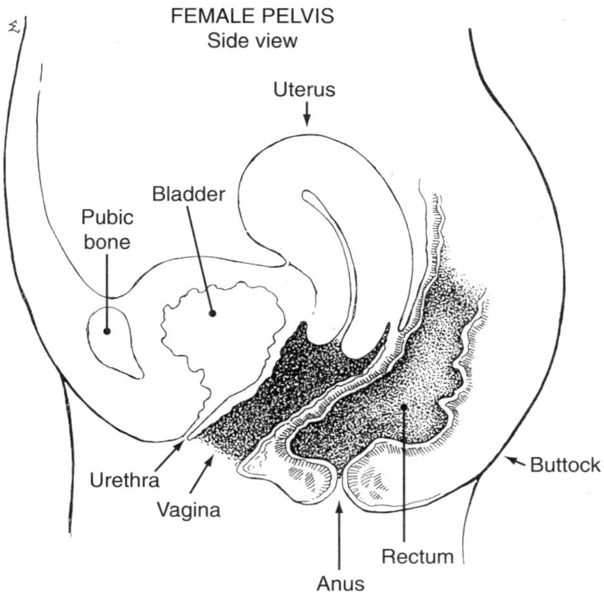

Figure 1.

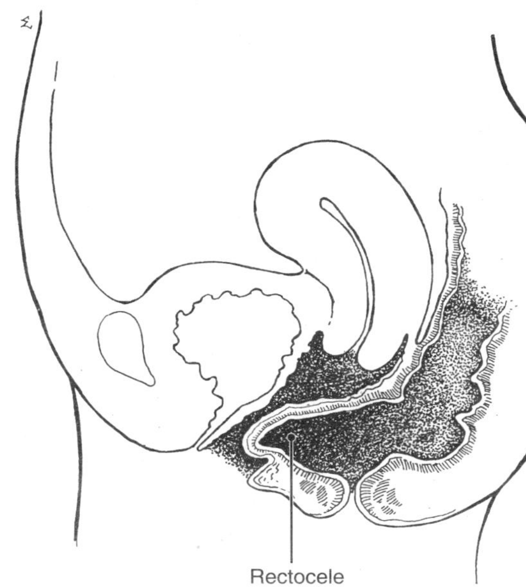

Figure 2. The bulge in the back wall of the vagina that is next to the rectum is called a *rectocele*. This bulge is corrected by the operation.

COMMON SIGNS AND SYMPTOMS

- There is a bulge on the back side of the vagina.
- When you strain during a bowel movement, this bulge enlarges, making it difficult to have a proper bowel movement.

DIAGNOSIS

- Usually, the diagnosis can be made by taking a detailed history and doing a thorough physical examination of this area of your body.
- The bulge in the back part of the vagina becomes more obvious when "pushing down" as though having a bowel movement. Sometimes the bulge becomes large enough that it comes out the opening of the vagina.
- Barium may be placed in your rectum and special x-rays taken. This will make it possible to see more clearly where the area of weakness is and where the repair needs to be done.
- Probes (something like an enema tip) are placed inside your vagina and anus. From the tip of these probes, harmless, painless sound waves are aimed at the area of the rectocele and also at your sphincter muscles. The sound waves bouncing back (the echoes) from this area are seen as pictures on a television screen that show the tissues in the vagina and where they are weak. They also show the condition of the muscles of your anus. This information helps the surgeon determine how they will be repaired.

○ TREATMENT

- It has been determined that the back part of your vagina is weakened (you have a rectocele) and that it needs to be repaired.

PREOPERATIVE PREPARATION

- You will have an examination of your blood, urine, heart (EKG), and lungs (chest x-ray).
- You will be instructed on how to clean out your bowel.
- Do not eat or drink anything for 8 hours before the operation.
- Do not douche or place anything in your vagina on the day of the operation.
- You may be given medicine that will make you feel drowsy before you are brought to the operating room.

□ OPERATION

- You will be asleep for the operation or be offered a spinal type of anesthesia, which will numb the area.
- The incision will be at the back part of the opening of your vagina as well as inside the vagina.
- You will not need a blood transfusion.
- The operation usually takes about 2 hours.

POSTOPERATIVE CARE

- You will be taken to a recovery room. When your blood pressure, pulse, and breathing are stable, you will be taken to a regular hospital room.

- There will be a catheter in your bladder for a day or so. This will make it easier for the urine to drain from the bladder.
- Pain will be controlled with medicine.
- That evening you will be helped to sit up in bed and on the next day to get out of bed.
- Your diet will be as you tolerate it.
- You should be able to go home in about 2 or 3 days.
- As with any operation, complications are always possible. With this type of operation, they can include bleeding, infection, separation of the wound, and possibly others.
- Arrangements will be made for your medicine and follow-up office visit. The stitches will be absorbed and do not require removal.

✣ HOME CARE

- You may walk about as you wish, even climb stairs, but don't overdo things.
- Do not douche or place anything in your vagina until we discuss it during your follow-up office visit. A sanitary pad can be used for any light drainage that may occur.
- Don't lift anything heavier than 5 pounds. Ask someone to do it for you.
- Be careful that you do not become constipated.
  - Include enough roughage and plenty of liquids in your diet.
  - You may need a mild laxative (example: milk of magnesia).
- You may shower as you wish. Avoid bathing for 2 weeks. Soaking this area too soon may not be desirable.
- Take medicine as prescribed for your pain.
- Engaging in sexual intercourse too soon can be harmful to your recovery. If you wish, let's talk about this during your follow-up visit.
- You may return to work when you feel up to it.

✆ CALL OUR OFFICE IF

- You do not have a bowel movement in a 36-hour period.
- The incision becomes red or swollen, or there is drainage from it.
- You develop a temperature higher than 100°F.
- You have any questions.

RECTOVAGINAL FISTULA (HIGH):
Transabdominal Repair

△ GENERAL INFORMATION

A rectovaginal fistula is an abnormal connection between the rectum and the vagina (Figs. 1 and 2). Correcting this condition can be a challenging problem for the following reasons: There are a number of causes; it can produce a variety of symptoms; there can be associated conditions that interfere with the treatment; and finally, there are a number of ways to repair it.

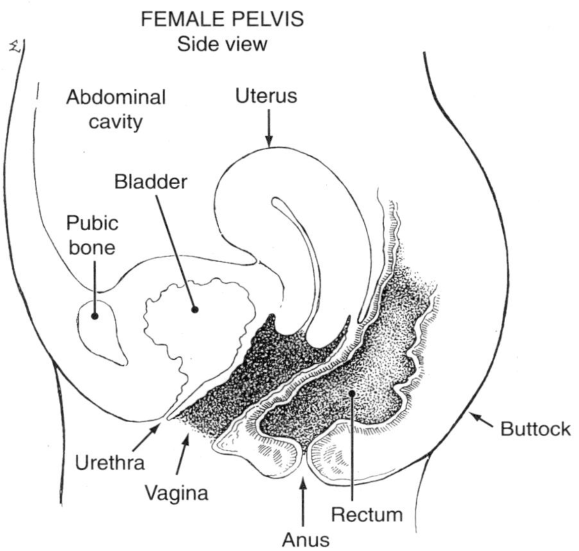

Figure 1. Normal female pelvic anatomy.

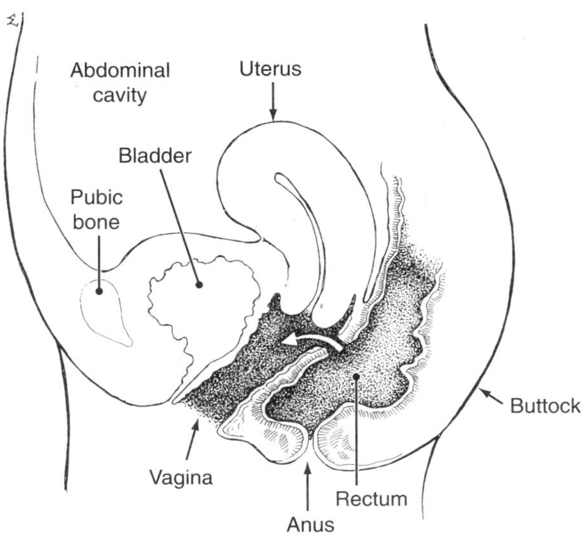

Figure 2. The operation to close an abnormal connection between the rectum and a point high in the vagina *(curved white arrow)* usually needs to be done through the abdomen. It cannot be done easily and properly from below.

COMMON SIGNS AND SYMPTOMS

- Most of the signs and symptoms are the result of feces coming into the vagina and the weakness of the damaged anal sphincter, which is no longer leakproof.
- The symptoms can include the following:
  - Flatus (gas) and stool in the vagina.
  - Foul discharge from the vagina.
  - Infection of the vagina.
  - Possible diarrhea, bleeding from the rectum, mucous discharge, anal spasm, and abdominal pain.

DIAGNOSIS

A detailed history will be taken to help determine the cause of the fistula and to help with the decision on the best treatment. A common history is one of a difficult delivery and tear of the tissue in the area.

- Sometimes the symptoms are strongly suggestive of a rectovaginal fistula, but nothing is seen on the physical examination. A blue dye is placed in the rectum and a tampon in the vagina. In 20 minutes, the tampon is removed. A blue stain on the tampon is evidence of a connection between the rectum and the vagina.
- *Proctoscopy*: This is done with a hollow instrument as big around as a dust mop handle that contains a magnifying lens and a light. While you lie on your side, the proctoscope is inserted gently into the rectum for a thorough examination.
- *Colonoscopy*: This is done with an optical instrument that is smooth, flexible, and as big around as your little finger, and that has a light at the tip. During the procedure, you will be given medicine that will make you feel drowsy. The tip of the instrument will be introduced gently through the anus and advanced until your entire large bowel is examined. If any suspicious tissue is seen, a small piece of it can be taken (a *biopsy*) for laboratory examination.
- *Ultrasonography*: This test uses a probe (something like an enema tip) that is placed inside the anus. From the tip of the probe, painless and harmless sound waves are sent out to the surrounding tissue. The sound waves bouncing back (the echoes) can be seen as pictures on a screen. They can show tears or scars of the sphincter muscle, even though the skin over this area looks normal.

○ TREATMENT

- The treatment for rectovaginal fistula is an operation. The choice of operation depends on the fistula's causes, location, and size; the types and seriousness of symptoms; the condition of the tissue around the fistula; associated problems that need to be taken care of; and the age and general condition of the individual.
- Generally, the techniques of repair involve an approach either from the abdomen or from the

bottom (the *perineum*). Very occasionally, both techniques may need to be used at the same time.

After careful consideration of all factors, the recommendation is that your repair be done through the abdomen.

PREOPERATIVE PREPARATION

- You will have an examination of your blood, urine, heart (EKG), and lungs (chest x-ray).
- You will be instructed on how to clean out your bowel.
- Do not eat or drink anything for 8 hours before the operation.
- Do not douche or use a tampon on the day of the operation.

□ OPERATION

- You will be asleep for the operation.
- The incision will be in your lower abdomen.
- The operation usually takes about 3 hours.

POSTOPERATIVE CARE

- You will be taken to a recovery room and observed. When your blood pressure, pulse, and breathing are stable, you will be taken to a regular hospital room.
- You may have a thin plastic tube in your nose for a few days.
- There will be a catheter in your bladder for a few days to empty the urine. This is more comfortable for you and helps with the healing.
- Pain will be controlled with medicine.
- That evening you will be helped to sit up in bed and on the next day to get out of bed.
- When your bowels start working, the tube in your nose will be removed and you will be started on a liquid to soft diet.
- You should be able to go home in 3 to 6 days.
- Arrangements will be made for your medicine, follow-up office visit, and stitch removal.
- As with any operation, complications are always possible. With your type of operation, they can include infection, break-down of the repair, blood clots, pneumonia, and possibly others.

✚ HOME CARE

- You may walk about as you wish, even climb stairs, but don't overdo things.
- Take medicine as prescribed for you.
- You will be given an appropriate diet to follow during your convalescence. This will include plenty of roughage and liquids in your diet to help prevent constipation. You may need to use a stool softener.
- Do not douche or use a tampon until after we discuss this during your postoperative office visit. A sanitary napkin should be sufficient for the expected vaginal discharge.
- Don't lift anything heavier than 5 pounds. Ask someone to do it for you.
- Engaging in sexual intercourse too soon can be harmful to your recovery. If you wish, let's talk about this during your follow-up visit.
- You may return to work when you feel up to it.

✆ CALL OUR OFFICE IF

- The incision becomes red or swollen, or there is drainage from it.
- You develop a temperature higher than 100°F.
- You do not have a bowel movement for 36 hours.
- You have any questions.

RECTOVAGINAL FISTULA (LOW): Transvaginal Repair

△ GENERAL INFORMATION

A *rectovaginal fistula* is an abnormal connection between the rectum and the vagina (Figs. 1 and 2). Correcting this condition can be a challenging problem for the following reasons: There are a number of causes; it can produce a variety of symptoms; there can be associated conditions that interfere with treatment; and finally, there are a number of ways to repair it.

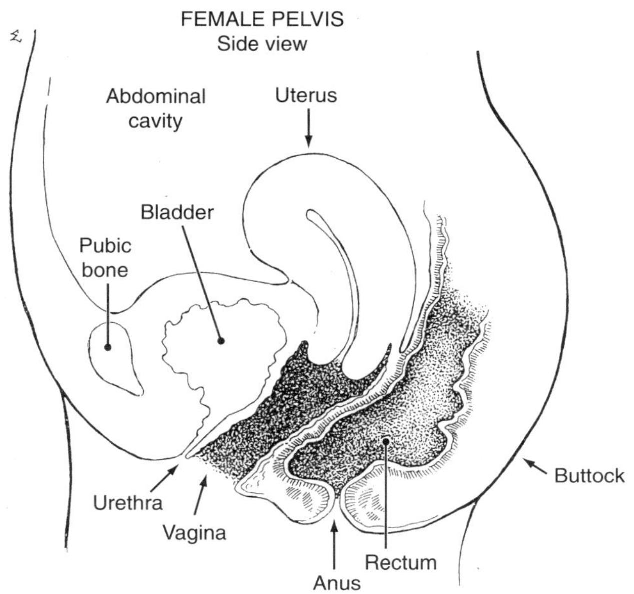

Figure 1. Normal female pelvic anatomy.

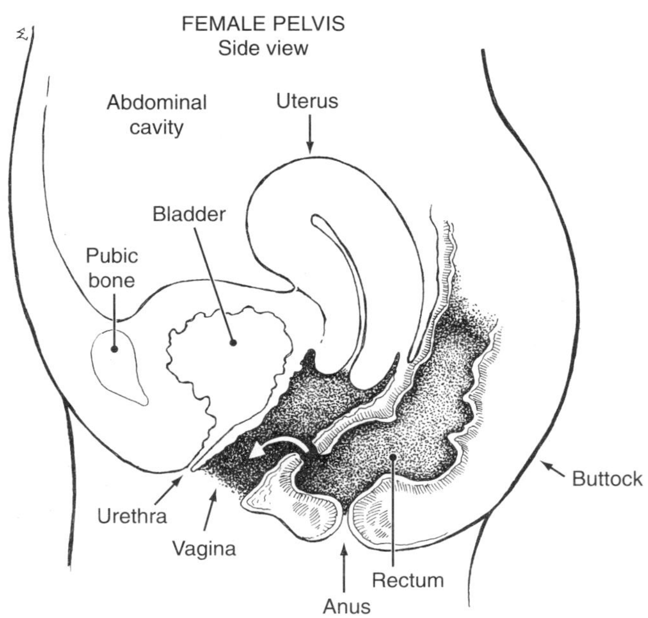

Figure 2. The operation to close an abnormal connection between the rectum and a point low in the vagina *(curved white arrow)* is done from below, with no need for an abdominal incision.

COMMON SIGNS AND SYMPTOMS

- Most of the signs and symptoms are the result of feces coming into the vagina and the weakness of the damaged anal sphincter, which is no longer leakproof.
- The symptoms can include the following:
  - Flatus and stool in the vagina.
  - Foul discharge from the vagina.
  - Infection of the vagina.
  - Possible diarrhea, bleeding from the rectum, mucous discharge, anal spasm, and abdominal pain. These, however, may result from a disease of the bowel that caused the fistula in the first place.

DIAGNOSIS

- A detailed history is taken because such information helps determine the cause of the fistula. In addition, it can help with the decision on the best treatment. For example, patients may report a history of a difficult, delivery and tear of the tissue in the area. Perhaps the seriousness of the tear was not recognized, or the tear was repaired but became infected. Rectovaginal fistulas are also common in patients with chronic colon conditions (example: Crohn's disease).
- Sometimes the symptoms are strongly suggestive of a rectovaginal fistula, but nothing is seen. A blue dye can be placed in the rectum and a tampon in the vagina. In 20 minutes, the tampon is removed. Blue staining of the tampon is evidence of a connection between the rectum and the vagina. There are a number of other clues and findings.
- *Proctoscopy:* This procedure is done with a hollow instrument the size of a dust mop handle that has magnifying lenses and a light in it. While you lie on your side, the proctoscope is lubricated and inserted gently into the rectum for a thorough examination.
- *Colonoscopy:* This procedure is done if disease of the bowel is suspected. An optical instrument that is smooth, flexible, and as big around as your little finger, and that has a light at its tip is inserted gently into your anus and then advanced until your entire large bowel is examined. If suspicious tissue is seen, a small piece of it can be taken (a *biopsy*) for laboratory examination. During the procedure you will be given medicine that will make you feel drowsy.
- *Ultrasonography:* This test uses a probe (something like an enema tip) that is placed inside the anus. From the tip of the probe, painless and harmless sound waves are sent out to the surrounding tissue. The sound waves bouncing back (the echoes) can be seen as pictures on a screen. They can show tears or scars of the sphincter muscle, even though the skin over this area looks normal. This is an important test. Many women who have a rectovaginal fistula also have a seriously scarred and weakened sphincter muscle. In such instances, just repairing the hole between the rectum and the vagina will not necessarily give a good result; fecal fluid still may

occasionally get past the weak sphincter and stain the underclothing.

THERAPY

There are a variety of treatments for rectovaginal fistula. Which one is best depends on the fistula's cause, location, and size; the number, types, and seriousness of symptoms; the condition of the tissue around the fistula; any associated problem that needs to be taken care of; and the age and general condition of the individual.

Generally, the techniques of repair involve an approach from the abdomen or from the vagina. Very occasionally, both techniques may need to be used at the same time.

After careful consideration of all factors, the recommendation is that you have the repair performed through the vagina. The reasons for this recommendation have been discussed with you.

PREOPERATIVE PREPARATION

- You will have an examination of your blood, urine, heart (EKG), and lungs (chest x-ray).
- You will be instructed on how to clean out your bowel.
- Do not eat or drink anything for 8 hours before the operation.
- Do not douche or use a tampon on the day of the operation.
- Shower or bathe as usual on the morning of the operation.
- You may be given medicine that will make you feel drowsy before you are brought to the operating room.

□ OPERATION

- You will be asleep for the operation.
- The incision will be in your vagina only. If the anal sphincter also needs to be repaired, the incision will also be around the anus. This will be discussed with you in detail before anything is planned or done.
- The operation usually takes about 3 hours.

POSTOPERATIVE CARE

- You will be taken to a recovery room and observed. When your blood pressure, pulse, and breathing are stable, you will be taken to a regular hospital room.
- You may have a thin plastic tube in your nose. It goes down into your stomach to suck up the air you swallow. It will be removed when your bowels start working.
- There will be a catheter in your bladder for a few days to empty the urine. This is more comfortable for you and helps with the healing.
- Pain can be controlled with medicine. The nurse will give it to you, or you can give yourself a preset amount of pain medicine when you feel you need it with a device connected to the tubing giving you intravenous fluids. This is called *patient controlled analgesia* (PCA).
- That evening after the operation you will be helped to sit up in bed and on the next day to get out of bed.
- When your bowels start working, the tube in your nose will be removed and you will be started on a liquid diet. This will be increased as you tolerate it.
- You should be able to go home in 3 to 6 days.
- Arrangements will be made for your medicine, follow-up office visit, and stitch removal.
- As with any operation, complications are always possible. With this type of operation, they can include infection, break-down of the repair, blood clots, pneumonia, and possibly others.

✚ HOME CARE

- You may walk about as you wish, even climb stairs, but don't overdo things.
- Take medicine as prescribed for your pain.
- You will be given an appropriate diet to follow during your convalescence.
- Be careful that you do not become constipated.
  - Include enough roughage and plenty of liquids in your diet.
  - You will be instructed on the use of a stool softener and possibly a mild laxative (example: milk of magnesia).
- Do not use a douche or tampon until after we discuss this during your postoperative office visit. A sanitary napkin should be sufficient for the expected vaginal discharge.
- Don't lift anything heavier than 5 pounds. Ask someone to do it for you.
- Engaging in sexual intercourse too soon can be harmful to your recovery. If you wish, let's talk about this during your follow-up visit.
- You may return to work when you feel up to it, but let's talk about it first during a follow-up office visit.

✆ CALL OUR OFFICE IF

- You develop any unusual signs or symptoms.
- The incision becomes red or swollen, or there is drainage from it.
- You develop a temperature higher than 100°F.
- You do not have a bowel movement in 24 hours.
- You have any questions.

RENAL ARTERY STENOSIS

△ GENERAL INFORMATION

There are many causes of *hypertension* (high blood pressure). The most common cause for which something physical can be done to correct the problem is narrowing *(stenosis)* of the artery to one or both kidneys. When the blood flow to a kidney is reduced, a number of chemical changes take place in the body that produce substances that raise the blood pressure.

An artery can be blocked in a number of ways. By far, the most common are cholesterol deposits *(atheroma)* in the wall of the artery and thickening of the artery *(hyperplasia)* so that it becomes narrower (Fig. 1).

COMMON SIGNS AND SYMPTOMS

- There may be an abrupt onset of high blood pressure. (Ordinary high blood pressure has a more gradual course.)
- There may be a peculiar humming sound (a *bruit*) heard with the stethoscope over the kidney area. It is produced by the jet of blood passing through the narrowed artery.

DIAGNOSIS

- Anyone having the abrupt appearance of high blood pressure, especially a child, adolescent, or pregnant woman, and having a humming sound over the kidney area should be suspected of having narrowing of the renal artery as the cause of the high blood pressure.
- *Renin assay*: This blood test can show whether the cause of the high blood pressure is narrowing of the renal artery.
- *Doppler ultrasound*: Harmless sound waves are aimed at the arteries to the kidney. The sound waves bouncing back (the echoes) from this area are seen as pictures on a screen. This is a convenient and painless way to see if there are any abnormalities in the artery to the kidney.
- *Arteriography*: Dye is injected into the aorta and pictures taken as the dye flows from the aorta into the renal arteries. It is the most accurate way to show the location of the narrowing and how extensive it is.

○ TREATMENT

The best treatment is to somehow get blood into the kidney through the narrowed artery. This involves an operation in which one or more of the following needs to be done:

- Place a bypass tube that bridges over the narrowed area to get blood from the normal part of the artery into the kidney.
- Remove the narrowed part of the artery and reconnect the normal cut ends.
- Place a tiny catheter with a small balloon attached to it in the artery. When the balloon reaches the narrow area, it is inflated to stretch the artery.
- Do a plastic operation on the artery to correct the narrowing.
- If possible, remove what is narrowing the artery.
- As a last resort, remove the kidney and the vessels because the artery and its branches are too badly damaged to correct.

After careful consideration of all factors, it is recommended that you have an operation to correct your problem.

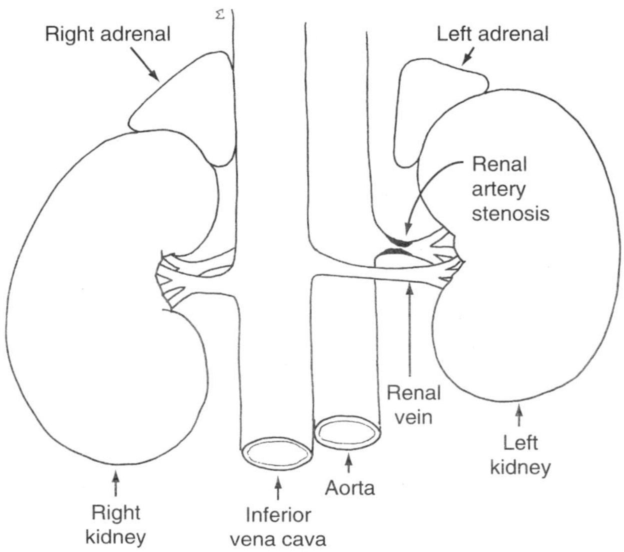

Figure 1. This is one type of renal stenosis.

PREOPERATIVE PREPARATION

- In addition to the tests already mentioned, your heart (EKG) and lungs (chest x-ray) will be examined.
- Special attention will be paid to the condition of other major vessels in the body, especially the aorta and the vessels to the legs and the brain.
- Do not eat or drink anything for 8 hours before the operation.
- Shower as usual on the morning of the operation.
- You may be given medicine that will make you feel drowsy before you are brought to the operating room.

□ OPERATION

- You will be asleep for the operation.
- You will not receive a blood transfusion unless it is absolutely necessary.
- The operation usually takes about 3 hours.

POSTOPERATIVE CARE

- You will be taken to a recovery room and observed. When your blood pressure, pulse, and breathing are stable, you will be taken to a regular hospital room.
- You will have a thin plastic tube in your nose. It goes down to your stomach to suck up the air you swallow. It will be removed when your bowels start working.

- Pain will be controlled with medicine.
- That evening you will be helped to sit up in bed and on the next day to get out of bed.
- After the tube in your nose is removed, your diet will be as you tolerate it.
- You will be able to go home as soon as your blood pressure is under satisfactory control.
- Arrangements will be made for your medicines, follow-up office visit, and stitch removal.
- As with any operation, complications are always possible, some of them serious. With your type of operation, they can include bleeding, pneumonia, infection, heart problems, clotting in the artery, and possibly others. Also, sometimes the blood pressure does not come down right away or completely.

✚ HOME CARE

- You may walk about as you wish, even climb stairs, but don't overdo things.
- Unless advised otherwise, you may shower as you wish with any dressings on or off. After you dry yourself, replace any dressings with clean, dry ones.
- Be certain to take all the medicines prescribed for you.
- Eat as you wish.
- Do not drive a car unless you can move freely and without pain and are not taking medicines that decrease your alertness.
- You may resume sexual activity whenever you wish.
- You may return to work when you feel up to it, but first let's talk about it during your follow-up visit.

✆ CALL OUR OFFICE IF

- You develop any unusual signs or symptoms.
- The incision becomes red or swollen, or there is drainage from it.
- You develop a temperature higher than 100°F.
- You have any questions.

△ GENERAL INFORMATION

Many thousands of women and men have cosmetic surgery of the nose. Because it occupies the center of the face, a nose that is too dominant, is misshapen, or is just not appropriate for the face can greatly affect a person's appearance.

The anatomy of the nose differs from person to person. Also, each nose has its own contours and proportions. This means that when choosing a plastic surgeon for rhinoplasty, it is wise to look for someone who has a continuing interest, specific training, and appropriate experience and who has demonstrated clinical skills in performing this operation. Getting an opinion from two plastic surgeons is appropriate.

CANDIDATES FOR RHINOPLASTY

By far, most persons have this operation for cosmetic improvement. For this reason, you should be sure you are having the operation because *you* want it, not because of someone else's desires or concerns.

First, the surgeon and you should discuss at least the following:

- What the problem is and what can be done about it.
  - The expected (not guaranteed) results.
  - Realistic expectations for the result.
  - The possibility that both your and the surgeon's expectations will not be realized.
  - The possible complications.

○ TREATMENT

- There are a number of specific and unique problems with each nose (Fig. 1). Each problem requires a different operative technique to correct it.
- Your particular problem, or combination of problems, as well as the method necessary to correct it will be discussed with you.

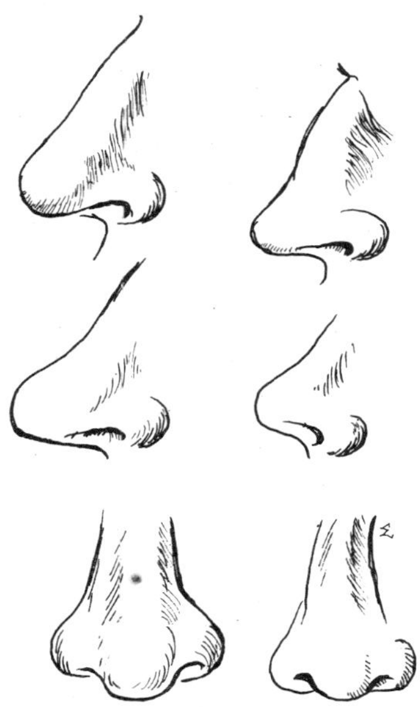

Figure 1. Illustrated are a few examples of noses whose appearance can be changed favorably by rhinoplasty.

PREOPERATIVE PREPARATION

- A detailed history will be taken and a physical examination will be carried out as it applies to your face, with particular emphasis on the nose.
- It will be necessary to make sure that you don't have any significant illness that would affect your ability to have the operation safely.
- There are some general medical conditions that affect the nose and the tissues inside it. These will be looked for and evaluated thoroughly before anything further is done.
- A number of photographs will be taken of you (with special emphasis on the nose) from several angles.
- You may be shown a gallery of photos of other patients to give you an example *(only)* of the possible outcome.
- Do not take aspirin or medicines containing aspirin, mood-altering drugs, garlic, vitamin E, multivitamins, or alcohol or smoke for 10 days before the operation.
- Shower or bathe as usual the morning of the operation.
- Thoroughly remove all makeup from your face, especially mascara.
- You will be given medicine that will make you feel drowsy before you are brought to the operating room.

□ OPERATION

- The operation will be done under local or general anesthesia. If it is done under local anesthesia, the entire nose will be made numb. Also, you will be given medicine that will keep you very drowsy.
- During the operation, you may feel some tugging but no pain.
- The operation usually takes 1 to 2 hours.
- Many patients have little memory of the operation itself.

POSTOPERATIVE CARE

- You will be taken to a recovery room. When your blood pressure, pulse, and breathing are stable and you are completely alert, you should be able to go home that same day with a responsible adult.
- You will have a firm, rigid dressing over your nose and a gauze dressing under the openings to collect any discharge.

✚ HOME CARE

- Restrict your activity only to things that are essential. Do not engage in any strenuous activity.
- During the day, keep your head elevated in either a sitting position or a reclining chair.
- During sleep, have two pillows under your head.
- Change the dressing at the tip of your nose as necessary. There will be some bloody drainage for 1 to 2 days.
- Take medicines as prescribed for pain.

- Do not blow your nose. Wipe or dab gently with tissue if necessary.
- Sneeze with your mouth open.
- It is easier to eat soft to liquid foods.
- Do not lift anything heavier than 5 pounds. Ask someone to do it for you.
- Do not bend over at the waist; bend at the knees.
- Do not remove the splint over the nose.
- If you use ice to help with any swelling around the eyes, be careful that the nose splint dressings do not get wet. The splint will be removed in about 1 week.
- Usually there are crusts of blood and other secretions in the nostrils. These can be softened by applying an antibiotic ointment with a cotton swab and gently removed.
- Avoid frequent or prolonged telephone conversations.
- You may brush your teeth gently with a soft brush. Avoid manipulating the upper lip.
- Wash your face carefully to avoid getting the dressings wet.
- Take baths until the dressings are removed.
- Do not wash your hair unless someone can do it for you and it is certain you will not get the nasal dressings wet.
- Avoid pullover clothing such as sweaters, T-shirts, or turtleneck sweaters.
- Do not swim for 4 to 6 weeks after the dressings are removed.
- Do not wear eyeglasses that rest on the nose for 4 to 6 weeks. You'll be shown how they can be supported by being taped to your forehead. You may wear contact lenses in 2 to 3 days.
- After the dressings and splint are removed, you may gently cleanse the skin of your nose with a mild soap or Vaseline lotion.

✆ CALL OUR OFFICE IF

- You have unusual signs or symptoms.
- There is bleeding from the nose.
- You develop a temperature higher than 100°F.
- You have any questions.

△ GENERAL INFORMATION

A mass in the *scrotum* (the sac behind the penis) can be a number of things. Because such a mass can either be something not to worry about or something that can be very serious, it is wise to see a doctor if such a condition is present.

The *testicle* is the organ that is most easily felt in the sac. All the normal structures in the scrotum are not easily felt unless something is wrong with them.

COMMON SIGNS AND SYMPTOMS

- There may be no symptoms at all, except that a mass may be present on the testicle or the entire testicle may be enlarged.
- Sometimes the entire scrotum is swollen so that a normal testicle inside it cannot be felt.
- Often, the mass in the testicle hurts; even the entire testicle may hurt.
- The mass or swelling can be there for quite a while, or it can appear almost overnight and be very painful.
- Very rarely, the entire scrotum (both right and left sides) is swollen.

DIAGNOSIS

Different problems can produce different symptoms and different findings on examination. The most important things are the history and the physical examination of the scrotum. Sometimes it is impossible to determine what is inside the scrotum just by examining it with the hands; some other tests may be necessary, including the following:

- *Transillumination*: The examining room is darkened and a bright focused light is placed directly on the skin of the scrotum. If the swelling in the scrotum is just clear fluid, the light usually goes through the thin skin of the scrotum and comes out through the other side, allowing the outline of the mass to be seen. If the fluid is something dense like blood or there is a solid mass, the light will not come through at all.
- *Ultrasound*: Harmless sound waves are aimed at the area of your scrotum. The sound waves bouncing back (the echoes) from this area are seen as a picture on a screen. This is a painless and convenient way to examine organs and tissues inside the scrotum.

The following are some of the possible diagnoses (Fig. 1):

- *Hernia*: A portion of the intestine has come through an opening in the muscle (the hernia) and traveled down toward the scrotum, usually the upper part of it. Most of the time, this mass goes away when the person lies down. This can occur at any age.
- *Tumor*: Usually, a mass can be felt on the testicle. The mass may enlarge gradually and not hurt. Sometimes, however, it occurs in a few hours and is very painful. This happens because of bleeding

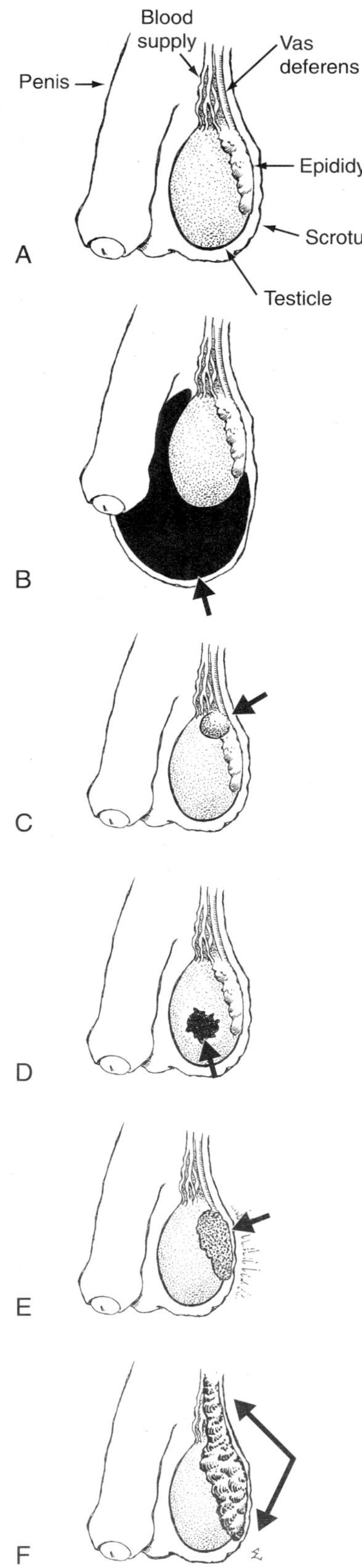

Figure 1. *A*, Normal contents of scrotum; *B*, hydrocele; *C*, spermatocele; *D*, cancer; *E*, acute epididymitis; *F*, chronic epididymitis.

within the tumor. In these circumstances, the testicle will be tender. Tumors are most commonly seen in younger men.

- *Hydrocele*: This is caused by too much fluid forming around the testicle and ballooning out the scrotum. Most of the time, the reason is not known. Sometimes fluid comes from an irritated testicle. Hydrocele can occur at any age but is most common in older adults.
- *Epididymitis*: This is an infection of the epididymis (the sperm is stored here) that spreads usually from an infection in the prostate, bladder, or penis. The skin of the scrotum is swollen, and the testicle is so tender that the person walks with a waddle so that the legs do not touch or bump the scrotum.
- *Spermatocele*: When a duct becomes blocked so that the sperm can't get past, the accumulated sperm forms a swelling (a *cyst*). It is usually the size of a cherry or cranberry.
- *Varicocele*: This is formed by the dilated veins that drain the testicle (like the varicose veins that drain the leg). These dilated veins in the scrotum feel like a "bag of worms" and occur more often on the left side.
- *Torsion of the testicle*: The testicle can suddenly twist on itself so that the veins cannot easily drain the blood from it. This causes the testicle to become swollen and very painful. An immediate operation is necessary; otherwise the testicle may become gangrenous and die.
- *Mumps orchitis*: This condition is uncommon. It is seen mostly in adolescents and young adults a week or so after the mumps start. The testicle is large and very tender.

Finally, even with all of these tests, it is sometimes not possible to make an exact diagnosis without performing an operation to open the scrotum and look inside. Sometimes the diagnosis and the treatment have to be done at the same time in the operating room while you are asleep.

The most likely diagnosis and the way to treat it will be explained to you in detail before anything is planned or done.

SEBACEOUS CYST

△ GENERAL INFORMATION

The human skin has several types of very tiny glands just under its surface. One such type is the sweat gland; another is the oil *(sebaceous)* gland that puts out very tiny amounts of very thick oils. Sometimes, the very tiny pore that lets these oils come to the surface gets plugged. Because the gland keeps on producing the oily material, it becomes enlarged. When it is large enough that you can feel it, it is called a *sebaceous cyst*. The material in it gradually becomes thick, has a cheese-like appearance, and has a sweaty odor (Fig. 1).

- A sebaceous cyst can stop growing when it is pea-sized or it can continue to grow until it is as big as a golf ball.
- Sebaceous cysts are not cancerous, and they never become cancerous.

COMMON SIGNS AND SYMPTOMS

- Sebaceous cysts usually appear as a smooth, dome-shaped growth in the skin, most commonly in the head and neck and upper back.
- They do not hurt unless they are infected.

DIAGNOSIS

- Usually, the diagnosis can be made by taking the history and doing a careful examination of the lump.

○ TREATMENT

- Removing the sebaceous cyst by an operation is the only way to cure the problem.

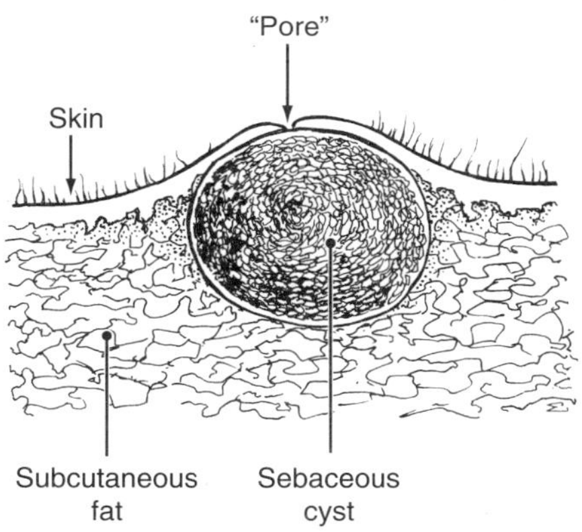

Figure 1. Usually a sebaceous cyst is removed entirely, including the "sac" that is part of it.

PREOPERATIVE PREPARATION

- Do not eat or drink anything for 4 hours before the operation.

□ OPERATION

- The skin over the sebaceous cyst will be painted with an antiseptic solution and surrounded with towels.
- A very fine, short needle will be used to inject an anesthetic around the area so that it will become completely numb.
- A cosmetic incision will be made and the cyst removed entirely.
- The operation usually takes less than 30 minutes.
- The incision will be closed in a similar cosmetic manner.
- If the cyst is infected and red and full of pus, then the wise thing is to simply make a small incision and let the pus out. A few weeks later, when things have quieted down and the sebaceous cyst is much smaller, it can be totally excised as described above.

POSTOPERATIVE CARE

- You should be able to go home directly after the operation.
- Arrangements will be made for your follow-up office visit and stitch removal.

✙ HOME CARE

- Resume your usual activities.
- You may shower as you wish with any dressings on or off.
  - There may be narrow strips of tape across the incision. It's all right if they get wet. They will be removed in the doctor's office.
  - After you dry yourself, replace any dressings with clean, dry ones.
- Pain is minimal and can be controlled with over-the-counter medicine.

✆ CALL OUR OFFICE IF

- The incision becomes red or swollen, or there is drainage from it.
- You develop a temperature higher than 100°F.
- You have any questions.

△ GENERAL INFORMATION

Shoulder pain can have many causes. Most commonly, however, it is the result of inflammation and swelling due to overuse, stress, strain, or trauma. But sometimes there is no apparent cause. The most commonly involved tissue is the rotator cuff, which is made up of a group of tendons from four muscles. These four muscles start at the shoulder blade *(scapula)* and then attach around the humerus (the upper arm bone) to form a cuff at the shoulder joint. Over the rotator cuff muscles is the *acromion*, which is a bone that sticks out from the upper part of the shoulder blade. In between the acromion and the rotator cuff is a *bursa*, which is a lubricating sac that provides a smooth gliding surface between the rotator cuff and the acromion bone (Fig. 1). With inflammation or trauma in this area, there is swelling of the tissue, which prevents the rotator cuff from sliding normally underneath the acromion.

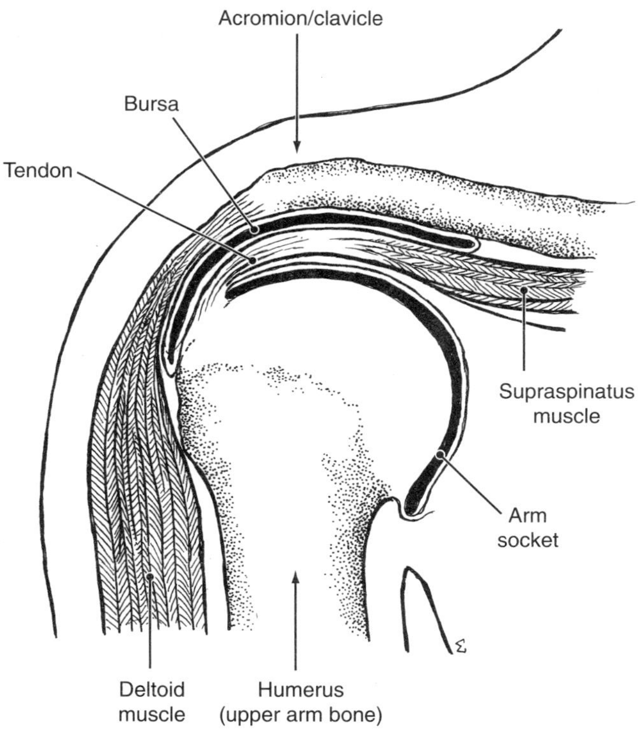

Figure 1.

COMMON SIGNS AND SYMPTOMS

- The most common symptom is pain, particularly when the arm is raised to shoulder level or above.

DIAGNOSIS

The diagnosis is made by taking a detailed history and performing a thorough physical examination.

- Regular x-rays of the shoulder do not show the rotator cuff but can help in evaluating other possible causes of your shoulder pain, such as arthritis or calcium deposits.
- A local anesthetic may be injected into the space between the rotator cuff and the acromion. If this reduces the pain, it is a strong sign that there is bursitis and inflammation of the rotator cuff.
- Arthrogram: This is performed by injecting a special dye into the shoulder joint and then taking x-rays to see if the rotator cuff is damaged.
- MRI (magnetic resonance imaging): No x-rays are used with this technique; instead, it is done with harmless magnetic fields and radio waves. A computer develops the pictures to show organs from several angles. This can help determine if the rotator cuff is torn.

○ TREATMENT

The initial treatment for bursitis or tendinitis of the shoulder includes some or all of the following:

- Rest by avoiding activities and motions that cause pain.
- Medications that reduce inflammation may help relieve pain.
- Cortisone injections may be used to relieve severe inflammation.
- Physical therapy is helpful, particularly in patients who have significant stiffness of the rotator cuff tendons. You can learn these exercises so that you can do them on a daily basis without supervision by a therapist.
- Surgical treatment is indicated in fewer than 10% of patients with bursitis and tendinitis. The aim of surgery is to increase the space between the rotator cuff tendons and the acromion bone. This operation can be done through a regular incision or with an arthroscope, which is an instrument about as thick as a pencil.

After careful consideration of all factors, the recommendation is that you have an operation to correct your shoulder bursitis.

PREOPERATIVE PREPARATION

- Stop all aspirin-containing medications and any other anti-inflammatory medications (examples: Motrin or ibuprofen) at least 7 days before the operation. If pain medication is necessary, use Extra-Strength Tylenol.
- You will have an examination of your blood, urine, heart (EKG), and lungs (chest x-ray).
- Do not eat or drink anything for 8 hours before the operation.
- Shower or bathe as usual on the morning of the operation.
- You may be given medicine that will make you feel drowsy before you are brought to the operating room.

□ OPERATION

- The choice of anesthetic will be discussed with you beforehand.

Arthroscopic Surgery. The arthroscope is inserted into the shoulder joint through several very small incisions around your shoulder. The joint, and especially the rotator cuff tendons, is inspected carefully to see if a tear is present. The acromion is exposed and the undersurface made flat and smooth. Other corrections are made as necessary.

Open Surgery. A 2-inch incision is made at the outer edge of the shoulder, and the undersurface of the acromion is removed, so that it is flat and smooth. Other corrections are made as necessary.

- Either operation usually takes about 1½ hours.

POSTOPERATIVE CARE

- You will be taken to a recovery room and observed. When your blood pressure, pulse, and breathing are stable and you are completely alert, you should be able to go home that same day with a responsible companion.
- Your arm will be in a sling.
- Your pain will be controlled with medicine.
- Move your fingers, wrist, and elbow as much as possible to help reduce swelling and stiffness.
- Arrangements will be made for your medicine, follow-up office visit, and stitch removal.
- As with any operation, complications are always possible. With this type of operation, they can include bleeding, separation of the incision, and possibly others.

✚ HOME CARE

- You may walk about as you wish, even climb stairs.
- If you had open surgery, your arm will remain in a sling until it is determined when you can begin moving it. Shoulder motion can begin immediately following arthroscopic surgery, although this will be painful for the first few weeks.
- Take medicine as prescribed for your pain.
- Do not drive a car if your arm cannot move freely and without pain or if you are taking medicines that decrease your alertness.
- Physical therapy is an essential part of your recovery, so begin it as soon as possible after your operation. Your ability to flex the shoulder joint will be regained over the first 4 weeks. A strengthening program will be arranged for you.
- Returning to work depends on your job responsibilities. Let's discuss this during your follow-up office visit.

✆ CALL OUR OFFICE IF

- There is excessive bleeding, swelling, redness, or drainage from the surgical area.
- You experience an increase in your pain or pain that is not relieved by your prescription medication.
- You develop a temperature higher than 100.5°F.
- You develop numbness or tingling in your arm or hand.
- You have any questions.

SHOULDER: Rotator Cuff Tear

△ GENERAL INFORMATION

The *humerus* is the upper arm bone. When the ball of the humerus (the humeral head) and the socket into which it fits (the *glenoid*) cannot stay in their normal relationship, the shoulder is unstable (Fig. 1). Because this joint has more motion than any other joint in the body, it is not unusual for it to become unstable. Instability of the shoulder joint, or inability to keep the ball and socket reduced (in place), most commonly occurs when the ball slides out of the front part of the shoulder. This most often happens when the elbow is held away from the side and the hand is pointing up or turned outward. This sliding of the humerus out of the front part of the socket accounts for well over 90% of all instability problems of the shoulder. Most commonly, a significant traumatic event occurs (for example, the person falls on the side of the shoulder, tries to make a tackle, makes a rebound while the arm is pulled back, or falls while skiing) that forces the arm farther backward, externally rotates it, and causes the shoulder to dislocate. Assistance is often required to get the shoulder reduced. After reduction, a short period of immobilization is followed by a rehabilitation program.

Unfortunately, the chance of having a recurrent dislocation increases with the activity level and the age of the patient. Younger patients, such as teenagers, who continue to participate in sports have a greater than 90% chance of redislocating their shoulder.

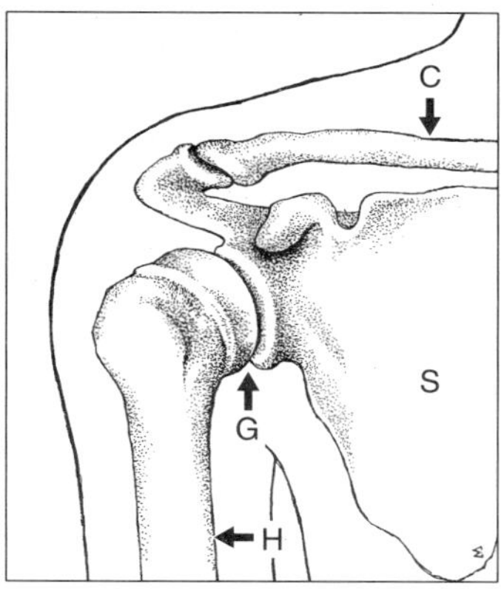

Figure 1. View of the shoulder joint without the rotator cuff (the shoulder joint capsule) in place. G, Glenoid fossa; S, scapula (shoulder blade); C, clavicle (collarbone); H, humerus.

COMMON SIGNS AND SYMPTOMS

- There is a history of instability of the joint when the arm is elevated away from the body and the arm and hand are turned to outward. The pain usually goes away once the acute dislocation is corrected and after a short period of immobilization.
- With each dislocation, there again is discomfort for a short period of time. Patients who have persistent pain may have a more unusual problem, such as a tear in the rotator cuff muscles or the lining (capsule) of the shoulder (Fig. 2).

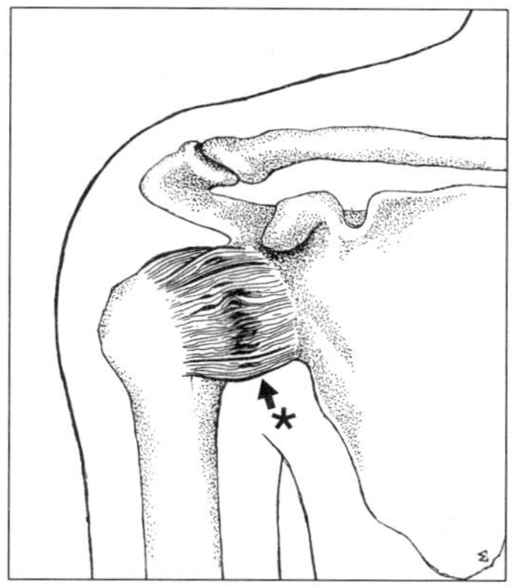

Figure 2. The asterisk indicates the torn rotator cuff.

- Patients avoid maximum arm elevation and external rotation.

DIAGNOSIS

- The diagnosis is best made by a careful, detailed history and a thorough physical examination.
- The history includes a substantial traumatic event with the arm positioned away from the patient's side and rotated externally. Less commonly, the history is one of repetitive activities that stretch the front of the shoulder, leading to instability.
- The arm will be placed in a position that will cause a feeling of apprehension that the shoulder may come out of place. In this position, gentle force on the posterior aspect of the arm in a forward direction will increase the apprehension, while pushing the humerus posteriorly from the anterior position will decrease it.
- Plain x-rays often show characteristic findings. Calcification at the front and lower aspect of the socket (glenoid) is also suggestive of anterior instability. Less commonly seen are loose pieces of tissue *(loose bodies)*.

○ TREATMENT

- A first-time dislocation is treated with a period of immobilization followed by a rehabilitation program. The period of immobilization may have little or no effect on the risk of recurrence and is primarily used to help lessen the pain from the dislocation.
- Physical therapy is directed toward improving the strength and function of the rotator cuff as well as the muscles that control the shoulder blade. Strengthening these muscles may reduce or eliminate the episodes of instability.
- An operation is recommended in the following circumstances:
  - There is recurrent dislocation (generally, three or more episodes of instability per year).
  - Dislocation occurs at rest or during sleep.
  - In some situations, for a first-time dislocation; for example, to avoid having an athlete miss two sports

seasons or a worker's not being able to perform job responsibilities.

After careful consideration of all factors, the recommendation is that you have an operation to correct your chronic shoulder instability.

PREOPERATIVE PREPARATION

- You will have an examination of your blood and urine. You may also have an examination of your heart (EKG) and lungs (chest x-ray).
- Do not eat or drink anything for 8 hours before the operation.
- If you need to take daily medicines, you may do so with a small sip of water on the morning of the operation.
- Stop all aspirin-containing medications or other anti-inflammatory medications, such as Motrin or ibuprofen, at least 7 days before the operation. If pain medication is necessary, use Extra-Strength Tylenol.
- Shower (and shave) as usual on the morning of the operation.
- You may be given medicine that will make you feel drowsy before you are brought to the operating room.

□ OPERATION

- The operation can be performed on an outpatient basis.
- You will be asleep for the operation.
- The operation can be done arthroscopically, although it may need to be converted to an open procedure, or it can be done through an open surgical incision from the start. All three techniques can be successful. The technique chosen will be discussed with you beforehand.
- *Arthroscopy* is done with an instrument called an *arthroscope* that is about as thick as a pencil and has a light and a magnifying lens. One arthroscope is inserted through a tiny incision in the front of the shoulder and another in the back of the joint. This allows visualization of the area that has been injured by the instability to repair the injured tissue.
- In the vast majority of patients who dislocate their shoulder, the cartilage edge of the glenoid (the *labrum*) will have torn away from the socket. The capsule and lining of the shoulder joint are attached to this tissue. To stabilize the shoulder, the labrum is repaired by placing it back against the rim of the socket, deepening the socket, and securing the capsule of the shoulder joint appropriately.
- *Open surgery* is performed through a 3-inch incision made in the crease next to the axilla (armpit). With careful dissection, the lining of the joint is exposed and then opened. The labrum that is torn away from the rim of the socket is repaired so that it is in a normal position again.
- The operation usually takes about 1½ hours.

POSTOPERATIVE CARE

- You will be taken to a recovery room and observed. When your blood pressure, pulse, and breathing are stable and you are completely alert, you should be able to go home that same day with a responsible adult.
- There will be a bandage over the incision, and your arm will be in sling.
- An ice pack may be applied to the site of the operation to minimize swelling and reduce pain.
- Your pain will be controlled with medicines that you take by mouth. A prescription for pain medicine will be given to you. If you have a history of problems with certain pain medicines, please discuss this with the surgeon before your operation.
- As with any operation, complications are always possible. Although they are uncommon with this type of operation, they can include damage to the nerves in this area that raise the arm or bend the elbow, separation of the incision, infection, excessive stiffness, and possibly others. Your shoulder may develop symptoms of instability despite the operation. This happens in fewer than 5% of patients who undergo this type of operation.

✙ HOME CARE

- You may walk about as you wish, even climb stairs, but don't overdo things.
- The dressing should be kept clean and dry. You will be informed when the dressing can be changed. If you would like to take a shower, the entire area should be covered with plastic and sealed with tape so that the incision does not get wet.
- Place an ice pack on your shoulder for 30 minutes three times a day for the first 3 days.
- Move your fingers, wrist, and elbow as much as possible to help reduce swelling and stiffness.
- You should keep the sling or immobilizer on at all times until directed by the surgeon to do otherwise.
- If physical therapy is recommended, this should be started as soon as possible after the operation. In general, it is possible to move your arm into a handshake position or to elevate your arm to the level of your shoulder after the operation without risking damage to the stabilization. Even so, your restrictions will be reviewed with you following the operation.
- Do not drive until we have discussed this during your follow-up office visit.
- You may return to work when you feel comfortable. Simple activities such as writing are allowed as tolerated. Other activities will be discussed with you during your follow-up office visit. A return to full activity without restrictions may take up to 6 months following your operation.

✆ CALL OUR OFFICE IF

- You experience excessive bleeding, redness, or drainage from the surgical area.
- You experience severe pain, an unexpected increase in your pain, or pain that is not relieved by your prescription medicines.
- You have a temperature higher than 100°F.
- You have numbness or tingling in the arm or hand.
- You experience trouble breathing or heart palpitations.
- You have any questions.

△ GENERAL INFORMATION

Some people with cirrhosis of the liver develop an accumulation of fluid in their abdomen (called *ascites*). Usually, this can be made to go away with medical treatment, which consists of adjusting the diet and medication. With time, however, such medical treatment may stop working; the fluid will reaccumulate and the abdomen will become larger and larger.

COMMON SIGNS AND SYMPTOMS

- The abdomen becomes large and round. Sometimes it looks as large as in a full-term pregnancy.
- There is some difficulty with breathing.
- The legs become swollen.

DIAGNOSIS

- The history (of cirrhosis), the findings on physical examination, the laboratory tests, and the clinical course are the most important ways to make the diagnosis.

○ TREATMENT

- The initial treatment should be medical because often this relieves the problem. Sometimes, however, it is not helpful, or it helps for a while but then the fluid reaccumulates.
- The fluid can be removed easily with a syringe and needle, and you will feel much better. Many times this is done as part of medical treatment and to obtain a sample of the fluid. But, there are two serious drawbacks to continued use of this method:
  - This fluid in the abdomen has a lot of valuable protein in it that you need, so you cannot afford to have it removed and thrown away.
  - It will quickly reaccumulate.
- The best treatment at this stage is an operation to drain the fluid from the abdomen into a vein in the general circulation.

After careful consideration of all factors, the recommendation is that you have such an operation.

PREOPERATIVE PREPARATION

- If you have any other medical problems, they will be looked into also, so that you can be in the best possible condition for the operation.
- Do not eat or drink anything for 8 hours before the operation.
- Shower as usual on the morning of the operation.
- You may be given medicine that will make you feel drowsy before you are brought to the operating room.

□ OPERATION

- This operation is done with either a general anesthetic to put you to sleep or a local anesthetic and some medicine to keep you drowsy. The choice will be discussed with you beforehand.
- This operation involves placing a device about the size of a cigarette lighter under the skin in your lower chest. This device has a one-way valve and a thin plastic tube at each end. One tube is placed in the abdomen that contains the fluid; the other tube is placed under the skin and connected to a vein in the neck. This is called a *shunt*. The one-way valve lets the fluid go only from the abdomen into the vein.
- The operation usually takes about 2 hours.

POSTOPERATIVE CARE

- You will be taken to a recovery room and observed. When your blood pressure, pulse, and breathing are stable, you will be taken to a regular hospital room.
- There will be a snug binder around your abdomen that helps to keep the fluid flowing into the tube.
- You will be shown how to press on the pump every so often to help move the fluid along.
- Pain can be controlled with medicine.
- That evening you will be helped to sit up in bed and on the next day to get out of bed.
- You will be able to go home after your condition is stable.
- As with any operation, complications are always possible. With this type of operation, they can include infection, bleeding, clogging of the shunt, kidney problems, and possibly others.

✚ HOME CARE

- You may walk about as you wish, even climb stairs.
- Take the medicines and follow the diet prescribed for you while you were in the hospital.
- You may shower as you wish and with any dressings on or off.
  - There may be narrow strips of tape across the incision. It's all right if they get wet; they will be removed in the doctor's office.
  - After you dry yourself, replace any dressings with clean, dry ones.
- Be careful that you do not become constipated.
  - Include enough roughage and plenty of liquids in your diet.
  - You may need a mild laxative (example: milk of magnesia).
- You may drive your car when you feel up to it but not if you are taking medicine that reduces your alertness.
- You may resume sexual activity whenever you choose.
- You may return to work when you feel up to it, but let's talk about it first during your follow-up office visit.

✆ CALL OUR OFFICE IF

- You develop any unusual signs or symptoms.
- Your abdomen begins to swell again.
- You develop a temperature higher than 100°F.
- You have any questions.

△ GENERAL INFORMATION

Basal cell cancer is a new, uncontrolled growth of the skin. Fortunately, it usually grows slowly and almost never spreads *(metastasizes)* to different areas of the body. Basal cell cancer is seen most commonly in areas of the head and neck that have had chronic exposure to the sun. If treated early and properly, there's a very high chance for cure.

COMMON SIGNS AND SYMPTOMS

- The lesion usually is slightly raised, red to brown, and has smooth borders. Some lesions are ulcerated in their center. Occasionally, the lesion may bleed.

DIAGNOSIS

- Usually, the diagnosis can be made by taking a detailed history and doing a thorough physical examination.
- A small piece of the lesion is taken (called a *biopsy*) for examination in the laboratory.
- Sometimes, if the examination makes the diagnosis virtually certain, the entire lesion may be removed without a biopsy.

PREOPERATIVE PREPARATION

- Do not eat or drink anything for 8 hours before the operation.
- Shower (and shave) as usual that morning.
- You may be given medicine to make you feel drowsy before you are brought to the operating room.

□ OPERATION

- The lesion and the skin around it will be painted with an antiseptic solution and the area draped with sterile towels.
- The area around the lesion will be made numb with an anesthetic injected by a thin, short needle.
- The incision will be made along the skin creases so that it will show as little as possible afterward.
- During the operation, you may feel some tugging but no pain.
- After the cancer is removed, it sometimes is sent to the pathology laboratory. There the pathologist examines the margins to check that they are "clear" of the cancer. If this check is done, expect a 15- to 30-minute wait while you are on the operating table.
- A cosmetic closure will be made using fine suture material. Narrow strips of special tape will be applied across the incision to help reduce the tension on it.

POSTOPERATIVE CARE

- You will be taken to a recovery room. When your blood pressure, pulse, and breathing are stable and you are completely alert, you should be able to go home that same day with a responsible adult.
- Pain can be controlled with over-the-counter medicine.
- Arrangements will be made for your medicine, follow-up office visit, and stitch removal.

✣ HOME CARE

- Resume your usual activities.
- Unless instructed otherwise, you may shower as you wish with any dressings on or off.
  - There may be narrow strips of tape across the incision. It's all right if they get wet.
  - After you dry yourself, replace any dressings with clean, dry ones.
- Unless instructed otherwise, take care of the incision at a convenient time once a day as follows:
  - Remove the dressings.
  - If there are narrow strips of tape across the incision, do not pull them off. They will be removed at the doctor's office.
  - Touch the entire area of the incision with cotton swabs dipped in hydrogen peroxide.
  - Touch the incision again using ordinary rubbing alcohol.
  - You may be instructed to cover the incision with an antibiotic ointment.
  - Replace the dressings with clean, dry ones.

✆ CALL OUR OFFICE IF

- There is bleeding from the incision.
- The incision becomes red and swollen, or if there is drainage from it.
- You develop a temperature higher than 100°F.
- You have any questions.

△ GENERAL INFORMATION

This is a cancerous growth of the outer layer of the skin. It is seen most commonly in older persons who have a fair complexion and have been exposed to the sun over a long period of time. The areas most frequently affected are the scalp, neck, top of the ear, lower lip, and back of the arms and hands.

COMMON SIGNS AND SYMPTOMS

- The lesion usually begins as a small bump on the skin that is firm and red to red-brown or tan in color.
- There may be crusting on its surface. Later, a shallow ulcer may form in the center of the lesion.
- Occasionally the lesion may bleed.

DIAGNOSIS

- Although squamous cell cancer has a characteristic appearance, it still can be mistaken for other benign or malignant lesions. The only certain way to make the diagnosis is by examining a piece of it under the microscope. Two options are available:
  - **Excision Biopsy.** If the lesion is small enough, it is practical to excise all of it. If it is a cancer, this will constitute both the diagnosis and the treatment.
  - **Incision Biopsy.** For a larger lesion, a small piece of the lesion is removed for laboratory examination.
- With either of these techniques, the area around the lesion is swabbed with an antiseptic solution and surrounded with sterile towels. A very thin, short needle is used to inject an anesthetic around the lesion to make the area numb. The tissue is then obtained for diagnosis.

○ TREATMENT

These cancers will enlarge and possibly spread to other areas of the body if they are not removed. There are several ways to do this.

Surgery. The area containing the lesion is swabbed with an antiseptic solution and surrounded with sterile towels. A very fine short needle is used to inject an anesthetic that will make the area numb.

- A cosmetic incision will be made and the entire lesion removed in one piece along with some normal tissue around it.
- The incision will be closed in a cosmetic fashion.
- The *advantage* of this method of treatment is that all the borders and deep margins can be examined to be certain they are free of cancer.
- The *disadvantage* is that it requires an operation.

Electrodissection. This method is best used for small lesions that appear superficial. The area is prepared as above. The surface of the lesion is scraped or shaved off and the base burned with a special type of needle that transmits an electrical current.

- The *advantage* of this method is that the procedure can be done in the office with minimal equipment.
- The *disadvantages* are as follows:
  - The specimen is not removed, so the edges and deep margins cannot be examined under the microscope to be absolutely certain they are clear.
  - A scab forms over the burned area that must be taken care of until it heals over.
  - This procedure should be done only by someone who is very experienced in electrosurgery.

Chemosurgery. This method is best in the following situations:

- The cancer is one that has come back.
- The patient cannot afford to lose any more normal tissue than is absolutely necessary.
- The borders of the cancer are not clear, so when the lesion is examined it is difficult for the surgeon to know where to cut to get all of the cancer, but not too much normal tissue.
- The surrounding tissue has been damaged by previous irradiation and will not heal well if it is cut or stitched.
- The cancer is very close to, or actually in, the bone and cartilage.

This technique is used by specialists in dermatologic (skin) surgery. It is done as follows: A small area of the tumor is painted with a special solution that "pickles" this specific part of the tumor on the spot. The pickled area is removed and examined under the microscope. If any borders of this removed piece are positive for cancer, the tissue in this positive border area is treated in the same way by "pickling" and removing some of it. This is done as many times as necessary over a period of time in separate sessions until all of the removed pieces have negative borders.

- The *advantages* to this method are as follows:
  - It can be used for a cancer that is in a location in which it would be very difficult to remove properly any other way.
  - Very little normal tissue is removed.
- The *disadvantages* of this method are as follows:
  - It often requires a number of small operations.
  - Pain cannot be easily or completely controlled.
  - This technique should be used for the lesions described above and not for lesions that can easily be cut out and the skin brought together again.

X-ray therapy. This technique is useful when it would be difficult to cut out the cancer and bring the edges together without producing a noticeable deformity. This technique should not be used for lesions that can be removed easily and in areas in which the incision can be stitched together easily again.

After careful consideration of all factors, the recommendation is that you have an operation to remove your skin tumor. This is almost always an outpatient procedure.

PREOPERATIVE PREPARATION

- Do not eat or drink anything for 4 hours before the operation.

☐ OPERATION

- The operation will be done as already described.
- During the operation, you may feel some tugging but no pain.

POSTOPERATIVE CARE

- You will be taken to a recovery room and observed. When your blood pressure, pulse, and breathing are stable and you are completely alert, you should be able to go home that same day with a responsible adult.
- Arrangements will be made for your medicine, follow-up office visit, and stitch removal.

✚ HOME CARE

- Resume your usual activities.
- Take medicine as prescribed for your pain.
- Unless instructed otherwise, you may shower if you wish with the dressing on or off. After you dry the other parts of your body, take care of the incision as instructed for your specific situation.
- Do not drive if you are taking medicines that may decrease your alertness.

✆ CALL OUR OFFICE IF

- There is bleeding from the incision.
- The incision becomes red or swollen, or there is drainage from it.
- You develop a temperature higher than 100°F.
- You have any questions.

△ GENERAL INFORMATION

A skin graft is a piece of skin taken from one area of the body to cover an open wound in another area. There are several types of grafts (Fig. 1).

In a *split-thickness graft* only the superficial layers of the skin are used. This can be either a *thin split-thickness skin graft* (A) or *thick split-thickness skin graft* (B). If the graft includes all layers of the skin, it is called a *full-thickness skin graft* (C). Occasionally, the graft might include skin, hair, fat, and muscle. This is called a *myocutaneous graft* (D). Finally, the graft might include skin, hair, fat, muscle, and cartilage or bone. This is called a *composite graft* (E).

Stitches are needed to close the donor site (the area from which the skin graft is taken) of a full-thickness, myocutaneous or composite graft. The donor site for a split-thickness skin graft heals by itself, very much like a deep scrape wound.

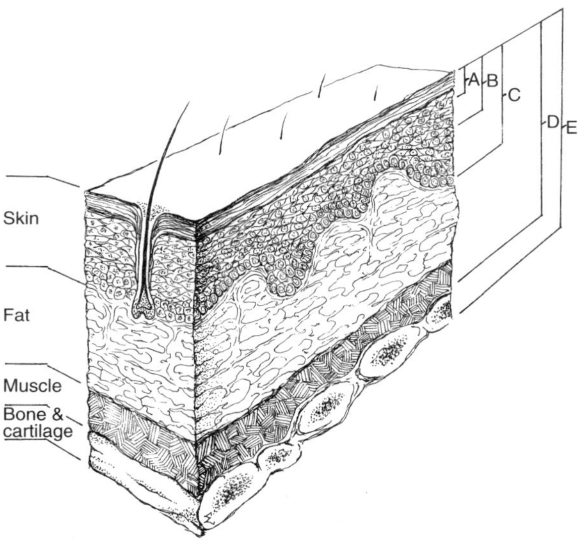

Figure 1.

GENERAL USES OF VARIOUS GRAFTS

- Full-thickness skin grafts are used to cover smaller wounds of the face and hands. The donor skin for the face usually is taken from behind the ear. For the fingers, the skin is usually taken from the hand itself.
- Thin split-thickness skin grafts usually are taken from the thigh or buttocks and occasionally the abdomen.

Each patient requires individual attention. The choice of the type of skin graft and other details will be discussed with you before anything is planned or done.

PREOPERATIVE PREPARATION

- The laboratory tests ordered before the operation will depend on your special circumstances. This will all be explained to you.
- Be certain to tell the doctor or nurse if you are taking any aspirin or similar medicines. They can increase bleeding during the operation, so you'll have to stop taking them 10 days before the procedure.
- Shower with a germicidal soap (example: Dial) the evening before and the morning of the operation.
- Do not eat or drink anything for 8 hours before the operation.
- You may be given medicine that will make you feel drowsy before you are brought to the operating room.

□ OPERATION

- You will lie on a comfortable table.
- Local or general anesthesia will be used, or a combination of local anesthesia and a medicine to make you feel drowsy during the operation. The choice of anesthetic will depend on the size and location of the grafted area and the location of the donor site.
- For skin grafting on the face, another medicine (epinephrine) is often added to the local anesthetic to reduce bleeding. This medicine can make your heart beat faster and cause you to perspire and feel hungry. This is normal.
- During the operation, you may feel some tugging but no pain.
- Sometimes the skin graft is taken with a special instrument (called a *dermatome*) that makes a loud noise and vibrates. This will last just a few seconds.

POSTOPERATIVE CARE

- If the operation is done under general anesthesia, you will be taken to a recovery room and observed. When your blood pressure, pulse, and breathing are stable and you are completely alert, you should be able to go home that same day with a responsible adult. Otherwise, you will be taken to a regular hospital room and remain in the hospital as long as necessary.
- Elaborate dressings are common after skin grafting procedures. Don't be alarmed.
- Occasionally, there may be some drainage or a collection of slightly bloody fluid in and around the dressings. This is expected.
- Numbness and even muscle weakness around the operated area can last for several hours. This is from the local anesthetic solution.
- Bruising around the area of the operation, especially with surgery around the face, is expected.
- As with any operation, complications are always possible. With this type of operation they can include bleeding, infection, loss of the skin graft, and possibly others.
- Arrangements will be made for your medicine, follow-up office visit, and stitch removal.

✚ HOME CARE

- Collection of blood under the skin graft is a major cause of loss of the skin graft. To minimize this risk:

- Keep the graft site elevated. Examples: *Head surgery*—sleep with the head raised on two or three pillows. *Arm*—use a sling or similar supporting device. *Leg*—lie down as much as possible and keep the leg raised above the level of the heart.
- Minimize movement of the graft site. Examples are: avoid unnecessary talking, eat a soft diet, restrict walking.
- Depending on the site of your skin graft, avoid bending down, standing excessively, sneezing, coughing, or straining to have a bowel movement.

- Keep the dressings dry.
- Take pain medicines as prescribed.
- Avoid situations that might raise your blood pressure and possibly trigger bleeding.

✆ CALL OUR OFFICE IF

- You have persistent weakness, especially with closure of the eyelids. This is most important.
- You develop any unusual signs or symptoms.
- The incision becomes red or swollen, or there is drainage from it.
- You develop a temperature higher than 100°F.
- You accidentally get the dressings wet.
- You have any questions.

△ GENERAL INFORMATION

Tumors of the small intestine are not common. However, because almost half of them are malignant, they must be investigated thoroughly.

COMMON SIGNS AND SYMPTOMS

When food reaches the small intestine it has the consistency of applesauce. Thus, a tumor has to almost completely block the intestine to cause symptoms.

- There may be cramping abdominal pain or bloating.
- Complete blockage may produce colicky pain and a distended abdomen.
- The tumor can bleed into the intestine itself. This blood then comes out with bowel movements. If the bleeding continues, it can lead to anemia and even to shock and require emergency attention.

DIAGNOSIS

- A detailed history and a thorough physical examination can be important and will be done. Unfortunately, it is still difficult to make the diagnosis just with these methods alone.
- *Abdominal x-ray*: This may show the distended intestine, but it will not usually show the cause of the obstruction.
- *Small bowel x-ray*: Contrast material is swallowed and x-rays are taken as it travels along the small intestine. Sometimes, this will show the point of the obstruction and perhaps even the cause of it.
- *CT scan (computed tomography scan):* This special x-ray machine is shaped like a huge doughnut. As you lie on the table inside the hole in the doughnut, x-rays are taken as very thin slices through the abdomen. This sometimes makes it possible to see fine details of organs and tissues in the abdomen and the probable cause of the problem.
- *Colonoscopy*: This can be useful if there is blood in the stool and it is not clear where it is coming from. Colonoscopy is done with an optical instrument with a light at its tip that is smooth, flexible, and as big around as your little finger. You will be given medicine that will make you feel drowsy during the procedure. The tip of the instrument will be lubricated and inserted gently in your anus and then into the large bowel to examine all of it. If the results of this examination are negative, it increases the chance that the problem is in the small intestine.
- The tumor may be found during an emergency exploratory operation in a patient who is hemorrhaging or has complete obstruction of the intestine.

○ TREATMENT

- Removing the part of the intestine with the tumor in it and the reconnecting the open ends is the only treatment that will take care of this condition.

PREOPERATIVE PREPARATION

- You will have an examination of your blood, urine, heart (EKG), and lungs (chest x-ray).
- Do not eat or drink anything for 8 hours before the operation. This, of course, will not be possible if the operation needs to be done right away.
- Shower (and shave) as usual on the morning of the operation.
- You will be given medicine that will make you feel drowsy before you are brought to the operating room.

□ OPERATION

- You will be asleep for the operation.
- The portion of the small intestine with the tumor in it will be removed and the intestine reconnected.
- You will not receive a blood transfusion unless it is absolutely necessary.
- The operation usually takes about 2 hours.

POSTOPERATIVE CARE

- You will wake up in a recovery room. When your blood pressure, pulse, and breathing are stable, you will be taken to a regular hospital room.
- You will have a thin plastic tube in your nose. It goes down to your stomach to suck up the air you swallow. It will be removed when your bowels start working.
- That evening you will be helped to sit up in bed and on the next day to get out of bed.
- Pain will be controlled with medicine.
- After the tube in your nose is removed, your diet will start with liquids and gradually be increased as tolerated.
- You should be able to go home in 4 to 6 days.
- Arrangements will be made for your medicine, follow-up office visit, and stitch or clip removal.
- As with any operation, complications are always possible. With your type of operation, they can include peritonitis, leakage from a stitched area, bowel obstruction, wound infection, and possibly others.

✣ HOME CARE

- You may walk about as you wish, even climb stairs.
- You may eat as you did before the operation.
- Take medicine as prescribed for your pain.
- Unless instructed otherwise, you may shower as you wish with any dressings on or off.
  - It's all right if the stitches, clips, or strips of tape across the incision get wet. They will be removed in the doctor's office.
  - After you dry yourself, replace any dressings with clean, dry ones.
- Driving a car with an automatic shift is not too demanding. But if you suddenly have to slam on the brakes or twist to turn the wheel, you may strain the

sutures or tear something. During the follow-up visit let's discuss when you can resume driving.
- You may resume sexual activity whenever you choose.
- You may return to work when you feel up to it, but let's talk about it first during your follow-up office visit.

✆ CALL OUR OFFICE IF

- You develop any unusual signs or symptoms.
- The incision becomes red or swollen, or there is drainage from it.
- You develop a temperature higher than 100°F.
- You have any questions.

△ GENERAL INFORMATION

- There are poisonous snakes in practically every state in the United States, although most are found in the southeastern and southwestern states.
- Approximately 45,000 persons are treated for snakebite each year.
- About 7,000 of these bites are presumed to be from poisonous snakes. Rattlesnakes are responsible for more than 50% of all poisonous bites.
- One-third of snake bites occur in children younger than 10 years of age, usually in an area around their house.
- About 98% of snake bites are on the legs.
- Only a dozen or so persons die each year from snake bite.
- A snake bite is a medical emergency.

DIAGNOSIS

- A detailed history and careful physical examination will be done to confirm that there actually has been a snake bite.
- If you can bring the snake carcass with you, it will be possible to determine whether it is poisonous or nonpoisonous. Otherwise, a description of the snake might be helpful.

Poisonous Snakes (Pit Vipers) (Fig. 1)

- Have a pit between the eyes and the nostrils.
- The pupil of the eye is in the shape of a slit.
- Have two fangs.
- On the underside of the tail area, the creases (plates) go all the way across.
  - The *one exception* to these rules is the coral snake:
  - It has round pupils.
  - It does not have fangs.
  - It is the only snake with red and yellow bands that are next to each other.

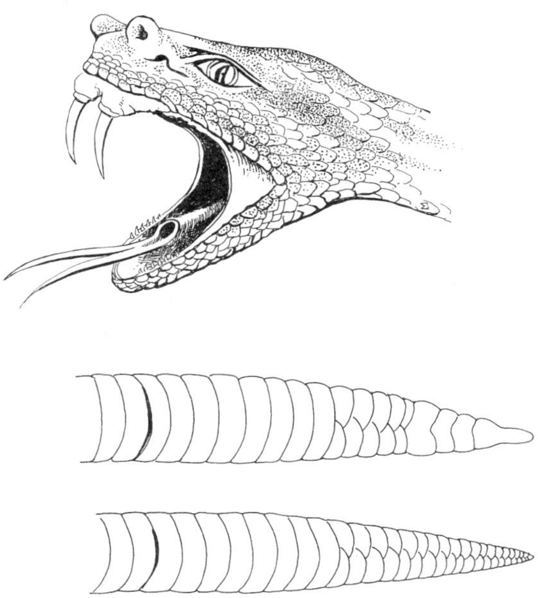

Figure 1.

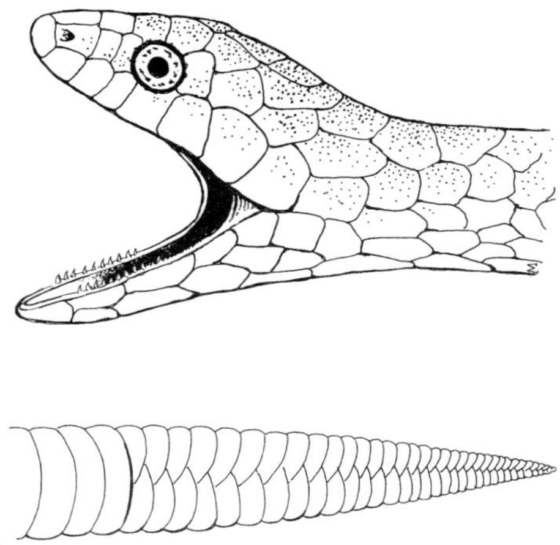

Figure 2.

Nonpoisonous Snakes (Fig. 2)

- Do not have a pit.
- Have round pupils.
- Do not have fangs; instead, they have a row of teeth.
- The creases (plates) on the underside are in two pieces.

- Pattern of bite marks:
  - Nonpoisonous snakes—usually in the shape of a U.
  - Poisonous snakes—one or two puncture wounds.
- Not all snake bites are accompanied by release of snake venom (poison) into the wound.
- Snake venom is a complex mixture of chemicals that can immediately cause a number of alarming and extremely serious reactions. Venom can affect the nerves, create problems with bleeding and clotting, and destroy red blood cells and tissue. Also, it contains a chemical that allows the poison to spread quickly.
- Treatment must be started right away.
- Treatment can begin while the patient is being transported to the emergency department. The bitten limb, however, should be kept still.
- Place a tourniquet that blocks blood flow in the veins but *not* the arteries (check the pulse) so as to slow down the spread of the poison. Do *not* release the tourniquet at intervals; the poison will escape. The tourniquet can be left on for up to 2 hours.
- Do not place cold packs on the extremity.
- Remove as much of the poison as possible. Cut through the fang marks with incisions about $\frac{1}{4}$ inch long and $\frac{1}{8}$ inch deep and apply mechanical suction. If necessary, the suction can be done with the mouth as long as there are no open sores in the mouth. Any swallowed poison is quickly neutralized by the acid in the stomach. If this is done right away, about 50% of the poison can be removed in 15 minutes.
- Neutralize the poison. Antidotes (antivenom) are available in many large emergency departments. Information about antivenom can also be obtained from the local zoo. You will receive a skin test dose of antivenom before receiving the full dose.

- Prevent or reduce the effect of the poison:
  - Give plasma, blood, and other fluids.
  - Treat any bleeding problems.
  - Supply enough oxygen.
  - Prevent complications.
  - Give strong antibiotics.
  - Treat for tetanus.
  - Treat vomiting or convulsions.
  - Closely watch the condition of the kidneys.
- The length of stay in the hospital depends on your clinical course.

SOMATOSENSORY-EVOKED POTENTIAL (SSEP) MONITORING

△ GENERAL INFORMATION

This procedure (commonly called *SSEP monitoring*) indicates how well your spinal cord and some of your nerves are working. It is often used to monitor the spinal cord and nerve function during a number of neurosurgical and spinal operations.

HOW SSEP MONITORING WORKS

- Our brain is constantly collecting information from the world around us.
- This information is gathered by "sensors" throughout our body, such as the skin, eyes, ears, and nose.
- When one of these sensors is stimulated, the information it receives is sent to the brain by way of a tiny electrical signal that travels along a nerve.
- We can measure these electrical signals as they travel along the nerve by placing small measuring electrodes near the nerve. We can also determine when the signal traveling along the nerve finally reaches the brain.
- These measurements allow the anesthesiologist and the surgeon to determine how powerful these signals are and how fast they are traveling. In turn, this information allows the doctors to know whether the nerves and spinal cord are operating normally.

WHEN IS SSEP NEEDED?

Spine

During an operation, your nerves, spinal cord, and certain parts of your brain work normally even though you are under anesthesia. Because of this, SSEP monitoring during an operation can tell the doctors whether the spinal cord and brain are working normally or are at risk for injury.

Most commonly, SSEP monitoring is used in major spine surgery such as correction of *scoliosis* (curvature of the spine) or repair of bones of the back (called *vertebrae*) that are broken or out of line. During these operations, the surgeon must move the vertebrae to correct the problem. However, this may put pressure on the spinal cord, which is surrounded and protected by these bones. Excessive pressure may cause temporary or permanent damage to the cord.

SSEP allows the anesthesiologist and surgeon to monitor spinal cord function constantly while the operation is going on. If too much pressure is put on the spinal cord, the doctors will know it and relieve it before any permanent damage is done. (Years ago the only option was to wait until the operation was complete and the patient was awake to find out if any damage was done, and then it was too late.) Simple back operations, such as removing a herniated disk or a laminectomy, pose little risk of injuring the spinal cord and so do not routinely need SSEP monitoring.

Brain

Many neurosurgical procedures (brain operations) put the areas of the brain that receive all these sensory signals at risk for injury. In these operations, SSEP monitoring can tell the neurosurgeon when these areas might be damaged so that dissection in this area can be avoided. Most commonly, the operations involve the blood vessels that supply the areas of the brain, that have to do with sensation. However, any type of brain surgery can benefit from SSEP monitoring.

Other Uses

Rarely, a vascular surgeon will ask for SSEP monitoring because the procedure that is planned may put the spinal cord at risk for injury. An example is repair of a large aortic aneurysm, during which the spinal cord might not receive enough blood.

THE PROCEDURE

SSEP monitoring requires stimulating a nerve and measuring the time it takes the electrical signal to travel along the spinal cord and into the brain. To stimulate the nerve, a tiny electrical shock is applied to the nerve. This shock is delivered by the SSEP machine through a small pad placed over the selected nerves in either your ankle or wrist. These pads will be placed before you go to sleep. Before the pads are applied, all the oil and dirt must be cleansed from the skin. This cleaning will require a strong soap (much like Lava soap) and some pretty firm scrubbing. Once in place, these pads will be tested to see that they are working properly. All you will feel is a little tingling (only a tiny electric current is needed for this).

Measuring the nerve signals started by the small electric shock requires that four to seven recording electrodes be placed on your back and scalp so that the signals can be picked up and recorded. These electrodes contain tiny needles that will be inserted while you are asleep. Your only knowledge that these electrodes were ever in place might be a spot of blood on your scalp. Sometimes it is necessary to place these recording needles while you are awake. The needles are so small, not much bigger than a hair, that most people are not bothered by their placement.

The actual recording occurs continuously during the operation while you are under general anesthesia. The anesthesiologist and surgeon are in constant communication so that any abnormal signal can be quickly noted and steps taken to avoid any harm.

RISKS

Every procedure has risks, including SSEP monitoring. The procedure itself is very safe. Just the same, however, because needles are used, there is a very small risk that the needle site might become infected or that the needle might break off in the skin. Because electric current is applied to the skin, there is also a very small risk of burning the skin under the pad. Even if these complications do occur, they are minor and temporary. The great benefit of SSEP monitoring far outweighs any of these very small risks.

The main difficulty with SSEP monitoring is that the only parts of the spinal cord and brain we can monitor are those areas that involve sensation. We cannot measure all of the areas of the nervous system that control movement, and because of this, we cannot measure how well the nerves that tell the muscles to move (called *motor nerves*) are working. Sometimes the SSEP signals are perfectly normal, yet none of the motor nerves works. In other words, the person may be paralyzed but still have normal sensation. Usually, any pressure on the spinal cord that is strong enough to hurt the motor nerves can also injure the sensory nerves. Therefore, the SSEP signals almost always change when the motor nerves are being hurt. The doctors who do this type of monitoring realize its limitations and so never rely only on this monitoring to make sure the spinal cord is working. Oftentimes during a major spine operation, the anesthesiologist will lighten the anesthetic enough that the doctors can ask the patient to move his or her feet or hands to make certain the motor nerves are working.

SSEP monitoring has been a great advance in surgery and has allowed patients to have more complicated operations with less risk of suffering serious injury to the spinal cord or brain.

△ GENERAL INFORMATION

Spinal stenosis is a condition in which the spinal cord or one of its branches is squeezed or pinched as it passes through a narrow *(stenosed)* area. On the back of the vertebrae that make up the spine, there is a canal *(spinal canal)* that is about as big around as a fountain pen. The spinal cord runs through this canal from the brain to the waist. Spinal nerves connected to it along the way carry all sensations (e.g., pain, heat, cold) from the body back to the brain. Sometimes, one of these nerves traveling to the spinal cord through the opening between the vertebrae becomes pinched. This produces pain in the area associated with that nerve (Fig. 1).

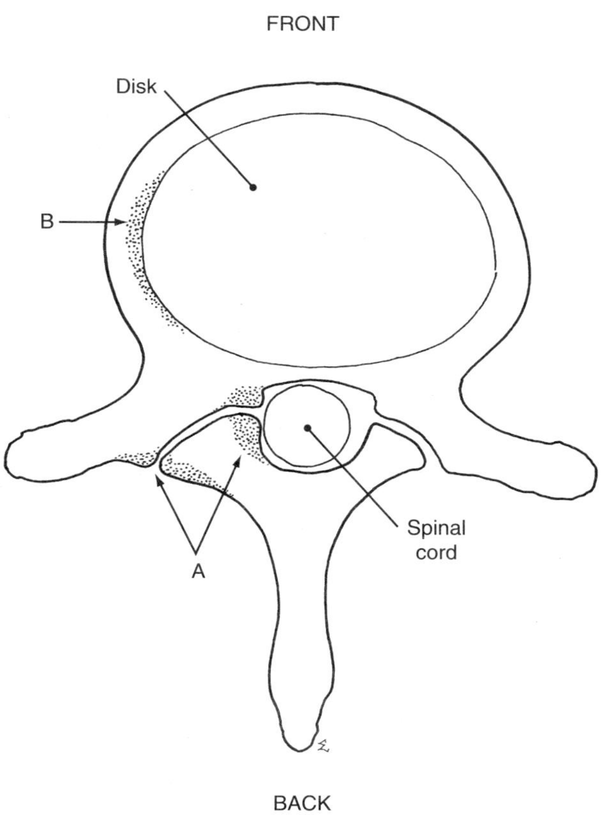

Figure 1. A vertebra as seen from the top. Areas where changes that can contribute to spinal stenosis are stippled. They can include overgrowth of bone at the facets (A) and degeneration around the disk (B).

COMMON SIGNS AND SYMPTOMS

- The typical patient has gradual onset of back pain.
  - Early on, the pain is relieved by rest.
  - Along with the pain, there may be "pins and needles" sensation of the legs, but after a while the pain becomes constant.
  - There may be some difficulty in urinating or moving the bowels.
  - Finally, weakness of the legs may develop in addition to the pain.

DIAGNOSIS

The following tests are commonly necessary to arrive at an accurate diagnosis:

- *CT scan (computed tomography scan)*: These special x-rays are taken as very thin slices through the area of the spine thought to be the cause of the problem. They make it possible to see the fine details in and around the spine and the nerves passing through the various openings.
- *MRI (magnetic resonance imaging)*: No x-rays are used with this technique. Instead, it is done with harmless magnetic fields and radio waves. A computer develops the pictures to show organs from several angles. It is especially useful for examining nerves, blood vessels, and bone tissue.
- X-rays of your spine from various angles can provide valuable information.

○ TREATMENT

- The initial treatment should aim at relieving symptoms by trying to widen—even if it's just a little—the narrowed area so that the nerve is not pinched. This can include the following:
  - Changing the type and amount of physical activity.
  - Applying mild traction to your spine at intervals to widen the stenosed area.
  - Wearing a firm, sponge rubber collar to limit twisting and turning of your neck.
- If such measures do not work, then an operation should be seriously considered.
- An operation should be performed in the following circumstances:
  - If muscle weakness develops, a sign that the nerve to that muscle might die permanently.
  - If the pain is continuous and nothing makes you comfortable except for strong pain medicines.
  - If you simply cannot carry out your activities.

After the most careful consideration of all factors, the recommendation is that you have an operation for your spinal stenosis.

PREOPERATIVE PREPARATION

- You will have an examination of your blood, urine, heart (EKG), and lungs (chest x-ray).
- Do not eat or drink anything for 8 hours before the operation.

□ OPERATION

- You will be asleep for the operation.
- The incision will be over the area of the spine with the stenosis.
- The operation usually takes about 3 to 4 hours.

POSTOPERATIVE CARE

- You will be taken to a recovery room and observed. When your blood pressure, pulse, and breathing are stable, you will be taken to a regular hospital room.

- Pain will be controlled with medicine.
- On the next day you will be helped to sit up in bed and on the following day to get out of bed.
- The surgeon and the rest of the hospital team will start working with you early on the various stages of your recovery.
- As with any operation, complications are always possible. With this type of operation they can include blood clots, bleeding, infection, damage to the cord or one of its branches, and possibly others.
- It is impossible to assure you that everything will be perfectly well after the operation. Many patients get dramatic relief of pain and soon. Others have some remaining pain. Very rarely, there is little relief of pain.
- You should be able to go home in about 1 week.
- Arrangements will be made for your medicine, follow-up office visit, and stitch removal.

✚ HOME CARE

- Continue with the physical exercise program started while you were in the hospital.
- Take the pain medicines prescribed for you.
- Eat as you wish, but include plenty of roughage and liquids in your diet to help prevent constipation.
- Unless instructed otherwise, you may shower as you wish.
- Arrangements can be made for a home visiting nurse if one is needed.
- Do not drive a car until we first talk about it.

✆ CALL OUR OFFICE IF

- The incision becomes red or swollen, or there is drainage from it.
- You develop a temperature higher than 100°F.
- You have any questions.

△ GENERAL INFORMATION

The spleen is located in the left upper part of the abdomen. It is slightly soft and normally about the size of a soft drink can (Fig. 1). Sooner or later, all your blood passes through the spleen, which is made up of tissue put together like a very fine sponge. The blood goes in and out of the channels in this spongy tissue. As it does this, the blood is cleansed of older and weaker red and white blood cells, platelets (involved with blood clotting), and whatever else is not healthy and should not be in the blood stream. Even so, removal of the spleen usually does not create serious problems in adults.

Sometimes the spleen loses its ability to perform its functions properly:

- It removes cells before they are old.
- It removes cells faster than you can make new ones.
  - If it removes red blood cells too fast, you can become anemic (too few red blood cells).
  - If it removes the platelets too fast, there may be problems with blood clotting.

The spleen can do quite a number of things that can make a person sick. In addition, however, the spleen itself can be the only organ that is diseased.

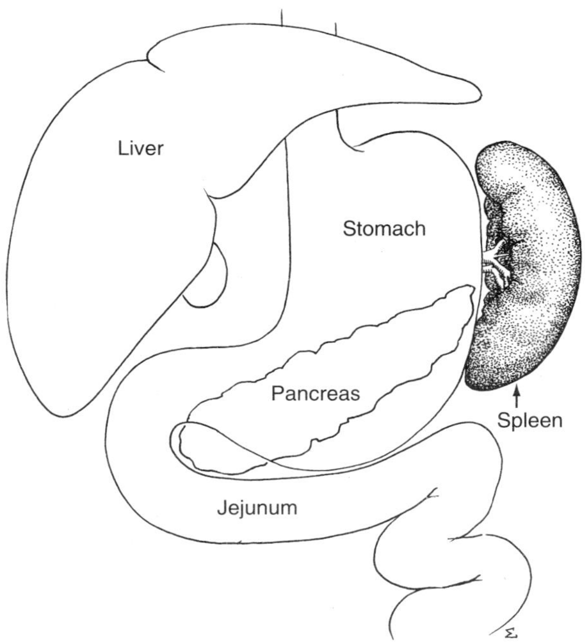

Figure 1. The spleen and its relationship to other organs in the abdomen.

COMMON SIGNS AND SYMPTOMS

- If the disease happens to be one that causes the spleen to become large, then a mass can be felt in the left part of the upper abdomen.
- If there is anemia, the skin is pale.
- There may be bruises because of poor blood clotting.
- The spleen can do a number of harmful things yet still be normal in size and appearance.

DIAGNOSIS

There are a number of tests available to find out how and why the spleen is creating a problem. Which tests are used, and how and when they are used, depend on what disorder of the spleen is suspected. These tests are usually done by a hematologist, who is a specialist in diseases of the blood.

○ TREATMENT

- There are several medical treatments for these splenic-blood conditions, and often they work well. Sometimes, however, the condition responds for a while and then comes back. Different medicines can then be tried.
- Every once in a while, the spleen continues to cause harm and must be removed.

After careful consideration of all factors, the recommendation is that you have your spleen removed.

PREOPERATIVE PREPARATION

- The goal is to get you in the best possible shape for the operation.
- Some tests may need to be done to help the surgeon know whether there are other problems inside the abdomen that need to be taken care of.
- *CT scan (computed tomography scan)*: These special x-rays are taken by a machine that is shaped like a huge doughnut. You will lie on a table inside the hole in the "doughnut." The x-rays are taken as very thin slices through the area of the abdomen, including the spleen. This makes it possible to see the fine details in the spleen and nearby organs and tissues.
- Do not eat or drink anything for 8 hours before the operation.
- Shower or bathe as usual on the morning of the operation.
- You may be given medicine that will make you feel drowsy before you are brought to the operating room.

□ OPERATION

- You will be asleep for the operation.
- You will not receive a blood transfusion unless it is absolutely necessary. You may receive a transfusion of platelets.
- The operation usually takes about 2 hours.

POSTOPERATIVE CARE

- You will wake up in a recovery room. When your blood pressure, pulse, and breathing are stable, you will be taken to a regular hospital room.
- You may have a thin plastic tube in your nose. It goes down to your stomach to suck up the air you swallow. It will be removed when your bowels start working.

- That evening you will be helped to sit up in bed and on the next day to get out of bed.
- Pain will be controlled with medicine. The nurse will give it to you, or you can give yourself a preset amount of pain medicine when you feel you need it. This is done by a method called patient controlled analgesia (PCA), in which you control the amount of pain medication with a device that is connected to the tubing giving you intravenous fluids.
- You will be given an incentive spirometer. Breathing into this as you are instructed will help you expand your lungs and reduce the risk of developing pneumonia.
- When the tube in your nose is removed, you will be started on a liquid diet. This will be increased as you tolerate it.
- You should be able to go home in about 3 to 5 days.
- Arrangements will be made for your medicine, follow-up office visit, and stitch or clip removal.
- As with any operation, complications are always possible. With this type of operation they can include lung infection, bleeding, pneumonia, blood clots, and possibly others.

✣ HOME CARE

- Continue with the program started while you were in the hospital.
- You may walk about as you wish, even climb stairs, but don't overdo things.
- Take medicine as prescribed for your pain.
- Unless instructed otherwise, you may shower as you wish with any dressings on or off.
  - There may be narrow strips of tape across the incision. It's all right if they get wet; they will be removed in the doctor's office.
  - After you dry yourself, replace any dressings with clean, dry ones.
- Include enough roughage and plenty of liquids in your diet to help prevent constipation. You may need a mild laxative (example: milk of magnesia).
- Driving a car with an automatic shift is not too demanding. But if you suddenly have to slam on the brakes or twist to turn the steering wheel, you may get into an accident or strain the sutures or tear something. During your follow-up visit, let's discuss when you can resume driving.
- You may resume sexual activity whenever you choose.
- You may return to work when you feel up to it, but let's talk about it first during your follow-up office visit.

✆ CALL OUR OFFICE IF

- The incision becomes red or swollen, or there is drainage from it.
- You develop a temperature higher than 100°F.
- You have any questions.

△ GENERAL INFORMATION

Before starting therapy for most cancers, it is necessary to know the extent of the cancer. That's why patients have various tests done before treatment is started. This process is called *staging*. Staging is particularly important for certain cancers because the treatment varies so much, depending on where the cancer is located.

METHODS OF STAGING

When the cancer affects the abdomen, there are a number of staging methods that can be used.

Imaging

- *CT scan (computed tomography scan)*: These special x-rays are taken by a machine that is shaped like a huge doughnut. You will lie on a table inside the hole in the "doughnut." The x-rays are taken as very thin slices through any area of the body, in this instance the abdomen. This makes it possible to see the fine details of organs and tissues in the abdomen.
- *MRI (magnetic resonance imaging)*: No x-rays are used with this technique. Instead, the imaging is done with harmless magnetic fields, radio waves, and computers. A computer develops the pictures to show organs from several angles. It is especially valuable for examining your blood vessels, nerve tissue, and bones.
- *PET scan (positron emission tomography scan)*: This is a very sophisticated way of not only seeing a mass but also being able to tell how much "biologic activity" there is in the mass. This provides information on how fast the tumor is growing.
- *Ultrasound*: Harmless sound waves are aimed at the various areas of your abdomen. The sound waves bouncing back (the echoes) from this area are seen as a picture on a screen. Ultrasound is a convenient and painless way to examine organs and tissues inside your abdomen.

Endoscopy

- *Esophagogastroduodenoscopy*: This is an examination of your esophagus, stomach, and duodenum. It is done with an optical instrument that is smooth, flexible, has a light at its tip, and is as big around as your little finger. Your mouth and throat will be sprayed with an anesthetic to make them numb and you will be given medicine to make you feel drowsy. The instrument will be inserted gently into your mouth, down your esophagus, and into the stomach and then the duodenum. All these areas will be examined carefully.
- *Colonoscopy*: This instrument is very much like the one used to examine the esophagus and stomach. Again, medicine will be given to make you feel drowsy, and the lubricated instrument will be inserted gently through the anus into the rectum and then the entire colon so that it can be examined carefully.
- *X-rays*: These can provide valuable information on the organs inside the abdomen.

Interventional Radiology

- The skin over the abdominal mass is prepared with an antiseptic solution and injected with an anesthetic to make it numb.
- A special needle is introduced through the numbed skin and advanced down into the mass. As everything is watched on the ultrasound or x-ray screen, a piece is taken (a *biopsy*) for examination in the laboratory.

Laparoscopy

- Laparoscopy is performed with an optical instrument about as big around as your little finger that has a light at its tip. It is introduced into the abdomen through a tiny incision in the navel. Organ tissue inside the abdomen can be looked at directly (but not from all sides) by this technique. However, the tissue cannot truly be felt.

LAPAROTOMY

Laparotomy (opening the abdomen) is reserved for those situations in which the tissue has to be felt, sizable biopsies need to be taken, and organs need to be removed or repositioned.

- You will have an examination of your blood, urine, heart (EKG), and lungs (chest x-ray).
- Do not eat or drink anything for 8 hours before the operation.
- You may be given medicine that will make you feel drowsy before you are brought to the operating room.

□ OPERATION

- You will be asleep for the operation.
- The abdomen will be opened and a thorough and systematic examination made both by sight and by feel. A biopsy of relevant tissue will be performed.
- On occasion, it may be necessary to remove an organ (example: the spleen) or to reposition organs (example: the ovaries) because this will help with the medical or x-ray treatment of your problem.
- The operation usually takes about 2 hours.

POSTOPERATIVE CARE

- You will be taken to a recovery room and observed. When your blood pressure, pulse, and breathing are stable, you will be taken to a regular hospital room.
- Pain will be controlled with medicine.
- That evening you will be helped to sit up in bed and on the next day to get out of bed.
- You should be able to go home in several days.
- Arrangements will be made for your medicine, follow-up office visit, and stitch removal.
- As with any operation, complications are always possible. With this type of operation, they can include bleeding, pneumonia, wound infection, bowel obstruction, and possibly others.

✚ HOME CARE

- You may walk about as you wish, even climb stairs, but don't overdo things.

- Eat whatever you wish, but include plenty of roughage and liquids in your diet to help prevent constipation.
- Unless instructed otherwise, you may shower as you wish with any dressings on or off. After you dry yourself, replace any dressings with clean, dry ones.
- Do not drive a car unless you can move freely and without pain and are not taking medicines that decrease your alertness.
- You may resume sexual activity whenever you choose.
- You may return to work when you feel up to it.

✆ CALL OUR OFFICE IF

- You develop any unusual signs or symptoms.
- The incision becomes red or swollen, or there is drainage from it.
- You develop a temperature higher than 100°F.
- You have any questions.

△ GENERAL INFORMATION

Cancer of the stomach is a new growth that starts in the lining of the stomach. It is most common in older men.

COMMON SIGNS AND SYMPTOMS

The signs and symptoms of stomach cancer depend on its location and size and may include belching; pain under the breast bone; a mildly full feeling, especially after meals—even small ones; loss of appetite, nausea, and even vomiting; weight loss; anemia; and weakness and fatigue. If the cancer has spread to other organs, the symptoms may come from these other organs.

DIAGNOSIS

- You will have an examination of your blood, urine, heart (EKG), and lungs (chest x-ray).
- *Stomach x-rays*: Barium (it looks and flows like buttermilk) is swallowed, and x-ray pictures are taken as it flows down the esophagus, into the stomach, and then out into the duodenum. This can show the size and location of the tumor.
- *Gastroscopy*: This is done with an optical instrument (a *gastroscope*) that has a light at its tip, is smooth and flexible, and is about as big around as your little finger. Your mouth and throat will be sprayed with an anesthetic to make them numb. You will be given medicine to make you feel drowsy. The instrument will be passed gently down your esophagus and into your stomach and then a short distance past the stomach. All these areas will be examined carefully, and if anything suspicious is seen, a piece will be taken (a *biopsy*) for laboratory examination.
- *CT scan (computed tomography scan)*: These x-rays are taken in a special way as very thin slices through the area of the abdomen. This makes it possible to see the fine details in the abdomen—in this instance the stomach, liver, and surrounding tissue.

○ TREATMENT

The treatment for cancer of the stomach is an operation to remove the part of the stomach affected by the cancer as well as the lymph nodes draining this area and to reconnect the cut ends (Fig. 1).

After careful consideration of all factors, it is recommended that you have such an operation.

PREOPERATIVE PREPARATION

- You will have an examination of your blood, urine, heart (EKG), and lungs (chest x-ray).
- The goal is to get you in the best possible condition for this major operation.
- Do not eat or drink anything for 8 hours before the operation.
- You may be given medicine that will make you feel drowsy before you are brought to the operating room.

□ OPERATION

- You will be asleep for the operation.
- The incision will be in your upper abdomen.
- The operation usually takes about 3 hours.

POSTOPERATIVE CARE

- You will be taken to a recovery room and observed. When your blood pressure, pulse, and breathing are stable, you will be taken to a regular hospital room.
- You will have a thin, plastic tube in your nose. It will be removed as soon as your bowels start working.

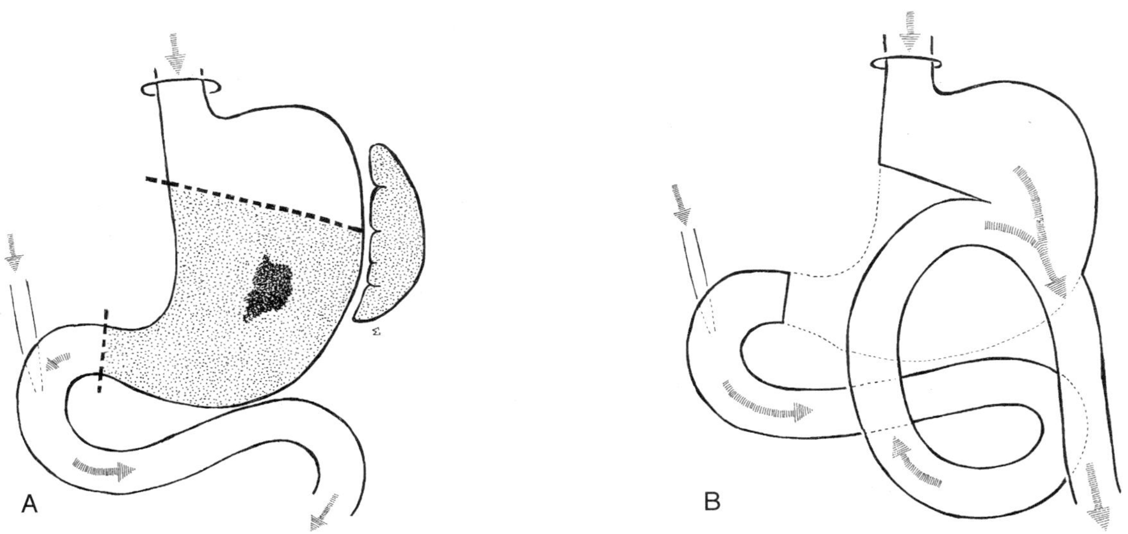

Figure 1. The choice of operation for cancer of the stomach depends on a number of things, including the size of the cancer and its location within the stomach. *A,* One common type of operation is shown. The position of the stomach *(stippled area)* with the cancer in it *(dark area)* is removed along the dashed lines. In this instance, the spleen to the right of the stomach is also removed. *B,* The cut end of the stomach is reconnected to the small intestine as shown. The arrows in *A* and *B* show the route of food and of bile.

- That evening you will be helped to sit up in bed and on the next day to get out of bed.
- Pain will be controlled with medicine.
- You will be given an incentive spirometer. Breathing into this as you are instructed will help you expand your lungs and reduce the risk of developing pneumonia.
- After the tube in your nose is removed, your diet will be liquids; more solid foods will be added as you tolerate them.
- As with any operation, complications are always possible. With this type of operation, they can include bleeding, leakage where the stomach is reconnected, pneumonia, heart problems, blood clots, and possibly others.
- You should be able to go home in about 1 week.
- Arrangements will be made for your medicine, follow-up office visit, and stitch removal.

✣ HOME CARE

- Continue with the program started while you were in the hospital.
- You may walk about as you wish, even climb stairs, but don't overdo things.
- Take the medicines prescribed for you.
- Follow the diet outlined for you.
- Unless instructed otherwise, you may shower as you wish with any dressings on or off. After you dry yourself, replace any dressings with clean, dry ones.
- Do not drive a car unless you can move freely and without pain and are not taking medicines that reduce your alertness.
- You may resume sexual activity whenever you choose.
- You may return to work when you feel up to it.

✆ CALL OUR OFFICE IF

- The incision becomes red or swollen, or there is drainage from it.
- You develop a temperature higher than 100°F.
- You have any questions.

STOMACH ULCER

△ GENERAL INFORMATION

Stomach ulcers are seen mostly in older persons and more often in men. They differ from the more common ulcers of the *duodenum* (the part of the intestine just past the stomach). For example, although stomach ulcers are one-fifth as common as duodenal ulcers, they cause one-half of the deaths from ulcers. There are many theories on what causes stomach ulcers.

COMMON SIGNS AND SYMPTOMS

- Loss of appetite.
- Vague pain in the upper abdomen.
- Weight loss because of pain associated with eating.

DIAGNOSIS

Anyone who has the above history and symptoms might have a stomach ulcer. Further information can be obtained from the following procedures:

- *Stomach x-rays (upper GI series)*: Barium is swallowed and x-rays taken as it goes down the esophagus, into the stomach and then out to the duodenum. This examination may show the ulcer, but too often it cannot reliably tell the difference between a plain ulcer and a cancer-related ulcer.
- *Gastroscopy*: This is done with an optical instrument with a light at its tip that is smooth, flexible, and as big around as your little finger. After your mouth and throat are sprayed with an anesthetic to make them numb, you will be given some medicine to make you drowsy. The instrument will then be inserted gently into your esophagus and stomach and then into the duodenum so that all these areas can be thoroughly examined. Several tiny pieces will be taken of the stomach ulcer (a *biopsy*) and sent to the laboratory for examination to be certain it is just an ulcer and not an ulcer in a cancerous tumor.

○ TREATMENT

- A stomach ulcer responds less well to medical ulcer therapy than a duodenal ulcer, and if it does respond, two times out of three, the ulcer comes back. Just the same, it is reasonable to give a 6- to 10-week trial of intensive medical therapy.
- If there is a recurrence, and especially if there is a second recurrence, an operation should be done.
- An operation is strongly advised if the ulcer does not even begin to respond to medical treatment.
- An emergency operation must be done if the ulcer bleeds a lot or makes a hole through the stomach.

PREOPERATIVE PREPARATION

- You will have an examination of your blood, urine, heart (EKG), and lungs (chest x-ray).
- Do not eat or drink anything for 8 hours before the operation.
- Shower as usual on the morning of the operation.
- You may be given medicine that will make you feel drowsy before you are brought to the operating room.

□ OPERATION

- The aim of the operation is to remove the part of the stomach with the ulcer in it and then to reconnect your stomach (Fig. 1).
- You will be asleep for the operation.
- You will not receive a blood transfusion unless it is absolutely necessary.
- The operation usually takes about 2½ hours.

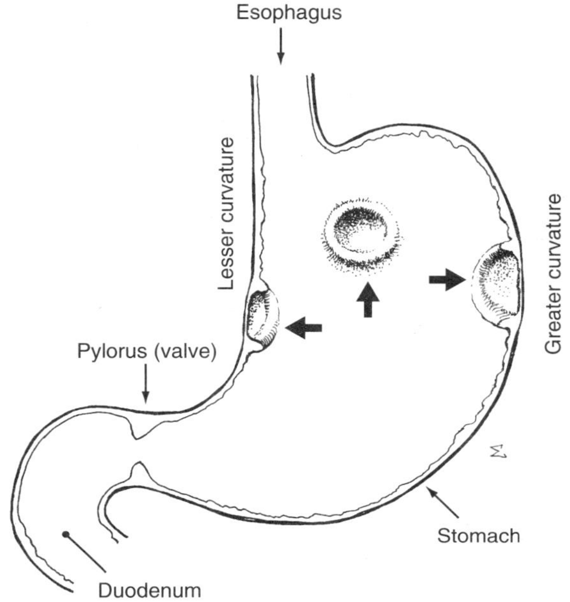

Figure 1. Several possible locations of stomach ulcer *(bold arrows)* are shown. The location of the ulcer plus other medical considerations determine the type of operation that is best to correct the problem.

POSTOPERATIVE CARE

- You will wake up in a recovery room. When your blood pressure, pulse, and breathing are stable, you will be taken to a regular hospital room.
- You will have a thin plastic tube in your nose. It goes down to your stomach to suck up the air you swallow. It will be removed when your bowels start working.
- That evening you will be helped to sit up in bed and on the next day to get out of bed.
- Pain can be controlled with medicine. The nurse will give you, or you can give yourself, a preset amount of pain medicine when you feel you need it. This type of pain relief, called patient-controlled analgesia (PCA) uses a device that releases the medicine into the tubing giving you intravenous fluids.
- You may be given an incentive spirometer. Breathing into this as you are instructed will help expand your lungs and reduce your risk of developing pneumonia.
- After the tube in your nose is removed, you will be started on a liquid diet. This will be increased to solid foods as you tolerate them.
- As with any operation, complications are always possible. With this type of operation, they can include failure of the stomach to empty properly,

bleeding, infection, leakage from the reconnected stomach, heart problems, bowel obstruction, and possibly others.
- You should be able to go home in about 5 days.
- Arrangements will be made for your medicine, follow-up office visit, and stitch or clip removal.

✚ HOME CARE

- Continue with the program started while you were in the hospital.
- You may walk about as you wish, even climb stairs, but don't overdo things.
- Take medicine as prescribed for your pain.
- You will be given a suggested diet to follow during your convalescence.
- Be careful that you do not become constipated.
  - Include enough liquid in your diet.
  - You may need a mild laxative (example: milk of magnesia).
- Unless instructed otherwise, you may shower as you wish and with any dressings on or off.
  - There may be narrow strips of tape across the incision. It's all right if they get wet; they will be removed in the doctor'soffice.
  - After you dry yourself, replace any dressings with clean, dry ones.
- Driving a car with an automatic shift is not too demanding. But if you suddenly have to slam on the brakes or twist to turn a wheel, you may strain the sutures or tear something. During your follow-up visit, let's discuss when you can resume driving.
- You may resume sexual activity whenever you choose.
- You may return to work if you feel up to it, but let's talk about it first during your follow-up office visit.

✆ CALL OUR OFFICE IF

- You develop any unusual signs or symptoms.
- The incision becomes red or swollen, or there is drainage from it.
- You develop a temperature higher than 100°F.
- You have any questions.

△ GENERAL INFORMATION

X-rays of the stomach usually are taken when there is reason to suspect something is wrong with the stomach. Among these reasons are the following:

- Pain in the upper part of the abdomen that appears to be caused by an ulcer.
- Blood in the stool that is found either by the patient or by the doctor during a routine physical examination.
- Feeling full after even a small meal.
- The stomach feels full for a long time after a meal as though the stomach is not emptying properly.
- Loss of appetite.
- Loss of weight.
- Frequent belching or even vomiting, especially after eating.
- Something is known to be wrong with the stomach and is being treated; the x-rays are done to check on the patient's progress.

HOW AN X-RAY OF THE STOMACH WORKS

If you were to have an x-ray of your abdomen right now—just as you are—the x-rays would pass right through all the soft tissue and the x-ray picture would be very dark. You would not be able to see any of the stomach. Barium, however, shows up on the x-rays. If barium is placed in the stomach, it will show the outline of the stomach that will make it possible to see the following:

- If there is an ulcer (a crater), this will fill with barium and will show up as a white area.
- If there is a growth on the wall of the stomach, the barium won't be able to fill this spot, and it will appear as a black area (Fig. 1).

PREPARATION FOR STOMACH X-RAY

- Do not eat or drink anything after midnight before the day of the examination. On the morning of the examination, do not drink any fluid (or even chew gum). Swallowing creates a lot of saliva, which sticks to the lining of your stomach and interferes with how well the barium can show fine details in the stomach.

THE PROCEDURE

- You will be asked to remove your outer clothing and will be given a long gown to wear.
- You will lie on an x-ray table. The x-ray films are located inside the table, just under your abdomen. The x-ray machine is right over your stomach.
- The table will be shifted to the upright position with you on it. You will be in a standing position.
- You'll be given a large glass of barium (it has the color and consistency of buttermilk) and asked to take a number of swallows.
- X-rays will be taken of the barium as it travels down your esophagus and into the stomach.
- Next, you will be asked to drink the rest of the glass of barium. Your stomach now will have a fair amount of barium in it. The radiologist will be looking at where the barium goes and where it cannot go.

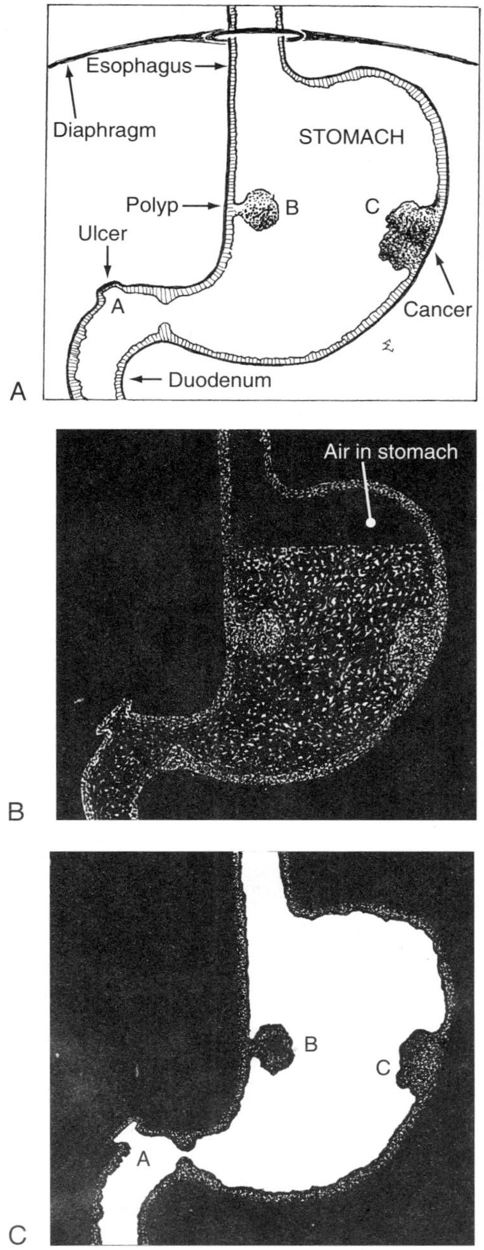

Figure 1. *A*, A stomach with a polyp (B) and a cancer (C) shown inside it and an ulcer (A) shown in the duodenum. *B*, The appearance of the stomach on an ordinary x-ray. *C*, The appearance of the stomach, the duodenum, and the three lesions (A–C) as seen on x-ray after barium is swallowed.

- Sometimes during the examination you will be asked to swallow a "fizzy" drink. It produces gas that stretches the stomach, making it easier to see details.
- The table will be adjusted so that it is flat. You'll be lying on your back.
- The radiologist will press down on your stomach to

help the barium get into all the nooks and crannies so that all areas inside the stomach can be examined.

- You will be asked to turn from side to side and even onto your stomach. This helps the barium reach all parts of your stomach so that no area is missed.
- During this time, the table and the x-ray machine over you will sometimes move in several directions.
- Next, the radiologist will watch the barium as it leaves the stomach to enter the duodenum. This is the area where most ulcers occur, so the duodenum will be examined with special care.
- The examination is now over and you will be free to go about your business.
- You are encouraged to drink a lot of fluids and possibly take a mild laxative.
- The barium will color your stools slightly white for the next day or two.

The x-rays that were taken will all be assembled and examined by the radiologist. The findings will be reported to your personal physician.

SUBCLAVIAN STEAL SYNDROME

△ GENERAL INFORMATION

In the *subclavian steal syndrome*, a person becomes dizzy and feels faint because the blood that is in the vessel that goes to the brain is "stolen" by the blood vessel that goes to the arm. To understand how this happens, you need to look at the illustration (Fig. 1) and explanations.

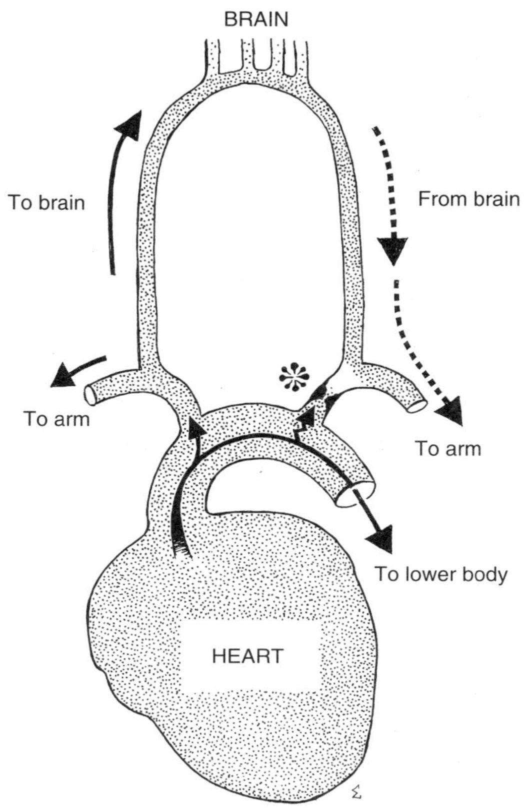

Figure 1. Occasionally, the artery to the arm is narrowed from cholesterol deposits *(asterisk)* and has reduced the amount of blood to the arm. Thus, when the arm on this side is used it needs more blood. This causes the blood in the vessels to the brain to flow away from the brain *(dashed line)* so that blood can flow in the arm artery, thereby "stealing" blood from the brain. The operation changes things so that enough blood can get to the arm without stealing it from the brain.

The heart pumps blood that goes out through the aorta (as big around as a mop handle) and its branches. There are three branches from the aorta that themselves give off a number of branches. The important ones here are the four branches taking blood to the brain: the right *common carotid artery* and the right *vertebral artery*. Similar vessels are on the left side. They all connect at the bottom of the brain (the *circle of Willis*) and from there, give off branches to different parts of the brain. Then there are the right and left *subclavian arteries*, which supply blood to the arms.

Once in a while, a blockage develops. Because blood cannot get to the arm the normal way, the arm artery (the *subclavian* artery) "steals" blood from the *vertebral* artery on that side that normally would have blood in it flowing toward the brain. This happens because the blood in the right side goes up to the circle of Willis, and instead of all of the blood going to the brain, some of it goes down the wrong way in the left vertebral artery to take blood to the left subclavian artery and the arm.

COMMON SIGNS AND SYMPTOMS

Such "stealing" of blood from the brain produces the following symptoms:

- Lightheadedness and a spinning sensation. Also, there is weakness and a "pins and needles" sensation in the arm, leg, or face.
- Difficulty with the eyes and with speaking and occasionally unconsciousness.
- The symptoms usually are brought on by exercising the affected arm.

DIAGNOSIS

- Usually, the diagnosis can be made by taking a detailed history and doing a thorough physical examination.
- The blood pressure in the affected arm usually is lower than in the opposite arm.
- One purpose of the examination is to make certain that the symptoms are not caused by some other disease.
- *Doppler ultrasound*: Harmless sound waves are aimed at the blood vessels in this area. The sound waves bouncing back (the echoes) from this area are seen as a picture on a screen. Ultrasound is a convenient and painless way to examine the blood vessels in this area for any blockage and determine its location and extent.
- *Arteriography*: Dye is injected into the arteries to see if there is an obstruction, and if so where it is located and how bad it is. Also, the neighboring arteries can be examined to see how they contribute to the problem and how they might help solve it.

○ TREATMENT

For a verified diagnosis of subclavian steal syndrome, the treatment is an operation to get enough blood to the arm so that it does not have to "steal" it from the vertebral artery. Usually, this is done by placing a bypass graft from the carotid artery of the aorta to the subclavian artery.

After careful consideration of all factors, the recommendation is that you have an operation to correct your problem.

PREOPERATIVE PREPARATION

- An examination of your blood, urine, heart (EKG), and lungs (chest x-ray) will be done.
- Do not eat or drink anything for 8 hours before the operation.

- Shower (and shave) as usual on the morning of the operation.
- You may be given medicine that will make you feel drowsy before you are brought to the operating room.

☐ OPERATION

- You will be asleep for the operation.
- The incision will be just above your clavicle (collar bone).
- The operation usually takes about 2 hours.

POSTOPERATIVE CARE

- You will wake up in a recovery room. When your blood pressure, pulse, and breathing are stable, you will be taken to a regular hospital room.
- That evening you will be helped to sit up in bed and on the next day to get out of bed.
- Pain can be controlled with medicine.
- You should be able to go home in about 3 to 5 days.
- As with any operation, complications are always possible. With this type of operation, they can include bleeding, clotting of the bypass vessels, infection, heart problems, and possibly others.
- Arrangements will be made for your medicine, follow-up office visit, and stitch removal.

HOME CARE

- Resume your usual activities.
- You may walk about as you wish, even climb stairs, but don't overdo things.
- Eat as you wish.
- Take medicine as prescribed for your pain.
- Unless instructed otherwise, you may shower as you wish with any dressings on or off.
  - There may be narrow strips of tape across the incision. It's all right if they get wet; they will be removed in the doctor's office.
  - After you dry yourself, replace any dressings with clean, dry ones.
- Driving a car with an automatic shift is not too demanding. But if you suddenly have to slam on the brakes or twist to turn a wheel, you may strain the sutures or tear something. During the follow-up visit, let's discuss when you can resume driving.
- You may resume sexual activity whenever you choose.
- You may return to work when you feel up to it, but let's talk about it first during your follow-up office visit.

CALL OUR OFFICE IF

- You develop any unusual signs or symptoms.
- The incision becomes red or swollen, or there is drainage from it.
- You develop a temperature higher than 100°F.
- You have any questions.

△ GENERAL INFORMATION

The diaphragm is a sheet of muscle about as thick as ten sheets of this paper. It separates the heart and lungs in the chest cavity from the organs in the abdominal cavity. A *subphrenic abscess* is a localized collection of pus right under the diaphragm and touching it (Fig. 1).

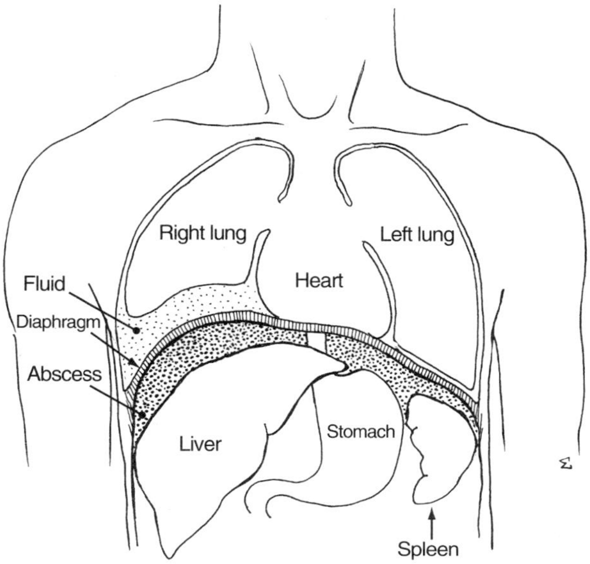

Figure 1. A subphrenic abscess can occur anywhere under the diaphragm. Most often, however, it is found under the right diaphragm (and on top of the liver).

COMMON SIGNS AND SYMPTOMS

The signs and symptoms of a subphrenic abscess are caused by the effects of the pus on the diaphragm and surrounding structures. They can include some of the following:

- Fever that goes sharply up and down ("spikes") along with shaking chills and sweating.
- Fast pulse.
- Pain, tenderness, and some redness of the skin on the left or right side of the abdomen.
- Pushing up of the diaphragm because of the pus under it.
- Chest pain.
- Shortness of breath.
- Fluid in the chest.
- Hiccoughs.

DIAGNOSIS

- The diagnosis can often be made by taking a careful history, doing a thorough physical examination, and evaluating the laboratory reports.
- In most cases, subphrenic abscess occurs as a complication of an abdominal operation or is due to a hole in the intestine caused by an illness or injury.
- You will have some or all of the following tests.
- *Chest x-ray*: This may show an elevation of the diaphragm, fluid in the chest, or an inflamed lung just above the diaphragm or other problems under the diaphragm.
- *Ultrasound*: Harmless sound waves are aimed at the area of your diaphragm. The sound waves bouncing back (the echoes) from this area are seen as a picture on a screen. Ultrasound is a convenient and painless way to examine organs and tissues inside this area of your body.
- *CT scan (computed tomography scan):* These special x-rays are taken by a machine that is shaped like a huge doughnut. You will lie on a table inside the hole in the "doughnut" and x-rays are taken as very thin slices through the area of the diaphragm. This makes it possible to see the fine details in and around the diaphragm.
- *Aspiration*: A needle may be inserted in the presumed abscess to determine its nature and to take a sample from it or remove all of it.

○ TREATMENT

If a subphrenic abscess is not treated or does not respond to the treatment given, there is a high risk of death. The treatment can be given in two ways:

Catheter Drainage

- You will lie on a table and be given medicine to make you feel drowsy.
- The skin over the abscess will be painted with an antiseptic solution and made numb.
- A thin plastic tube will be placed through the numbed skin and into the abscess cavity and as much of the pus will be removed as possible.

Advantages of This Method

- An operation and incision are not necessary.

Disadvantages of This Method

- The pus may be too thick to come out through the tube.
- There may be more than one cavity (like soap bubbles) and it may not be possible to drain all of them.
- It doesn't correct the cause of the abscess.
- This method is not effective if the abscess is caused by a fungus.
- There is a risk that the needle may pass through noninfected areas and infect them also.

Operation

Advantages of This Method

- Everything can be seen clearly and cleaned more thoroughly and some risks avoided.

Disadvantages of This Method

- It is an operation.

After careful consideration of all factors, the recommendation is that you have an open drainage of your subphrenic abscess.

PREOPERATIVE PREPARATION

- Do not eat or drink anything for 8 hours before the operation.

- You may be given medicine that will make you feel drowsy before you are brought to the operating room.

☐ OPERATION

- You will be asleep for the operation.
- The incision will be just under the last ribs and over the area of the abscess.
- The operation usually takes about 2 hours.

POSTOPERATIVE CARE

- You will be taken to a recovery room and observed. When your blood pressure, pulse, and breathing are stable, you will be taken to a regular hospital room.
- There will be a plastic tube coming from your abdomen to the outside to drain additional fluid present.
- You may have a thin plastic tube in your nose for a day or two.
- That evening you will be helped to sit up in bed and on the next day to get out of bed.
- You will be given an incentive spirometer. Breathing into this as you are instructed will help you expand your lungs and reduce the risk of developing pneumonia.
- Pain will be controlled with medicine.
- Arrangements will be made for your medicine, follow-up office visit, and stitch removal.
- As with any operation, complications are always possible, some of them serious. With this type of operation, they can include bleeding, the persistence or recurrence of the abscess, bowel obstruction, pneumonia, fluid in the chest, liver abscess, wound infection, and possibly others.

✚ HOME CARE

- You may walk about as you wish, even climb stairs, but don't overdo things.
- Take medicine as prescribed for your pain.
- Be certain to take any antibiotics prescribed for you.
- Unless instructed otherwise, you may shower if you wish with any dressings on or off.
  - There may be narrow strips of tape across the incision. It's all right if they get wet, they will be removed in the doctor's office.
  - After you dry yourself, replace any dressings with clean, dry ones.
- Arrangements can be made for a home visiting nurse if one is needed.
- Do not drive until we talk about it during your follow-up office visit.
- You may return to work when you feel up to it, but let's first talk about it during a follow-up office visit.

✆ CALL OUR OFFICE IF

- The incision becomes red or swollen, or there is drainage from it.
- You develop a temperature higher than 101°F.
- You have any questions.

△ GENERAL INFORMATION

The sympathetic nervous system is a group of nerves that carry sensations back to the spinal cord from areas inside the body. They also help regulate how blood flows in the body by changing the size of the blood vessels.

The sympathetic nerves originate in the spinal cord and extend to various parts of the body. Once these fibers leave the spinal cord, they form large groupings that are called ganglia. Three important ones are as follows:

- *Stellate ganglion*: This is located at the base of the neck and supplies the head, neck, and arms.
- *Celiac plexus ganglia*: These are located deep in the pit of the stomach and supply the organs of the abdomen.
- *Lumbar ganglia*: Located deep in the lower back region, these supply the legs (Fig. 1).

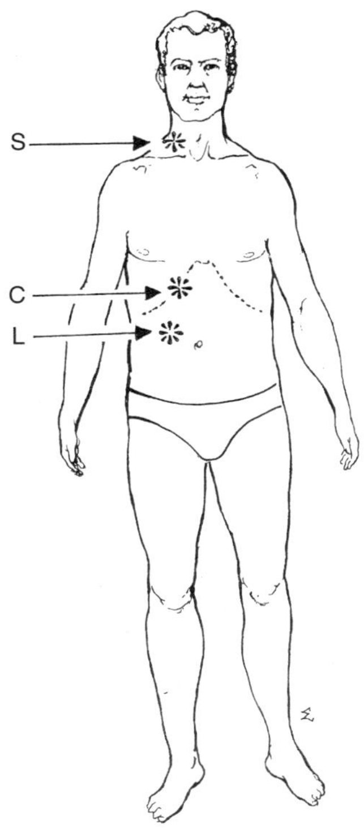

Figure 1. Three ganglia commonly used to obtain a sympathetic nerve block are the stellate (S), the celiac (C), and the lumbar (L).

HOW THE BLOCKS ARE PERFORMED

Sympathetic nerve blocks generally are performed by anesthesiologists with special interest and skill in pain management. Usually, the block is done by injecting a local anesthetic around a group of sympathetic nerves, ganglia, or nerve groupings associated with the painful area.

For all blocks, it is important that you do not eat or drink anything for 4 hours before the procedure.

STELLATE GANGLION BLOCK

A stellate ganglion block is done for several reasons:

- Relief of pain in the arm due to injury (often called *reflux autonomic dystrophy*).
- Relief of pain in the head and neck area due to herpes zoster infection.
- Relief of pain after chest surgery that does not respond to the usual therapy.

The person performing the block is thoroughly acquainted with the location of the ganglia deep in the neck, even though these ganglia cannot be felt.

- You will lie on your back on a comfortable table.
- The skin around the lower neck on the side that is affected will be swabbed with an antiseptic solution and surrounded with sterile towels.
- A short fine needle will be used to inject an anesthetic solution in the skin to make it numb.
- A special needle is placed through the numbed skin in the lower part of the neck and advanced down to the ganglia.
- The local anesthetic is slowly and gently injected over a period of several minutes.
- You should experience pain relief within several minutes after the injection.

The side effects of a stellate ganglion block are drooping of the eyelid or hoarseness lasting for about 4 hours.

After the procedure is completed, you will be observed. When your blood pressure, pulse, and breathing are stable, you should be able to leave with a responsible adult.

CELIAC PLEXUS BLOCK

A celiac plexus block is usually done for relief of pain originating in the abdomen, most commonly from cancer of organs in the upper abdomen, especially the pancreas.

- You will be positioned on a comfortable table face down with a pillow under your stomach.
- The skin over your back will be swabbed with an antiseptic solution and surrounded with sterile towels. A short, fine needle will be used to inject a small amount of anesthetic in the skin to make it numb.
- One or two special needles are placed through the numbed skin in the back next to the spine and directed down to the celiac ganglia. A special x-ray machine will be used to be certain the needle is accurately placed and that the anesthetic is injected into the correct area.
- If the procedure is done for relief of pain, disappearance of the pain shortly after the injection means the needle is in the correct position. If the injection is done for another reason, a fall in blood pressure often indicates correct placement of the needle.
- After the procedure is completed, you will be observed for several hours. When your blood pressure, pulse, and breathing are stable, you should be able to leave the hospital with a responsible adult.

- As with any procedure, complications are always possible. For this procedure, they can include temporary lowering of the blood pressure. If some of the local anesthetic enters the blood stream, you may experience a ringing in the ears or even pass out for several seconds. This loss of consciousness can sometimes be accompanied by temporary jerking movements of the arms or legs.

Note: The anesthetic solution that is injected usually gives temporary relief, very much like the local anesthetic used by dentists. If there is satisfactory relief of pain with such medication, a solution can be injected that gives much longer-lasting relief, often 2 to 6 months. In such instances, the drug injected destroys the nerve tissue rather than just temporarily anesthetizing it. Before any such step is taken, however, there will be much more detailed discussion with you.

LUMBAR BLOCK

Like a stellate block, a lumbar block can be used to treat pain from a herpes infection or sympathetic dystrophy of the leg. Also, it can be used to determine if a patient with problems with the leg arteries would benefit from a sympathectomy.

- You will lie face down on a comfortable table with a pillow under your stomach.
- Your back will be swabbed with an antiseptic solution and surrounded with sterile drapes.
- A very fine needle will be used to inject an anesthetic in the skin over the ganglion to make it numb.
- A special needle will be passed through the numbed skin and advanced down to the ganglion.
- After the needle is checked with x-rays to be certain it is in the correct position, the injection of medicine will be started slowly and given over a few minutes time.
- The skin over the leg usually feels warm in about 5 minutes. Although uncommon, as with any procedure, complications are always possible. For this procedure they can include unintentional injection of the drug into the blood vessel. Occasionally, the thigh becomes numb temporarily, which makes it difficult to know if the injection is successful.
- You will be observed, and when your blood pressure, pulse, and breathing are stable, you should be able to go home with a responsible adult.

As you can see, sympathetic nerve blocks can be very valuable in helping with conditions that do not respond to any other therapy.

△ GENERAL INFORMATION

Very few people besides doctors and nurses have ever heard of T tubes, let alone know much about them. However, for those who need them, they can be very important and sometimes even life saving.

WHAT ARE T TUBES?

- They are thin-walled rubber tubes that are in the shape of a T. Like the letter T, they have one long arm and two short arms.
- The tubes vary in size from that of thin spaghetti to large macaroni.

WHERE AND HOW ARE THEY USED

- They are used in the common bile duct, which drains bile from the liver and gallbladder into the small intestine (the *duodenum*) (Fig. 1).

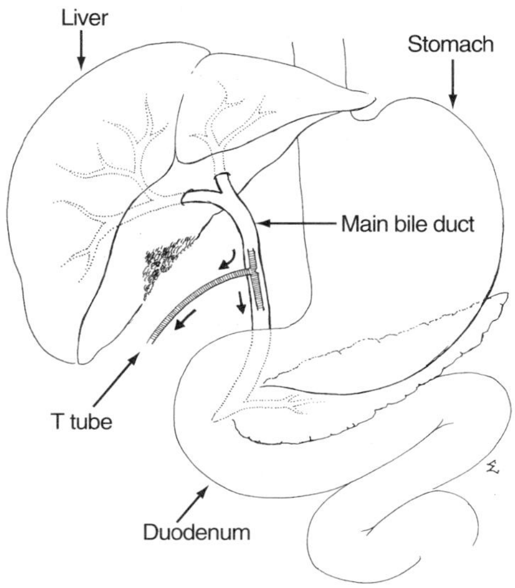

Figure 1. Usually a T tube is placed in the common bile duct.

- Normally the common bile duct is about the size of a pencil. However, if it is blocked, it can swell to two to three times this size.
- During an operation, the common bile duct may need to be opened to look for and remove gallstones that may have lodged in it. When this is completed, the opening cannot be closed in a leak-proof manner. The bile continues to leak out and accumulates under the liver or in other parts of the body where it can cause an infection.
- For this reason, the T tube is placed in the common duct so that the short arms are inside the duct and the long arm comes out through a very small hole in the skin. This long arm is connected to a small bag that collects the bile.

WHEN AND WHY THEY ARE USED

- So that bile can come straight to the outside and be collected in a small plastic bag. This is safer than having it leak inside the body and possibly cause an infection.
- So that one of the short arms of the T tube can act as a support for the suture line if the common duct has to be divided and reconnected.
- In a week or so, the long arm of the T-tube is used to inject dye into the common duct and take x-ray pictures of it to see the following:
  - How well the common duct is healing.
  - Whether there is a leak.
  - Whether fluid can enter into the duodenum easily.
  - Whether there are any stones still in the duct.
  - If the x-rays show good results, the T tube can easily be removed.
- If the x-rays show that stones are still present in the common bile duct, the T tube is removed, leaving a tunnel where the long arm came to the outside. With x-ray guidance, a special wire can be passed through the tunnel and into the common duct and the stones fished out.

HOW DOES ONE TAKE CARE OF A T TUBE?

- The long arm of the T tube is taped as well as stitched to the skin so that it won't accidentally come loose.
- You'll be shown how to change dressings and how to empty the bile from the small plastic bag. It's easy.
- Unless instructed otherwise, you may shower as you wish with any dressings on or off.
  - There may be narrow strips of tape across the incision. It's all right if they get wet. They will be removed in the doctor's office.
  - After you dry yourself, replace any dressings with clean, dry ones.
  - Incidentally, before you enter the shower, you can tape the bag to your body so that it won't dangle.

HOW LONG DOES IT STAY IN?

- This depends on why it was put in.
- Under the usual circumstances, it is removed within 2 or 3 weeks.
- In a few instances, it needs to stay in for several months.

HOW IS IT REMOVED?

- It's simple. The anchoring stitches are snipped and the tube slips right out in a few seconds.
- The hole in the skin closes by itself in several days.

✆ CALL OUR OFFICE IF

- The tube slips out. Don't panic, but call the doctor promptly so that something can be done before the hole closes. If the doctor cannot be reached, go to the closest hospital emergency room.
- You develop a temperature of higher than 101°F or shaking chills.
- You develop abdominal pain or vomiting.
- The T tube stops draining.
- You develop any unusual signs or symptoms.
- You have any questions.

TEMPORAL ARTERY BIOPSY

△ GENERAL INFORMATION

The *temporal artery* is as big around as a piece of spaghetti and is located just in front of your ear (Fig. 1). A *biopsy* involves taking a piece of this artery to make a diagnosis of certain illnesses that affect blood vessels (commonly arteritis).

The reasons the temporal artery is chosen for the biopsy are the following:

- It's easy to reach.
- If part of it is removed, you won't miss it.
- The temporal artery is just as likely to be involved with arteritis as any other artery.

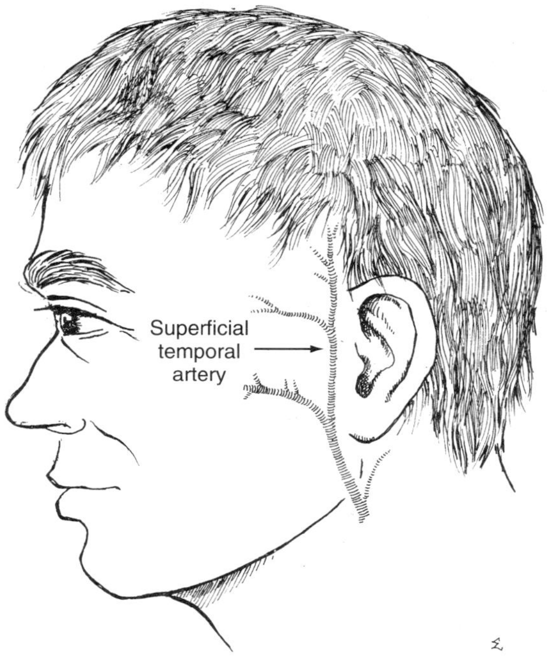

Figure 1. The superficial temporal artery is located just in front of the ear. Removing a short piece of it (a *biopsy*) does not produce any undesirable effect.

COMMON SIGNS AND SYMPTOMS

Usually the main symptoms are aching and stiff muscles. The problem can be present for a long time, or it may come on rather abruptly.

- Additional symptoms include headache, cramps of the jaw or tongue when chewing, eye problems, scalp tenderness, and sore throat.
- Many muscles and joints may ache.
- There can be fever, constant fatigue, and loss of appetite and weight.
- These symptoms are most often seen in older persons.

DIAGNOSIS

- A number of blood tests will be performed. Some results may be positive; a number of them may be negative. There is no one blood test that can definitely make the diagnosis. Even if a lot of the test results are negative, that does not mean that a biopsy of the artery will not show the disease.
- The specific diagnosis can be made only by a microscopic examination of a portion of the artery. Even then, however, there may be disease of the arteries but no evidence of it in the particular artery on which the biopsy was performed. So, even if the biopsy results are negative, there is still a 10% or greater chance that the disease can be diagnosed by taking a biopsy of the opposite artery.

○ TREATMENT

The treatment of the condition is medical. The purpose of the biopsy is to establish the diagnosis so that treatment can be given in a more confident and specific manner.

PREOPERATIVE PREPARATION

- Do not eat or drink anything for 6 hours before the operation.

□ OPERATION

- The operation will be done under local anesthesia.
- The area in front of your ear will be painted with an antiseptic solution and draped with towels.
- A very fine, short needle will be used to inject an anesthetic solution in the skin over the artery to make it completely numb.
- A ½-inch cosmetic incision will be made in a natural crease just in front of your ear and a short length of the artery removed.
- During the operation, you may feel some tugging but no pain.
- There will be a cosmetic closure.

POSTOPERATIVE CARE

- You will be taken to a recovery room. When your blood pressure, pulse, and breathing are stable, you should be able to go home with a responsible escort.
- Arrangements will be made for your medicine, follow-up office visit, and stitch removal.

✚ HOME CARE

- Resume your usual activities.
- You may shower as you wish with any dressings on or off.
  - There may be narrow strips of tape across the incision. It's all right if they get wet. They will be removed in the doctor's office.
  - After you dry yourself, replace any dressings with clean, dry ones.

✆ CALL OUR OFFICE IF

- You develop any unusual signs or symptoms.
- The incision becomes red or swollen, or there is drainage from it.
- You develop a temperature higher than 100°F.
- You have any questions.

△ GENERAL INFORMATION

Tennis elbow (the medical term is *lateral epicondylitis*) is the most common painful condition of the elbow. Inflammation or tearing of the muscle that is attached to the *lateral* (outside) *epicondyle* (bony knob at elbow) will cause pain, making it hard to grip, turn the hand, or swing your arm as you would during the backhand stroke of tennis. A small muscle called the *extensor carpi radialis brevis*, which is used to extend the wrist is most commonly involved in this condition (Fig. 1).

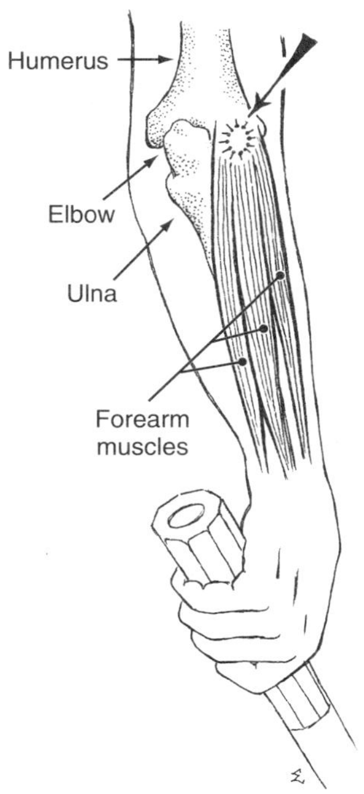

Figure 1. Anatomy of the elbow and forearm muscles as they relate to tennis elbow. Maximum pain usually is experienced at the lateral epicondyle of the humerus *(bold arrow)*.

COMMON SIGNS AND SYMPTOMS

The pain of epicondylitis usually has a gradual onset. The condition is often caused by a sudden change in activity level, such as playing an excessive amount of tennis or other racquet sports on a weekend, or repetitive use of the arm at work. At first, the pain may occur only following activities that involve the elbow, wrist, and hand, but if the condition progresses, pain may be present at rest and also when trying to sleep. A simple hand shake or lifting of a briefcase can be extremely painful.

DIAGNOSIS

- The diagnosis is made by taking a detailed history of the symptoms and doing a thorough physical examination of the elbow.
- The pain can be reproduced by pressing the area of the muscle just beyond the epicondyle.
- Extension of the wrist against resistance or extension of the third (long) finger will also reproduce symptoms.
- X-rays are used to rule out other conditions such as arthritis or loose pieces of tissue in the joint. Epicondylitis can lead to calcification at the origin of the tendon in some patients, which can be seen on the x-ray.
- Specialized tests such as a magnetic resonance imaging (MRI) scan are rarely used to evaluate this condition.

○ TREATMENT

- The activity that is causing the epicondylitis, such as playing tennis, lifting a briefcase, or certain work-related movements, must be avoided until the pain is under control. Sometimes just switching hands is enough to rest the affected elbow.
- An elbow support, often called a counterforce brace, is useful in reducing the pain. The support is placed just beyond the area of pain, and by applying pressure to this area of the muscle, it reduces the stresses across the inflamed or partially torn muscle origin.
- A splint to immobilize the wrist may be used early in the treatment of epicondylitis to help rest the muscles of the elbow.
- Anti-inflammatory medications such as ibuprofen (Motrin) are commonly used to reduce inflammation and alleviate pain.
- When anti-inflammatory medicines are ineffective or the early treatment program is unsuccessful in relieving the pain of epicondylitis, a cortisone injection may be given. A small amount of cortisone is injected at the site of the epicondylitis. Two or three injections of cortisone may be necessary before resolution of this condition.
- It is important to realize that this condition may take 6 to 12 months to resolve.
- An operation is indicated for those patients (fewer than 5%) who have failed to respond to appropriate treatment, including rest and elbow support, medications, and cortisone injections, over a period of 6 months and continue to have discomfort that interferes with their recreational or employment activities.

After careful consideration, it is recommended that your epicondylitis be treated by an operation.

PREOPERATIVE PREPARATION

- You will have an examination of your blood, urine, heart (EKG), and lungs (chest x-ray).
- Do not eat or drink anything for 8 hours before the operation.
- If you must take medicines daily, you may take yours with a small sip of water on the morning of the operation.
- Stop all aspirin-containing medications and anti-inflammatory medications such as Motrin or

Ibuprofen, at least 7 days prior to the operation. If pain medication is necessary, use Extra-Strength Tylenol.
- Shower as usual on the morning of the operation.
- You may be given medicine that will make you feel drowsy before you are brought to the operating room.

□ OPERATION

- The operation for lateral epicondylitis is performed on an outpatient basis.
- Most commonly, the patient is put to sleep for this operation although occasionally, a regional nerve block with sedation may be used. The choice will be discussed with you beforehand.
- A short incision is made on the outer aspect of the elbow.
- The area involved with epicondylitis is consistently located at the extensor carpi radialis brevis muscle.
- The affected tissue is removed.
- The fascia (strong tissue) of the muscle is reattached to the remaining small segment of tissue left on the epicondyle at the time of exposure. The skin is then closed in a cosmetic fashion. After a dressing is applied to the incision site, the elbow and wrist are splinted. The splint will be left on for 3 to 7 days to help alleviate discomfort.
- The operation usually takes about 1½ hours.

POSTOPERATIVE CARE

- You will be taken to a recovery room and observed. When your blood pressure, pulse, and breathing are stable and you are completely alert, you should be able to go home that same day with a responsible adult.
- Your pain will be controlled with medications that you take by mouth. If you have a history of problems with certain pain medications, be certain to tell this to the doctors and nurses before the operation.
- Arrangements will be made for your medicine, follow-up office visit, and stitch removal. Additionally, arrangements will be made for your physical therapy.

✚ HOME CARE

- You may walk about as you wish, even climb stairs.
- Take medicine as prescribed for your pain.
- Your diet may be as you tolerate it.
- Your arm and hand should be elevated as much as possible during the first 48 hours after your operation. When sitting or lying down, the operated elbow should be elevated above the level of your heart. An ice pack should be applied to the operated elbow for 30 minutes three times a day to minimize swelling and reduce pain.
- Your dressing should be kept clean and dry until removed. When taking a shower or bath, a plastic bag can be placed around the entire arm and sealed at the top with tape.
- It is important to move your fingers as much as possible and as much as your dressing will allow, to help reduce swelling and stiffness of the fingers and hand.
- Driving your car is not recommended until your bandage and splint have been removed from your operative arm and you can use the hand without difficulty. This may take 10 to 14 days or longer. Driving with only one hand is discouraged.
- After your dressing and splint have been removed, you will need physical therapy to regain the full use of your hand and arm. You may receive instructions on this during your office visit along with supplemental educational materials, or a trained physical therapist will work with you to maximize your recovery from this type of surgery. Therapy will include a program to regain the flexibility of your elbow, wrist, and hand. When your recovery from your operation allows, you can undertake a gradual strengthening program that includes elbow and wrist exercises. Treatments such as ultrasound may be helpful but generally are not recommended until 6 weeks after your operation to allow normal healing of the operative site.
- After you have recovered from the operation and regained some elbow and wrist strength, you may be able to resume activities you engaged in before the onset of your condition. The key is to improve the way the elbow is used, including conditioning the elbow as well as the rest of your body, and to avoid a sudden increase in the use of the elbow without preparing for such activity. At work, alternating hands so that both elbows share the work is useful. Keeping the elbows close to the side of the body will also minimize the risk of epicondylitis. If you must engage in repetitive activities in which the arm is lifted to shoulder height or above, a support or raised surface should be used to minimize the time spent performing these activities with the elbow away from the side.
- For sports such as tennis, it is important to learn and maintain correct technique. This may require the assistance of a knowledgeable professional in your sport. It is important to perform warm-up exercises, including stretching of the elbow, wrist, and hand, as well as cool-down exercises such as stretching after participation in the sport. Applying an ice pack to the area of the elbow most commonly affected is also helpful. Equipment used during the sport, such as a tennis racquet, must be carefully selected for the weight and grip size that best suits your size, strength, and abilities.

✆ CALL OUR OFFICE IF

- The area of the incision becomes swollen or red and warm, or there is drainage from it.
- You develop a temperature higher than 100.5°F.
- You develop numbness and tingling in the hand.
- You have any questions.

△ GENERAL INFORMATION

The testicles are located in separate pockets in the *scrotum* (the "sac" under the penis). The surface of the testicle is free, smooth, and slippery except for part of one side where blood and other vessels enter and leave it. Once in a great while, the testicle twists on itself (this is called a *torsion*). This torsion chokes off the vessels in the testicle (Fig. 1). It is thought that a testicle that is not adequately anchored to the side of the scrotum is more likely to experience torsion.

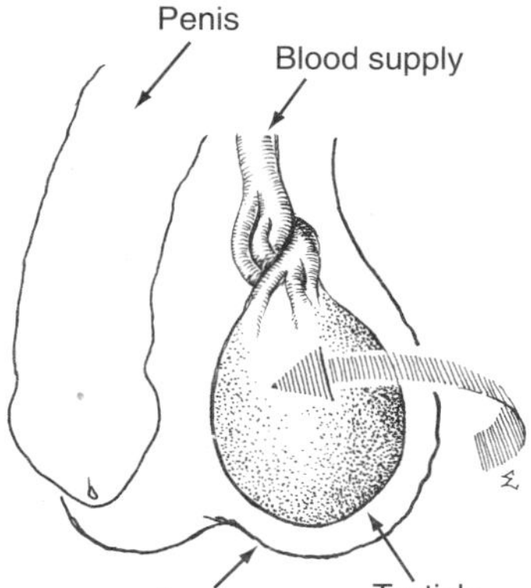

Figure 1. The testicle can twist in either a clockwise or a counterclockwise direction. For this reason experience and skill are needed to "untwist" the testicle in the correct direction when trying to do it from the outside and thus avoid an emergency open operation.

COMMON SIGNS AND SYMPTOMS

Most of the signs and symptoms are the result of not enough blood getting to or leaving the testicle.

- There can be sudden pain, or the pain can come on gradually and then become much worse. The scrotum may become enlarged and red, and its wall may be filled with fluid.
- There is nausea and vomiting.
- The affected testicle may be higher than the other.
- The testicle is extremely tender when touched.
- There may be fever.

DIAGNOSIS

There are a number of conditions that resemble testicular torsion for which the treatment is quite different. For this reason, you will be asked for a detailed history and have a thorough physical examination.

- *Doppler ultrasound*: Harmless and painless sound waves are aimed at your scrotum. The sound waves bouncing back (the echoes) from this area are seen as a picture on a screen. Doppler ultrasound is a convenient way to examine and evaluate blood flow of the testicles.
- *Radionuclide scan*: A tiny amount of radioactive material is injected into your vein, and a machine will record whether it reaches your testicle normally, poorly, or not at all.

○ TREATMENT

Proper treatment requires prompt diagnosis and correction because the longer the blood supply to the testicle remains choked off, the greater the risk that the testicle will develop gangrene and die. *Note*: It is important for you to understand that if the testicle becomes gangrenous, it will need to be removed. It will not come back to life, and leaving it could cause serious complications.

- An attempt is made to untwist the testicle by hand. You will receive pain medicine, if necessary, before this is tried. If it is successful, then nothing more is necessary at this particular time.
- There is a tendency for torsion to happen again. For this reason, even if the twisted testicle is successfully untwisted by hand from the outside, it is advisable that you have an operation soon after the first episode. During this operation, both testicles are stitched to the scrotum to prevent them from twisting.
- If it is not possible to untwist them by hand, an emergency operation is necessary. (The testicle can be saved 85% of the time if it is untwisted within 6 hours. It can be saved only 10% of the time if it remains twisted for longer than 24 hours.)
- If the testicle is successfully untwisted from the outside and you are to have an operation later, you will need to be prepared for it.

PREOPERATIVE PREPARATION

- You will have an examination of your blood and urine and possibly of your heart (EKG) and lungs (chest x-ray).
- Do not eat or drink anything for 8 hours before the operation.
- Shower as usual the morning of the operation.
- You may be given some medicine to make you feel drowsy before you are brought to the operating room.

□ OPERATION

- You will be asleep for the operation.
- The incision will be over the scrotum.
- The testicle will be untwisted and several stitches placed to hold it in proper position.
- The operation usually takes about 1 hour or so, depending on what needs to be done.
- You will be taken to a recovery room and observed until your blood pressure, pulse, and breathing are stable and you are completely alert. Whether you can go home that same day or must stay in the hospital a day or so will depend on the extent of the operation.
- Pain will be controlled with medicine.
- You may have a scrotal suspensory support.
- Arrangements will be made for your medicine, follow-up office visit, and stitch removal.
- As with any operation, complications are always possible. With this type of operation, they can

include infection, death of the testicle even though at the time of the operation it appeared as if it could survive, and possibly others.

HOME CARE

- Lie down as much as possible; this will help decrease any swelling of the scrotum and testicle.
- You may eat as you did before the operation.
- You may shower if you wish. After you dry yourself, replace any dressings with clean, dry ones.
- Wearing jockey-type underwear may be more comfortable.
- Be careful that you do not become constipated.
  - Include enough roughage and plenty of liquids in your diet.
  - You may need a mild laxative (example: milk of magnesia).
- Engaging in sexual intercourse too soon can be harmful to your recovery. If you wish, let's talk about this during your follow-up visit.
- You may return to work when you feel up to it.

CALL OUR OFFICE IF

- You develop any unusual signs or symptoms.
- The incision becomes red or swollen, or there is drainage from it.
- You develop a temperature higher than 100°F.
- You have any questions.

TESTICLE, UNDESCENDED (CRYPTORCHIDISM): Adult

△ GENERAL INFORMATION

Before birth, a boy's testicles are located high in the abdomen, right by the kidneys. Shortly before birth, the testicle, along with the blood vessels and the tube that eventually carry sperm, travels downward and comes through a hole in the groin to enter the *scrotum* (the sac under the penis).

Once in about 25 births, the testicle doesn't quite reach the scrotum. This is called an *undescended testicle* (the medical term is *cryptorchidism*). Most (but not all) such testicles will come down into the scrotum within a year. Very few descend after 1 year, and some never will. About 90% of children with an undescended testicle also have a hernia. Very rarely, neither testicle will be in the scrotum at birth.

The reason why the testicle does not descend into the scrotum is not clearly known, but it probably relates to hormone levels.

CONCERNS

- The testicle does best in the cooler surroundings of the scrotum rather than in the warmer environment of the groin or the abdomen. If the testes remain out of the scrotum in a warm environment, the cells that will eventually make sperm (and allow a man to father a child) will decrease after 2 years.
- Testicles that remain undescended have a higher risk of becoming cancerous later in life.
- An undescended testicle located in the groin is at greater risk of being injured. Also, it has have a higher risk of *torsion* (twisting).

DIAGNOSIS

- A detailed history and a careful physical examination will be done, especially of the scrotum and its contents.
- *Ultrasound*: Harmless sound waves are aimed at the area of your scrotum. The sound waves bouncing back (the echoes) from this area are seen as a picture on a screen. Ultrasound is a convenient and painless way to examine organs and tissues inside this area of your body.
- *CT scan (computed tomography scan)*: These special x-rays are taken by a machine that is shaped like a huge doughnut. You will lie on a table inside the hole in the "doughnut" while x-rays are taken as very thin slices through the area of the scrotum, groin, and abdomen. This test is done to get the most reliable information on the location of the testicle, which may be very small. Such information can make it easier to find the testicle at the time of an operation.

○ TREATMENT

When treating an adult with an undescended testicle, several things must be taken into consideration.

Sperm. A testicle that is not in the scrotum by about 2 years of age starts losing its ability to make sperm; it probably cannot make any sperm at all if it remains undescended to age 12 years.

Hormones. The ability of the testicle to make hormones is not affected by its location. Incidentally, one normal testicle in the scrotum is more than enough to make the necessary amount of hormone.

Cancer. The risk of cancer is higher in an undescended testicle than in a testicle that has come down into the scrotum normally. There is evidence that even if an undescended testicle is brought down into the scrotum after the age of 12 years, the risk of it developing cancer is the same as if it remained undescended. Of course, if the testicle is in the scrotum, a cancer developing in it can be felt or seen. This is not possible if it is undescended.

So, given the concerns about sperm, hormones, cancer, and appearance, the following are the general guidelines for treatment of an undescended testicle:

- Bring an undescended testicle into the scrotum by the age of 2 years. This will result in the least harm to the testicle.
- For children aged 2 to 12 years, it still is advisable to bring the testicle down into the scrotum, even though it may not function normally.
- A testicle that is not in the scrotum by age 40 years may look fairly normal (although it usually is smaller), but it cannot make sperm. It may still make hormones but the risk of developing cancer is increased.
- The recommendation is that such a testicle be looked for and removed, primarily to eliminate the risk of cancer. However, even when the initial decision is to locate the testicle and bring it down to the scrotum, the testicle when found may be so small (say the size of a pea) that it would not make much sense to do the extra surgery to bring it down into the scrotum. The wise and correct thing would be to remove it.
- If desired, a plastic prosthesis shaped like a testicle can be placed in the scrotum.
- After the age of 40 years, it may be that the risk of an operation to find and remove an undescended testicle may be equal to the risk of leaving the testicle in place.

The above guidelines can be modified for several reasons, such as the following:

- There is an infertility problem and so a desire not to lose any chance whatever of providing sperm.
- There is a male hormone problem and the need not to lose a testicle that makes these hormones.
- A person is older than 40, and there is concern about cancer. The choice is to remove the testicle.

After a detailed discussion with you and careful consideration of all factors, the decision is that something be done about your undescended testicle, either bring it into the scrotum or find it and remove it.

PREOPERATIVE PREPARATION

- You will have an examination of your blood, urine, heart (EKG), and lungs (chest x-ray).
- Do not eat or drink anything for 8 hours before the operation.

- Shower as usual on the morning of the operation.
- You may be given medicine that will make you feel drowsy before you are brought to the operating room.

☐ OPERATION

- You will be asleep for the operation.
- The incision will be on the lower side of your abdomen. The testicle will be searched for and if the decision was to remove it, this will be done and the operation completed. *Note*: On occasion no testicle will be found.

If the decision is to bring the testicle down into the scrotum, this will be done if at all possible.

- The operation usually takes about 1 to 3 hours, depending on what is done.

POSTOPERATIVE CARE

- You will be taken to a recovery room and observed. When your blood pressure, pulse, and breathing are stable, you will be taken to a regular hospital room.
- That evening you will be helped to get out of bed and walk around.
- You should be able to go home in 1 or 2 days.
- Arrangements will be made for your medicine, follow-up office visit, and stitch removal.

✚ HOME CARE

- You may walk about as you wish, even climb stairs, but don't overdo things.
- You may eat as you did before the operation.
- Take medicine as prescribed for your pain.
- Unless instructed otherwise, you may shower if you wish with any dressings on or off.
  - There may be narrow strips of tape across the incision. It's all right if they get wet; they will be removed in the doctor's office.
  - After you dry yourself, replace any dressing with clean, dry ones.
- You may drive only if you are not taking medicines that will reduce your alertness.
- Engaging in sexual intercourse too soon can be harmful to your recovery. If you wish, let's talk about this during your follow-up visit.
- You may return to work when you feel up to it.

✆ CALL OUR OFFICE IF

- You develop any unusual signs or symptoms.
- The incision becomes red or swollen, or there is drainage from it.
- You develop a temperature higher than 100°F.
- You have any questions.

TESTICLE, UNDESCENDED (CRYPTORCHIDISM): Infant

△ GENERAL INFORMATION

Before birth, a boy's testicles are located high in the abdomen, right by the kidneys. Shortly before birth, the testicle, along with the blood vessels and the tube that eventually carry sperm, travels downward and comes through a hole in the groin to enter the *scrotum* (the sac under the penis).

Once in about 25 births, the testicle doesn't quite reach the scrotum. This is called an *undescended testicle* (the medical term is *cryptorchidism*). Most (but not all) such testicles will come down into the scrotum within a year. Very few descend after 1 year, and some never will. About 90% of children with an undescended testicle also have a hernia. Very rarely, neither testicle will be in the scrotum at birth.

The reason why the testicle does not descend into the scrotum is not clearly known, but it probably relates to hormone levels.

CONCERNS

- The testicle does best in the cooler surroundings of the scrotum rather than in the warmer environment found in the groin or the abdomen. If the testes remain out of the scrotum in a warm environment, the cells that will eventually make sperm (and allow a man to father a child) will decrease after 2 years.
- Testicles that remain undescended have a higher risk of becoming cancerous later in life.
- An undescended testicle located in the groin is at greater risk of being injured. Also, it has a higher risk of *torsion* (twisting).

DIAGNOSIS

- A detailed history and a careful physical examination will be done and especially of the scrotum and its contents.
- Most children who are thought to have undescended testicles do not actually have this problem. What they have is a very strong muscle reflex that easily and quickly pulls (retracts) the testicles up and out of the scrotum when the scrotum is touched. This is not a serious problem and no treatment is necessary. It simply is necessary to be certain it is a *retractile* testicle rather than an *undescended* testicle. Such patients should be followed regularly. Over time, 20% of such patients will require an operation to keep the testicle in the scrotum.

○ TREATMENT

Hormone Injections. Such treatment will bring the testicle down in about 25% of infants. The chance is 50% if both testicles are undescended. You may discuss with your pediatrician when or if such treatment could be given.

Surgical Treatment. This involves an operation in which the testicle is freed and brought down to the scrotum. At the same time, any associated hernia can be repaired.

Keep in mind that if the choice is for an operation, your son will get the most benefit if it is done by the age of 2 years. Any harm that may come to the testicle because of waiting too long is not reversible, even if after the delay, the testicle is brought down.

After careful consideration of all factors, the recommendation is that your son should have an operation (called an *orchidopexy*) to correct the problem.

PREOPERATIVE PREPARATION

- Do not let your son eat or drink anything for 6 hours before the operation.
- Very rarely, the testicle is located so high it cannot be brought down in one operation, and another operation may be required at a later time. Also very rarely, the testicle is found but it is not developed and is the size of a small pea. It cannot be brought down, but even if it could, it would not do any good because it won't function normally. What can or should be done if these unusual circumstances develop will be discussed with you.

□ OPERATION

- The operation will be done under general anesthesia.
- Tissues that are keeping the testicle from coming down will be cut, freeing the testicle so that it can be placed in the scrotum.
- The operation usually takes about 1 hour.

POSTOPERATIVE CARE

- Your son will be taken to a recovery room and observed. When his blood pressure, pulse, and breathing are stable, and he is completely alert, you should be able to take him home on that same day.
- Arrangements will be made for your son's medicine and follow-up office visit. The stitches will dissolve by themselves.
- As with any operation, complications are always possible, some of them serious. With this type of operation, they can include the testicle's becoming scarred and not growing, infection, bleeding, and possibly others.

✚ HOME CARE

- Allow the child to be active. However, avoid contact sports, play with straddle toys, and similar activities for 2 weeks.
- You will be instructed on how to bathe your child and take care of the incision.

✆ CALL OUR OFFICE IF

- The scrotum swells or becomes blue.
- The incision becomes red or swollen, or there is drainage from it.
- He develops a temperature higher than 100°F.
- You have any questions.

△ GENERAL INFORMATION

Cancer of the testicle is the most common tumor in men aged 18 to 35 years. The cause of the cancer in your testicle is not known. There are two main types of testicle cancer: *seminoma* and *nonseminomatous germ cell tumor*. The treatment for each type is quite different.

COMMON SIGNS AND SYMPTOMS

- A painless firm mass or swelling is felt in one of the testicles inside the scrotum (the sac beneath the penis). Usually, the mass can be easily felt.
- Often, there is a fullness or heaviness on one side of the scrotum. Rarely, a minor injury to the testicle will cause the cancer in it to bleed, producing swelling and pain.
- Rarely, the first signs and symptoms a person has are those caused by the spread of the tumor to the lungs or lymph nodes.

DIAGNOSIS

- Usually, the diagnosis can be made by taking a detailed history, doing a thorough physical examination, and considering the laboratory reports.
- Examination of the scrotum will reveal a firm mass in the involved testicle.
- Blood is drawn for tumor marker levels (AFP = alpha-fetoprotein and beta-hCG = beta human chorionic gonadotropic hormone), which may be elevated with cancer of the testicle.
- *Ultrasound*: Harmless sound waves are aimed at the area of your scrotum. The sound waves bouncing back (the echoes) from this area are seen as a picture on a screen. Ultrasound is a convenient and painless way to examine organs and tissues inside this area of your body.

After careful consideration of all factors, and especially the fact that there is a high probability that you have cancer of the testicle, it is recommended that your testicle be removed, both to confirm the probable diagnosis of cancer and also to allow intelligent planning of further therapy.

Note: It is important to realize that it is not possible to be absolutely certain of the diagnosis of cancer of the testicle before the operation. Cutting or placing a needle into the testicle to remove a small piece of it (a *biopsy*) poses a serious risk of spreading the cancer to the surrounding tissue, thus making it incurable. The technique of performing an operation to both make the diagnosis and remove the cancerous testicle will be thoroughly explained to you before anything is planned or done. In the hands of an experienced urologist, it is very rare that a normal testicle is removed in error.

PREOPERATIVE PREPARATION

- You will have an examination of your blood, urine, heart (EKG), and lungs (chest x-ray).
- If any other medical problems are present, they will be corrected as much as possible before the operation.
- Do not eat or drink anything for 8 hours before the operation.
- Shower or bathe as usual on the morning of the operation.
- You may be given medicine that will make you feel drowsy before you are brought to the operating room.

□ OPERATION

- You will be asleep during the operation, or offered a spinal type of anesthetic. The choice will be discussed with you beforehand.
- An incision is made in the groin and the testicle is removed through this incision. The entire testicle is sent to the pathologist for careful study and histologic diagnosis and confirmation of testicular cancer (Fig. 1).
- The operation usually takes about 1 hour.

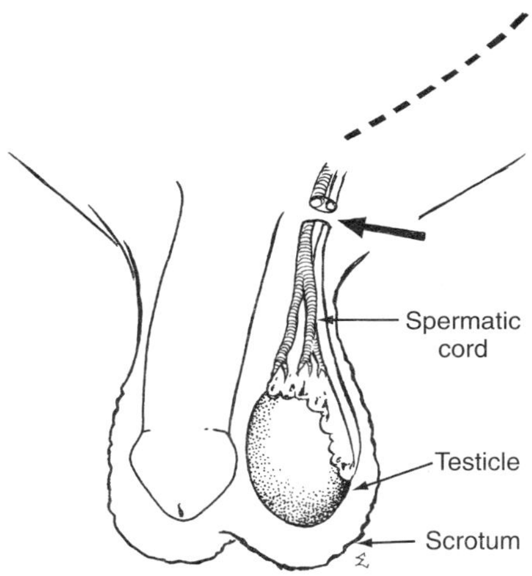

Figure 1. The spermatic cord contains the artery, vein, and the vas deferens (sperm travels through it). The radical orchiectomy is performed through the incision shown *(dashed line)*. The testicle and a portion of the cord are removed by a division marked by the solid arrow.

POSTOPERATIVE CARE

- You will be taken to a recovery room and observed. When your blood pressure, pulse, and breathing are stable, you will be either transferred to a regular hospital room or sent home with a responsible adult.
- There will be a gauze dressing over the incision that can be removed the following morning.
- You will have moderate pain over the next few days but will be given medicine to control this.

✚ HOME CARE

- That evening you may sit up in bed and the next day get out of bed.
- You may walk about as you wish, even climb stairs, but don't overdo things.
- Eat as you wish.

- You may take a shower if you wish (but not a tub bath) with any dressings on or off.
  - There may be narrow strips of tape across the incision. It's all right if they get wet; they will be removed in the doctor's office.
  - After you dry yourself, replace any dressings with clean, dry ones.
- Take medicine as prescribed for your pain.
- You should not drive a car too soon. Let's talk about it during your follow-up office visit.
- Because engaging in sexual intercourse too soon after the operation can be harmful to your recovery, it is recommended that you do not do so for 2 weeks after the operation.
- You should be able to perform light office work in 1 to 2 weeks or strenuous activity in 3 to 4 weeks.
- As with any operation, complications are always possible. The complications associated with this type of operation include infection, bleeding, and possibly others. Occasionally, the scrotum will become enlarged and filled with blood (a *hematoma*). It may take up to 6 weeks before the swelling goes down, but this should not lead to any further difficulties.
- Your sex life should not be changed by having one testicle removed. Your ability to father children can be determined by having an analysis of your semen. If you wish, let's talk about this.

✆ CALL OUR OFFICE IF

- You develop any unusual signs or symptoms.
- The incision becomes red or swollen, or there is drainage from it.
- You develop a temperature higher than 100°F.
- You have any questions.

FURTHER TREATMENT

Further treatment will depend on the type of tumor that was removed, how extensive it was, and where it may have spread.

- If the cancer is a seminoma, and is small and is not found to have spread, you will most likely receive radiation therapy to the lymph nodes draining the testicle. If the seminoma is extensive, but still has not spread, the primary treatment may be chemotherapy. More tests will be needed before the decision can be made. There will be a full discussion with you about this before anything is planned or done.
- If the cancer is found to be a nonseminomatous germ cell tumor, and appears to be confined to the testicle, you may require a retroperitoneal lymph node resection (surgical removal of the lymph nodes in the back of your abdomen) in order to improve your chances of cure. Any decision or recommendation will be discussed with you before anything is planned or done.

TESTICLE CANCER: Retroperitoneal Lymph Node Dissection

△ GENERAL INFORMATION

In some patients with cancer of the testicle, the cancer is of the type and the conditions are such that the best chances for cure are to remove the testicle and the lymph nodes that drain the testicle. This is your situation.

The testicles are the two egg-shaped structures in the scrotum (the sac under the penis). Cancer of the testicle is the most common type of cancer in men aged 18 to 35 years. There are two main types of cancer of the testicle: *seminoma* and *nonseminomatous germ cell tumor.*

The treatment for seminoma is removal of the testicle followed by either chemotherapy or x-ray treatment to the lymph nodes draining the testicle. The treatment for nonseminomatous germ cell tumor of the testicle that does not appear to have spread to other organs besides the lymph nodes is an operation to remove the testicle and the lymph nodes draining it. You had your testicle removed and it is the type that has the best chance of being cured by an operation that goes by the long name of retroperitoneal lymph node dissection.

PREOPERATIVE PREPARATION

Before any preparations are made for an operation, studies need to be done to be as certain as possible there is no cancer elsewhere in the body. Some or all of the following tests will be performed:

- You will have an examination of your blood, urine, heart (EKG), and lungs (chest x-ray).
- CT scan (computed tomography scan): These special x-rays are taken by a machine that is shaped like a huge doughnut. While you lie on a table inside the hole in the "doughnut," x-rays are taken as very thin slices through the entire abdomen. This makes it possible to see the fine details in the tissues and organs in the abdomen.
- *MRI (magnetic resonance imaging)*: No x-rays are used with this technique; instead, it is done with harmless magnetic fields and radio waves. A computer develops the pictures to show organs from several angles. It is especially useful for examining blood vessels and their relationship to tissues and organs that are important in this operation.
- Blood will be drawn for tumor marker levels (AFP = alpha-fetoprotein and beta-hCG = beta-human chorionic gonadotropic hormone) that may be elevated with cancer of the testicle and can be used as a gauge now and during your follow-up observations.
- Any important medical conditions present will be corrected as much as possible before the operation.
- Shower or bathe as usual on the morning of the operation.
- You may be given medicine that will make you feel drowsy before you are brought to the operating room.

□ OPERATION

- You will be asleep for the operation.
- Your abdomen will be scrubbed with an antiseptic solution and surrounded with sterile drapes.
- The incision will run up and down in your abdomen. The lymph nodes will be removed and sent to the laboratory for detailed and careful examination (Fig. 1).
- You will not receive a blood transfusion unless it is absolutely necessary.
- The operation usually takes about 4 hours.

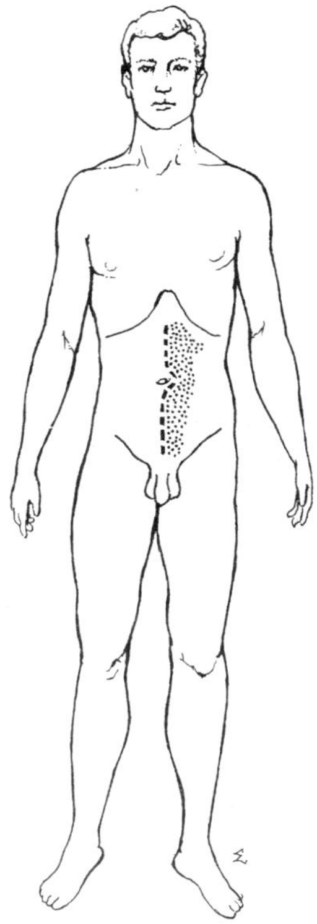

Figure 1. Usually the incision for this operation is made up and down on the abdomen *(dashed line)*. The lymph nodes removed are indicated by the stippled area.

POSTOPERATIVE CARE

- You will be taken to a recovery room and observed. When your blood pressure, pulse, and breathing are stable, you will be taken to a regular hospital room.
- There will be a thin catheter in your penis to drain the urine from your bladder.
- You may have a thin plastic tube in your nose. It goes down to your stomach to suck up the air you swallow. It will be removed when your bowels start working.
- Pain can be controlled with medicine. The nurse will give it to you, or you can give yourself a preset amount of pain medicine when you feel you need it.

This type of pain relief, called patient-controlled analgesia (PCA), uses a device that releases the medicine into the tubing giving you intravenous fluids.
- That evening you will be helped to sit up in bed and on the next day to get out of bed.
- You will be given an incentive spirometer. Breathing into this as you are instructed will help you expand your lungs and reduce the risk of developing pneumonia.
- You will have some special stockings on to help prevent the formation of blood clots.
- When your bowels start working, the tube in your nose will be removed and you will be started on a liquid diet that will be increased as you tolerate it.
- You should be able to go home in 4 to 7 days.
- Arrangements will be made for your medicine, follow-up office visit, and stitch or clip removal.
- As with any operation, complications are always possible. With your type of operation, they can include infection, bleeding, blood clots, bowel obstruction, and fluid in the abdomen. A small percentage of patients have a loss of ejaculation during sexual intercourse. This is due to the dissection of the nerve fibers running through the lymph nodes. The ability to have an erection and an orgasm will remain unchanged.

✣ HOME CARE

- Continue with the program started while you were in the hospital.
- You may walk about as you wish, even climb stairs, but don't overdo things.
- Take medicine as prescribed for your pain.
- You may eat as you wish but be careful that you do not become constipated. Include enough roughage and plenty of liquids in your diet. You may need some help with a mild laxative (example: milk of magnesia).
- Unless instructed otherwise, you may shower if you wish with any dressings on or off.
  - There may be narrow strips of tape across the incision. It's all right if they get wet; they will be removed in the doctor's office.
  - After you dry yourself, replace any dressings with clean, dry ones.
- Driving a car with an automatic shift may not seem to be too demanding. However, if you may have to slam on the brakes or twist to turn the steering wheel, you can strain your sutures or tear something. During your follow-up visit, let's discuss when you can resume driving.
- Because engaging in sexual intercourse too soon after the operation could be harmful to recovery, it is recommended that you not do so for 3 to 4 weeks after the operation.
- You should be able to return to light office work in 2 to 3 weeks and more strenuous activity in 4 to 5 weeks. Let's talk about it during your follow-up office visit.

✆ CALL OUR OFFICE IF

- You develop any unusual signs or symptoms.
- The incision becomes red or swollen, or there is drainage from it.
- You develop a temperature higher than 100°F.
- You have any questions.

TETANUS

GENERAL INFORMATION

Tetanus (lockjaw) is an infection that is produced by bacteria (called *Clostridium tetani*). These bacteria grow in conditions in which there is a low level of oxygen. They produce a poison *(toxin)* that affects the nervous system (and so is called a *neurotoxin*).

These bacteria are found in many places, but especially in the soil and in the intestines of both humans and animals. Addicts who use dirty needles are a source of infection.

COMMON SIGNS AND SYMPTOMS

- Irritability. There are muscle spasms of the head and neck.
- Difficulty in swallowing (because of the spasms).
- Stiffness of the jaw ("lockjaw").
- The muscles of the chest become so stiff, that it is difficult to breathe.
- Any stimulation—even turning on a light in the room or jarring the bed—can throw the whole body into violent spasm.

TREATMENT: Prophylaxis

- The recommendation for prophylaxis against tetanus depends on:
  - The condition of the wound and how prone it is to develop tetanus (see Table below).
  - Whether the individual has had a tetanus shot in the past *(immunization)*.
- Regardless of what type of immunization a person had in the past, *all* wounds need to be treated as soon as possible. Special attention should be paid to removing dead or badly bruised tissue and thoroughly rinsing the wound. This is particularly important in wounds that are at risk of developing tetanus, which include the following:
  - Wounds with dirt in them.
  - The injury occurred in a barnyard, stable, or other place that might contain manure.

TREATMENT: Acute Tetanus Infection

- Admit to the hospital and place in a dark, quiet room
- Give medicine to relax the muscles.
- If necessary, place a tube down the trachea to improve breathing.
- Give antibiotics to help prevent infection by other types of bacteria.
- Give tetanus immune globulin.

PROGNOSIS

- The earlier the symptoms appear after the injury, the worse the prognosis.
- Very few patients with severe spasms survive.
- Drug addicts who develop tetanus have a very high death rate.

Features of the Wound	More Prone to Develop Tetanus	Less Prone to Develop Tetanus
Age of wound	Longer than 6 hours	Less than 6 hours
Appearance	Jagged	Clean cut or scrape
Depth	More than ¼ inch	Less than ¼ inch
How it happened	Torn, crushed, burned	By sharp knife, glass
Signs of infection	Yes	No
Badly bruised tissue present	Yes	No
Dead tissue present	Yes	No
Dirt, feces, etc., in wound	Yes	No

	More Prone to Develop Tetanus		Less Prone to Develop Tetanus	
History of immunization	Give toxoid	Give tetanus immune globulin	Give toxoid	Give tetanus immune globulin
Don't know, or incomplete	Yes	Yes	Yes	Yes
Immunized	No*	No	No†	No

*Yes, if more than 5 years since last dose.
†Yes, if more than 10 years since last dose.

△ GENERAL INFORMATION

The chest contains a left and right lung with the heart in the middle. Normally, the lungs fit snugly against the ribs and expand inside the chest wall as the chest itself expands. In other words, the lungs, which are elastic like a rubber balloon, simply follow the chest as it swells out and then goes down.

COMMON SIGNS AND SYMPTOMS

Sometimes, fluid will form between the lungs and the chest wall (Fig. 1). This fluid can be blood, serum, pus, or lymph, and it can be evidence of a disease process.

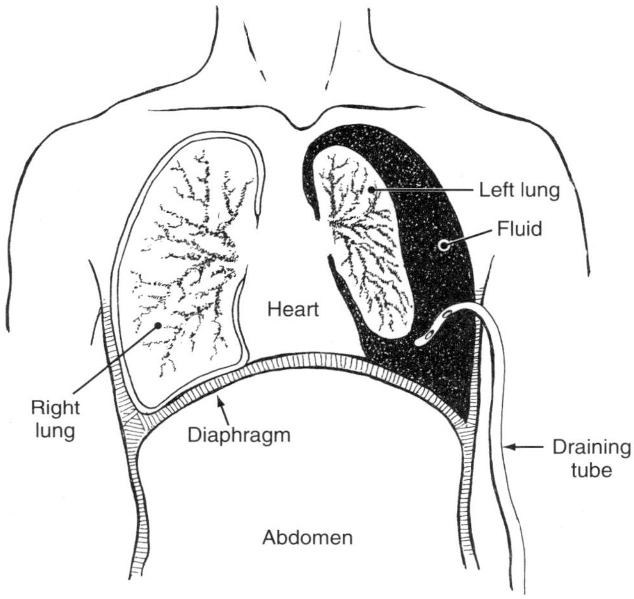

Figure 1.

Whatever the type of fluid present and the reason why it formed, it presses on the lung itself and will not let it expand properly. When the lung cannot expand properly, it cannot take in the right amount of oxygen and you become short of breath, especially while working or walking.

○ TREATMENT

Before treatment can be started, it is necessary to find out the nature of the fluid. A sample is removed by a technique called *thoracentesis*, which can be done in the doctor's office or at the bedside.

THE THORACENTESIS

- X-rays of your chest will show exactly where the fluid is located. This will help the physician know where to go to drain it.
- You will be properly positioned for this procedure.
- The area over the fluid in the chest will be painted with an antiseptic solution and draped. A fine needle will be used to inject an anesthetic in the skin to make it completely numb.
- The exact procedure to be done will depend on the reason for it. For example:
  - **To obtain fluid for laboratory examination:** A needle is placed through the numbed skin and into the fluid in the chest. A syringe full of fluid will be obtained for laboratory examination. This will show whether it is caused by an infection, irritation from an injury, or possibly even cancer.
  - **For immediate relief of symptoms:** The needle is placed through the numbed area in the skin and as much fluid as possible is removed. This technique is simple and can be done in a short while. However, not all of the fluid can be removed by this technique. Still, the rest of it may be expected to go away after treatment is started.
  - **For continuous removal of fluid:** The procedure is the same as above except that the tube will be left in the chest cavity and connected to a special collecting bottle. You will need to stay in the hospital until all of the fluid is removed and it is clear that it will not come back again.

POSTOPERATIVE CARE

- A chest x-ray may be taken after the thoracentesis to check the condition of the lungs.
- If you are to go home the same day, you will do this after your blood pressure and pulse are stable and your breathing is improved. You must be accompanied by a responsible adult.
- If the drainage tube is left in place, you will be taken to a hospital room.
- The tube attached to the draining bottles will be quite long so that you can move about some.
- Pain will be controlled with medicine.
- You will be able to eat as you wish.
- You will be able to go home when the chest fluid problem is under control.
- Arrangements will be made for your medicine and follow-up office visit.
- As with any operation, complications are always possible. With your type of operation, they can include infection, bleeding, puncture of the lung, heart problems and possibly others.

✚ HOME CARE

- Resume activities as before but avoid doing too much too soon.
- You may shower or bathe as before.
- Eat as you wish, but be careful that you do not become constipated.
  - Include enough roughage and liquid in your diet.
  - You may need a mild laxative (example: milk of magnesia) in 2 or 3 days.
- Driving your car may be important to you, but when you can do this safely depends on the procedure you had, the medicines you are taking, and your

condition in general. During your follow-up visit, let's discuss when you can resume driving.
- You may resume sexual activity whenever you choose.
- You may return to work when you feel up to it, but let's talk about it first during your follow-up office visit.

✆ CALL OUR OFFICE IF

- You develop shortness of breath or any unusual signs or symptoms.
- You develop a temperature higher than 101°F.
- You have any questions.

△ GENERAL INFORMATION

The nerves and blood vessels to and from the arm must first pass under the *clavicle* (the collar bone) before they can get to where they're going. But there are also ribs and muscles under the clavicle, and the space left for the passage of the nerves and blood vessels can sometimes be very small (Fig. 1).

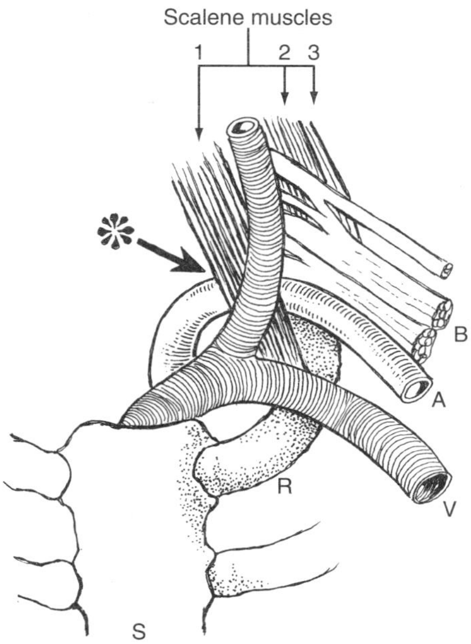

Figure 1. There are some variations in the abnormalities that trap the blood vessels and nerves to produce this syndrome. A common one is shown (asterisk). The structures shown are artery (A); brachial plexus (nerves to the arm) (B); vein (V); rib (R); sternum (breastbone) (S); and the scalene muscles.

A number of conditions can cause this tight squeeze, including:

- An extra rib or a crooked rib that gets in the way of the nerves and vessels.
- The muscles under the rib are not quite in their correct position or are overdeveloped and so can sometimes press on the nerves and vessels.
- The arm has to carry a heavy load which pulls the clavicle down. This makes the space under the ribs smaller so the nerves and blood vessels are squeezed.
- About 75% of persons with this syndrome are older women.

COMMON SIGNS AND SYMPTOMS

From Squeezed Nerves

- Pain, "pins and needles," or numbness over the fingers and hand.
- Later, the muscles become weak and may even get smaller.

From Squeezed Blood Vessels

- Pain, cold fingers, weakness in the arm or hand, all made worse by cold. There may be swelling and a blue color of the fingers and hand.

DIAGNOSIS

- Usually the diagnosis can be made by taking a detailed history, doing a thorough physical examination, and carefully considering the laboratory reports.
- A number of tests will be done first to establish the diagnosis of thoracic outlet syndrome. Great care will be taken to be certain that the symptoms are not caused by some other disease that can produce some of these same symptoms.
- Finally, no one single test is 100% accurate.

Some tests that help make the diagnosis if they are positive include the following:

- The person takes a deep breath, pulls the neck back and turns the head toward the affected arm. This partially closes the space under the clavicle and makes the pulse in the wrist weaker.
- The pulse is taken as the person throws the shoulder back and downward (like an exaggerated version of the military "attention" position). This will squeeze the artery to the arm and make the pulse weaker.
- The pulse is taken as the arm is pulled up and back as far as possible. This will make the pulse weaker.
- X-ray of the neck and chest may show abnormalities of the ribs and/or other bones.
- *MRI (magnetic resonance imaging)*: No x-rays are used with this technique. Instead, harmless magnetic fields and radio waves are used. A computer develops the pictures to show bones, vessels, and muscles from several angles. It is especially valuable for examining blood vessels and nerve tissue.
- *Arteriogram*: Dye is injected into the artery and x-ray pictures are taken as the dye flows through the artery. This helps show where and how much an artery might be squeezed.
- *Phlebogram*: Dye is injected into the arm vein and x-ray pictures are taken of the dye as it flows through the vein being squeezed as it passes under the clavicle. This gives a good idea of how narrow the area might be.

○ TREATMENT

- Except in instances where the artery is blocked or there is damage to the nerve, the initial treatment should be medical and include the following:
    - Losing weight.
    - Improving poor posture.
    - Strengthening the shoulder muscles.

These methods are helpful in at least half of those affected, especially overweight, middle-aged persons with poor posture.

- An operation should be considered if there is no improvement after 4 months on the above program.

After careful consideration of all factors, the recommendation is that you have an operation to try to correct your problem. The reasons for this recommendation have been explained to you.

PREOPERATIVE PREPARATION

- In addition to the above tests, you will have an examination of your blood, urine, heart (EKG), and lungs (chest x-ray).
- Do not eat or drink anything for 8 hours before the operation.
- Shower as usual on the morning of the operation.
- You will be given medicine that will make you feel drowsy before you are brought to the operating room.

☐ OPERATION

- You will be asleep for the operation.
- The operation consists of removal of the first rib through an incision in the axilla (arm pit) or above the clavicle.
- You will not need a blood transfusion.
- The operation usually takes about 2 hours.

POSTOPERATIVE CARE

- You will wake up in a recovery room. When your blood pressure, pulse, and breathing are stable, you will be taken to a regular hospital room.
- That evening you will be helped to sit up in bed and on the next day to get out of bed.
- Pain will be controlled with medicine.
- Your diet will be as you tolerate it.
- You should be able to go home in 2 or 3 days.
- Arrangements will be made for your medicine, follow-up office visit, and stitch removal.
- As with any operation, complications are always possible, some of them serious. With your type of operation, they can include injury to the nerve or artery, an opening into the chest cavity, bleeding, pneumonia, only partial relief of the problem, and possibly others.

✚ HOME CARE

- You may walk about as you wish, even climb stairs, but don't overdo things.
- Favor the arm on the side of the operation until we discuss this during the follow-up office visit.
- You may shower as you wish and with any dressings on or off.
  - There may be narrow strips of tape across the incision. It's all right if they get wet. They will be removed in the doctor's office.
  - After you dry yourself, replace any dressings with clean, dry ones.
- Driving a car with an automatic shift may not seem too demanding, but if you suddenly have to slam on the brakes or twist to turn the wheel, you may strain the sutures or tear something. During your follow-up visit, let's discuss when you can resume driving.
- You may return to work when you feel up to it, but let's discuss this first during your follow-up office visit.

✆ CALL OUR OFFICE IF

- You develop any unusual signs or symptoms.
- The incision becomes red or swollen, or there is drainage from it.
- You develop a temperature higher than 100°F.
- You have any questions.

△ GENERAL INFORMATION

Each leg has two sets of veins that drain blood from the legs back up to the heart and lungs. One set is the *superficial* veins just under the skin (they are the ones you see on the surface of your leg). The other set is the *deep* veins (they run up and down deep in the center of the leg) (Fig. 1).

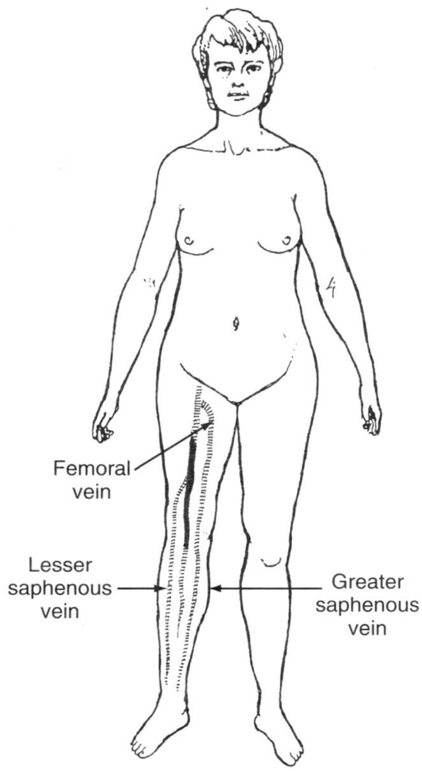

Figure 1. The greater saphenous vein and the lesser saphenous vein (the superficial veins) drain into the femoral vein (the deep vein). If the femoral vein clots, the drainage of blood from the leg then depends on the greater saphenous vein.

These two systems of veins connect with each other at various points along the length of the leg.

The superficial veins have one-way valves that let the blood go only in one direction—up toward the heart and lungs. If these valves break down (for example, during pregnancy or in persons who have to stand for long periods of time), the blood doesn't move very well in just one direction. This causes the veins to swell up, a condition called *varicose veins*. People sometimes wear elastic stockings to keep these veins from swelling. They are not often a serious problem.

The deep veins in the leg don't need any valves or any support from elastic stockings. Every time you move your legs or feet, the muscles around these deep veins squeeze the veins, which forces the blood to go upward towards the heart and lungs.

A *thrombus* (clot) forming in the deep veins can be a serious thing.

CAUSES OF THROMBUS FORMATION

People undergoing operations are susceptible to having the blood in the veins clot abnormally due to the following:

- **Stasis** (the blood is standing still): The veins expand some during anesthesia. When water runs through a garden hose and then the same amount runs through a fire hose, it won't flow as fast or with as much force in the larger hose. Similarly, the flow of blood is slower in the expanded veins, and this slow flow predisposes to clotting.
- **Immobility**: As mentioned before, the leg muscles are relaxed during an operation, so they don't squeeze the veins to make the blood move along as fast as before. This too predisposes to clotting.
- **Intimal injury** (injury to the lining of the vein): The expansion of the veins causes small tears in the lining of the vein so that the surface becomes a little rough (this is all microscopic). Injury to the lining can also occur with excessive handling of a vein. A rough surface in the lining of a vein encourages clots to form.
- **Hypercoagulability** (the blood clots too easily): Certain chemical changes take place in the blood during anesthesia and operations that make it clot more easily. Certain illnesses can do the same thing.

COMPLICATIONS OF THROMBUS

- The clot blocks off the leg veins and just stays there. The result can be a swollen leg because blood cannot move forward. Most of the time this can be treated. Sometimes however, it can be severe and even permanent.
- Part of the clot can break off and go up into the lungs and plug the vessels in the lungs. This is called a *pulmonary embolus*. At least 50,000 people in this country die each year from a pulmonary embolus.

Who Is at Greater Risk?

- It is valuable to know which conditions have a high, medium, or low risk of clot formation. Some circumstances that carry a higher risk are older age, longer operation, previous clotting problems, obesity, cancer, trauma, bone operations on the legs and pelvis, and lower abdominal operations.

PREVENTION

There are several ways to help prevent clot formation:

Discourage Stasis

- Fitting your legs and thighs with air stockings ("boots"). They are connected to an air compression machine, and while you are asleep, they gently squeeze your legs for 15 seconds every minute or so, to help push the blood along (as your leg muscles normally would squeeze the deep veins).
- Having you move your legs as soon as possible after the operation.

Avoid Injury to the Veins

- Gentle handling of the tissue, especially large veins, during the operation helps to prevent the roughening of the lining of these veins that predisposes clots to form.

Treat Hypercoagulability

- Sometimes, blood-thinning medicines are given before, during, and after the operation. Which medicine is used, how much is used, and for how long depends on the special circumstances of the patient and on the operation.
- The principal purpose is to make the blood thin enough that it won't clot too fast, but not make it so thin that you will bleed abnormally during the operation. Blood-thinning medications have been used in thousands of patients and are quite safe.

Of course, these precautions do not always work, but they are the best way to keep the risk of blood clots forming to an absolute minimum. This explanation may help you to better understand some of the things that will be done in association with your operation.

THYROGLOSSAL DUCT CYST

△ GENERAL INFORMATION

When an embryo in the mother's womb is not much bigger than your thumb, the thyroid gland begins to form from tissue near the back of the tongue. From there, it gradually moves down and by the time of birth it is in the middle of the neck. Once in a great while, however, this tissue doesn't move down the way it should, and a very thin tube (a *duct*) is left that extends from the back of the tongue down to the middle of the front of the neck.

This duct can sometimes swell with fluid, producing a lump (called a *cyst*). Usually, the cyst is not much bigger around than a nickel. The name for this condition is *thyroglossal duct cyst* (*thyro* = thyroid; *glossal* = tongue; *duct* = tube; *cyst* = cavity). It is seen most commonly in children under 10 years of age (Fig. 1).

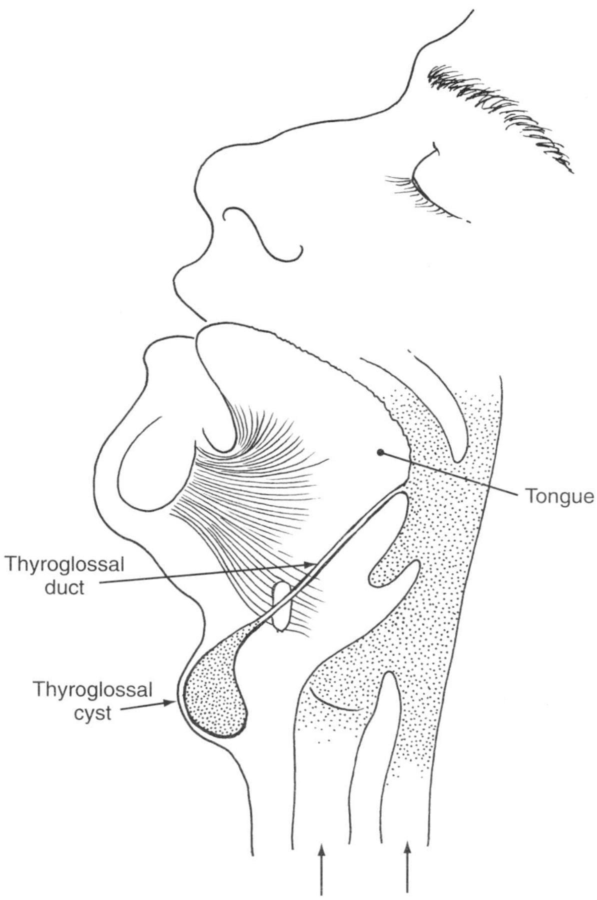

Figure 1. Side view of head and neck with a thyroglossal duct cyst.

COMMON SIGNS AND SYMPTOMS

- There is a mass in the middle of the front part of the neck, just above the Adam's apple.
- The mass is smooth, round, not too hard, can be moved somewhat, and usually does not hurt.

DIAGNOSIS

- Usually, the diagnosis can be made by taking a detailed history and doing a thorough physical examination.
- **Ultrasound**: Harmless sound waves are aimed at the neck. The sound waves bouncing back (the echoes) from inside the organs and tissues in the neck are seen as a picture on a screen. This is a convenient and painless way to examine organs and tissues inside the neck. Finding a mass in the shape of a sphere that is filled with fluid is usually enough to make the diagnosis.

○ TREATMENT

Although a thyroglossal duct cyst may sometimes go away by itself, an operation is usually advised because

- It may become infected.
- It may get bigger and become unsightly.
- It might, instead, be something more serious.

PREOPERATIVE PREPARATION

- You will have an examination of your blood and urine and possibly the lungs (chest x-ray), and heart (EKG).
- Do not eat or drink anything for 8 hours before the operation.
- Shower as usual on the morning of your operation.
- You may be given medicine that will make you feel drowsy before you are brought to the operating room.

□ OPERATION

- You will be asleep for the operation.
- The incision will be made from side-to-side over the mass in a cosmetic manner so that it will show as little as possible afterwards. It will be closed in the same cosmetic manner.
- The operation usually takes about 2 hours.

POSTOPERATIVE CARE

- You will wake up in a recovery room. When your blood pressure, pulse, and breathing are stable and you are completely alert, you should be able to go home that same day with a responsible adult. Sometimes it is necessary to remain in the hospital until the next day.
- There will be a small dressing over the incision.
- Pain will be controlled with medicine.
- Arrangements will be made for your medicine, follow-up office visit, and stitch removal.

✚ HOME CARE

- You may resume your usual activities.
- You may walk about as you wish, even climb stairs.
- You will have a slightly sore throat while swallowing for a few days.
- You may eat as you did before the operation.
- Unless instructed otherwise, you may shower as you wish with any dressings on or off.

- There may be narrow strips of tape across the incision. It's all right if they get wet; they will be removed in the doctor's office.
- After you dry yourself, replace any dressings with clean, dry ones.

✆ CALL OUR OFFICE IF

- The incision becomes red or swollen, or there is drainage from it.
- You develop a temperature higher than 100°F.
- You have any questions.

△ GENERAL INFORMATION

The thyroid gland is located in the neck on each side of the *trachea* (windpipe) and just behind the *larynx* (voice box). It produces thyroid hormone, which regulates your metabolism, or energy level.

Sometimes, growths or nodules can occur in the thyroid. Most are benign; however, some nodules are cancerous and the cancer can spread outside the gland. The cause of your nodule is not known.

COMMON SIGNS AND SYMPTOMS

- Often, there are no symptoms at all. The nodule is discovered by chance while you are dressing or taking a shower, or maybe your doctor found it during a routine examination. Sometimes, the first thing noticed is the swelling that causes the thyroid to stick out.

DIAGNOSIS

- A detailed history and a thorough physical examination are essential.

Some or all of the following tests may be necessary:

- *Ultrasound*: Harmless sound waves are aimed at the thyroid gland and surrounding tissue. The sound waves bouncing back from this area (the echoes) are seen as a picture on a screen. This is a convenient and painless way to see whether the nodule is solid or is filled with fluid (a *cyst*).
- *Biopsy*: The skin over the nodule is prepared with an antiseptic solution and then made numb. A needle is then passed through the numb skin and inserted into the nodule to remove the fluid if it is a cyst, or if it is solid to obtain a tiny piece of it (a *biopsy*) for laboratory examination.
- *Thyroid scan*: A very small amount of harmless radioactive solution is injected into your vein. It is quickly taken up by any part of the thyroid gland that is working. You will lie on a table as a special detector passes over your thyroid and records which areas of your thyroid work and which do not. This test helps find the abnormal areas.
- *CT scan (computed tomography scan)*: Special x-rays are taken as very thin slices through the area of the thyroid and surrounding tissue. This makes it possible to see the size and shape of the thyroid.

The biopsy of the nodule in your thyroid showed that it is cancer, specifically, papillary cancer. This is the most favorable type of cancer that is found in the thyroid. When treated properly, there is a very high cure rate.

○ TREATMENT

The treatment for your condition is an operation. The side of your thyroid gland with cancer in it as well as most of the opposite side of the thyroid will be removed. In addition, if any lymph nodes appear to be involved with the cancer, they will also be removed (Fig. 1).

PREOPERATIVE PREPARATION

- You will have an examination of your blood, urine, heart (EKG), and lungs (chest x-ray).
- Do not eat or drink anything for 8 hours before the operation.

□ OPERATION

- You will be asleep for the operation.
- A cosmetic side-to-side incision will be made in the lower part of your neck.
- The operation usually takes about 2 hours.

POSTOPERATIVE CARE

- You will be taken to a recovery room and observed. When your blood pressure, pulse, and breathing are stable, you will be taken to a regular hospital room.
- That evening you will be able to get out of bed with assistance.
- You will have a sore throat and possibly a raspy voice. This should be temporary.
- As with any operation, complications are always possible. Although they are uncommon with this type of operation, they can include hoarseness and a low calcium level. Usually these are temporary, but once in a great while they may be permanent. There are ways to treat these. Rarely, bleeding can occur postoperatively.
- An estimate of your chances of cure can be made only after all the test results are back.
- You should be able to go home in 1 or 2 days.

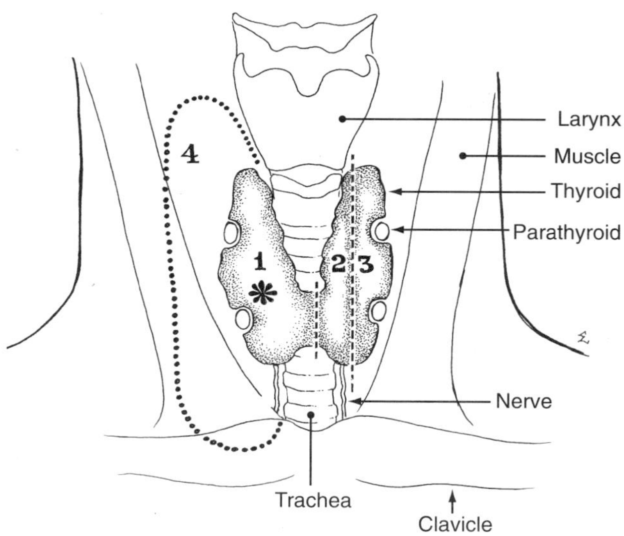

Figure 1. The extent of an operation for papillary cancer of the thyroid *(asterisk)* depends on a number of factors. There can be removal of only one lobe of the thyroid (area 1), removal of the lobe with cancer and at least half of the opposite lobe (area 2), or a total thyroidectomy (areas 1–3). Sometimes all of the lymph node–bearing tissue on the side of the neck with the cancer needs to be removed (area 4). The parathyroid glands are not purposely removed.

- Arrangements will be made for your medicine, follow-up office visit, and stitch removal.

✣ HOME CARE

- You may walk about as you wish and even climb stairs, but don't overdo things.
- You may eat as you wish.
- Be certain to take the medicines prescribed for you.
- Unless instructed otherwise, you may shower if you wish with any dressings on or off. After you dry yourself, replace any dressings with clean, dry ones.
- Do not drive a car unless you can move freely and without pain and are not taking any medicines that decrease your alertness.
- You may return to work when you feel up to it.

✆ CALL OUR OFFICE IF

- You develop any unusual signs or symptoms.
- The incision becomes red or swollen, or there is drainage from it.
- You develop a temperature higher than 101°F.
- You have any questions.

△ GENERAL INFORMATION

Amputation of the toe may be needed for several reasons, including the following:

- A severe cut or crushing injury to the great toe.
- Decreased circulation to the toes as a result of diabetes, hardening of the arteries *(atherosclerosis)*, or blood clots blocking the arteries.

COMMON SIGNS AND SYMPTOMS

- The common symptom is pain.
- If the circulation to the toe is severely decreased, the pain is worse when the foot is elevated.
- The toe may become cool; there may also be a change in color.

DIAGNOSIS

- The diagnosis usually can be made by taking a detailed history and doing a careful physical examination with particular attention to the color, pulses, sensation, and overall appearance of the toe.
- *Plethysmography*: This test measures the blood flow to the toe. This is helpful in determining the extent of the problem and at what level the amputation should be carried out.

PREOPERATIVE PREPARATION

- You will have an examination of your blood, urine, heart (EKG), and lungs (chest x-ray).
- Do not eat or drink anything for 8 hours before the operation.
- Shower or bathe as usual on the morning of the operation, if this is possible.
- You may be given medicine that will make you feel drowsy before you are brought to the operating room.

□ OPERATION

- This operation commonly is done by making the toe area numb as well as giving you some medicine to make you feel drowsy. However, it can be done with you totally asleep. The choice of the anesthetic will be discussed with you beforehand.
- The operation generally takes about 1 hour.

POSTOPERATIVE CARE

- You will be taken to a recovery room and observed. When your blood pressure, pulse, and breathing are stable and you are completely alert, you should be able to go home that same day with a responsible adult.
- You will be instructed on how to wear either a wooden shoe or a removable brace.
- Most persons can bear weight on their foot right after the operation but you may have to use crutches for a period of time.
- Arrangements will be made for your medicine, follow-up office visit, and stitch removal.
- As with any operation, complications are always possible. With your type of operation, they can include infection and the need to re-operate at a higher level because your circulation is not good enough to heal the wound or because the disease has progressed.

✚ HOME CARE

- Take it easy for the first week or so.
- When sitting, if possible keep the foot level with your thigh. This will probably be more comfortable and also help keep the swelling down.
- You will be instructed on when and how much weight you should bear on your foot.
- Keep the dressing dry. You can sponge bathe or bathe in the tub with your leg hanging out.
- Take medicine as prescribed for your pain.
- Include enough roughage and plenty of liquids in your diet to help prevent constipation.
- Driving a car with an automatic shift may not seem too demanding, but if you suddenly have to slam on the brakes you may not be able to do so and may get into an accident. Let's talk about when you can resume driving at your follow-up visit.
- You may return to work when you feel up to it, but let's talk about it first during a follow-up office visit.

✆ CALL OUR OFFICE IF

- The incision becomes red or swollen, or there is drainage from it.
- You develop a temperature higher than 100°F.
- You have any questions.

△ GENERAL INFORMATION

Most people who fracture a toe tell of dropping a heavy object on it or of striking the bare toe against a relatively immovable object such as a night stand, chair, or wall. You look down and there you have it; a bulging toe and indescribable pain.

COMMON SIGNS AND SYMPTOMS

- Signs and symptoms include swelling, a bluish color around the toe, and pain. Sometimes the person can't put on his or her shoe or even walk on the foot.

DIAGNOSIS

- Sometimes the toe may look terrible but is not actually broken. Therefore, it usually is necessary to obtain an x-ray to verify that the toe is fractured.

○ TREATMENT

- Fortunately, even if the toe is broken, an operation is rarely needed.
- Simple fractures can usually be treated by taping the toe to the unbroken toe next to it. This type of treatment generally is not recommended when more than one toe is broken.
- Some severe fractures involving multiple toes may require that pins be placed across the fracture to hold the fragments in the correct position.
- Your fracture needs to be corrected by an operation.

PREOPERATIVE PREPARATION

- You will have an examination of your blood and urine and, depending on your general health, an examination of your heart (EKG) and lungs (chest x-ray).
- Do not eat or drink anything for 8 hours before the operation.
- You may be given medicine that will make you feel drowsy before you are brought to the operating room.

□ OPERATION

- The extent of the operation depends on the severity of the fractures.
- Generally, this operation is done with a spinal type anesthesia or a general anesthesia.
- On occasion, the bones can be straightened out by simple manipulation without the need for an incision and then held in a position as is appropriate.
- Less commonly, a small incision must be made to actually see the fragments as they are being straightened by the surgeon.
- The operation usually takes about 1 hour.

POSTOPERATIVE CARE

- You will be taken to a recovery room and observed. When your blood pressure, pulse, and breathing are stable and you are completely alert, the chances are good that you will be able to go home the same day with a responsible adult. If the operation was more extensive, you will need to stay in the hospital for a day or two.
- Arrangements will be made for your medicine, crutches if needed, and the follow-up office visit.

✚ HOME CARE

- The degree of activity allowable will depend on the extent of the fractures and the type of operation necessary to correct the problem. You will be given instructions on this before you leave the hospital.
- Sit with your foot elevated on one pillow. This will help lessen the pain and also any swelling.
- If the pins that were used to keep your toes in alignment are protruding, the foot will need to be kept dry until the pins are removed in 3 to 6 weeks. Generally, during this time you will wear a wooden shoe or a small walking brace.

✆ CALL OUR OFFICE IF

- There is reduced feeling in the toes or there is a change in the normal color of the toes or foot.
- There is any drainage around a pin site.
- You develop a temperature higher than 100°F.
- You have any questions.

△ GENERAL INFORMATION

The tonsils are glands that are found on each side of the back part of the throat (Fig. 1). For the first 18 months of life, the tonsils help the body fight off infection, but they are no longer needed after the age of about 2 years.

Usually the tonsils are big as a plum pit, but they can be larger, especially when infected. Tonsils that have been infected repeatedly can become quite large (Fig. 2). They also provide a home for infectious organisms that can infect your throat when your resistance is low. Sometimes, tonsils get large enough to interfere with breathing, causing loud snoring as well as breath-holding episodes (called *apnea*). Frequent bacterial infections or tonsillitis cause many missed work days.

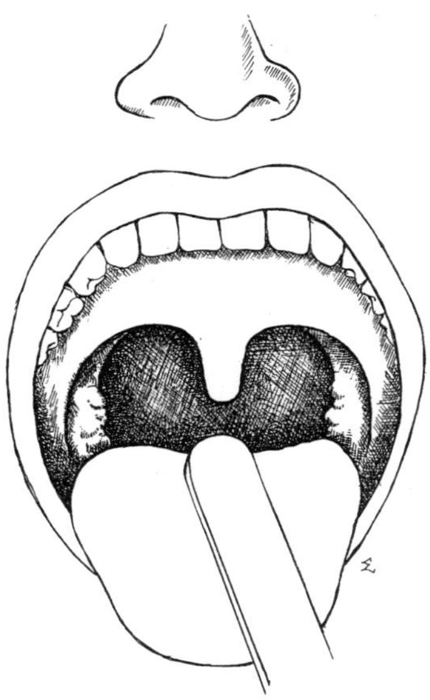

Figure 1. Relatively normal-sized tonsils.

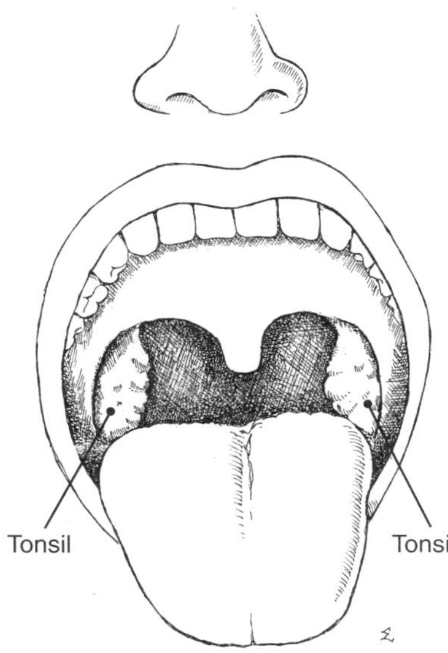

Figure 2. Abnormally large tonsils.

COMMON SIGNS AND SYMPTOMS

The tonsils become enlarged and infected much more commonly in children. However, a few individuals persist in having infected, enlarged tonsils, even into adulthood.

DIAGNOSIS

- The diagnosis requires taking a detailed history to be certain of the cause of the symptoms. Most of the time, large swollen tonsils are due to infection. In adults, however, it is important to make sure that the swelling is not due to a tumor of the tonsil, especially when only one is enlarged.
- Swelling of the lymph nodes in the neck (along with the swollen tonsils) should not automatically be assumed to be from the infected tonsil. Removing a tiny piece of a suspiciously enlarged lymph node (a *biopsy*) can easily be done with a needle as an office procedure.

○ TREATMENT

- The treatment of infected tonsils *(tonsillitis)* generally is medical and consists of a 10- to 14-day course of antibiotics. Sometimes in more resistant cases, an even stronger antibiotic for up to 4 weeks may be necessary.
- An operation to remove the tonsils is indicated in the following circumstances:
  - There are repeated tonsillar infections (four to five times a year) and many missed days of work or school.
  - A history of peritonsillar abscess: This is a collection of pus behind the tonsil.
  - Enlarged tonsils causing very loud snoring, often accompanied by breath-holding.
  - Suspicion of cavernous growth.

After careful consideration of all factors, the recommendation is that you have your tonsils removed.

PREOPERATIVE PREPARATION

- You will have appropriate laboratory studies performed.
- Do not eat or drink anything for 8 hours before the operation.
- You may be given medicine that will make you feel drowsy before you are brought to the operating room.

□ OPERATION

- The operation can be done under local anesthesia with heavy sedation, or it can be done with you asleep. The choice will be discussed with you beforehand.
- The operation generally takes less than 1 hour.

POSTOPERATIVE CARE

- You will be taken to a recovery room and observed. When your blood pressure, pulse, and breathing are stable, you will be taken to the outpatient recovery area.
- Your throat will be quite sore, and you may have some pain shooting up toward your ear.
- You will be given pain medicine as you need it.
- You will be given popsicles and juices in the holding area. When you are able to take these fluids, you will be able to go home with a responsible adult.
- Because of the sore throat you won't feel like taking anything by mouth. Even so, you must drink fluids; otherwise you can become dehydrated and this can cause fever.
- Arrangements will be made for your medicines and follow-up office visit.

✚ HOME CARE

- Rest as much as possible and avoid any strenuous activity.
- Speaking will be somewhat painful. This is expected. Not speaking too much will give the back of your throat some rest.
- Don't lift anything over 5 pounds. Ask someone to do it for you.
- Generally, the pain in your throat may get worse before it gets better. The pain medicine will greatly help with the pain but may not make it go away completely.
- You will have bad breath from scabs where the tonsils were removed. These scabs fall off in about 7 to 10 days, and your breath odor will return to normal. Do not gargle, as this will hurt and may cause bleeding.
- Because of the throat pain, eating may not be possible right away. Just the same, you must take in some nourishment. *Favor*: clear liquids such as water, apple juice, Gatorade, and popsicles. *Avoid*: citrus juices, and carbonated beverages (colas) because they may cause increased pain and throat irritation.
- After a few days, start trying foods that are easy to swallow. *Favor*: Jell-O, soft noodles, warm broths, pudding, yogurt, and ice cream. *Avoid*: steamy, hot, or spicy foods or hard, crunchy foods.
- To avoid constipation, be sure you include plenty of liquids in your diet. You may need some help with a mild laxative (example: milk of magnesia).
- You may return to work when you feel up to it. Most adults need about 1 week to recuperate and start back on a more normal diet.

✆ CALL OUR OFFICE IF

- There is any bleeding other than blood-tinged saliva after the first 2 days, because this can be an emergency. If you cannot reach the doctor promptly, have someone take you to the hospital emergency room.
- You develop a temperature higher than 101°F.
- You have any questions.

△ GENERAL INFORMATION

The tonsils are glands that are found on each side of the back part of the throat (Fig. 1). For the first 18 months of life, the tonsils help the body fight off infection, but they are no longer needed after the age of about 2 years.

Usually, tonsils are about as big as a plum pit, but they can be larger, especially if infection is present. Tonsils that repeatedly become infected can become quite large (Fig. 2). The tonsils also provide a home for bacteria that can infect the throat when a person's resistance is low. They also can get so large that they can interfere with a child's normal, clear breathing, causing loud snoring and even episodes of breath-holding (called *apnea*) during sleep.

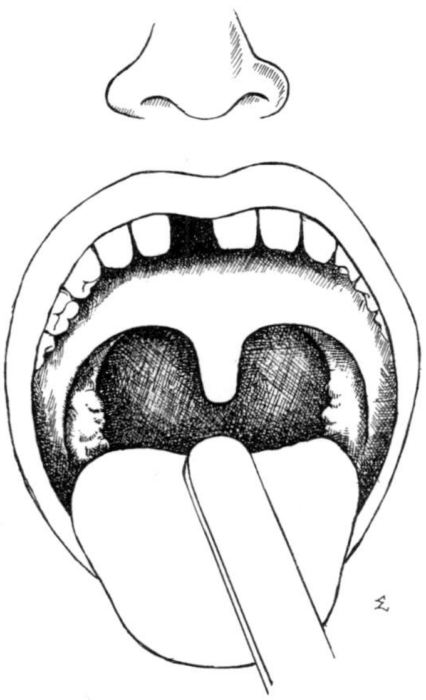

Figure 1. Relatively normal-sized tonsils.

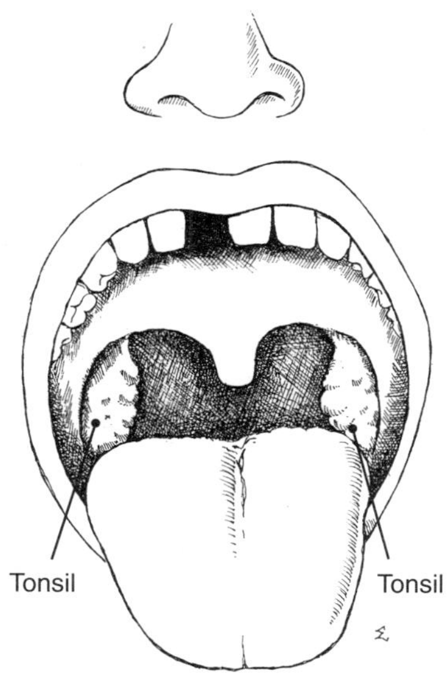

Figure 2. Abnormally large tonsils.

COMMON SIGNS AND SYMPTOMS

Swollen tonsils are rather common in children as they tend to get colds frequently. Tonsils in children can swell with the slightest infection, then return to normal size when the illness goes away. However, some children's tonsils remain swollen and flare up most of the time, causing problems such as the following:

- Frequent sore throats that last longer than usual.
- Ear infections.
- Difficulty in breathing because of the enlargement of this tissue in the back of the throat.
- Occasional formation of abscesses, or pockets of pus, next to the tonsil.
- Poor eating because of soreness.

DIAGNOSIS

- The diagnosis can be made by taking a detailed history and doing a thorough physical examination. Occasionally, laboratory tests are needed.

○ TREATMENT

- The initial treatment for tonsillitis is antibiotic therapy. Only tonsillitis caused by bacteria will get better with the appropriate antibiotic. Sometimes, two or even three different antibiotics need to be tried in very resistant cases. Tonsillitis caused by a virus (the same cause of colds) has the same symptoms as bacterial tonsillitis but won't necessarily go away with antibiotics.

An operation to remove the tonsils is appropriate in the following circumstances:

- Frequent infections that cause absences from school.
- Symptoms such as loud snoring and breath-holding during sleep.
- Repeated ear infections in association with the recurrent tonsillitis.

After careful consideration of all factors, the recommendation is that your child have a tonsillectomy.

PREOPERATIVE PREPARATION

- Unless instructed otherwise, your child should not eat or drink anything for 8 hours before the operation.
- Medicine may be given to your child before the operation to reduce anxiety and also to reduce the amount of saliva in the throat.

□ OPERATION

- The operation will be done under general anesthesia. Your child will be completely asleep and will not feel any pain during the operation.
- After the tonsils are removed, the adenoid tissue in the back of the nose will be evaluated. If it is enlarged and interfering with normal breathing through the nose, or repeatedly becomes infected, it too will be removed.
- The operation generally takes about 1 hour.

POSTOPERATIVE CARE

- Your child will be taken to a recovery room until the blood pressure, pulse, and respirations are stable and then transferred to the outpatient surgical area.
- The child will be watched carefully to be certain there is no bleeding and that breathing is normal.
- Your child will be given fluids or a popsicle.
- Pain will be controlled with medicine.
- As with any operation, complications are always possible. While they are uncommon with this operation, they can include bleeding, a sore throat for 1 to 2 weeks, and occasionally a change in the voice, which lasts as long as the pain is present, but then goes away.
- You should be able to take your child home that same day.
- Arrangements will be made for pain medicine, any antibiotics, and the follow-up office visit.

✣ HOME CARE

- Restrain your child from too much activity and rough play. Your child should probably not go to school for 1 week and should be closely observed in case any bleeding occurs.
- Your child will have a sore throat and an earache. Generally, these will get worse before they get better.
- Give your child medicines for pain as directed. It is better if this medicine is given along with food.
- The pain medicine will greatly help with the pain but will not make it go away completely. Because of the sore throat, eating may not be possible right away. Just the same, be certain the child drinks enough fluids to avoid dehydration. *Favor*: clear liquids such as water, apple juice, Gatorade, and popsicles. *Avoid*: citrus juices and carbonated beverages (colas) because they may cause increased pain and throat irritation.
- After a few days, start offering easy-to-swallow foods, such as Jell-O, soft noodles, warm broth, pudding, yogurt, and ice cream. *Avoid*: steamy, hot, spicy, or hard, crunchy foods.
- Your child may bathe or shower as desired.
- There may be a bad odor from the mouth or nose due to scabs in the surgical area. This is not an infection and will go away in 1–2 weeks as the tissues heal.

✆ CALL OUR OFFICE IF

- There are any unusual signs or symptoms.
- There is any bleeding other than blood-tinged saliva for the first 2 days.
- If there is bleeding that is bright red or with blood clots, this can be an emergency. If you cannot reach a doctor, promptly take your child to the hospital emergency room.
- Your child develops a temperature higher than 101°F.
- You have any questions.

△ GENERAL INFORMATION

A *tracheostomy* is an opening made directly through the skin and into the *trachea* (windpipe) in the front of the neck. There are three main reasons for doing a tracheostomy:

- There is a blockage in the mouth, throat, or voice box that prevents air flow from the lungs to the outside. Blockage is sometimes caused by swelling from infection or cancer of the throat. It is often not possible to put such patients to sleep in the operating room in the regular manner unless they have a tracheostomy tube. In such situations, tracheostomy simply allows the air from the lungs to exit directly out the front of the neck, bypassing the blockage.
- Some patients who have weak or diseased lungs or a brain injury or who are recovering from major surgery may need assistance with breathing. When such patients are on a ventilator (breathing machine) for more than a week or so, they may require a tracheostomy so that they'll be more comfortable. Also, mucus in the lungs is easier to suction out through a tracheostomy tube.
- Injury to the face or neck may cause so much swelling in the mouth or throat that a tracheostomy is needed in order to breathe. A tracheostomy may also be required for an operation to repair broken facial bones.

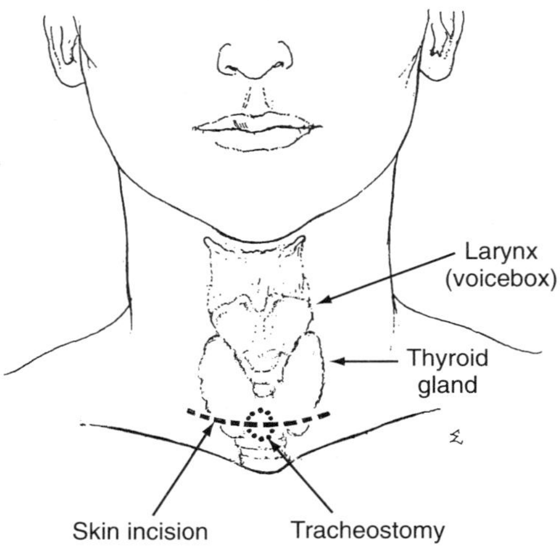

Figure 1.

WHEN TO DO A TRACHEOSTOMY

Considerable experience is needed to know when the patient should have a tracheostomy. As a rule, if there is a serious question about whether or not the patient needs a tracheostomy, it is safer to perform the tracheostomy.

□ OPERATION

- The operation is often done under local anesthesia.
- The front part of the neck is swabbed with antiseptic solution and the area surrounded with sterile towels. A thin needle is used to inject an anesthetic solution into the skin in the middle of the front of the neck about an inch above the breastbone.
- An incision about one-half inch long is made in the numbed skin over the trachea (Fig 1).
- An opening as big around as the tip of your little finger is made in the trachea and a special type of curved tube (a *tracheostomy tube*) is placed inside the trachea (Fig 2).

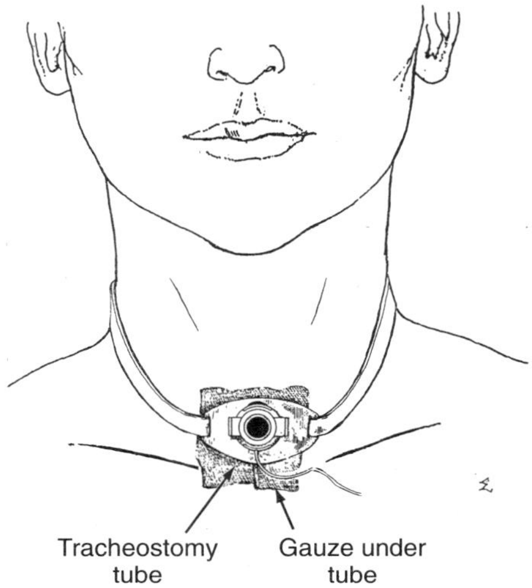

Figure 2.

POSTOPERATIVE USE

Once the tracheostomy is performed, a number of things can be done:

- A tracheostomy tube can be used to suck out accumulating mucus.
- An oxygen tube can be placed in front of the tracheostomy so that extra oxygen can go in.
- The tracheostomy tube can be hooked up to a ventilator.

✣ HOME CARE

- If you have to go home with a tracheostomy tube, you will be shown how to keep it clean. Most of the time, you will be able to cough out the mucus from your lungs. If not, a suction machine can help you. It is best if a family member can learn to help you care for your tracheostomy tube.
- When the tube is opened directly to the outside, the person cannot speak because the breath goes straight out through the hole and not through the voice box as it does normally. However, in some cases, speaking is possible by simply placing a finger over the hole and forcing the air to come out the normal way through the mouth. For patients who need a tracheostomy for longer periods of time, there are various models of tracheostomy tubes that have valves that allow them to speak freely.

REMOVING THE TUBE

In many instances, the tracheostomy tube is temporary. Once the surgery is completed and the patient is stronger, it can be removed. When the tracheostomy tube is no longer needed, it takes just a few minutes to slip it out of the neck. The hole in the trachea closes by itself in several days.

TRANSESOPHAGEAL ECHOCARDIOGRAPHY

△ GENERAL INFORMATION

Before a major operation, most patients have tests to evaluate their physical condition, especially the heart and lungs.

During the operation, wires are taped to certain areas of the body so that the anesthesiologist can monitor your heart, lungs, blood pressure, and oxygen level.

In certain situations, it is especially important that your heart be watched even more closely. Transesophageal echocardiography is a way to do that.

WHAT IS ECHOCARDIOGRAPHY?

- This technique uses ultrasound.
- In ultrasound, harmless, painless sound waves are aimed at soft tissue in your body (in this instance, the heart and the vessels going to and coming from it). The sound waves bouncing back (the echoes) from the heart and vessels are seen as moving pictures on a screen. This is a very valuable way to examine organs or tissues as they are working.
- The closer the organ being examined to the source of the sound waves, the sharper the picture.
- In the chest, the esophagus is located right behind the heart. So the sound waves are sent out from inside the esophagus. That's how this technique gets its long name: *trans* = through; *esophageal* = esophagus (your swallowing tube); *echo* = sound waves bouncing back; *cardio* = heart, *graphy* = picture. The procedure commonly is called TEE.

WHAT CAN TEE SHOW?

- It can show how well the heart is contracting before, during, and right after an operation.
- The heart valves can be observed as they open and close to see if any abnormality is present.
- The vessels coming to and leaving the heart can be watched and the blood flow through them estimated.

WHO CAN BENEFIT FROM TEE?

- Patients having heart vessel operations such as coronary artery bypass or heart valve replacement, or repair of an aneurysm of the aorta.
- Patients having major operations in which there is an underlying heart problem and there is a need for especially careful monitoring of the heart.
- Patients in whom an echocardiogram done from the outside will not be satisfactory. An example might be a person who is very obese.
- Patients who already have a satisfactory echocardiogram from outside the chest before the operation but need to have the heart watched during the operation as well. It is not practical or possible to do it from outside the chest during the operation.

THE PROCEDURE

- The TEE probe is smooth and flexible and about as big as the tip of your little finger.
- The TEE probe is placed down your esophagus only after you are completely asleep. After the probe is in the esophagus, it is positioned so that the part that sends out the sound waves is right behind your heart.
- After the TEE probe is in place, the anesthesiologist connects it to the ultrasound machine and is then ready to monitor your heart and blood vessels.
- *Note*: TEE should not be performed if you have problems swallowing liquids or solid food or if you have had an operation on your esophagus. If you are informed by the anesthesiologist that a TEE will be done during the operation, report any problems you have had with swallowing.
- After the TEE probe is removed, you may have some discomfort in your throat for a day.

POSSIBLE COMPLICATIONS

- As with any procedure, complications are always possible. They are rare with TEE but can include injury to the lining of the esophagus or even making a hole in it and causing infection.

This explanation of transesophageal echocardiography will help you better understand the sophisticated techniques that sometimes are used to make an operation safer.

△ GENERAL INFORMATION

The tendons that *flex* (bend) your fingers into your palm travel through a series of pulleys (which make up a tunnel) in the palm and finger. These help keep the tendons in their place so they can efficiently bend your fingers. Sometimes a nodule or knot can form on one of these tendons. This usually occurs in the lower part of the palm. When the fingers flex and the tendon is pulled proximally toward the elbow, this knot can catch on one of the pulleys. This causes a clicking and catching, or "triggering," of the fingers (Fig. 1).

The cause of trigger finger is not truly known. It occurs in *tendinitis* (swelling and inflammation of the tendons) and can be aggravated by activities that require repetitive flexion of the fingers (overuse).

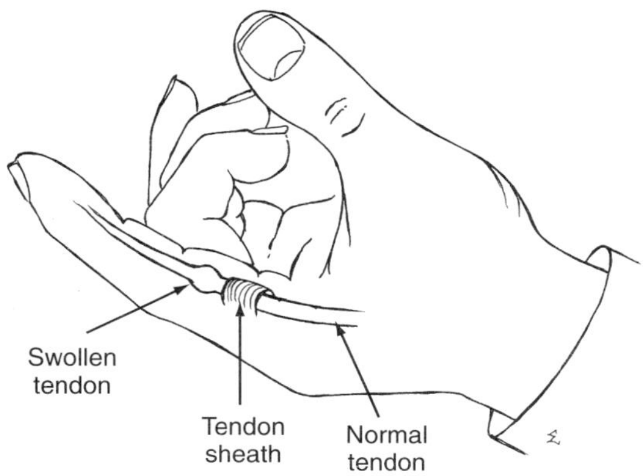

Figure 1. Occasionally, the swollen area of the tendon gets stuck ("lockage") in the sheath. When it lets go, the finger pops into a straight position.

COMMON SIGNS AND SYMPTOMS

- Mild trigger fingers cause a sensation of catching in the fingers although there is full motion. Although the problem is actually in the distal (lower part) palm, the catching or triggering is experienced in the middle finger joint (between the first joint and the base of the finger).
- In some cases, the finger can lock in the flexed (bent) position. Often one has to manually straighten out the finger with the opposite hand.

DIAGNOSIS

- The diagnosis is rather straightforward. Catching or locking is often obvious.
- You may be asked to bend and extend your fingers while the doctor palpates (feels) the distal palm, where the locking actually occurs. Often a nodule can be felt; this region can be tender when pressure is applied.
- More complicated studies are not needed to establish the diagnosis.

○ TREATMENT

- Mild cases of catching that do not limit activities or cause discomfort do not require formal treatment.
- Many cases with true catching and locking can be treated successfully without an operation. Cortisone can be injected into the tendon sheath to shrink the nodule, which will stop the triggering.
- When injections do not eliminate the triggering, and symptoms are bothersome enough, an operation may be indicated. This consists of simply releasing the pulley in the distal palm. The nodule will then shrink as it is no longer being irritated by the pulley. Release of this one pulley does not lead to loss of motion or function of the finger, as not all of the pulleys are needed for normal hand function.

PREOPERATIVE PREPARATION

- Do not eat or drink anything for 8 hours before the operation.
- You may need an examination of your blood and heart (EKG) before the operation.
- Shower or bathe as usual on the morning of the operation.

□ OPERATION

- The operation usually is done under local anesthesia. The palm area over the nodule is made numb by injecting anesthetic medicine into it with a fine needle.
- During the operation, you may feel some tugging but no pain.
- After the first pulley is released you will be asked to move your fingers and make a fist on the operating room table. This will not hurt. It must be done to be certain that there is no longer any catching or triggering and that the release is complete before the short skin incision is closed.

POSTOPERATIVE CARE

- You should be able to go home directly after the operation.
- Arrangements will be made for your medicine, follow-up office visit, and stitch removal.
- You will be asked to flex and extend your fingers after surgery to keep them loose and prevent them from becoming stiffer.
- As with any operation, complications are always possible. Although they are uncommon with this type of operation, they can include injury to the nerve or blood vessels of the fingers. Also, the finger can swell and become stiff after this operation.

✣ HOME CARE

- Resume your usual activities as much as possible.
- You will be asked to keep your dressing and incision dry until the stitches are removed (usually 7 to 14 days after the operation).

- If you need to shower or bathe, one way to protect the hand and dressings from getting wet is to put your entire arm in a small trash bag and completely seal it with tape at the open end. Repeat this with a second bag over the first one.
- You may ask to see a physical therapist to have supervised exercise sessions. This will help you regain all of your finger motion. The therapist will also treat any swelling that develops after the operation.

✆ CALL OUR OFFICE IF

- You develop any unusual signs or symptoms.
- The incision becomes red or swollen, or there is drainage from it.
- You develop a temperature higher than 100°F.
- You develop progressive or worsening swelling in your fingers or they become stiff.
- You have any questions.

TUBAL LIGATION (TUBAL STERILIZATION)

△ GENERAL INFORMATION

A sterilization operation on a woman is done in the following circumstances:

- There is a medical reason for it.
  - An illness that will be made worse by a pregnancy.
  - Inability to take contraceptive medicines.
  - There is a present or potential psychiatric reason not to become pregnant.
- There is a personal reason for it.
  - Does not wish to have more children.
  - Does not wish to use, or is not able to reliably practice, other types of birth control.
  - The sex partner refuses to use, or does not reliably practice, birth control.

BEFORE ANYTHING IS PLANNED

- You should be absolutely certain you wish to have a sterilization operation.
- You should be aware that, although there is no legal requirement that your husband also sign the authorization for your operation, you will be strongly urged to get his signature also.
- You should realize that this is meant to be *permanent* sterilization.
- Although there are operations to reconnect your tubes if you change your mind later, they are not minor operations. Also they are not always successful, and they increase the risk of tubal pregnancy.
- You should not think that if you change your mind and the tubes cannot be reconnected, you can always have in vitro fertilization with an embryo transfer. Those are complicated procedures that have varying success rates.
- You should be fully informed of the failure rate of tubal sterilization.
- You should be fully informed of the possible complications of tubal sterilization.
- You will need to participate in a discussion of alternative methods of contraception.
- If the reasons for your request are psychiatric or medical, there will need to be a letter stating this from your doctor.

TIMING

To Be Done at the Time of Delivery

- The sterilization operation should be planned well in advance of your anticipated date of delivery.
- If a cesarean section (C-section) is planned, then the sterilization should be done at the same time.
- If it is to be done following natural childbirth, then it should take place within 6 to 36 hours after delivery.
- If there's anything unusual about your delivery that would increase the risk of sterilization at that particular time, then the surgery should be postponed.
- In women who have heart disease, serious high blood pressure, kidney disease, or acute toxemia, the sterilization operation should be postponed; doing it along with the delivery may increase the risk of complications following the delivery.

Delayed Tubal Ligation

- If none of the above applies to you, then the operation can be done at a convenient time. This is an outpatient procedure.

PREOPERATIVE PREPARATION

For Sterilization at the Time of Natural Childbirth

- The usual preparations for natural childbirth.

For Sterilization Not Associated with Childbirth

- A detailed history and a thorough physical examination will be done.
- An examination of your blood, urine, heart (EKG), and lungs (chest x-ray) will be done.
- The operation is best done between your menstrual periods.
- Do not eat or drink anything for 8 hours before the operation.
- Shower as usual on the morning of the operation.
- You may be given medicine that will make you feel drowsy before you are brought to the operating room.

□ OPERATION

Done at the Time of Delivery

- The tubes will be divided in a manner known to be the most successful (Fig. 1).

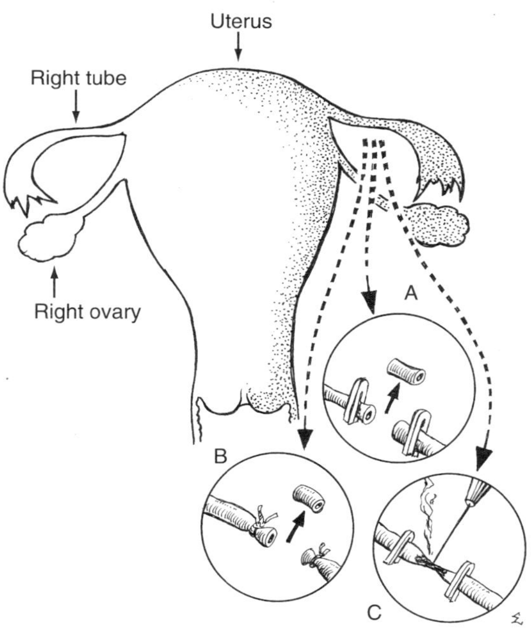

Figure 1. The fallopian tube can be interrupted in several ways: clipping with removal of a short segment of it (A); ligation and division (B); or clipping and burning the tube with an electrical current (C).

Not Associated with Childbirth

- The operation will be done under general anesthesia.
- The operation is straightforward and usually takes about 1 hour.

POSTOPERATIVE CARE

Done at the Time of Delivery

- Your care will be part of that given after a normal delivery.

Not Associated with Delivery

- You will wake up in a recovery room. When your blood pressure, pulse, and breathing are stable and you are completely alert, you should be able to go home that same day with a responsible adult.

✣ HOME CARE

- Return to your previous activities as you tolerate them.

✆ CALL OUR OFFICE IF

- You develop any unusual signs or symptoms.
- You develop a temperature higher than 100°F.
- You have any questions.

TUBAL LIGATION: Reversal (Tubal Sterilization: Reversal)

△ GENERAL INFORMATION

This is an operation to reconnect the *fallopian tubes* (which were intentionally divided for purposes of birth control) so that it is again possible for an egg from a woman's ovary to travel toward and reach the uterus.

Normally, once a month an egg *(E)* is released from the ovary *(O)* (Fig. 1). The egg finds its way to the opening (the *fimbria*) *(F)* of the fallopian tube. Once inside the fallopian tube *(T)*, the egg moves toward the cavity of the uterus. If there is sperm *(S)* in the uterus, the egg and sperm may unite. This united egg and sperm is called a zygote *(Z)*. The zygote develops into an *embryo* that attaches to the inside of the uterus (implants), and if all goes well, starts growing. Over 9 months it develops into a full-term baby.

A way for a woman to avoid becoming pregnant is to prevent the egg and sperm from reaching each other. One method is to divide the fallopian tube (called *tubal sterilization*). The fallopian tube can be interrupted in several ways: It can be divided; a piece of it can be removed; it can be tied; it can be burned. Several of the above can be done at the same time.

At a later time and for a number of reasons, a woman may wish to again be able to become pregnant in the normal way. Generally, two options are available:

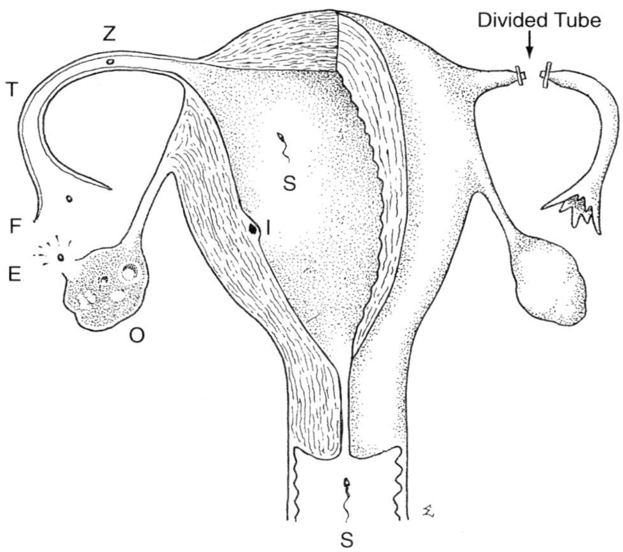

Figure 1.

In vitro Fertilization. In this modest but specialized operation, an egg that is just ready to be released is removed from the ovary and placed in a nourishing solution along with sperm from the partner. If the egg and sperm unite and form an embryo, it is inserted into the woman's uterus (by another modest operation) in the hope that it will implant and start a pregnancy.

Reversal of Sterilization. This is an operation in which an interrupted tube is reconnected (Fig. 2). Because the tunnel in the fallopian tubes is small (about the size of the lead in a pencil) and there is scarring from the method used to interrupt the fallopian tube, the operation to reconnect it is delicate and requires skill and experience. It is performed by specialists in the field. For the above reasons, it must be realized that, for any chance of a successful pregnancy, it is necessary to have an egg, a sperm, and a way for them to meet.

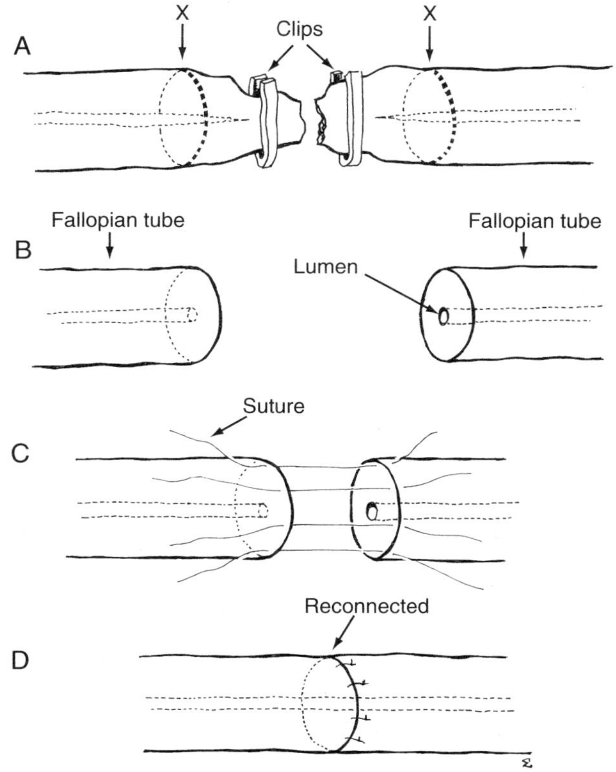

Figure 2. *A*, The clipped, divided, scarred ends of the fallopian tubes are cut across what appears to be normal tissue (X). *B*, The divided ends are examined to see if they are open. *C*, Very fine suture material is used to reconnect the open ends of the tube. *D*, The reconnected tube.

Sperm. Is sperm of the proper quality available? There are tests that can determine this.

Egg. Is an egg available? We cannot assume that this is true just because ovaries are present. A number of tests are available to determine this. Some of the methods are as simple as charting your daily temperature, while others may require serial blood hormone tests and ultrasound examinations during one menstrual cycle.

Fallopian Tubes. Are the tubes in good enough condition to be reconnected? Special, somewhat involved types of x-rays are used to determine this. Occasionally, a surgical procedure called a *laparotomy* is required.

Answers to these questions will help the gynecologist

decide whether to recommend in vitro fertilization or to attempt to reconnect the fallopian tubes.

All factors were carefully considered, the most important being which method will give you the best chance of becoming pregnant. The recommendation for you is that an attempt be made to reconnect your fallopian tubes.

PREOPERATIVE PREPARATION

- You will have an examination of your blood, urine, heart (EKG), and lungs (chest x-ray).
- Do not eat or drink anything for 8 hours before the operation.
- Do not douche or use a tampon on the day of the operation.
- You may be given medicine that will make you feel drowsy before you are brought to the operating room.

□ OPERATION

- You will be asleep for the operation.
- If possible, a "bikini" incision will be used unless you have had a previous lower abdominal incision that runs in an up and down direction.
- The operation will be done with magnifying lenses.
- Extremely fine suture material (as fine as a hair) will be used.
- During the operation, a small tube may be temporarily placed in your uterus through the vagina. This will be used to inject some fluid into the uterus to see if it can come out of the opened fallopian tubes.
- You will not need a blood transfusion.
- The operation generally takes 2 to 3 hours.

POSTOPERATIVE CARE

- You will be taken to a recovery room and observed. When your blood pressure, pulse, and breathing are stable, you will be taken to a regular hospital room.
- Your diet will be as you tolerate it.
- Pain can be controlled with medicine.
- You should be able to go home in about 2 days.
- Arrangements will be made for your medicine, follow-up office visit, and stitch or clip removal.
- As with any operation, complications are always possible. With your type of operation, they can include infection, bleeding, and possibly others.

✚ HOME CARE

- You may walk about as you wish, even climb stairs, but don't overdo things.
- Eat as you wish.
- Do not douche or use a tampon on the day of the operation.
- Drive as you wish but not if you are taking medicines that may decrease your alertness.
- You may resume sexual activity after the first menstrual period.
- You may return to work when you feel up to it.

✆ CALL OUR OFFICE IF

- You develop any unusual signs or symptoms.
- The incision becomes red or swollen, or there is drainage from it.
- You develop a temperature higher than 100°F.
- You have any questions.

FOLLOW-UP CARE

It is important to remember that there is no assurance that because your fallopian tubes have been reconnected, you will have no difficulty in becoming pregnant. If you are having difficulty, a repeat examination of the tubes can confirm that they are open. However, there are several reasons why you may not be able to become pregnant. One also must be alert to the possibility (15 to 20%) of developing a tubal pregnancy. If there are any questions about this, be certain to discuss them further with us.

TUBAL PREGNANCY (ECTOPIC PREGNANCY)

△ GENERAL INFORMATION

A normal pregnancy starts when the egg from the ovary travels down the *fallopian tube* of the uterus. This tube is as thick around as a pencil with a tunnel in it the size of the lead in a pencil. The egg reaches the uterus to meet the sperm coming up from the opening of the uterus (the *cervix*). Then the fertilized egg develops roots in the lining of the uterus (implants) and starts to grow.

Sometimes, however, the egg gets stuck as it comes down the tube. The much smaller sperm from the other end keeps on wiggling up the tube and fertilizes the egg right there in the tube. When this happens, the pregnancy starts in the tube and the egg begins to develop and grow in this very narrow area. This is a *tubal pregnancy* (also called an *ectopic pregnancy*). It is a serious problem because there is so little space for growth that the fallopian tube can burst (Fig. 1).

Some of the causes of tubal pregnancy:

- Previous pelvic infection causing scarring of the fallopian tube.
- A previous tubal pregnancy.
- Endometriosis.
- Pelvic surgery.

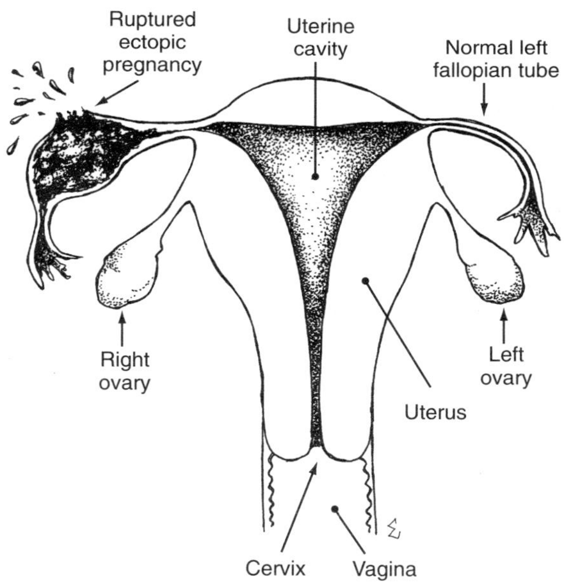

Figure 1. The most dangerous complication of tubal pregnancy is hemorrhage from rupture of the tube containing the pregnancy.

COMMON SIGNS AND SYMPTOMS

- There is little or no menstrual bleeding 2 to 4 weeks after a missed period.
- There is light stabbing pain in the right or left side of the lower abdomen that may last just a short while. Soon, however, the pain becomes sharp, severe, and persistent.
- An extremely tender mass might be felt in the right or left side of the lower abdomen.
- If the cervix is jiggled during a vaginal examination, there is extreme pain because this also jiggles the tubes.
- If a tube ruptures:
  - The pain spreads throughout the entire abdomen.
  - There is dizziness, shock, fainting, and a very fast pulse.
  - The bowel slows down or stops working entirely.

DIAGNOSIS

A woman who is young enough to have children and has some of the less serious signs and symptoms should be suspected of having an ectopic pregnancy. The way to establish the diagnosis is to promptly perform some of the following tests:

- Take the history and do a thorough examination with a focus on the gynecologic organs.
- Take blood for an emergency blood test, pregnancy test, and other hormone tests.
- *Ultrasound*: Harmless sound waves are aimed at the area of the pelvis. The sound waves bouncing back (the echoes) from this area are seen as a picture on a screen. Ultrasound is a quick and painless way to examine the pelvic organs.
- *CT scan (computed tomography scan)*: These special x-rays are taken by a machine that is shaped like a huge doughnut. You will lie on a table inside the hole in the "doughnut." These x-rays are taken so that they show up as very thin slices through the area of the uterus, fallopian tubes, and ovaries. This makes it possible to see the fine details of these organs.
- *Culdocentesis*: A needle is inserted into the abdominal cavity through the uppermost part of the vagina (which is very close to the ovary and the tube). If blood is withdrawn by the needle, this is evidence of a ruptured ectopic pregnancy.
- *Laparoscopy*: This is done with a *laparoscope* while the patient is asleep. The laparoscope is a tube with lenses in it and a light at its tip and is about as thick as your little finger. It is inserted into the abdomen through a tiny incision in your navel. The entire pelvis can be examined directly.
- *Note*: Sometimes there is just not enough time to do all these tests. If the patient is rapidly getting worse, an emergency operation will be necessary. The operation can both make the diagnosis and treat the problem.

○ TREATMENT

- The treatment of tubal pregnancy is an operation.

PREOPERATIVE PREPARATION

- An examination of your blood, urine, heart (EKG), and lungs (chest x-ray) will be done. Fluids through the veins will have been started when you were admitted to the hospital.

☐ OPERATION

- You will be asleep for the operation.
- The aim will be to stop the bleeding and, if possible, to remove the ectopic tissue while saving all or most of the tube. The ovary is rarely removed.
- A blood transfusion may be necessary.

POSTOPERATIVE CARE

- You will be taken to a recovery room and observed. When your blood pressure, pulse, and breathing are stable, you will be transferred to a regular hospital room.
- Pain will be controlled with medicine.
- Soon you will be helped to sit up in bed and then to get out of bed.
- Your diet will be as you tolerate it.
- You should be able to go home in several days.
- Arrangements will be made for your medicine, follow-up office visit, and stitch or clip removal.
- As with any operation, complications are always possible. With this type of operation, they can include infection, injury to the colon or bladder, clotting problems, and possibly others.

✣ HOME CARE

- You may walk about as you wish, even climb stairs, but don't overdo things.
- You may eat as you wish.
- Unless advised otherwise, you may shower if you wish with any dressings on or off. After you dry yourself, replace any dressings with clean, dry ones.
- Include plenty of roughage and liquids in your diet to help prevent constipation.

✆ CALL OUR OFFICE IF

- The incision becomes red or swollen, or there is drainage from it.
- You develop a temperature higher than 100°F.
- You have any questions.

△ GENERAL INFORMATION

Some individuals have loose skin and fat that hangs across the lower abdomen (a *panniculus*) that looks something like an apron (Fig. 1). A panniculus can be the result of a number of things.

- Being overweight and then going on a diet and losing that weight. The skin and fat across the abdomen become loose and sag.
- Multiple pregnancies.
- Simple relaxation of the tissue.

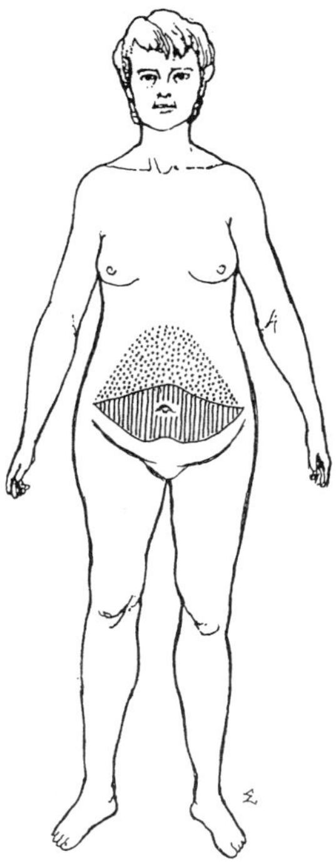

Figure 1. The excess skin and fat to be removed are indicated by the vertical lines. The stippled area is undercut so that cut ends can be brought together without tension.

COMMON SIGNS AND SYMPTOMS

- The panniculus is large, unwieldy, and interferes with daily activities.
- It is difficult to dress attractively.
- It is difficult to carry out personal hygiene.
- There is constant moisture and irritation of the skin on the undersurface of the panniculus.
- It limits one's personal and social life.

DIAGNOSIS

- Usually, the diagnosis can be made by taking a detailed history and doing a thorough physical examination.
- The surgeon will make certain that this appearance is from a fatty apron and not fat inside the abdomen or a hernia sticking out.

○ TREATMENT

- Taking off more weight won't reduce the size of the apron very much. In fact, it might make it even more flabby.
- A panniculus that looks like an apron is not suitable for treatment by liposuction.
- An operation to remove this extra skin and fat is the best treatment for this condition.

PREOPERATIVE PREPARATION

- You will have an examination of your blood, urine, heart (EKG), and lungs (chest x-ray).
- Starting 1 week before the operation, shower with an antibacterial soap (example: Dial).
- If the skin under the panniculus is red and raw, keep some soft cotton cloth there to allow some air to circulate to help keep it dry.
- Do not eat or drink anything for 8 hours before the operation.
- Shower as usual on the morning of the operation.
- You may be given medicine that will make you feel drowsy before you are brought to the operating room.

□ OPERATION

- You will be asleep for the operation.
- As much skin and fat will be removed to eliminate the panniculus (apron) yet leave enough tissue so that it can be brought together looking smooth and without tension (Fig. 2).
- You will not receive a blood transfusion unless it is absolutely necessary.
- The operation usually takes about 2 hours.

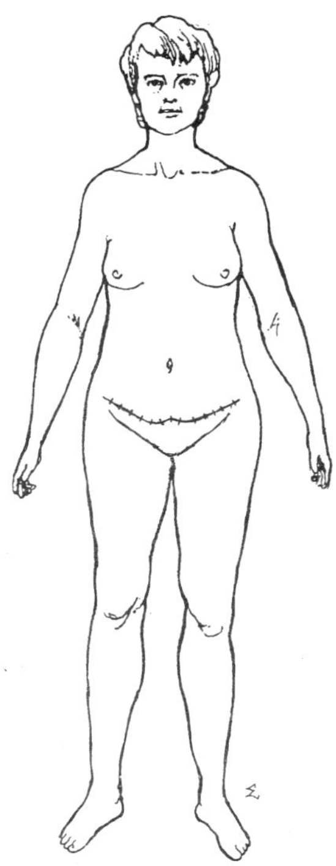

Figure 2. Results of the completed operation. When necessary, a "new" umbilicus is fashioned.

POSTOPERATIVE CARE

- You will wake up in a recovery room. When your blood pressure, pulse, and breathing are stable, you will be taken to a regular hospital room.
- There will be a small plastic tube from the wound to drain any fluid that might form inside.
- A girdle or abdominal binder may be placed at the end of the operation.
- That evening you will be helped to sit up in bed and on the next day to get out of bed.
- You will be shown how to take care of this draining tube; it's easy. The draining tube usually is removed after a few days.
- As with any operation, complications are always possible. With your type of operation, they can include bleeding, wound infection, blood clots in your lungs, heart problems, and possibly others.
- You should be able to go home in 1 to 2 days.
- Arrangements will be made for your medicine, follow-up office visit, and stitch removal.

✚ HOME CARE

- Resume your usual activities.
- You may walk about as you wish, even climb up stairs, but don't overdo things.
- Take medicine as prescribed for your pain.
- You may eat as you did before the operation.
- Be careful that you do not become constipated.
  - Include enough roughage and liquid in your diet.
  - You may need a mild laxative (example: milk of magnesia).
- Unless instructed otherwise, you may shower as you wish with any dressings on or off.
  - There may be narrow strips of tape across the incision; it's all right if they get wet. They will be removed in the doctor's office.
  - After you dry yourself, replace any dressings with clean, dry ones.
- Your incision and the muscles of the abdomen may ache, especially at the end of the day and after you have been standing for a long period. You can support them by wearing a girdle or similar garment that is snug (but not too tight). Wearing it over a cotton undergarment is easier on your incision and the stitches.
- Driving a car with an automatic shift is not too demanding, but if you suddenly have to slam on the brakes or twist to turn the wheel, you may strain the sutures or tear something. During the follow-up visit, let's discuss when you can resume driving.
- You may resume sexual activity whenever you choose.
- You may return to work when you feel up to it.

✆ CALL OUR OFFICE IF

- The incision becomes red or swollen, or there is drainage from it.
- You develop a temperature higher than 100°F.
- You have any questions.

ULCERATIVE COLITIS: Colectomy, Rectal Mucosectomy, and Ileal Pouch–Anal Anastomosis

△ GENERAL INFORMATION

Ulcerative colitis is a serious inflammatory condition of the lining of the large bowel that causes it to bleed very easily. It also can cause problems elsewhere in the body. This condition usually develops slowly, but occasionally it can come on abruptly and be very severe. Mostly, however, it is a chronic condition with ups and downs. The cause of ulcerative colitis is not known.

COMMON SIGNS AND SYMPTOMS

The symptoms depend on how active the disease is, how much of the large bowel is involved, and how long the disease has been present. The most common symptoms are as follows:

- Abdominal pain from the inflamed bowel.
- Bleeding: This can be mucus, mucus with blood, or just blood. Sometimes the bleeding can be very severe.
- Diarrhea: There may be four to six bowel movements a day. Rarely, they can be much more numerous.
- Other symptoms include fever; weight loss; arthritis-like pains in the wrists, ankles, and knees; eye problems; spine problems; and stomach ulcers.

DIAGNOSIS

- Usually the diagnosis can be made by taking a detailed history, doing a thorough physical examination, and carefully considering the laboratory reports.
- Ulcerative colitis must be distinguished from other conditions associated with diarrhea or bleeding from the rectum. These include hemorrhoids, cancer, and diarrhea from amebic and *Salmonella* infections.
- Because ulcerative colitis almost always involves the rectum, it can often be diagnosed by proctoscopy. A *proctoscope* is a hollow tube about as big around as a dust mop handle that has lenses in it and a light at its tip. While you lie on your side, the lubricated instrument is inserted gently into your rectum and a careful examination done. If necessary a small piece of tissue (a *biopsy*) is taken (this does not cause any pain) for laboratory examination.
- *Colonoscopy*: This is done with an optical instrument that is smooth, flexible, and as big around as your little finger and has a light at its tip. During colonoscopy, you will be given medicine that will make you drowsy. The tip of the instrument is lubricated and then gently inserted into your anus. It can be used to inspect your entire large bowel. Colonoscopy helps determine how much of the large bowel is involved and the seriousness of the condition.

○ TREATMENT

- At the beginning, the treatment always should be medical (except for certain emergency situations).
- About 50% of individuals with ulcerative colitis will respond to some degree to medical therapy.

It is generally agreed that an operation is necessary for at least the following conditions:

- The ulcerative colitis has been present and active for more than 15 years.
- It simply does not respond to any type of medical treatment.
- There are several worrisome abnormal changes (seen under the microscope) in the biopsy tissue.
- Cancer is present in the area of colon that also has ulcerative colitis.
- The ulcerative colitis has caused serious problems in organs other than the large bowel.

In the following situations there is a high risk that the person will die unless the colon is removed right away:

- Massive bleeding that will not slow down.
- Formation of a hole in the colon.
- Massive infection of the colon.

Several operations are possible for ulcerative colitis, depending on many factors:

- **Option 1.** All of the colon and rectum is removed, and the end of the small intestine is brought out through an opening in the side of the abdomen (an *ileostomy*) so the stool can be collected in a bag.
- **Option 2.** The same as Option 1 except that the stool is collected in a natural pouch made from your small intestine. This pouch remains inside your abdomen, but there is an opening to the outside. The pouch needs to be emptied with a catheter several times a day.
- **Option 3.** All of the colon and rectum are removed, and a natural pouch is created from small bowel that stays inside your abdomen. The end of the small bowel is brought down below and connected to your anus. The pouch collects the stool (it has the consistency of applesauce) until it becomes full. It then empties through your anus. This method requires a lot of intensive retraining of the sphincter in your anus so that you can control the frequent soft stools.
- **Option 4.** The colon is removed and the small bowel connected directly to the rectum. This operation can be used only if the rectum is not involved with ulcerative colitis.

Each of these operations has important advantages and disadvantages, and each must be carefully matched to the individual patient's problem and general condition.

Each operation may affect your sex life. This will be discussed with you.

After very careful consideration of all factors, it is recommended that you have an operation as described in Option 3 (Figs. 1 and 2).

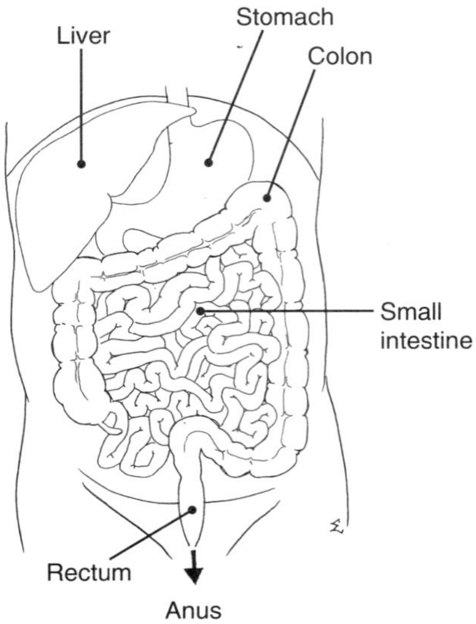

Figure 1. Normal relationships among the small intestine, colon, rectum, and anus.

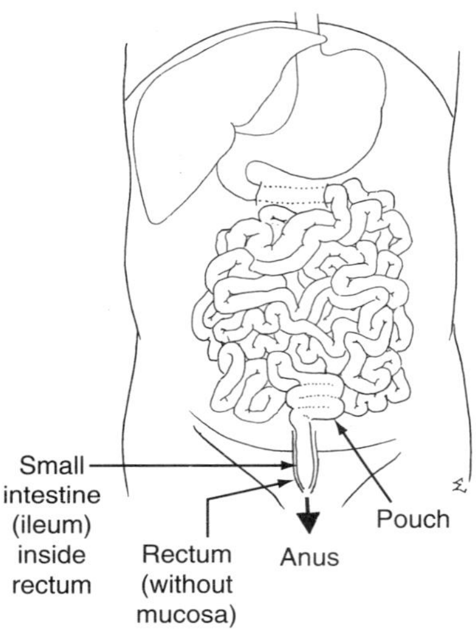

Figure 2. The entire colon is removed, but only the mucosa (the lining) of the rectum is removed; the muscles of the rectum and the anus (the sphincter) are left in place. A pouch for temporary collection of stool is fashioned almost at the end of the small intestine (the ileum). The end of the small intestine is positioned inside the rectum (whose muscles, along with those of the anus, are left intact).

An ileostomy (a bypass) is also performed so that stool will collect in a bag on your side for several weeks instead of the stool passing over the new connection between the ileum and the anus. When everything has healed, the ileostomy will be closed and you will have bowel movements in the normal way.

The advantages to this operation are that the disease is eliminated, there is no permanent opening of intestine on your side, and there are fewer limitations on your lifestyle.

PREOPERATIVE PREPARATION

- You will have an examination of your blood, urine, heart (EKG), and lungs (chest x-ray).
- Do not eat or drink anything for 8 hours before the operation.
- Shower as usual on the morning of the operation.
- You may be given medicine that will make you feel drowsy before you are brought to the operating room.

☐ OPERATION

- You will be asleep for the operation.
- You will not receive a blood transfusion unless it is absolutely necessary.
- The operation usually takes about 4 hours.

POSTOPERATIVE CARE

- You will wake up in a recovery room. When your blood pressure, pulse, and breathing are stable, you will be taken to a regular hospital room.
- You will have a thin plastic tube in your nose. It will be removed when your bowels start working.
- There will be a small plastic tube in your bladder for a few days. This makes it easier for you to pass your urine and for the nurses to measure how much you are putting out.
- Pain can be controlled with medicine. The nurse will give it to you, or you can give yourself a preset amount when you feel you need it. This type of pain relief, called patient-controlled analgesia (PCA), uses a device that releases the medicine into the tubing giving you intravenous fluids.
- That evening you will be helped to sit up in bed and on the next day to get out of bed.
- After the tube in your nose is removed, you will be started on a diet that will be carefully worked out for you by the dietitian.
- As with any operation, complications are always possible, some of them serious. With your type of operation, they can include bleeding, bowel obstruction, infection and abscess formation, blood clots, and possibly others.
- You should be able to go home in about 10 days.
- Arrangements will be made for your medicine, follow-up office visit, stitch or clip removal, and conferences with the ostomy nurse and the dietitian.

✚ HOME CARE

- Continue with the program started while you were in the hospital.
- You may walk about as you wish, even climb stairs, but don't overdo things.
- Follow the diet guidelines given to you.
- Take medicine as prescribed for your pain.
- You will be advised regarding when you may begin taking showers.
- Arrangements can be made for a home visiting nurse if one is needed.
- Do not drive a car or return to work until we first discuss it during your office visit.

✆ CALL OUR OFFICE IF

- You develop any unusual signs or symptoms.
- You develop abdominal cramps or bloating.
- The incision becomes red or swollen, or there is drainage from it.
- You develop a temperature higher than 100°F.
- You have any questions.

ULCERATIVE COLITIS: Proctocolectomy with Ileostomy (Koch Pouch)

△ GENERAL INFORMATION

Ulcerative colitis is a serious inflammatory condition of the lining of the large bowel that causes it to bleed very easily. It also can cause problems elsewhere in the body. This condition usually develops slowly, but occasionally it can come on abruptly and be very severe. Mostly, however, it is a chronic condition with ups and downs. The cause of ulcerative colitis is not known.

COMMON SIGNS AND SYMPTOMS

The symptoms depend on how active the disease is, how much of the large bowel is involved, and how long the disease has been present. The most common symptoms are as follows:

- Abdominal pain from the inflamed bowel.
- Bleeding: This can be mucus, mucus with blood, or just blood. Sometimes the bleeding can be very severe.
- Diarrhea: There may be four to six bowel movements a day. Rarely, they can be much more numerous.
- Other symptoms include fever; weight loss; arthritis-like pains in the wrists, ankles, and knees; eye problems; spine problems; and stomach ulcers.

DIAGNOSIS

- Usually the diagnosis can be made by taking a detailed history, doing a thorough physical examination, and carefully considering the laboratory reports.
- Ulcerative colitis must be distinguished from other conditions associated with diarrhea or bleeding from the rectum. These include hemorrhoids, cancer, and diarrhea from amebic and *Salmonella* infections.
- Because ulcerative colitis almost always involves the rectum, it can often be diagnosed by proctoscopy. A *proctoscope* is a hollow tube about as big around as a dust mop handle that has lenses in it and a light at its tip. While you lie on your side, the lubricated instrument is inserted gently into your rectum and a careful examination done. If necessary a small piece of tissue (a *biopsy*) is taken (this does not cause any pain) for laboratory examination.
- *Colonoscopy*: This is done with an optical instrument that is smooth, flexible, and as big around as your little finger and has a light at its tip. During the colonoscopy, you will be given medicine that will make you drowsy. The tip of the instrument is lubricated and then gently inserted into your anus. It can be used to inspect your entire large bowel. Colonoscopy helps determine how much of the large bowel is involved and the seriousness of the condition.

○ TREATMENT

- At the beginning, the treatment always should be medical (except for certain emergency situations).
- About 50% of individuals with ulcerative colitis will respond to some degree to medical therapy. Unfortunately, most will eventually require an operation of one type or another.

It is generally agreed that an operation is necessary for at least the following conditions:

- The ulcerative colitis has been present and active for more than 15 years.
- It simply does not respond to any type of medical treatment.
- There are several worrisome abnormal changes (seen under the microscope) in the tissue that has been biopsied.
- Cancer is present in the area of colon that also has ulcerative colitis.
- The ulcerative colitis has caused serious problems in organs other than the large bowel.

In the following situations there is a high risk that the person will die unless the colon is removed right away:

- Massive bleeding that will not slow down.
- Formation of a hole in the colon.
- Massive infection of the colon.

Several operations are possible for ulcerative colitis, depending on many factors:

- **Option 1.** All of the colon and rectum is removed, and the end of the small intestine is brought out through an opening in the side of the abdomen (an *ileostomy*) so the stool can be collected in a bag.
- **Option 2.** The same as Option 1 except that the stool is collected in a natural pouch made from your small intestine. This pouch remains inside your abdomen, but there is an opening to the outside. The pouch needs to be emptied with a catheter several times a day.
- **Option 3.** All of the colon and rectum are removed and a natural pouch is created from small bowel that stays inside your abdomen. The end of the small bowel is brought down below and connected to your anus. The pouch collects the stool (it has the consistency of applesauce) until it becomes full. It then empties through your anus. This method requires a lot of intensive retraining of the sphincter in your anus so that you can control the frequent soft stools.
- **Option 4.** The colon is removed and the small bowel connected directly to the rectum. This operation can be used only if the rectum is not involved with ulcerative colitis.

Each of these operations has important advantages and disadvantages, and each must be carefully matched to the individual patient's problem and general condition.

Each operation may affect your sex life. This will be discussed with you.

After very careful consideration of all factors, it is

recommended that you have an operation as described in Option 2 (Figs. 1 and 2).

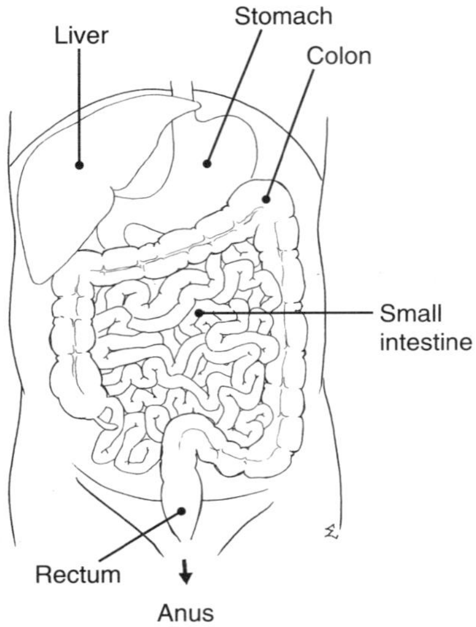

Figure 1. Normal relationships among the small intestine, colon, rectum, and anus.

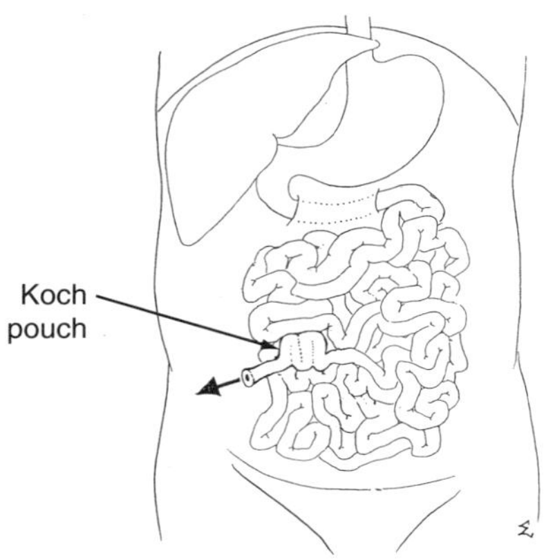

Figure 2. The entire colon, rectum, and anus are removed. A pouch (Koch pouch) for temporary collection of stool is fashioned almost at the end of the small intestine (the ileum). The end of the ileum is brought to the outside (as an ileostomy).

This operation provides the best chance of getting rid of your colon problem, of your coming through the operation safely, and of making it possible for you to live as normal a life as possible.

PREOPERATIVE PREPARATION

- You will have an examination of your blood, urine, heart (EKG), and lungs (chest x-ray).
- Do not eat or drink anything for 8 hours before the operation.
- Shower as usual on the morning of the operation.
- You may be given medicine that will make you feel drowsy before you are brought to the operating room.

☐ OPERATION

- You will be asleep for the operation.
- You will not receive a blood transfusion unless it is absolutely necessary.
- The operation usually takes about 3 hours.

POSTOPERATIVE CARE

- You will wake up in a recovery room. When your blood pressure, pulse, and breathing are stable, you will be taken to a regular hospital room.
- You will have a thin plastic tube in your nose. It will be removed when your bowels start working.
- There will be a small plastic tube in your bladder for a few days. This makes it easier for you to pass your urine and for the nurses to measure how much you are putting out.
- Pain can be controlled with medicine. The nurse will give it to you, or you can give yourself a preset amount when you feel you need it. This type of pain relief, called patient-controlled analgesia (PCA), uses a device that releases the medicine into the tubing giving you intravenous fluids.
- That evening you will be helped to sit up in bed and on the next day to get out of bed.
- The hospital support team of doctors and nurses will start working with you early to show you how the ileostomy works and how to learn to take care of it.
- After the tube in your nose is removed, you will be started on a diet that will be carefully worked out for you by the dietitian.
- As with any operation, complications are always possible, some of them serious. With your type of operation, they can include bleeding, bowel obstruction, infection and abscess formation, blood clots, and possibly others.
- You should be able to go home in about 1 week.
- Arrangements will be made for your medicine, follow-up office visit, and stitch or clip removal.

HOME CARE

- Continue with the program started while you were in the hospital.
- You may walk about as you wish, even climb stairs, but don't overdo things.
- Follow the diet guidelines given you.
- Take medicine as prescribed for your pain.
- You will be advised on when you may start taking showers.
- Arrangements can be made for a home visiting nurse if one is needed.
- Do not drive or return to work until we first discuss it during your office visit.

✆ CALL OUR OFFICE IF

- You develop any unusual signs or symptoms.
- You develop abdominal cramps or bloating.
- The incision becomes red or swollen, or there is drainage from it.
- You develop a temperature higher than 100°F.
- You have any questions.

ULCERATIVE COLITIS: Total Colectomy with Ileorectal Anastomosis

△ GENERAL INFORMATION

Ulcerative colitis is a serious inflammatory condition of the lining of the large bowel that causes it to bleed very easily. It also can cause problems elsewhere in the body. This condition usually develops slowly, but occasionally it can come on abruptly and be very severe. Mostly, however, it is a chronic condition with ups and downs. The cause of ulcerative colitis is not known.

COMMON SIGNS AND SYMPTOMS

The symptoms depend on how active the disease is, how much of the large bowel is involved, and how long the disease has been present.

The most common symptoms are as follows:

- Abdominal pain from the inflamed bowel.
- Bleeding: This can be mucus, mucus with blood, or just blood. Sometimes the bleeding can be very severe.
- Diarrhea: There may be four to six bowel movements a day. Rarely, they can be much more numerous.
- Other symptoms include fever; weight loss; arthritis-like pains in the wrists, ankles, and knees; eye problems; spine problems; and stomach ulcers.

DIAGNOSIS

- Usually the diagnosis can be made by taking a detailed history, doing a thorough physical examination, and carefully considering the laboratory reports.
- Ulcerative colitis must be distinguished from other conditions associated with diarrhea or bleeding from the rectum. These include hemorrhoids, cancer, and diarrhea from amebic and *Salmonella* infections.
- Because ulcerative colitis almost always involves the rectum, it can often be diagnosed by proctoscopy. A *proctoscope* is a hollow tube about as big around as a dust mop handle that has lenses in it and a light at its tip. While you lie on your side, the lubricated instrument is inserted gently into your rectum and a careful examination done. If necessary a small piece of tissue (a *biopsy*) will be taken (this does not cause any pain) for laboratory examination.
- *Colonoscopy*: This is done with an optical instrument that is smooth, flexible, and as big around as your little finger and has a light at its tip. During colonoscopy, you will be given medicine that will make you drowsy. The tip of the instrument is lubricated and then gently inserted into your anus. It can be used to inspect your entire large bowel. Colonoscopy helps determine how much of the large bowel is involved and the seriousness of the condition.

○ TREATMENT

- At the beginning, the treatment always should be medical (except for certain emergency situations).
- About 50% of individuals with ulcerative colitis will respond to some degree to medical therapy. Unfortunately, most will eventually require an operation of one type or another.

It is generally agreed that an operation is necessary for at least the following conditions:

- The ulcerative colitis has been present and active for over 15 years.
- It simply does not respond to any type of medical treatment.
- There are several worrisome abnormal changes (seen under the microscope) in the tissue that has been biopsied.
- Cancer is present in the area of colon that also has ulcerative colitis.
- The ulcerative colitis has caused serious problems in organs other than the large bowel.

In the following situations there is a high risk that the person will die unless the colon is removed right away:

- Massive bleeding that will not slow down.
- Formation of a hole in the colon.
- Massive infection of the colon.

Several operations are possible for ulcerative colitis, depending on many factors:

- **Option 1.** All of the colon and rectum is removed, and the end of the small intestine is brought out through an opening in the side of the abdomen so the stool can be collected in a bag.
- **Option 2.** The same as Option 1 except that the stool is collected in a natural pouch made from your small intestine. This pouch remains inside your abdomen, but there is an opening to the outside. The pouch needs to be emptied with a catheter several times a day.
- **Option 3.** All of the colon and rectum are removed and a natural pouch is created from small bowel that stays inside your abdomen. The end of the small bowel is brought down below and connected to your anus. The pouch collects the stool (it has the consistency of applesauce) until it becomes full. It then empties through your anus. This method requires a lot of intensive retraining of the sphincter in your anus so that you can control the frequent soft stools.
- **Option 4.** The colon is removed and the small bowel connected directly to the rectum. This operation can be used only if the rectum is not involved with ulcerative colitis.

Each of these operations has important advantages and disadvantages, and each must be carefully matched to the individual patient's problem and general condition. Each operation may affect your sex life. This will be discussed with you.

After very careful consideration of all factors, the recommendation is that you have an operation as described in Option 4 (Figs. 1 and 2).

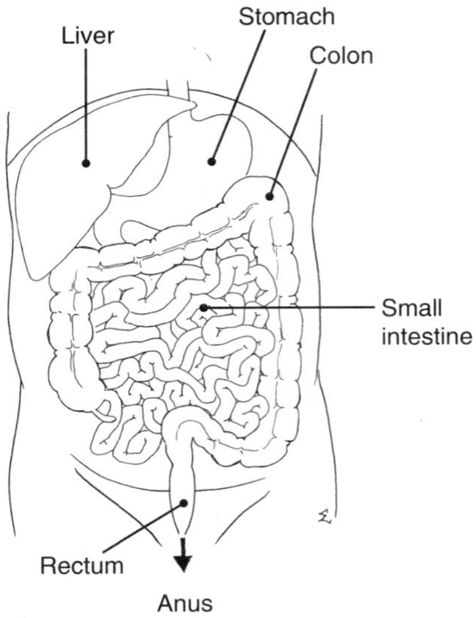

Figure 1. Normal relationships among the small intestine, colon, rectum, and anus.

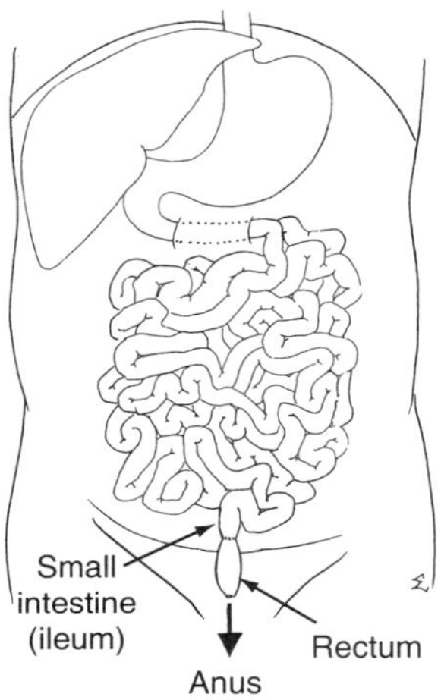

Figure 2. All of the colon is removed, and the small intestine (the ileum) is connected to the rectum.

PREOPERATIVE PREPARATION

- You will have an examination of your blood, urine, heart (EKG), and lungs (chest x-ray).
- Do not eat or drink anything for 8 hours before the operation.
- Shower as usual on the morning of the operation.
- You may be given medicine that will make you feel drowsy before you are brought to the operating room.

This operation has the best chance of getting rid of your colon problem, of your coming through the operation safely, and of making it possible for you to live as normal a life as possible.

☐ OPERATION

- You will be asleep for the operation.
- You will not receive a blood transfusion unless it is absolutely necessary.
- The operation usually takes about 3 hours.

POSTOPERATIVE CARE

- You will wake up in a recovery room. When your blood pressure, pulse, and breathing are stable, you will be taken to a regular hospital room.
- You will have a thin plastic tube in your nose. It will be removed when your bowels start working.
- There will be a small plastic tube in your bladder for a few days. This makes it easier for you to pass your urine and for the nurses to measure how much you are putting out.
- Pain can be controlled with medicine. The nurse will give it to you, or you can give yourself a preset amount when you feel you need it. This type of pain relief, called patient-controlled analgesia (PCA), uses a device that releases the medicine into the tubing giving you intravenous fluids.
- That evening you will be helped to sit up in bed and on the next day to get out of bed.
- The hospital support team of doctors and nurses will start working with you early to help solve any problems with control of your bowels.
- After the tube in your nose is removed, you will be started on a diet that will be carefully worked out for you by the dietitian.
- As with any operation, complications are always possible, some of them serious. With your type of operation, they can include bleeding, bowel obstruction, infection and abscess formation, blood clots, and possibly others.
- You should be able to go home in about 1 week.
- Arrangements will be made for your medicine, follow-up office visit, and stitch or clip removal.

✣ HOME CARE

- Continue with the program started while you were in the hospital.
- You may walk about as you wish, even climb stairs, but don't overdo things.
- Follow the diet guidelines given you.
- Take medicine as prescribed for your pain.
- Unless instructed otherwise, you may shower as you wish with any dressings on or off.
  - There may be narrow strips of tape across the incision. It's all right if they get wet. They will be removed in the doctor's office.
  - After you dry yourself, replace any dressings with clean, dry ones.
- Arrangements can be made for a home visiting nurse if one is needed.
- Do not drive a car or return to work until we first discuss it during an office visit.

✆ CALL OUR OFFICE IF

- You develop any unusual signs or symptoms.
- You develop abdominal cramps or bloating.
- The incision becomes red or swollen, or there is drainage from it.
- You develop a temperature higher than 100°F.
- You have any questions.

△ GENERAL INFORMATION

Ultrasound was first used about 50 years ago, but in recent years significant technical improvements have greatly increased and improved the way it can be used in the treatment of problems in almost all areas of the body. It normally is used in gynecology, cardiology, urology, and the intestinal tract. It also is used in blood vessel work, in the liver and gallbladder, and for other problems in the abdomen and in the breast. It also is used to guide needles when obtaining a biopsy through the skin or through tubes positioned in various areas of the body as well as by the surgeon in the operating room. Ultrasound itself is totally painless and harmless.

WHAT IS ULTRASOUND?

Sound is produced by vibration (called cycles). These cycles can range from 1 per second to many times more than this. Ultrasound is defined as more than 20,000 cycles per second and when used medically, it is usually over 1 million cycles per second. Sound waves at 20,000 cycles per second or higher cannot be heard.

Sound travels through different tissues at different rates. For example, it travels through fat, water, and soft tissue at about the same rate, which is four times faster than it travels through air. In bone, however, sound travels 10 times faster than in air. These differences in the rate at which sound travels through different tissues and in how much is bounced back are called the *acoustic mismatch*. It is the contrast produced by this mismatch that allows us to see different types of tissue.

THE APPARATUS

An important part of the ultrasound apparatus is the device that is placed over the area being examined. This is called a *transducer*. There are a number of different sizes and shapes of transducers depending on what is being examined (Fig. 1). These transducers give out the sound and also collect whatever sound bounces back to them. The echoes bouncing back are analyzed by the machine and displayed on the screen as a picture. How many or how few echoes are seen from an organ or tissue as compared to an organ or tissue next to it is referred to as *echogenicity*. An area being examined can have no echoes at all and be much darker, or it can have the same number of echoes as the surrounding tissue and thus cannot easily be seen as separate from that tissue. Finally, an organ can produce a lot of echoes and be bright and easily seen when compared with tissue next to it. There are many grades of dark and bright. For this reason, bone (having a lot of echoes) is seen more clearly when it is next to muscle or fat (few echoes). For the same reason, it is more difficult to distinguish fat from muscle, which have almost the same echogenicity.

HOW ULTRASOUND IS PERFORMED

- Most ultrasound is done by placing the transducer over the area being examined.
- No special preparation is necessary.
- You will lie on a comfortable table.
- For examinations done through the skin, the skin surface is lightly covered with a lubricant so that the transducer can glide more easily.
- The transducer will be passed in a number of directions over the area being examined, and the findings will be observed on a screen. What is seen on the screen can be printed for a permanent record.
- Ultrasound can be used in the office, in the clinic, or in the operating room.

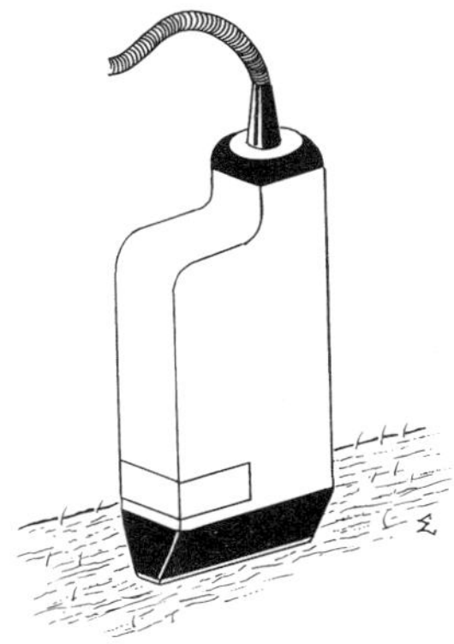

Figure 1. A commonly used transducer.

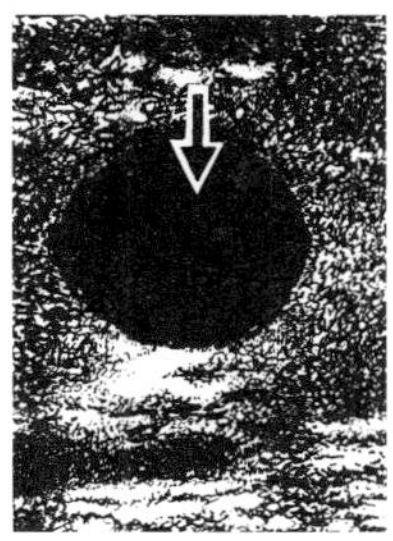

Figure 2. A characteristic ultrasound of a simple cyst of the breast *(arrow)*. It has sharp, well-defined borders; no echoes inside it indicates no masses present inside the cyst; it shows enhancement of echoes in the tissue on the opposite side (below) the cyst.

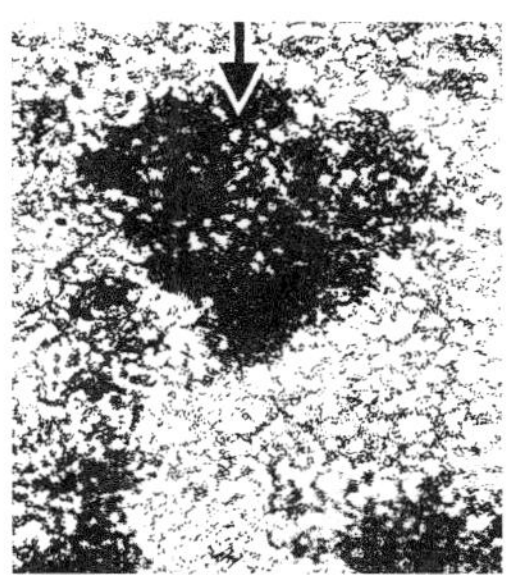

Figure 3. Ultrasound of a suspicious breast mass. The arrow points to a cancer. It has irregular, indistinct margins. There are mixed echoes inside the mass.

There are many examples of how an ultrasound picture can look, depending on what is being examined and the patient's problem. Examples of how two different masses in a breast might appear are shown in Figures 2 and 3.

How the ultrasound findings will be used will be thoroughly discussed with you.

△ GENERAL INFORMATION

Leakage of urine during exercise or when coughing, laughing, or sneezing is a common complaint among women. There can be a number of causes of urinary incontinence and until rather recently, most of these were poorly understood. As might be expected, the treatments were limited and the results discouraging. The situation has changed in the past few years and much can now be done for this distressing problem.

DIAGNOSIS

Proper treatment requires an accurate diagnosis. Some of the tests that may be necessary include the following:

- A detailed record of all of your symptoms.
- A thorough, focused physical examination of the pelvic area.
- Evaluation (generally by your primary physician) for any associated problems that may contribute to your urinary incontinence.
- An examination of your blood, urine, heart (EKG), and lungs (chest x-ray).
- Urodynamic testing: Your bladder and the reflexes that make it work will be studied in detail. These results will give important information to the doctor on the best way to treat your problem.
- You may have a special type of x-ray study of your rectum.

Quite often, women who have urinary leakage also have bulging in the vaginal area. This can have several causes:

- **Cystocele.** This is a loosening of the tissue between the front part of the vagina and the bladder, so that the bladder drops down and bulges in the vagina.
- **Rectocele.** This is a loosening of the tissue between the back part of the vagina and the rectum, causing the rectal tissue to bulge into the vagina.
- **Prolapse of the Uterus.** This is a loosening of the tissue that holds the uterus in the pelvis, causing the uterus to fall *(prolapse)* into the vagina.
- **Enterocele.** This is often seen in women who have had a hysterectomy. The sutured tissue in the pelvis has weakened, causing a hernia *(enterocele)* in the vaginal area.

If any of these vaginal bulges are present, it is usually advisable to correct them at the time of surgery for the urinary leakage.

○ TREATMENT

Based on the type and severity of leakage that is present and on the results of your tests, the recommendation is that you have a needle suspension procedure for your urinary incontinence.

PREOPERATIVE PREPARATION

- Do not eat or drink anything for 8 hours before the operation.

□ OPERATION

- This operation is performed mostly through the vagina, although you will also have a very small incision on your abdominal wall; it does not go down into your abdominal cavity. That's why this operation produces very little discomfort.
- The choice of general or spinal anesthesia will be discussed with you beforehand.
- An incision will be made in the vagina to place the stitches that will anchor the bladder to the abdominal wall, or the pubic bone.
- Your bladder will be looked into with a special lighted tube called a *cystoscope* to be certain the stitches are in the proper position.
- A *temporary* catheter will be placed in your bladder either through the normal opening of the bladder to the outside or through a tiny incision in your lower abdomen. This will be discussed with you beforehand.
- If you require any additional surgery to correct prolapse or bulging into the vagina, then this portion of the operation will be done also. This will be discussed with you in detail before the operation for your urinary incontinence.
- The operation generally takes about 2 hours.

POSTOPERATIVE CARE

- You will be taken to a recovery room and observed until your blood pressure, pulse, and breathing are stable and you are fully awake. Depending on the extent of the operation, you will either be taken to a regular hospital room or you will be able to go home that same day with a responsible adult.
- Pain will be controlled with medicine.
- Your diet will be as you tolerate it.
- While you are in the hospital, you will be observed to determine how well your bladder is emptying after the operation and whether you will need a catheter at home. For the first few days, your bladder will not empty completely but this will improve.
- The length of your hospital stay will depend on your general health and whether or not any additional surgery was done at the same time as the bladder surgery.
- As with any operation, complications are always possible. With this type of operation, they can include bleeding, infection, blood clots, control of your urine that is not entirely satisfactory, and possibly others.
- Arrangements will be made for your medicine, follow-up office visit, and stitch removal.

✢ HOME CARE

- You may walk about as you wish, even climb stairs, but don't overdo things.
- If you go home with a catheter, you will be given instructions on its care. It's not difficult.
- You will be given pain medications to use as you need them.

- You may shower as you wish but do not bathe until your doctor has given you permission.
- It is particularly important that you not lift anything heavier than 5 pounds. Ask someone to do it for you. Lifting could tear out the stitches that are holding everything in the proper position and affect the success of your operation.
- Include plenty of roughage and liquids in your diet to help avoid constipation. You may need some help with a mild laxative (example: milk of magnesia).
- Do not douche or place anything in your vagina. We can discuss when you may resume sexual intercourse.
- Do not drive a car until we have discussed it first at the office during your follow-up visit.

✆ CALL OUR OFFICE IF

- You have any difficulty with, or questions about your catheter (if you go home with one).
- You feel the need to urinate but are unable to empty your bladder.
- You have discomfort when you urinate or notice blood in your urine.
- You have any vaginal bleeding other than a little "spotting."
- The abdominal incision becomes red or swollen, or there is drainage from it.
- You develop a temperature higher than 100°F.
- You have any questions.

URINARY INCONTINENCE: Retropubic Urethropexy

△ GENERAL INFORMATION

Leakage of urine during exercise or when coughing, laughing, or sneezing is a common complaint among women. There can be a number of causes of urinary incontinence, and until rather recently most of these were poorly understood. As might be expected, the treatments were limited and the results discouraging. The situation has changed in the past few years, and much can now be done for this distressing problem.

DIAGNOSIS

Proper treatment requires an accurate diagnosis. Some of the tests that may be necessary include the following:

- A detailed record of all of your symptoms.
- A thorough, focused physical examination of the pelvic area.
- Evaluation (generally by your primary physician) for any associated problems that may contribute to your urinary incontinence.
- An examination of your blood, urine, heart (EKG), and lungs (chest x-ray).
- Urodynamic testing: Your bladder and the reflexes that make it work will be studied in detail. These results will give important information to the doctor on the best way to treat your problem.
- You may have a special type of x-ray study of your rectum.

Quite often, women who have urinary leakage also have bulging in the vaginal area. This can have several causes.

- **Cystocele.** This is a loosening of the tissue between the front part of the vagina and the bladder, so the bladder drops down and bulges in the vagina.
- **Rectocele.** This is a loosening of the tissue between the back part of the vagina and the rectum, causing the rectal tissue to bulge into the vagina.
- **Prolapse of the Uterus.** This is a loosening of the tissue that holds the uterus in the pelvis, causing the uterus to fall *(prolapse)* into the vagina.
- **Enterocele.** This is often seen in women who have had a hysterectomy. The sutured tissue in the pelvis has weakened, causing a hernia *(enterocele)* in the vaginal area.

If any of these vaginal bulges are present, it is usually advisable to correct them at the time of surgery for the urinary leakage.

○ TREATMENT

Based on the type and severity of leakage that is present and on the results of your tests, the recommendation is that you have a retropubic urethropexy procedure for your urinary incontinence.

PREOPERATIVE PREPARATION

- Do not eat or drink anything for 8 hours before the operation.

□ OPERATION

Whether the operation is performed through an incision on your abdomen or through the laparoscope, the steps for the operation are the same.

- The choice of general or spinal anesthesia will be discussed with you beforehand.
- The laparoscope is a smooth instrument about as big around as your little finger, that has magnifying lenses and a light in it. It is inserted through a tiny incision in your lower abdomen.
- Stitches will be placed on the right and left sides of the bladder to anchor it to either your abdominal wall or your pubic bone.
- Your bladder will be looked into with a special lighted tube called a *cystoscope* to be certain the stitches are in the proper position.
- A catheter will be placed in your bladder either through the normal opening of the bladder to the outside or through a tiny incision in your lower abdomen. This will be discussed with you beforehand.
- If you require any additional surgery to correct prolapse or bulging into the vagina, then this portion of the operation will be done also. This will be discussed with you in detail before the operation for your urinary incontinence.
- The operation generally takes about 2 hours.

POSTOPERATIVE CARE

- You will be taken to a recovery room and observed. When your blood pressure, pulse, and breathing are stable and you are fully awake, you will be taken to a regular hospital room.
- Pain will be controlled with medicine.
- Your diet will be as you tolerate it.
- While you are in the hospital you will be observed to determine how well your bladder is emptying after the operation and whether or not you will need a catheter at home. For the first few days, the bladder will not empty completely but this will improve.
- The length of your hospital stay will depend on your general health and whether or not any additional surgery was done at the same time as the bladder surgery.
- As with any operation, complications are always possible. With this type of operation, they can include bleeding, infection, blood clots, control of your urine that is not entirely satisfactory, and possibly others.
- Arrangements will be made for your medicine, follow-up office visit, and stitch removal.

✢ HOME CARE

- You may walk about as you wish, even climb stairs, but don't overdo things.
- If you go home with a catheter, you will be given instructions on its care. It's not difficult.
- You will be given pain medications to use as you need them.

- You may shower as you wish, but do not bathe until your doctor has given you permission.
- It is particularly important that you not lift anything heavier than 5 pounds. Ask someone to do it for you. Lifting could tear out the stitches that are holding everything in the proper position and affect the success of your operation.
- Include plenty of roughage and of liquids in your diet to help prevent constipation. You may need some help with a mild laxative (example: milk of magnesia).
- Do not douche or place anything in your vagina. We can discuss when you may resume sexual intercourse.
- Do not drive a car until we have discussed it first at the office during your follow-up visit.

✆ CALL OUR OFFICE IF

- You have any difficulty with, or questions about your catheter (if you go home with one).
- You feel the need to urinate but are unable to empty your bladder.
- You have discomfort when you urinate or notice blood in your urine.
- You have any vaginal bleeding other than a little "spotting."
- The incision becomes red or swollen, or there is drainage from it.
- You develop a temperature higher than 100°F.
- You have any questions.

△ GENERAL INFORMATION

Urodynamic testing is done to test a person's ability to control the bladder. This may be because of difficulty in holding the urine or in emptying the bladder, or both. This testing allows the doctors to identify the conditions under which a person leaks urine. It is also sometimes performed before an operation for a fallen (prolapsed) bladder or uterus, even if there is no bladder problem at present. This is because putting the prolapsed bladder back in its correct position will sometimes uncover hidden bladder problems that can be corrected at the time of the operation for the prolapse.

PREPARATION FOR THE TEST

- No special preparation is required on your part prior to this testing.
- You may shower or bathe as usual on the morning of the test.
- The entire procedure will take approximately 1 hour of your time, but only 20 to 30 minutes for the actual testing. The remainder involves getting you prepared for the test.
- This test may be performed even if you are having your menstrual period.
- This test is not painful. The only discomfort is having a full bladder during the testing. Occasionally, the catheter will cause some discomfort or burning. If this occurs, you will be given pain relief medicine specifically for the bladder.

THE TESTING

- You will be asked to empty your bladder.
- You will be given a single antibiotic tablet to help prevent any infection from occurring as a result of the testing.
- The testing will be performed either in a special chair designed for bladder testing or while you lie on a table as for a pelvic examination. You may also be asked to stand for a part of the testing.
- A very thin catheter will be placed into the bladder and a second catheter will be placed into either the vagina or the rectum (Fig. 1).
- Wires may be taped to the skin near your rectum. They will record the activity of your pelvic muscles during the test.
- Your bladder will be slowly filled with sterile water. The doctor or technician will ask you to state when you first have the urge to void, that is, when you feel as if your bladder is full and cannot hold any more water.
- You will then need to hold the water for a few minutes while the doctor or technician measures the pressure in your bladder and urethra. Also, you may be asked to cough several times or to perform other common stress activities such as bearing down, bouncing, or squeezing.
- Next, you will be asked to urinate while the catheters are still in place.

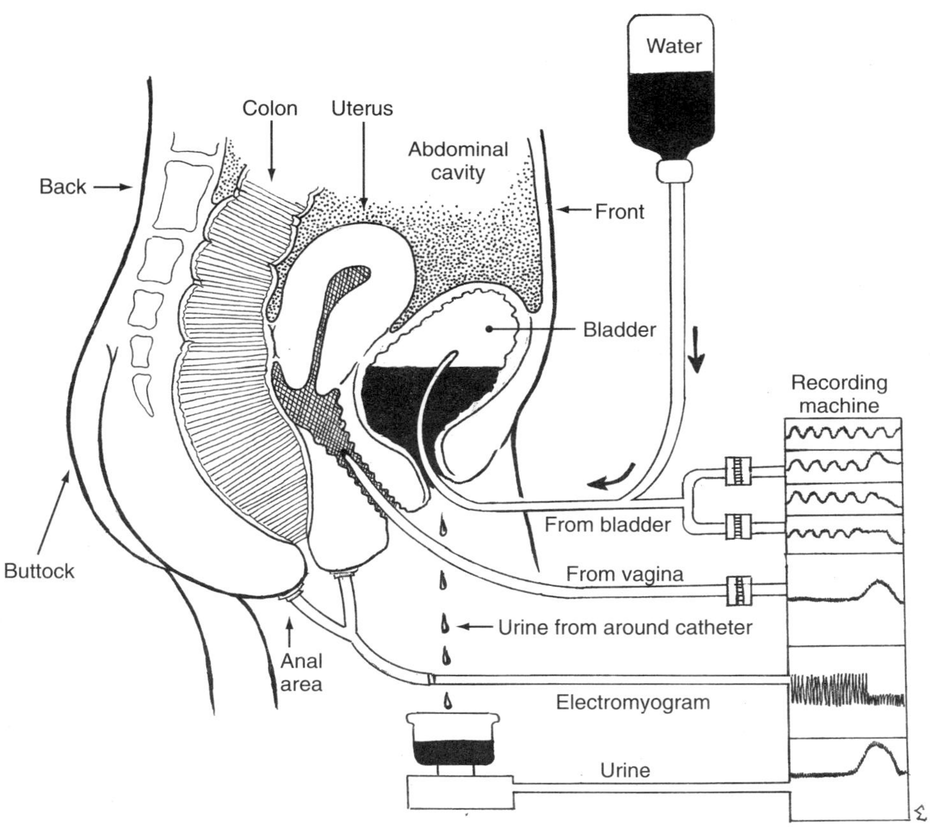

Figure 1. A catheter placed in the bladder measures the pressures and behavior of the muscles, bladder, and urethra (the channel from the bladder to the outside) as the bladder is stretched by the water flowing into it. A catheter in the vagina actually measures the pressure in the abdomen during this testing. You will be asked to urinate while the catheter is in your bladder. This urine is collected in the pan and measured. The wires attached to the skin of the buttocks record the behavior of the muscles in your pelvis during the various parts of this urodynamic testing.

- Some of the water placed in your bladder may leak during the course of this testing. Please do not worry about this, as the urine leakage problem is exactly what the doctor is trying to reproduce by testing. However, please do not voluntarily let go of the water until you have been requested to do so.

AFTER THE PROCEDURE

- The results of the tests may be discussed with you right after they are completed, or they may need to be analyzed further. If so, you will be asked to return to the office.

✆ CALL OUR OFFICE IF

- You experience persistent burning in your urethra following the test.
- You develop frequent and urgent urination.
- You develop a temperature higher than 100°F.
- You have any questions.

UTERUS CANCER: Radical Hysterectomy

△ GENERAL INFORMATION

Uterus cancer is a new, uncontrolled growth of the lining (called the *endometrium*) of the uterus. It is the most prevalent gynecologic cancer, most often seen in women between the ages of 50 and 70 years.

The cause is not truly known.

COMMON SIGNS AND SYMPTOMS

- Vaginal bleeding. This is particularly significant if it happens after the menopause. This can range from a light brown discharge to bright red liquid blood and even clots.
- It is important to realize that although cancer of the uterus occurs mostly in older women, it also can occur in women who are still menstruating. In these women, the menstrual bleeding may last too long, be too heavy, or be irregular.

DIAGNOSIS

- If anyone has the above history or symptoms, there should be concern about cancer of the uterus.
- The most commonly used method to make the diagnosis is by obtaining a small piece (a *biopsy*) of the endometrium.
- If the diagnosis is not entirely clear from the endometrial biopsy, the surest way to make the diagnosis is by scraping out the endometrium of the uterus (called a D&C for dilation and curettage) and examining this tissue under the microscope. This provides the diagnosis and shows in which part of the uterus the cancer is located.
- *CT scan (computed tomography scan)*: These special x-rays are taken by a machine that is shaped like a huge doughnut. You will lie on the table inside the hole in the "doughnut." The x-rays are taken as very thin slices through the lower abdomen. This makes it possible to see the fine details of the uterus, fallopian tubes, ovaries, and surrounding organs as well as the lymph nodes that drain these organs.

○ TREATMENT

- The primary treatment is an operation to remove the uterus, fallopian tubes, ovaries, and draining lymph nodes (Fig. 1). This is called a *radical hysterectomy*. Any additional treatment will depend on the findings in the removed uterus and associated tissue.

After careful consideration of all factors, the recommendation is that you have a radical hysterectomy.

PREOPERATIVE PREPARATION

- You will have an examination of your blood, urine, heart (EKG), and lungs (chest x-ray).
- Do not eat or drink anything for 8 hours before the operation.
- You will be given instructions on how to cleanse your bowels before the operation.
- Shower as usual on the morning of the operation.
- You may be given medicine that will make you feel drowsy before you are brought to the operating room.

□ OPERATION

- You will be asleep for the operation, or you may be offered a spinal type of anesthesia.
- You will not receive a blood transfusion unless it is absolutely necessary.
- The operation usually takes about 2 to 3 hours.

POSTOPERATIVE CARE

- You will be taken to a recovery room and observed. When your blood pressure, pulse, and breathing are stable, you will be taken to a regular hospital room.
- You may have a thin plastic tube in your nose. It goes down to your stomach to suck up the air you swallow. It will be removed when your bowels start working.
- There will be a thin catheter in your bladder; it will drain the urine for the first day or two.
- That evening you will be helped to sit up in bed and on the next day to get out of bed.
- Pain can be controlled with medicine. The nurse will give it to you, or you can give yourself a preset amount of pain medicine when you feel you need it. This type of pain relief, called patient controlled analgesia (PCA), uses a device that releases the medicine into the tubing giving you intravenous fluids.
- After the tube in your nose is removed, you will be started on a liquid diet and then given more solid foods as you tolerate them.
- You should be able to go home in about 1 week.
- Arrangements will be made for your medicine, follow-up office visit, and stitch or clip removal.

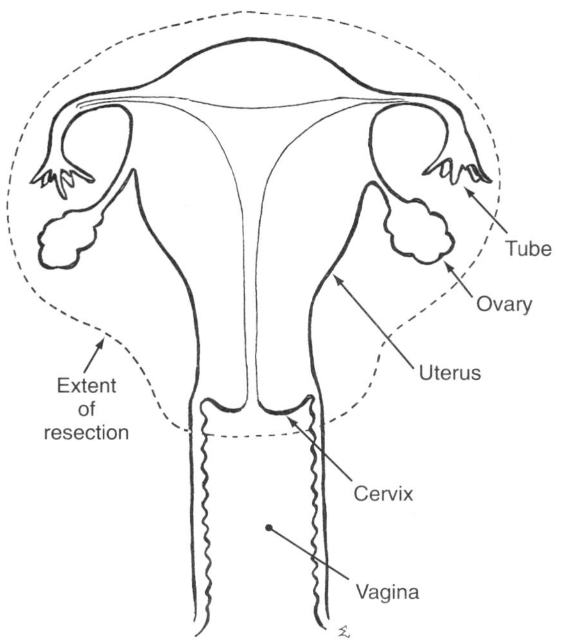

Figure 1. The tissue removed during an operation for cancer of the uterus is indicated by the dashed line. Usually it includes the uterus, tubes, ovaries, and surrounding lymph nodes as well as a segment of the upper vagina.

- As with any operation, complications are always possible. With this type of operation they can include infection, blood clots, bowel obstruction, and possibly others.

✣ HOME CARE

- Continue with the program started while you were in the hospital.
- You may walk about as you wish, even climb stairs.
- You may eat as you did before the operation.
- Unless instructed otherwise, you may shower as you wish and with any dressings on or off.
  - There may be narrow strips of tape across the incision. It's all right if they get wet. They will be removed in the doctor's office.
  - After your dry yourself, replace any dressings with clean, dry ones.
- Your incision and the muscles of the abdomen may ache, especially at the end of the day and after you have been standing for a long period. You can support them and be more comfortable by wearing a girdle that is snug (but not too tight). Wearing the girdle over a cotton undergarment is easier on your incision and the stitches.
- Be careful that you do not become constipated.
  - Include enough roughage and plenty of liquids in your diet.
  - You may need a mild laxative (example: milk of magnesia).
- Do not douche, use tampons, or engage in sexual intercourse until we talk about it when you come for your first follow-up office visit.
- Driving a car with an automatic shift may not seem too demanding, but if you suddenly have to slam on the brakes or twist to turn the steering wheel, you may not be able to do so or you may strain the sutures or tear something. During your follow-up visit, let's discuss when you can resume driving.

✆ CALL OUR OFFICE IF

- You develop any unusual signs or symptoms.
- The incision becomes red or swollen, or there is drainage from it.
- You develop a temperature higher than 100°F.
- You have any questions.

UTERUS FIBROIDS: Abdominal Hysterectomy

△ GENERAL INFORMATION

A *fibroid* of the uterus is an abnormal growth of the wall of the uterus. Fibroids are very common in adult women and can be as small as a pea or larger than a cantaloupe. There can be just one fibroid or there can be many. The cause of fibroids is not known.

COMMON SIGNS AND SYMPTOMS

- Often fibroids do not produce any symptoms. They are found during a routine pelvic examination.
- Any signs and symptoms are influenced by the size and location of the fibroids and whether or not a woman still has menstrual periods.
- The symptoms can include heavier menstrual flow; more frequent, longer, or premature menstrual periods; fullness in the pelvis or pressure on the bladder with more frequent urination; and painful or difficult bowel movements.
- Fibroids can increase in size shortly before the onset of menopause.
- Because of their location, they can cause an early miscarriage.

DIAGNOSIS

- A detailed history and a thorough pelvic examination are essential.
- *Ultrasound*: Harmless sound waves are aimed at the area of your pelvis. The sound waves bouncing back (the echoes) from this area are seen as a picture on a screen. Ultrasound is a convenient and painless way to examine the uterus, fallopian tubes, and ovaries.
- *CT scan (computed tomography scan)*: These special x-rays are taken as very thin slices through the area of your pelvis. This makes it possible to see the fine details of your uterus and other pelvic organs.
- *Laparoscopy*: This is done under general anesthesia with a rigid optical instrument that is as big around as your little finger and has a light at its tip. The instrument is inserted into the abdominal cavity through a tiny incision in your navel and the entire pelvic area is examined.

○ TREATMENT

The treatment depends on whether the fibroids produce symptoms and on the findings at the time the fibroids are examined directly. The treatment can be any of the following:

- Observation only for the time being.
- Stop any hormones that may be stimulating the fibroids to grow even larger.
- Burn the fibroids (if they are small and few) with a special electric needle introduced through the laparoscope. As the burn heals, the fibroid tissue shrinks to a scar.
- Cut out the fibroids but leave the uterus in place.
- An operation to remove the uterus, fallopian tubes, and ovaries.

After careful consideration of all factors, the recommendation is that you have an operation to remove your uterus, fallopian tubes, and ovaries through the abdomen (Fig. 1). The reasons for this recommendation have been explained to you.

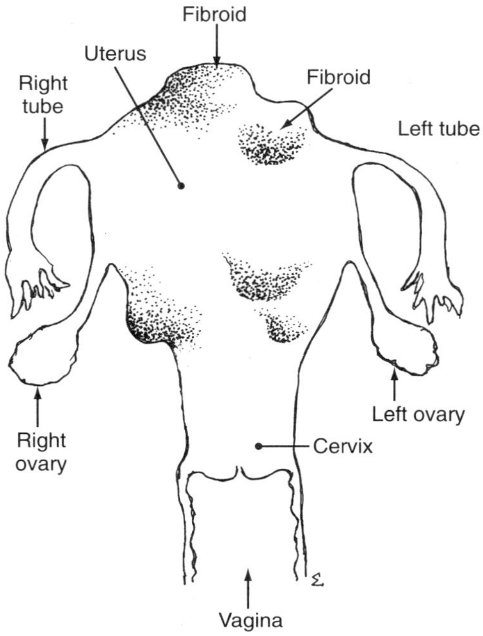

Figure 1. In this operation the uterus is removed and usually the two tubes and ovaries. Occasionally an ovary is left in place.

PREOPERATIVE PREPARATION

- You will have an examination of your blood, urine, heart (EKG), and lungs (chest x-ray).
- You will be instructed on how to cleanse your bowel before the operation.
- Do not eat or drink anything for 8 hours before the operation.
- Do not douche or use a tampon on the day of the operation.

□ OPERATION

- You will be asleep for the operation.
- The incision on the abdomen can be straight up and down or from side to side across the very lower abdomen (the "bikini" incision). Which type is more suitable will be discussed with you.
- The operation usually takes about 2 hours.

POSTOPERATIVE CARE

- You will be taken to a recovery room and observed. When your blood pressure, pulse, and breathing are stable, you will be taken to a regular hospital room.
- That evening you will be helped to sit at the bedside and the next morning to get out of bed.
- Pain will be controlled with medicine.

- You may have a thin, plastic tube in your nose. The tube will be removed as soon as your bowels start working. Your diet will then be increased as you tolerate it.
- You should be able to go home in about 2 to 4 days.
- As with any operation, complications are always possible, some of them serious. With this type of operation, they can include hemorrhage, injury to the ureters and bladder, infection, blood clots, and possibly others.
- Arrangements will be made for your medicine, follow-up office visit, and stitch removal.

✣ HOME CARE

- You may walk about as you wish, even climb stairs, but don't overdo things.
- Take medicine as prescribed for your pain.
- You may eat as you wish, but include plenty of roughage and liquids in your diet to help prevent constipation.
- Unless instructed otherwise, you may shower if you wish with any dressings on or off. After you dry yourself, replace any dressings with clean, dry ones.
- Do not douche or use a tampon until after we talk about this during the follow-up office visit. A sanitary napkin is best for the vaginal drainage usually seen after this operation.
- Don't lift anything heavier than 5 pounds. Ask someone to do it for you.
- Do not drive a car unless you can move freely and without pain and you are not taking medicines that decrease your alertness.
- Engaging in sexual intercourse too soon can be harmful to your recovery. If you wish, let's talk about this during your follow-up office visit.
- If your ovaries were removed, we can discuss your taking female hormones.
- You may return to work when you feel up to it.

✆ CALL OUR OFFICE IF

- The incision becomes red or swollen, or there is drainage from it.
- You develop excessive or bloody vaginal discharge or one with a strong odor to it.
- You develop a temperature higher than 100°F.
- You have any questions.

△ GENERAL INFORMATION

A *fibroid* of the uterus is an abnormal growth of the wall of the uterus. Fibroids are very common in adult women and can be as small as a pea or larger than a cantaloupe. There can be just one fibroid or there can be many. The cause of fibroids is not known.

COMMON SIGNS AND SYMPTOMS

- Often fibroids do not produce any symptoms. They are found during a routine pelvic examination.
- Any signs and symptoms are influenced by the size and location of the fibroids and whether or not a woman still has menstrual periods.
- The symptoms can include heavier menstrual flow; more frequent, longer, or premature menstrual periods; fullness in the pelvis or pressure on the bladder with more frequent urination; and painful or difficult bowel movements.
- Fibroids can increase in the size shortly before menopause.
- Because of their location, they can cause an early miscarriage.

DIAGNOSIS

- A detailed history and a thorough pelvic examination are essential.
- *Ultrasound*: Harmless sound waves are aimed at the area of your pelvis. The sound waves bouncing back (the echoes) from this area are seen as a picture on a screen. Ultrasound is a convenient and painless way to examine the uterus, fallopian tubes, and ovaries.
- *CT scan (computed tomography scan)*: These special x-rays are taken as very thin slices through the area of your pelvis. This makes it possible to see the fine details of your uterus and other pelvic organs.
- *Laparoscopy*: This is done under general anesthesia with a rigid optical instrument that is as big around as your little finger and has a light at its tip. The instrument is inserted into the abdominal cavity through a tiny incision in your navel and the entire pelvic area is examined.

○ TREATMENT

The treatment depends on whether the fibroids produce symptoms and on the findings at the time the fibroids are examined directly. The treatment can be any of the following:

- Observation only for the time being.
- Stop any hormones that may be stimulating the fibroids to grow even larger.
- Burn the fibroids (if they are small and few) with a special electric needle introduced through the laparoscope. As the burn heals, the fibroid tissue shrinks to a scar.
- Cut out the fibroids but leave the uterus in place.
- An operation to remove the uterus, fallopian tubes, and ovaries.

After careful consideration of all factors, the recommendation is that you have an operation to remove the fibroids but leave the uterus in place (Fig. 1). Some of the reasons for this recommendation are your strong desire to become pregnant. Also, the fibroids appear to be suitable for such treatment.

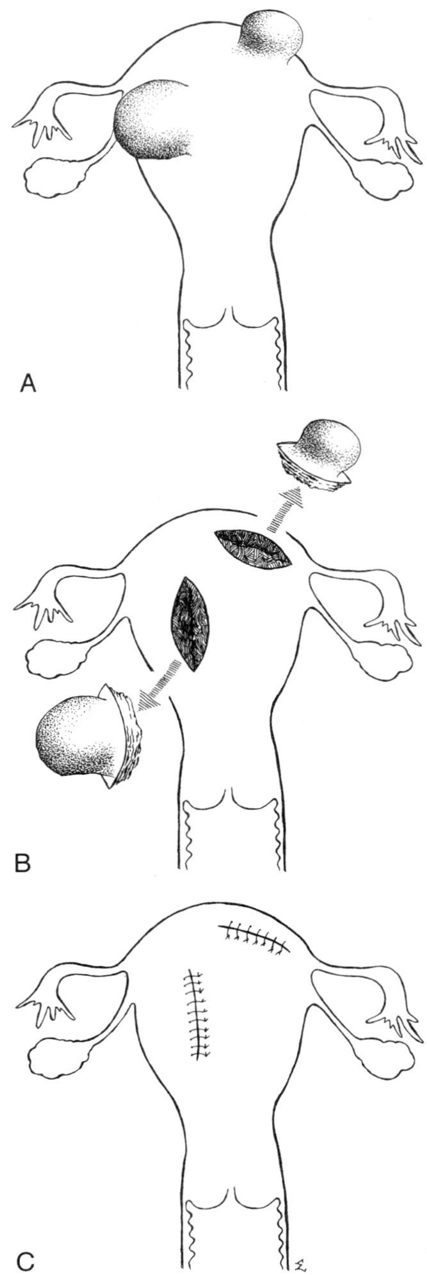

Figure 1. This operation is most suitable when the woman wants to keep her uterus and the fibroids are on the surface of the uterus but are too large to destroy with a laser beam *(A)*. Instead, the abdomen is opened, the fibroids are shelled out of the uterus *(B)*, and the incisions are closed *(C)*.

PREOPERATIVE PREPARATION

- You will have an examination of your blood, urine, heart (EKG), and lungs (chest x-ray).
- You will be instructed on how to cleanse your bowel before the operation.
- Do not eat or drink anything for 8 hours before the operation.
- Do not douche or use a tampon on the day of the operation.

☐ OPERATION

- You will be asleep for the operation.
- The incision on the abdomen can be straight up and down or from side to side across the very lower abdomen (the "bikini" incision). Which type is more suitable will be discussed with you.
- The operation usually takes about 2 hours.

POSTOPERATIVE CARE

- You will be taken to a recovery room and observed. When your blood pressure, pulse, and breathing are stable, you will be taken to a regular hospital room.
- That evening you will be helped to sit at the bedside and the next morning, to get out of bed.
- Pain will be controlled with medicine.
- You may have a thin, plastic tube in your nose. The tube will be removed as soon as your bowels start working. Your diet will then be increased as you tolerate it.
- You should be able to go home in about 2 to 4 days.
- As with any operation, complications are always possible, some of them serious. With this type of operation, they can include hemorrhage, injury to the ureters and bladder, infection, blood clots, and possibly others.
- Arrangements will be made for your medicine, follow-up office visit, and stitch removal.

✚ HOME CARE

- You may walk about as you wish, even climb stairs, but don't overdo things.
- Take medicine as prescribed for your pain.
- You may eat as you wish, but include plenty of roughage and liquids in your diet to help prevent constipation.
- Unless instructed otherwise, you may shower if you wish with any dressings on or off. After you dry yourself, replace any dressings with clean, dry ones.
- Do not douche or use a tampon until after we talk about this during the follow-up office visit. A sanitary napkin is best for the vaginal drainage usually seen after this operation.
- Don't lift anything heavier than 5 pounds. Ask someone to do it for you.
- Do not drive a car unless you can move freely and without pain and you are not taking medicines that decrease your alertness.
- Engaging in sexual intercourse too soon can be harmful to your recovery. If you wish, let's talk about this during your follow-up office visit.
- If your ovaries were removed, we can discuss your taking female hormones.
- You may return to work when you feel up to it.

✆ CALL OUR OFFICE IF

- The incision becomes red or swollen or there is drainage from it.
- You develop excessive or bloody vaginal discharge, or one with a strong odor to it.
- You develop a temperature higher than 100°F.
- You have any questions.

UTERUS FIBROIDS: Laparoscopic Laser Ablation

△ GENERAL INFORMATION

A *fibroid* of the uterus is an abnormal growth of the wall of the uterus. Fibroids are very common in adult women and can be as small as a pea or larger than a cantaloupe. There can be just one fibroid or there can be many. The cause of fibroids is not known.

COMMON SIGNS AND SYMPTOMS

- Often fibroids do not produce any symptoms. They are found during a routine pelvic examination.
- Any signs and symptoms are influenced by the size and location of the fibroids and whether or not a woman still has menstrual periods.
- The symptoms can include heavier menstrual flow; more frequent, longer, or premature menstrual periods; fullness in the pelvis or pressure on the bladder with more frequent urination; and painful or difficult bowel movements.
- Fibroids can increase in size shortly before the onset of menopause.
- Because of their location, they can cause an early miscarriage.

DIAGNOSIS

- A detailed history and a thorough pelvic examination are essential.
- *Ultrasound*: Harmless sound waves are aimed at the area of your pelvis. The sound waves bouncing back (the echoes) from this area are seen as a picture on a screen. Ultrasound is a convenient and painless way to examine the uterus, fallopian tubes, and ovaries.
- *CT scan (computed tomography scan)*: These special x-rays are taken as very thin slices through the area of your pelvis. This makes it possible to see the fine details of your uterus and other pelvic organs.
- *Laparoscopy*: This is done under general anesthesia with a rigid optical instrument that is as big around as your little finger and has a light at its tip. The instrument is inserted into the abdominal cavity through a tiny incision in your navel and the entire pelvic area is examined.

○ TREATMENT

The treatment depends on whether the fibroids produce symptoms and on the findings at the time the fibroids are examined directly. The treatment can be any of the following:

- Observation only for the time being.
- Stop any hormones that may be stimulating the fibroids to grow even larger.
- Burn the fibroids (if they are small and few) with a special electric needle introduced through the laparoscope. As the burn heals, the fibroid tissue shrinks to a scar.
- Cut out the fibroids but leave the uterus in place.
- An operation to remove the uterus, fallopian tubes, and ovaries.

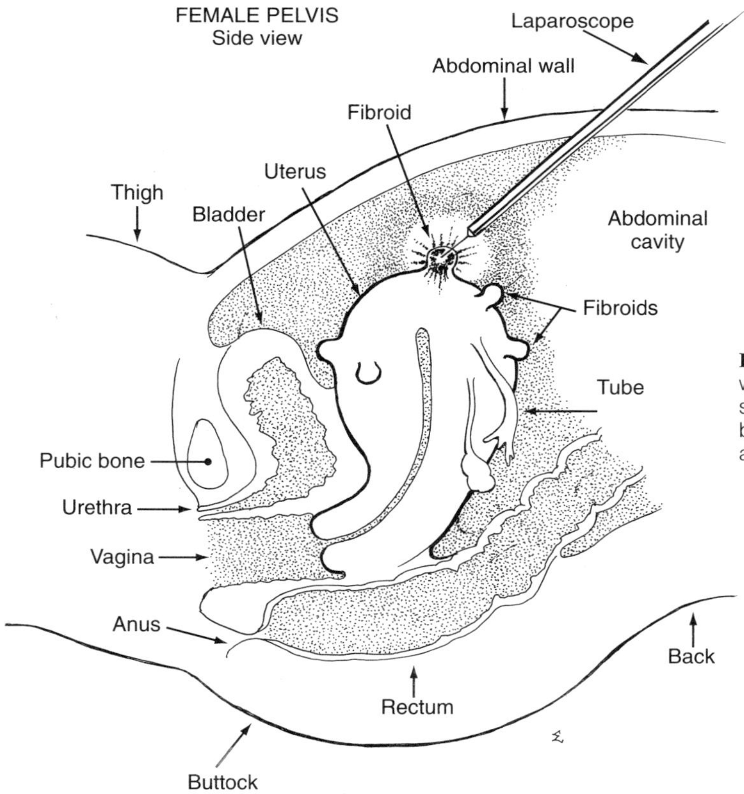

Figure 1. This operation is most suitable when the woman wants to keep her uterus and the fibroids on its surface are not too large. These fibroids are destroyed by a laser beam introduced into the abdomen through a laparoscope.

After careful consideration of all factors, the recommendation is that you have an operation to burn the small fibroids in your uterus. This is done with an electric needle introduced through a laparoscope (Fig. 1).

PREOPERATIVE PREPARATION

- You will have an examination of your blood, urine, heart (EKG), and lungs (chest x-ray).
- You will be instructed on how to cleanse your bowel before the operation.
- Do not eat or drink anything for 8 hours before the operation.
- Do not douche or use a tampon on the day of the operation.

□ OPERATION

- You will be asleep for the operation.
- Your abdomen will be swabbed with an antiseptic solution and draped with sterile sheets.
- Two laparoscopes will be introduced through tiny incisions in the abdomen. The electric needle is introduced through one of the laparoscopes and the fibroids burned as necessary.
- The operation usually takes about 2 hours.

POSTOPERATIVE CARE

- You will be taken to a recovery room and observed. When your blood pressure, pulse, and breathing are stable, you will be taken to a regular hospital room.
- That evening you will be helped to sit at the bedside and the next morning, to get out of bed.
- Pain will be controlled with medicine.
- You may have a thin, plastic tube in your nose. It will be removed as soon as your bowels start working. Your diet will be as you tolerate it.
- You should be able to go home in about 2 or 3 days.
- As with any operation, complications are always possible, some of them serious. With this type of operation, they can include hemorrhage, injury to the ureters and bladder, infection, blood clots, and possibly others.
- Arrangements will be made for your medicine, follow-up office visit, and stitch or clip removal.

✚ HOME CARE

- You may walk about as you wish, even climb stairs, but don't overdo things.
- Take medicine as prescribed for your pain.
- You may eat as you wish, but include plenty of roughage and liquids in your diet to help prevent constipation.
- Unless instructed otherwise, you may shower if you wish and with any dressings on or off. After you dry yourself, replace any dressings with clean, dry ones.
- Do not douche or use a tampon until after we talk about this during the follow-up office visit. A sanitary napkin is best for the vaginal drainage usually seen after this operation.
- Do not drive a car unless you can move freely and without pain and you are not taking medicines that decrease your alertness.
- Engaging in sexual intercourse too soon can be harmful to your recovery. If you wish, let's talk about this during your follow-up office visit.
- You may return to work when you feel up to it.

✆ CALL OUR OFFICE IF

- The incision becomes red or swollen, or there is drainage from it.
- You develop excessive or bloody vaginal discharge, or one with a strong odor to it.
- You develop a temperature higher than 100°F.
- You have any questions.

△ GENERAL INFORMATION

There are a number of reasons for wanting to remove a uterus. A common one is the presence of symptomatic fibroids. A *fibroid* of the uterus is an abnormal growth of the wall of the uterus. Fibroids are very common in adult women and can be as small as a pea or larger than a cantaloupe. There can be just one fibroid or there can be many. The cause of fibroids is not known.

COMMON SIGNS AND SYMPTOMS

- Often fibroids do not produce any symptoms. They are found during a routine pelvic examination.
- Any signs and symptoms that may be present are influenced by the size and location of the fibroids and whether or not a woman still has menstrual periods.
- The symptoms can include heavier menstrual flow; more frequent, longer, or premature menstrual periods; fullness in the pelvis or pressure on the bladder with more frequent urination; and painful or difficult bowel movements.
- Fibroids can increase in size shortly before menopause.
- Because of their location, they can cause an early miscarriage.

DIAGNOSIS

- A detailed history and a thorough pelvic examination are essential.
- *Ultrasound*: Harmless sound waves are aimed at the area of your pelvis. The sound waves bouncing back (the echoes) from this area are seen as a picture on a screen. Ultrasound is a convenient and painless way to examine the uterus, tubes, and ovaries.
- *CT scan (computed tomography scan)*: These special x-rays are taken as very thin slices through the area of your pelvis. This makes it possible to see the fine details of your uterus and other pelvic organs.
- *Laparoscopy*: This is done under general anesthesia with a rigid optical instrument that is as big around as your little finger and has a light at its tip. The instrument is inserted into the abdominal cavity through a tiny incision in your navel and the entire pelvic area is examined.

○ TREATMENT

The treatment depends on whether the fibroids produce symptoms and on the findings at the time the fibroids are examined directly. The treatment can be any of the following:

- Observation at regular intervals.
- Stop any hormones that may be stimulating the fibroids to grow even larger.
- Burn the fibroids (if they are small and few) with a special electric needle introduced through the laparoscope. As the burn heals, the fibroid tissue shrinks to a scar.
- Take out the fibroids but leave the uterus in place.
- An operation to remove the uterus, fallopian tubes, and ovaries. This usually is done through an abdominal incision. However, some women with fibroids who have had multiple pregnancies have relaxed tissue in the pelvis, especially in the vagina. This is an opportunity to remove the uterus through the vagina and at the same time tighten the vaginal tissue.
- Often, the structures in the upper part of the uterus can be dissected free with a *laparoscope*, an optical instrument that is as big around as your little finger and has a light at its tip. Two or three laparoscopes are placed in the abdomen through tiny incisions and the ovaries and upper part of the uterus dissected free. The surgeon then continues from below, removing the uterus through the vagina. After the uterus is removed, the excess relaxed vaginal tissue is trimmed and tightened.

After careful consideration of all factors, the recommendation is that you have an operation to remove your uterus, fallopian tubes, and ovaries through the vagina (Fig. 1).

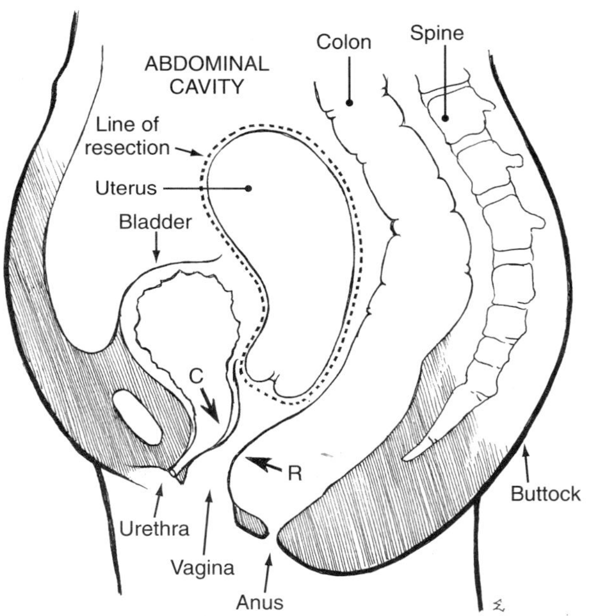

Figure 1. The dashed line indicates the border of resection of the uterus through the vagina. A cystocele (C) or rectocele (R) may also be repaired at this time.

PREOPERATIVE PREPARATION

- You will have an examination of your blood, urine, heart (EKG), and lungs (chest x-ray).
- You will be instructed on how to cleanse your bowel before the operation.
- Do not eat or drink anything for 8 hours before the operation.
- Do not douche or use a tampon on the day of the operation.

□ OPERATION

- You will be asleep for the operation.
- The uterus will be removed through the vagina.

- The excess relaxed vaginal tissue will be trimmed and then sewn together.

POSTOPERATIVE CARE

- You will be taken to a recovery room and observed. When your blood pressure, pulse, and breathing are stable, you will be taken to a regular hospital room.
- That evening you will be helped to sit at the bedside and the next morning, to get out of bed.
- Pain will be controlled with medicine.
- You may have a thin, plastic tube in your nose. It will be removed as soon as your bowels start working. Your diet will then be increased as you tolerate it.
- You should be able to go home in about 2 to 4 days.
- As with any operation, complications are always possible, some of them serious. With this type of operation, they can include hemorrhage, injury to the ureters and bladder, infection, blood clots, and possibly others.
- Arrangements will be made for your medicine, follow-up office visit, and stitch removal.

✚ HOME CARE

- You may walk about as you wish, even climb stairs, but don't overdo things.
- Take medicine as prescribed for your pain.
- You may eat as you wish. Include plenty of roughage and liquids in your diet to help prevent constipation.
- Unless instructed otherwise, you may shower if you wish with any dressings on or off. After you dry yourself, replace any dressings with clean, dry ones.
- Do not douche or use a tampon until after we talk about this during the follow-up office visit. A sanitary napkin is best for the vaginal drainage usually seen after this operation.
- Don't lift anything heavier than 5 pounds. Ask someone to do it for you.
- Do not drive a car unless you can move freely and without pain and you are not taking medicines that decrease your alertness.
- Engaging in sexual intercourse too soon can be harmful to your recovery. If you wish, let's talk about this during your follow-up office visit.
- If your ovaries were removed, we can discuss your taking female hormones.
- You may return to work when you feel up to it.

✆ CALL OUR OFFICE IF

- The incision becomes red or swollen, or there is drainage from it.
- You develop excessive or bloody vaginal discharge, or one with a strong odor to it.
- You develop a temperature higher than 100°F.
- You have any questions.

UTERUS FIBROIDS: Vaginal Hysterectomy, Laparoscopic-Assisted

△ GENERAL INFORMATION

A *fibroid* of the uterus is an abnormal growth of the wall of the uterus. Fibroids are very common in adult women and can be as small as a pea or larger than a cantaloupe. There can be just one fibroid or there can be many. The cause of fibroids is not known.

COMMON SIGNS AND SYMPTOMS

- Often fibroids do not produce any symptoms. They are found during a routine pelvic examination.
- Any signs and symptoms are influenced by the size and location of the fibroids and whether or not a woman still has menstrual periods.
- The symptoms can include heavier menstrual flow; more frequent, longer, or premature menstrual periods; fullness in the pelvis or pressure on the bladder with more frequent urination; and painful or difficult bowel movements.
- Fibroids can increase in size shortly before the onset of menopause.
- Because of their location, they may cause an early miscarriage.

DIAGNOSIS

- A pelvic examination by an experienced doctor can be quite reliable.
- *Ultrasound*: Harmless sound waves are aimed at the area of your pelvis. The sound waves bouncing back (the echoes) from this area are seen as a picture on a screen. Ultrasound is a convenient, painless, and harmless way to examine organs and tissues inside this area of your body.
- *CT scan (computed tomography scan)*: These special x-rays are taken by a machine that is shaped like a huge doughnut. You will lie on a table inside the hole in the "doughnut." The x-rays are taken as very thin slices through the area of your pelvis. This makes it possible to see the fine details of your uterus and other pelvic organs.
- *Laparoscopy*: This is done under general anesthesia with a rigid optical instrument that is as big around as your little finger and has a light at its tip. The instrument is inserted into the abdominal cavity through a tiny incision in your navel and the entire pelvic area examined.

○ TREATMENT

The treatment depends on whether the fibroids produce symptoms or on the findings at the time the fibroids are examined directly. The treatment can be any of the following:

- Observe the patient.
- Stop any hormones that may be stimulating the fibroids to grow even larger.
- Burn them (if small and few) with a special electric needle introduced through the laparoscope. As the burn heals, the fibroid tissue shrinks to a scar.
- Remove the fibroids but leave the uterus in place. This is for women who wish to try to become pregnant.
- An operation to remove the uterus, fallopian tubes, and ovaries. This usually is done through an abdominal incision. Some women with fibroids who have had multiple pregnancies have relaxed tissue in the pelvis, especially the vagina. This is an opportunity to remove the uterus through the vagina. At the same time the vaginal tissue can be tightened.
- The structures in the upper part of the uterus can often be dissected free with a *laparoscope,* an optical instrument that is as big around as your little finger and has a light at its tip. It is placed in the abdomen through a tiny incision, and the ovaries and upper part of the uterus dissected free. Then the surgeon continues from below, removing the uterus through the vagina. After the uterus is removed, the relaxed tissue is tightened.

After careful consideration of all factors, the recommendation is that you have an operation to remove your uterus and ovaries through the vagina with the help of a laparoscope (Fig. 1). The reasons for this recommendation have been explained to you.

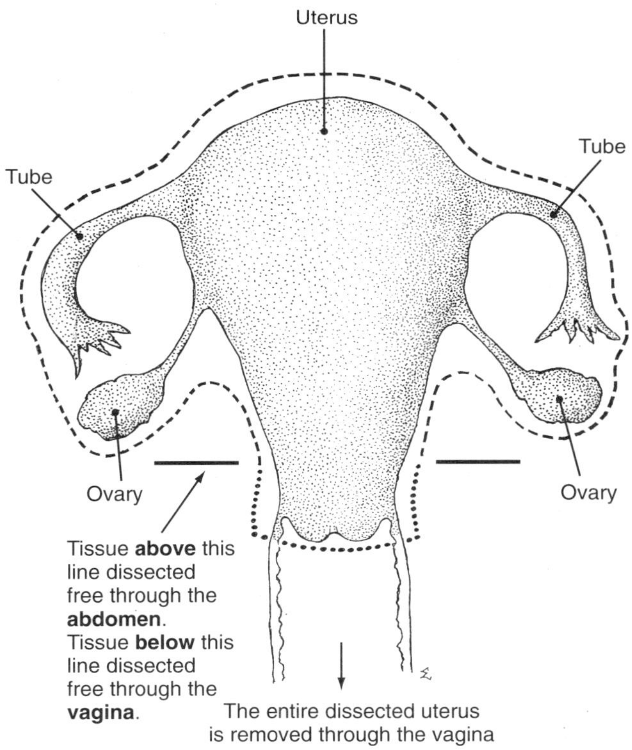

Figure 1. In this operation, the tubes, ovaries, and upper part of the uterus are dissected free *(dashed line)* with laparoscopes placed into the abdominal cavity through tiny incisions. The lower uterus is dissected free *(dotted line)* through the vagina. When all the dissection is completed, the entire specimen is removed through the vagina.

PREOPERATIVE PREPARATION

- You will have an examination of your blood, urine, heart (EKG), and lungs (chest x-ray). In addition to all the other tests, you will have a Papanicolaou (Pap) smear followed by a careful and thorough pelvic examination.
- You will be instructed on how to cleanse your bowel before the operation.
- Do not eat or drink anything for 8 hours before the operation.
- Do not douche or use a tampon on the day of the operation.
- Shower as usual on the morning of the operation.
- You may be given medicine that will make you feel drowsy before you are brought to the operating room.

□ OPERATION

- You will be asleep for the operation.
- Your abdomen will be swabbed with an antiseptic solution and draped with sterile sheets.
- Two laparoscopes will be introduced through tiny incisions in the abdomen and this part of the operation completed. Then the rest of the operation will be done through the vagina.
- You will not receive a blood transfusion unless it is absolutely necessary.
- The operation usually takes about 2 hours.

POSTOPERATIVE CARE

- You will be taken to a recovery room and observed. When your blood pressure, pulse, and breathing are stable, you will be taken to a regular hospital room.
- That evening you will be helped to sit at the bedside and the next morning, to get out of bed.
- Pain can be controlled with medicine. The nurse will give it to you, or you can give yourself a preset amount of pain medication when you feel you need it. This type of pain relief, called patient-controlled analgesia (PCA), uses a device that releases the medicine into the tubing giving you intravenous fluids.
- You may have a thin, plastic tube in your nose. It will be removed as soon as your bowels start working. Your diet will be as you tolerate it.
- You should be able to go home in about 4 days.
- As with any operation, complications are always possible, some of them serious. With this type of operation, they can include hemorrhage, injury to the ureters and bladder, infection, blood clots, and possibly others.
- Arrangements will be made for your medicine, follow-up office visit, and stitch removal.

✚ HOME CARE

- You may walk about as you wish, even climb stairs, but don't overdo things.
- Take medicine as prescribed for your pain.
- You may eat as you did before the operation.
- Be careful that you do not become constipated.
  - Include enough roughage and plenty of liquids in your diet.
  - You may need a mild laxative (example: milk of magnesia).
- You may shower if you wish with any dressings on or off.
  - There may be narrow strips of tape across the incision. It's all right if they get wet; they will be removed in the doctor's office.
  - After you dry yourself, replace any dressings with clean, dry ones.
- Do not douche or use a tampon until after we talk about it during the follow-up visit. A sanitary napkin is best for the drainage usually seen after this operation.
- Do not drive your car if you are taking medicine that reduces your mental alertness.
- Engaging in sexual intercourse too soon can be harmful to your recovery. If you wish, let's talk about this during your follow-up visit.
- You may return to work when you feel up to it.

✆ CALL OUR OFFICE IF

- The incision becomes red or swollen, or there is drainage from it.
- You develop excessive or bloody vaginal discharge, or one with a strong odor to it.
- You develop any new or unusual symptoms.
- You develop a temperature higher than 100°F.
- You have any questions.

△ GENERAL INFORMATION

The *uvula* is the structure that is located at the back of the soft palate (the floppy part at the back of the roof of the mouth) and hangs down at the back of your throat. The uvula is about 1 inch long, but in some people it is a lot longer and thicker. The tonsils in some adults can be quite enlarged owing to recurrent infections through the years. In addition, the soft palate can also be elongated and somewhat flabby. These excess throat tissues can be responsible for several problems.

COMMON SIGNS AND SYMPTOMS

- Snoring: These excess tissues in the back of the throat vibrate as the air to and from the lung passes by it. This produces loud snoring.
- Obesity can increase the amount of fatty tissue in your neck, throat, and chin.
- Facial and jaw structure can add to the crowding of all the internal throat tissues.
- A crooked nasal septum can prevent normal flow of air through the nose at night, causing mouth breathing.
- Breath-holding: This condition can progress over the years to the point where it causes gagging, gasping, and breath-holding (called *apnea*) while you sleep. Apnea can be dangerous because without regular breathing, your body does not get all the oxygen it needs. Also, the gasping often wakes you from a deep stage of sleep many times through the night so that you wake up feeling tired.

DIAGNOSIS

- The loud snoring is most often recognized by the spouse or bed partner of the patient.
- Often a tape recording of the snoring will also capture the gasping and the apnea.
- A sophisticated sleep study may be done at home or in a laboratory to monitor the level of oxygen in the blood, the heart rhythm, and brain activity.

○ TREATMENT

- In continuous positive airway pressure (CPAP), a machine gently pushes air through nose plugs or a face mask. If properly used every night, the CPAP machine can force air through the crowded tissue to allow you to breathe normally, quietly, and without apnea.
- For many patients, an operation is advisable:
  - Sometimes removal of the uvula alone is all that is needed.
  - For patients with large tonsils and a sagging palate, a tonsillectomy and a uvulopalatopharyngoplasty (UPPP) are necessary. UPPP involves removing the uvula and the sagging palate (Fig. 1).

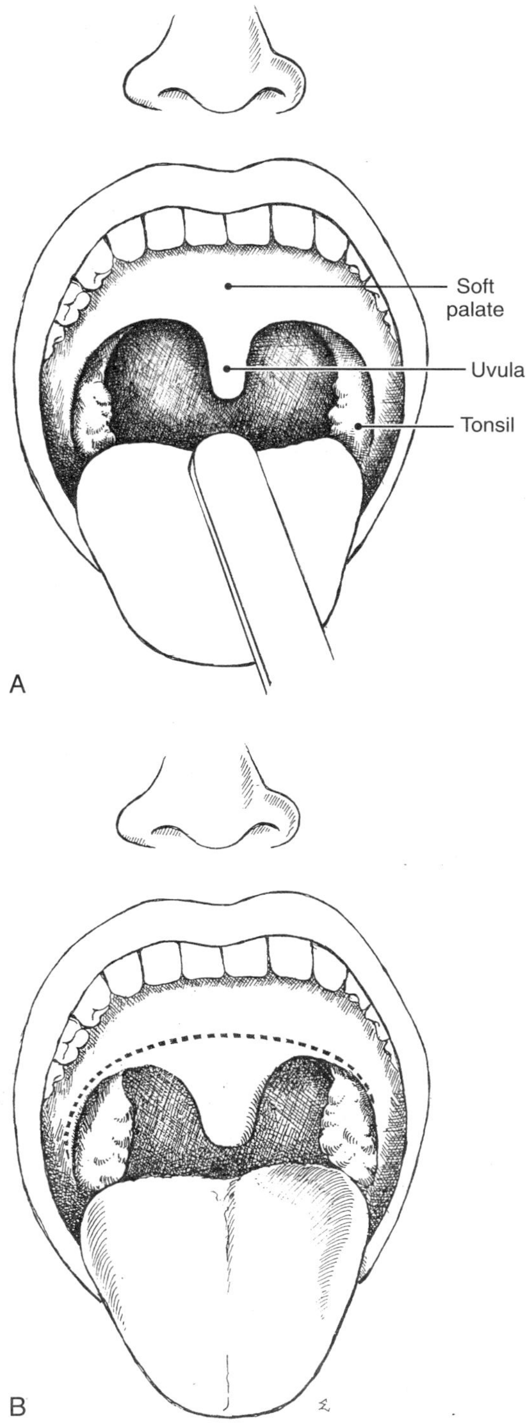

Figure 1. *A*, Typical normal anatomy. *B*, Thickened, wide uvula and large, floppy soft palate. The tonsils are also enlarged. In a UPPP, the uvula and a portion of the soft palate are removed *(dashed line)*. The enlarged tonsils are also removed at this time to tighten up the redundant tissue.

  - Often UPPP can be done in the office with a laser under local anesthesia, or it may be necessary for the patient to be asleep. The advantages and disadvantages of each technique will be discussed with you.

After careful consideration of all factors, the recommendation is that you have a UPPP under general anesthesia. The need for a tonsillectomy along with the UPPP will be discussed with you beforehand.

PREOPERATIVE PREPARATION

- You will have an examination of your blood, urine, heart (EKG), and lungs (chest x-ray).
- Do not eat or drink anything for 8 hours before the operation.

□ OPERATION

- You will be asleep for the operation.
- The operation usually takes about 1 hour.

POSTOPERATIVE CARE

- You will be taken to a recovery room and observed. When your blood pressure, pulse, and breathing are stable and you are completely alert, you should be able to go home that same day with a responsible adult.
- Pain will be controlled with medicine.
- The diet for the first 10 days should be liquids or soft foods that don't require much chewing.
- The stitches will dissolve or fall out by themselves in about 2 weeks.
- As with any operation, complications are always possible. With this type of operation, they can include bleeding, infection, and possibly others.
- Arrangements will be made for your medicine and follow-up office visit.

✣ HOME CARE

- You may walk about as you wish, even climb stairs, but don't overdo things.
- A small amount of blood-tinged saliva is common and may be noticed for a few days.
- Drink slowly and carefully for the first few days. Sometimes if you drink fast, liquids may come out of your nose. If this persists, be certain to mention it during your follow-up office visit.
- Most patients notice an immediate decrease in snoring and improvement in sleep. However, if after 4 to 6 weeks your previous symptoms return, be certain to mention this to us.
- Avoid doing a lot of talking for the first few days as this may put too much strain on your throat sutures.
- You may go back to work when you feel up to it.

✆ CALL OUR OFFICE IF

- You are having bleeding or cough up blood clots.
- You develop a temperature higher than 100°F.
- You have sleep apnea.
- You have any questions.

△ GENERAL INFORMATION

In this condition, the veins in the scrotum (the sac beneath the penis) that drain the testicle are distended and twisted. These veins normally are the size of spaghetti, but in the varicocele they may be as large as macaroni or even larger (Fig. 1). A varicocele reduces a person's fertility potential.

Although there are a few known causes of varicocele, most of the time the cause is not truly known. This is the situation with you.

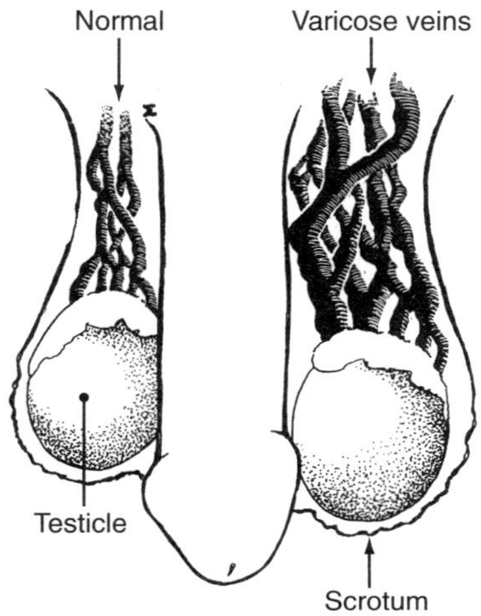

Figure 1.

COMMON SIGNS AND SYMPTOMS

- The scrotum feels heavy and may ache.
- The side of the scrotum involved is usually larger than the other.
- The dilated, twisted veins in the scrotum feel like a "bag of worms."

DIAGNOSIS

- Usually, the diagnosis can be made by taking a detailed history and doing a thorough physical examination.
- *Ultrasound*: Harmless sound waves are aimed at the area of your scrotum as well as the kidney. The sound waves bouncing back (the echoes) from this area are seen as a picture on a screen. Ultrasound is a convenient and painless way to look inside the scrotum to make certain the swelling is not from a tumor of the testicle.
- *Doppler ultrasound*: This works in the same way as regular ultrasound, but it gives more information about the blood vessels—whether they are actually physically blocked and if so, by what.

○ TREATMENT

- If one is certain that the swelling is a bunch of veins and nothing more than that, there is no reason to operate except for the sake of appearance, comfort, or concern about fertility.
- If it is not possible to be certain this is a harmless condition, then an operation is advisable.

After careful consideration of all factors, it is recommended that you have an operation for your condition. The reasons for this recommendation have been explained to you.

PREOPERATIVE CARE

- There will be an examination of your blood, urine, heart (EKG), and lungs (chest x-ray).
- Do not eat or drink anything for 8 hours before the operation.
- Shower as usual on the morning of the operation.
- You may be given medicine that will make you feel drowsy before you are brought to the operating room.

□ OPERATION

- You will be asleep for the operation.
- The incision will be made just above your groin. The abnormal veins will be tied off with care so as not to damage the testicle itself.
- The operation usually takes about 1 hour.

POSTOPERATIVE CARE

- You will wake up in a recovery room. When your blood pressure, pulse, and breathing are stable, you will be taken to a regular hospital room. You should be able to go home that same day. Otherwise, you may have to stay in the hospital overnight.
- There will be a snug bandage over the incision.
- Arrangements will be made for your medicine, follow-up office visit, and stitch removal.
- As with any operation, complications are always possible, some of them serious. With your type of operation, they can include bleeding, difficulty with urination, infection, and possibly others.

✚ HOME CARE

- Lie down as much as possible for the first 24 hours. This will help prevent swelling and make you more comfortable.
- You may eat as you did before the operation.
- Be careful that you do not become constipated.
  - Include enough roughage and liquid in your diet.
  - You may need a mild laxative (example: milk of magnesia).
- Unless instructed otherwise, you may shower if you wish with any dressings on or off.
  - There may be narrow strips of tape across the incision. It's all right if they get wet. They will be removed in the doctor's office.
  - After you dry yourself, replace any dressings with clean, dry ones.
- Wearing jockey-type shorts may help reduce any discomfort.

- The dilated veins in your scrotum will begin to shrink in about 6 weeks.
- Take medicine as prescribed for your pain.
- You may resume sexual activity whenever you choose.
- You may return to work when you feel up to it.

✆ CALL OUR OFFICE IF

- You develop any unusual signs or symptoms.
- You develop chills or a temperature higher than 100°F.
- You have any questions.

△ GENERAL INFORMATION

The two main systems of veins that drain blood from the leg are the *saphenous veins*, which you can see under the skin, and the deep veins inside the middle of the leg (Fig. 1).

The saphenous veins have valves that permit blood to go in only one direction—upward toward the heart. If these valves break down, the blood in the saphenous vein cannot move along and upward well enough, so the veins bulge and look twisted. These are called *varicose veins*. The veins deep in the leg do not have or need valves in them. They are surrounded and squeezed by the leg muscles so the blood in them has to move along. The two systems connect with each other.

Varicose veins occur most commonly in women (especially those who have had multiple pregnancies), in overweight persons, and in those who stand for long periods.

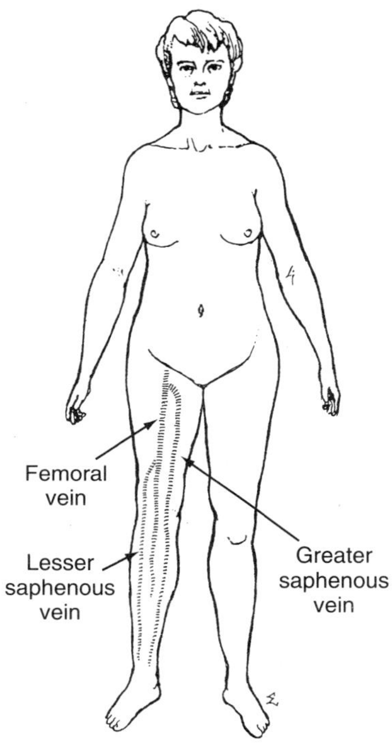

Figure 1. Usually it is the greater saphenous vein and the lesser saphenous vein and their branches that are varicosed and require treatment.

COMMON SIGNS AND SYMPTOMS

Because the blood in the varicose veins does not move along well enough, it doesn't carry away the waste products from the legs. Over a period of time, this can cause a number of problems, including

- Aching, heaviness, and cramping of the legs, which are made worse by standing for long periods of time.
- Skin rash, thin skin, and poor wound healing. Sometimes an ulcer will form just above the inner part of the ankle.
- Many persons are bothered by their unsightly appearance.

DIAGNOSIS

- Usually, the diagnosis can be made by taking a history and doing a physical examination.
- A number of simple tests can be done to be certain that the veins deep in the leg are open and working. This is important, because these deep veins are the ones that will do all the work if the saphenous veins are removed.
- *Venous Doppler ultrasound*: Harmless ultrasound waves are aimed at your legs. The waves bouncing back (the echoes) are seen as pictures on a screen. They can show if your deep veins are open.

○ TREATMENT

The ideal treatment is one that can do the following:

- Make it possible for the blood to flow normally.
- Relieve the heaviness and cramping in the legs.
- Prevent skin problems.
- Improve the appearance of the leg.

Nonsurgical Treatment

- Frequent elevation of the legs.
- Wearing elastic stockings. For many persons, this gives good relief and is all the treatment that is necessary.

Surgical Treatment

Injections of the Veins. A short very fine needle is used to inject a small amount of a very irritating solution into the vein. This causes the inside walls of the vein that is collapsed to stick to each other; no blood can flow through. These injections often need to be done a number of times.

- The *advantages* of this method are that no operation is necessary and it is good for small veins.
- The *disadvantages* are that the varicose veins tend to come back in 3 to 5 years; multiple visits and injections are needed; every so often, the irritating chemical leaks out of the vein and can cause a small ulcer in the skin; and it is not too good for treating large varicose veins.

Vein Stripping. In this operation, the entire saphenous vein is removed.

- The *advantages* of this method are that it is the most effective treatment, especially for larger varicose veins.
- The *disadvantages* are that it requires an operation and it is not too effective in removing the very small veins (even though it is safe to leave these).

After careful consideration of all factors, it is recommended that you have the operation to remove the veins that is commonly called vein stripping.

PREOPERATIVE PREPARATION

- An examination of your blood, urine, heart (EKG), and lungs (chest x-ray) will be done.
- Do not eat or drink anything for 8 hours before the operation.
- Shower as usual on the morning of the operation.

☐ OPERATION

- You will be asleep for the operation.
- A cosmetic incision will be made in your groin to locate the top end of the saphenous vein. Another incision will be made just above the ankle to locate the lower end of the vein. A special flexible wire will be inserted into the vein at the ankle and brought out of the top of the vein at the groin. This wire will be used to remove ("strip") the entire saphenous vein. Sometimes the vein is so twisted and crooked that the wire cannot follow the bends to reach the groin. In this case, very short cosmetic skin incisions can be made over the sharp bends to guide the wire past these twisted areas.
- The operation usually takes about 2 to 3 hours.

POSTOPERATIVE CARE

- You will be taken to a recovery room and observed. When your blood pressure, pulse, and breathing are stable, you will be taken to a regular hospital room.
- Your entire leg or legs will be bandaged.
- You will be gotten out of bed as soon as possible and every couple of hours asked to walk a few steps.
- Pain will be controlled with medicine.
- You should be able to go home in 1 to 2 days.
- Arrangements will be made for your medicine, follow-up office visit, and stitch removal.

✚ HOME CARE

- You should be up and walking a little every hour during the daytime. Otherwise, try to lie flat. Avoid sitting or standing whenever possible.
- Take medicine as prescribed for your pain.
- Sponge bathe as you wish.
- Include plenty of roughage and liquids in your diet to help prevent constipation.

✆ CALL OUR OFFICE IF

- There is bleeding through the bandages.
- You develop a temperature higher than 100°F.
- You have any questions.

△ GENERAL INFORMATION

Vasoligation is a simple, safe, and very reliable way to permanently prevent sperm from being able to get to the outside through the penis.

SOME DEFINITIONS

Testicles: These are two egg-shaped organs that lie in the *scrotum,* the sac behind the penis. The testicles make male hormones. They also make very young sperm by the millions.

Sperm: These are the microscopic cells that can fertilize the egg from a woman's ovary. They have a wiggly tail that helps them move. They are stored in the *epididymis,* which is attached to the testicle. Here the sperm mature and wait until they go to the outside during ejaculation.

Vas deferens: These are two tubes (one from each testicle) about the size of angel hair spaghetti. They carry the sperm to the urethra (the tunnel in the penis) so that the sperm can get to the outside.

Prostate: This gland is about the size of a walnut. It is located where the bladder opens into the *urethra,* the tunnel that carries urine to the outside. The prostate and the *seminal vesicles* right next to it secrete semen.

Semen: This is the slightly sticky white fluid that mixes with sperm and helps it get to the outside during ejaculation.

The vas deferens and the ducts from the prostate and the seminal vesicles connect to the urethra. During ejaculation the bladder sphincter closes tightly. This helps to direct the semen to the outside and prevents urine from mixing with the semen (Fig. 1).

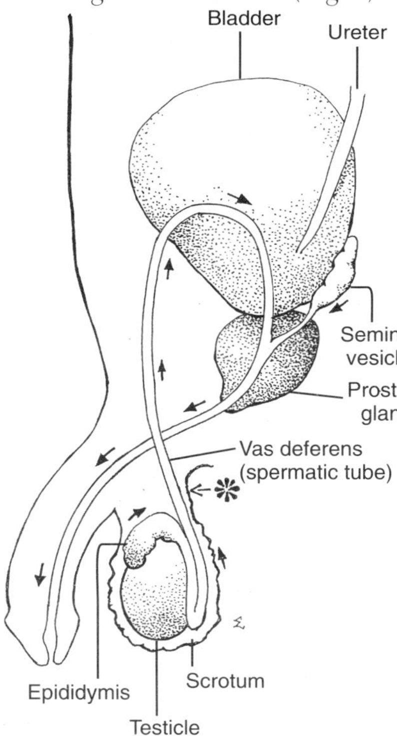

Figure 1. The vas deferens is usually ligated at a point indicated by the asterisk, preventing the sperm from going beyond this point.

VASOLIGATION

Vasoligation involves tying *(ligation)* of the two vas deferens so that sperm cannot leave the testicle. That's the only thing that is blocked. The male hormones made by the testicle are not affected at all. Also, semen continues to be made and comes out as before except it does not have sperm in it. You cannot tell the difference by just looking at the semen.

BEFORE THE VASOLIGATION

Although a vasoligation is easy, safe, and effective, it is a very important step. You should realize the following:

- You should consider a vasoligation as permanent. It will make you sterile, and you will not be able to father a child.
- A vasoligation is not meant to solve any sex problems you may have with your partner.
- You and your partner should clearly understand what a vasoligation means and what it involves.
- You should be certain you do not want to father any more children. Consider future possibilities that may make you change your mind; for example: you may remarry and want children following a divorce or death of your partner.
- Although there is an operation to reconnect the vas deferens, it is difficult, expensive, and by no means always successful.
- All of your male characteristics and sex drive will remain the same. The only change will be that your semen will not contain sperm.
- There is no evidence that vasoligation causes cancer.
- Some men (and women) feel that their sexual enjoyment is improved, because they can be more spontaneous without the need for prophylactic preparations and, of course, without the worry of a pregnancy.

PREOPERATIVE PREPARATION

- You will be given instructions on when to stop eating or drinking before the operation.
- Shower as usual on the morning of the operation and wash the scrotum thoroughly.

☐ OPERATION

- The operation will be done on an outpatient basis.
- The scrotum and groin area will be painted with an antiseptic solution and draped with sterile coverings.
- A very thin, short needle will be used to inject an anesthetic in the skin and upper part of the scrotum. This will make the area entirely numb.
- A tiny incision will be made in the skin of the upper part of the scrotum where the vas deferens is located. The vas deferens will be tied. Often, a short piece is removed for examination in the laboratory to be certain the correct tissue has been removed. The same will be done on the opposite side.
- A small stitch and bandage will be applied. Bring along a pair of jockey-type underwear. This provides support to the scrotum and helps keep the pain to a minimum.

- You will be taken to a recovery room. When your blood pressure, pulse, and breathing are stable and you are completely alert, you should be able to go home that same day with a responsible adult.
- As with any operation, complications are always possible. Although they are uncommon with your type of operation, they can include bleeding, infection, and possibly others.

✣ HOME CARE

- You may walk about, even climb stairs, but don't overdo things.
- For the first day, lie down as much as possible.
- For the first 24 hours, apply cold compresses to the scrotal area every 10 to 15 minutes while you are awake. This reduces the chance of bleeding and postoperative swelling. Commercial cold packs or simply a bag of frozen peas works well for this. Apply the cold pack on the outside of the undershorts and avoid direct contact with the scrotal skin.
- Keep the area dry for the first 24 hours after which you may shower as usual.
- Don't lift anything heavier than 5 pounds. Ask someone to do it for you.
- The small sutures used to close the skin are usually of the dissolving type and do not need to be removed.
- You may resume more strenuous activity, including sex, after 3 days but only as long as that activity does not cause discomfort.
  Note: It's *very important* to realize you still have sperm in your semen. It will take a number of ejaculations over several weeks before all the sperm leaves the tubes. Therefore, you'll be asked to supply a sample of your semen (you can collect it in a jar at home) for examination to see if it contains sperm. This will be done at 6 weeks and then at 12 weeks after the operation.
- It is safe to have sex without protection *only* after we demonstrate in the laboratory that no sperm are present in your semen.
- Until that time be certain to use birth control during sexual intercourse.
- You may experience some aching or pain in the testicles for a while. This usually gets better with time.

✆ CALL OUR OFFICE IF

- The scrotum becomes swollen.
- The incision becomes red or swollen, or there is drainage from it.
- You develop a temperature higher than 100°F.
- You have any questions.

△ GENERAL INFORMATION

When a man has an ejaculation, the creamy fluid that comes out of the penis (the *semen*) usually has sperm in it—by the thousands. It is this sperm that fertilizes the egg from the woman and that starts the pregnancy.

HOW SPERM GETS THERE

The sperm are manufactured in the *testicles* and mature in the *epididymis.* They then travel through the *vas deferens,* which is joined by small ducts coming from the *seminal vesicles.* Just before they empty into the urethra as it passes through the prostate gland. The seminal vesicles and prostate gland make the whitish fluid (the *semen*) that carries the sperm to the outside through the penis during ejaculation.

VASECTOMY

When a man has a vasectomy (also called *vasoligation*) the vas deferens is tied and divided. This prevents the sperm from reaching the outside. Everything else happens as before, including ejaculation of semen, except that there are no sperm in the semen. If there are no sperm that can get to the outside, then a man with a vasectomy cannot father a child.

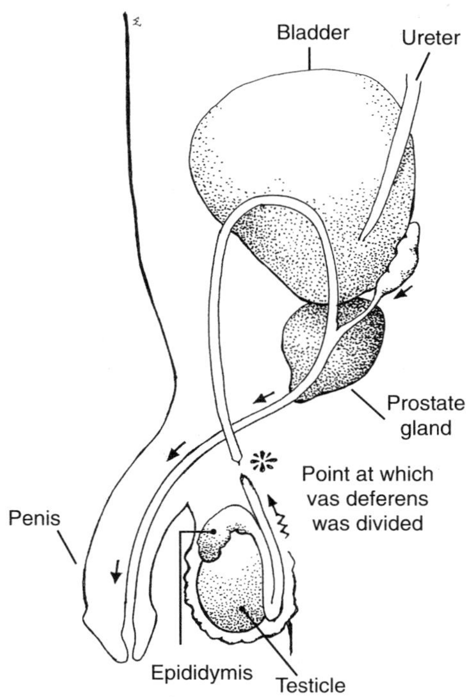

Figure 1. The asterisk shows the divided vas deferens (spermatic tube). The sperm cannot get past this point to reach the outside. In the repair, the divided ends of the spermatic cord are trimmed back to the normal tissue and reconnected. Now it is possible for the sperm to get to the outside.

VASECTOMY REVERSAL

Sometimes, however, circumstances change, and the man now wants very much to be able to father a child. For sperm to reach the outside, it is necessary to reconnect the vas deferens (the medical term for this operation is *vasovasostomy*).

Note: It is very important that you and your partner understand that, although the operation may proceed smoothly, that does not mean that the tunnel in the vas deferens (it is about as big as the thickness of a straight pin) will remain open as it is healing. Further, your testicle may no longer make any, sufficient, or good enough sperm. This is related to how long the sperm has been blocked: the longer the time since your vasectomy, the greater the risk of damage to the sperm. During the time the sperm were blocked, your body may have made substances, called *sperm immune antibodies,* that work against your sperm.

After careful consideration of all factors, the recommendation is that you have a vasectomy reversal. The reasons for this recommendation have been explained to you.

PREOPERATIVE PREPARATION

- You will have an examination of your blood.
- Do not take aspirin or aspirin-containing medicines for 1 week before the operation.
- Shower as usual on the morning of the operation.
- You may be given medicine that will make you feel drowsy before you are brought to the operating room.

□ OPERATION

- The operation may be done under local anesthesia. The skin over the scrotum will be made numb. You will be given medicine to make you feel drowsy or you will be asleep. The choice will be discussed with you beforehand.
- The incision will be over the scrotum.
- The blind ends of the vas deferens will be cut open and reconnected with extremely fine suture material (Fig. 1). An operating microscope will be used so that everything can be seen clearly and sewn as accurately as possible. It may be necessary to connect the vas deferens directly to the epididymis where the sperm is made.
- The operation usually takes about 2 hours.

POSTOPERATIVE CARE

- You will be taken to a recovery room and observed. When your blood pressure, pulse, and breathing are stable and you are completely alert, you should be able to go home that same day with a responsible adult.
- Arrangements will be made for your medicine and follow-up office visit. The stitches are the dissolving type.
- As with any operation, complications are always possible. With your type of operation, these can include bleeding, infection, and possibly others.

✣ HOME CARE

- Lie down as much as possible for the first day.
- Apply a cold pack on the scrotum (frozen peas in a plastic bag are a handy and effective way to do this). This will help keep down any swelling.
- Do not engage in strenuous activity for 2 weeks.
- Wearing jockey-type underwear may be more comfortable for you.
- You may shower if you wish in 48 hours.
- Don't lift anything heavier than 5 pounds. Ask someone to do it for you.
- You may resume sexual activity in 2 weeks. You may notice some blood in your semen. Don't worry; this is normal.

✆ CALL OUR OFFICE IF

- The scrotum swells and continues to do so.
- You develop any unusual signs or symptoms.
- The incision becomes red or swollen, or there is drainage from it.
- You develop a temperature higher than 100°F.
- You have any questions.

△ GENERAL INFORMATION

The inferior vena cava is a large vein (about as big around as a broom handle) in your abdomen and chest. It drains most of the blood from your legs and abdomen and takes it to the heart. The heart then pumps it into the tiny vessels of the lungs to get fresh oxygen and then out again into the general circulation.

Sometimes blood clots form in the veins of the legs and the vessels that drain into the inferior vena cava. Very rarely, one of the clots breaks off into the inferior vena cava and travels to the lungs. This broken-off clot is called an *embolus*. When such emboli reach the vessels in the lungs, they can't pass through them; they plug them up. If such a clot is big enough or if there are enough of the small clots, enough lung blood vessels are blocked so that blood cannot pass through to the lungs.

COMMON SIGNS AND SYMPTOMS

- Enough of these vessels are blocked to produce shortness of breath.
- The heart begins to tire out as it strains to pump blood through the blocked vessels.

DIAGNOSIS

- There will be a detailed history of your symptoms and complaints.
- The diagnosis should be suspected in a patient who has some of the above symptoms and is one who is prone to develop clots as follows:
  - Has been in bed for a long period of time and not moving the legs (thus not pumping blood out of them properly).
  - Has had an operation on the pelvis, which causes some of the veins there to form clots.
  - Has a blood problem of forming clots too easily.
- *X-rays* of the lungs will be done to look for lung tissue that is plugged and not working.
- *Lung scan*: These are studies that can show if blood and air are circulating through all parts of the lungs.
- *Angiograms*: X-rays are taken after dye is injected into the blood vessels to the lungs. The dye circulates through these vessels and can show the location of the clots. This method is very helpful but cannot always be done. Also, it has some risk associated with it.

○ TREATMENT

If these blood clots are not prevented from continuing to reach the lungs, the person may die.

- Early on, blood thinners can be given to prevent clots in the veins from getting larger.
- If blood thinners are successful in preventing a clot from getting larger, the body itself makes dissolving chemicals that sometimes slowly dissolve the clots already there.
- If such treatment with blood thinners is not successful, then an operation is advisable.
- Occasionally, special clot-dissolving medications may be necessary.
- Placing a filter in the vena cava is the safest and best treatment under these circumstances. A filter lets blood pass through it to continue to flow up the vena cava as it should. However, it prevents blood clots from passing through and going up the vena cava to the lungs.

PREOPERATIVE PREPARATION

- Do not eat or drink anything for 8 hours before the operation.
- You may be given medicine that will make you feel drowsy before you are brought to the operating room.

□ OPERATION

- The operation will be done under local anesthesia. Also, you will be given medicine that will keep you very drowsy during the procedure.
- The skin over a large vein in the neck will be painted with an antiseptic solution and surrounded with sterile towels. A thin needle will be used to inject an anesthetic in the skin over a large vein in the neck.
- A short incision will be made over this vein and a fine wire inserted into it. At the tip of this special wire is a gadget that unfolds like a spider web.
- The wire with this web is watched with x-rays as it is carefully pushed down the neck vein and into the vena cava in the abdomen. The web is positioned so that it lies below the kidney veins.
- At this point, the tiny web is unfolded. Blood can flow through the web but clots cannot get through (Fig. 1).
- The inserting wire is now disconnected from the web and slipped out.
- The procedure usually takes about 30 minutes.

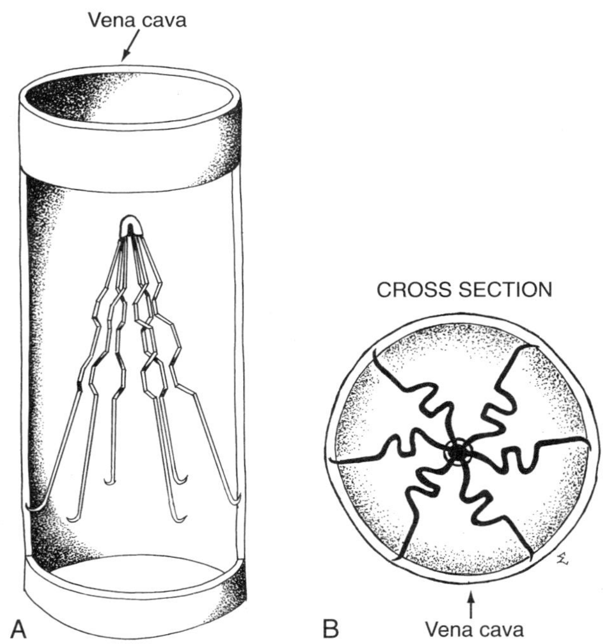

Figure 1. There are a number of designs of filters. The Greenfield filter *(A* and *B)* has had a high degree of success.

POSTOPERATIVE CARE

- You will be taken to a recovery room. As soon as your blood pressure, pulse, and breathing are stable, you will be taken to your regular hospital room.
- In the hospital room you will be helped to resume your previous activities.
- You will be receiving oxygen to help you with your breathing until you get over this acute phase.
- You will be started on blood thinners to keep new blood clots from forming.
- Your stay in the hospital will depend on how long it takes to clear up your other conditions.
- Arrangements will be made for your blood thinners (called *anticoagulants*), your first postoperative visit, and discussion of any further treatment.

✚ HOME CARE

- Resume your previous activities as discussed while you were in the hospital.
- You may walk about as you wish.
- You may be on a general diet.
- Shower or bathe as you wish.
- Elevate your legs at every opportunity during the day.

✆ CALL OUR OFFICE IF

- You have new or different shortness of breath.
- You cough up any blood-tinged mucus.
- Your legs swell.
- You develop a temperature higher than 100°F.
- You have any questions.

△ GENERAL INFORMATION

Villous adenoma is a growth found in the lining of the rectum or colon. It is soft and flat, often making it difficult to feel even as the examining finger passes over it during a routine rectal examination. There can be unsuspected cancerous changes in it, or there is a risk of cancer developing in it later. The cause of villous adenoma is not known.

COMMON SIGNS AND SYMPTOMS

- Many persons have no symptoms at all.
- There may be changes in bowel habits.
- There may be some blood in the stool or just mucus.
- There may be diarrhea.

DIAGNOSIS

- About one-third of villous adenomas can be reached with the examining finger.
- About 90% can be reached with a flexible sigmoidoscope.
- They may be as small as your little fingernail to the size of your palm.
- *Flexible sigmoidoscopy*: This is done with an instrument (a flexible sigmoidoscope) that is smooth, flexible, has lenses in it and a light at its tip, and is as big around as your little finger. It can be used to inspect the inside of the lower one-fourth of your bowel. This is an office procedure.
- *Colonoscopy*: This is done with an instrument that is similar to a flexible sigmoidoscope except that it is long enough to inspect your entire colon. Also, during the colonoscopy you will be given medicine that will make you feel drowsy. The tip of the instrument will be introduced through your anus gently and then advanced up the entire bowel, which will be examined for any abnormalities.
- *Barium enema*: Liquid barium is placed in the rectum (very much like a regular enema), and x-ray pictures are taken of the barium as it flows throughout the colon. A villous adenoma can show a characteristic picture.
- *Ultrasound*: A smooth, flexible instrument as thick as your little finger (an *ultrasound probe*) is lubricated and inserted through the anus and into the rectum. From the tip of the probe, harmless, painless sound waves are aimed at the villous adenoma in the wall of the rectum. The waves bouncing back (the echoes) are seen as pictures on a screen. This can help show how deeply the adenoma (and any cancer in it) penetrates the rectal wall.
- One of the most important responsibilities with a villous adenoma is to determine whether there is cancer in it (Fig. 1). Performing the usual biopsy (taking a piece the size of a small pea, for example) can be misleading. If such a piece is negative for cancer, it does not mean that no cancer is present in a different area of the adenoma. Even several biopsies can miss a cancerous area in the adenoma. For this reason, all of the adenoma must be removed so that it can be examined carefully in the pathology laboratory.

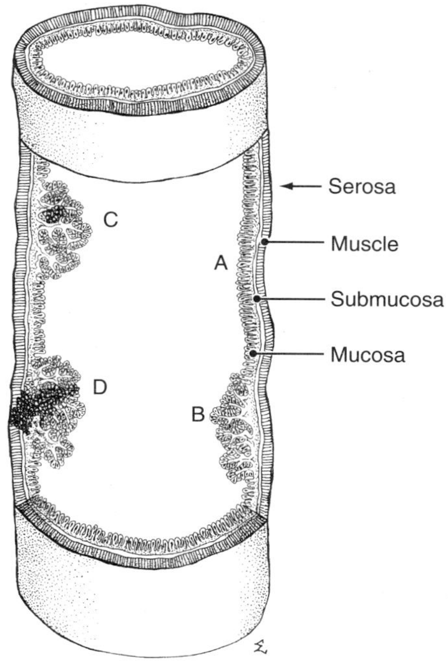

Figure 1. Segment of colon, showing normal anatomy (A); benign villous adenoma (B); villous adenoma with small, superficial cancer (C); and villous adenoma with deeply penetrating cancer (D).

○ TREATMENT

If all the villous adenoma can be removed through the anus and it is negative for cancer, then no further treatment is necessary at this time (Fig. 2).

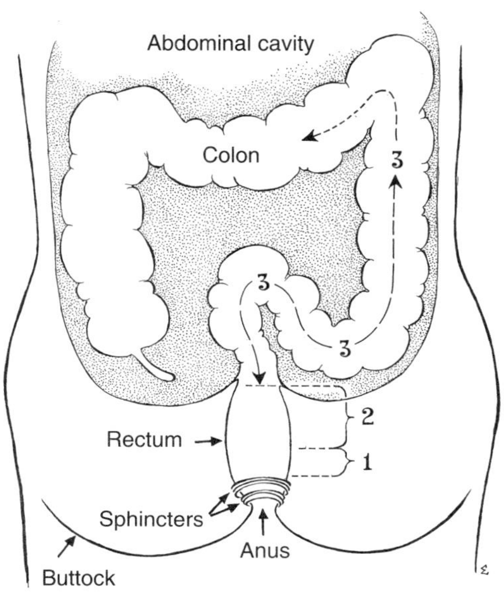

Figure 2. Colon and rectum, showing locations that may influence treatment: low rectum (1), mid and high rectum (2), and colon (3).

Many times, however, it just is not technically possible to remove completely and in one piece all of a suspicious adenoma through the anus for examination under the microscope. In such situations, it is wise to treat the adenoma as though it is cancerous even if the initial pea-sized biopsy done through the colonoscope is negative for cancer. The reasons for removing that part of the colon containing the villous adenoma are as follows:

- If cancer is later shown to be present in the removed colon, you will have had the proper treatment.
- If the removed adenoma was benign, you won't miss the extra colon.
- A lesion has been removed that could later become cancerous.

After careful consideration of all factors, the recommendation is that you have an operation to remove that part of your colon with the villous adenoma in it and to reconnect the divided colon so that you will have bowel movements as before (Figs. 3 and 4).

PREOPERATIVE PREPARATION

- You will have an examination of your blood, urine, heart (EKG), and lungs (chest x-ray).
- You will be instructed on how to clean out your bowel.
- Do not eat or drink anything for 8 hours before the operation.

☐ OPERATION

- You will be asleep for the operation.
- The operation usually takes about 2 hours.

POSTOPERATIVE CARE

- You will be taken to a recovery room and observed. When your blood pressure, pulse, and breathing are stable, you will be taken to a regular hospital room.
- You may have a thin plastic tube in your nose for several days.
- That evening you will be helped to sit up in bed and on the next day to get out of bed.
- Pain will be controlled with medicine.
- When your bowels start working, the tube in your nose will be removed and you will be started on a liquid diet. This will be increased to more solid food as you tolerate it.
- As with any operation, complications are always possible. With this type of operation, they can include pneumonia, blood clots, leakage where the bowel was reconnected, bowel obstruction, and possibly others.
- You should be able to go home in about 5 days.
- Arrangements will be made for your medicine, follow-up office visit, and stitch or clip removal.

✚ HOME CARE

- You may walk about as you wish, even climb stairs, but don't overdo things.
- Take medicine as prescribed for your pain.
- Eat as you wish.
- Unless instructed otherwise, you may shower if you wish and with any dressings on or off. After you dry yourself, replace any dressings with clean, dry ones.
- Include plenty of roughage and liquids in your diet to help prevent constipation.
- Do not drive a car unless you can move freely and without pain and are not on any medicines that decrease your alertness.
- You may return to work when you feel up to it.
- You may resume sexual activity whenever you choose.

✆ CALL OUR OFFICE IF

- The incision becomes red or swollen, or there is drainage from it.
- You develop a temperature higher than 100°F.
- You have any questions.
- You do not have a bowel movement for 36 hours.

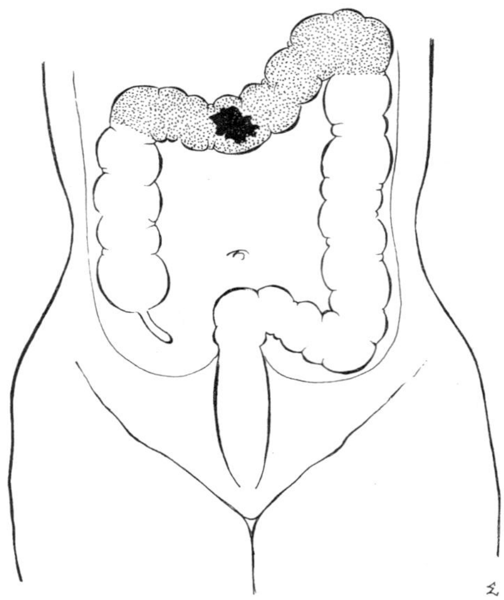

Figure 3. Possible location of villous adenoma *(dark area)* in the colon. The stippled area will be resected.

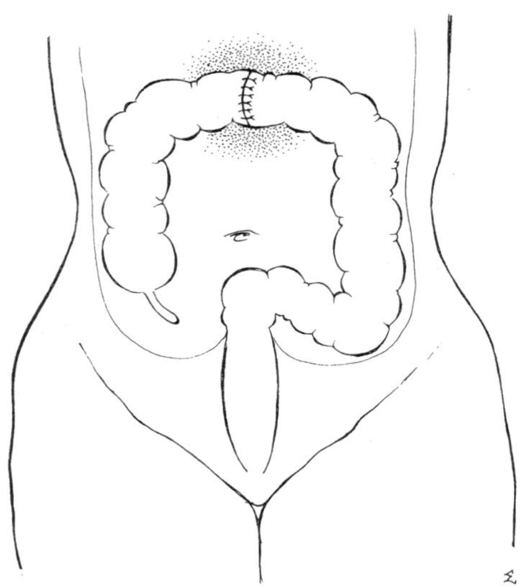

Figure 4. The divided ends of the colon have been reconnected.

VILLOUS ADENOMA: Diagnosis and Staging

△ GENERAL INFORMATION

Villous adenoma is a growth found in the lining of the rectum or colon. It is soft and flat, often making it difficult to feel even as the examining finger passes over it during a routine rectal examination. There can be unsuspected cancerous changes in it, or there is a risk of cancer developing in it later. The cause of villous adenoma is not known.

COMMON SIGNS AND SYMPTOMS

- Many persons have no symptoms at all.
- There may be changes in bowel habits.
- There may be some blood in the stool or just mucus.
- There may be diarrhea.

DIAGNOSIS

- About one-third of villous adenomas can be reached with the examining finger.
- About 90% can be reached with a flexible sigmoidoscope.
- They may be as small as your little fingernail to the size of your palm.
- *Flexible sigmoidoscopy*: This is done with an instrument (a flexible sigmoidoscope) that is smooth and flexible, has lenses in it and a light at its tip, and is as big around as your little finger. It can be used to inspect the inside of the lower one-fourth of your bowel. This is an office procedure.
- *Colonoscopy*: This is done with an instrument that is similar to a flexible sigmoidoscope except that it is long enough to inspect your entire colon. Also, during the colonoscopy you will be given medicine that will make you feel drowsy. The tip of the instrument will be gently introduced through your anus and then advanced up the entire bowel, which will be examined for any abnormalities.
- *Barium enema*: Liquid barium is placed in the rectum (very much like a regular enema), and x-ray pictures are taken of the barium as it flows throughout the colon. A villous adenoma can show a characteristic picture.
- *Ultrasound*: A smooth, flexible instrument as thick as your little finger (an *ultrasound probe*) is lubricated and inserted through the anus and into the rectum. From the tip of the probe, harmless, painless sound waves are aimed at the villous adenoma in the wall of the rectum. The waves bouncing back (the echoes) are seen as pictures on a screen. This can help show how deeply the adenoma (and any cancer in it) penetrates the rectal wall.
- One of the most important responsibilities with a villous adenoma is to determine whether there is cancer in it (Fig. 1). Performing the usual biopsy (taking a piece the size of a small pea, for example) can be misleading. If such a piece is negative for cancer, it does not mean that no cancer is present in a different area of the adenoma. Even several biopsies can miss a cancerous area in the adenoma.

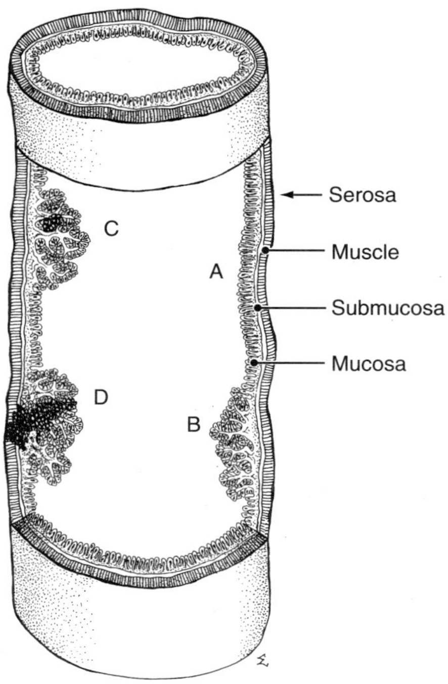

Figure 1. Segment of colon, showing normal anatomy (A); benign villous adenoma (B); villous adenoma with small, superficial cancer (C); and villous adenoma with deeply penetrating cancer (D).

For this reason, all of the adenoma must be removed so that it can be examined carefully in the pathology laboratory.

○ TREATMENT

For the above reasons, treatment needs to be in two parts.

Part I. If possible, remove the entire villous adenoma as one piece to see whether there is cancer in it.

Part II. Determine the type of operation to be performed if cancer is found in the villous adenoma, or if the adenoma cannot be removed beforehand to see whether cancer is present in it.

Part I

Preparation for Removal of Rectal Adenoma

- You will have an examination of your blood, urine, heart (EKG), and lungs (chest x-ray).
- You will be instructed on how to clean out your bowel.
- Do not eat or drink anything for 8 hours before the operation.

Removal of Adenoma

- You will be asleep for the operation.
- The villous adenoma will be removed from below (through the anus) as one piece and sent to the pathology laboratory for detailed examination. The results of these tests will not be known for several days.

Decision on Further Treatment

If no cancer is present, no further treatment is necessary.

If cancer is present, then a cancer operation is necessary. The nature of the operation will be determined by at least the following:

- The location of the cancer.
- The size of the cancer.
- How deeply the cancer penetrates into the wall of the rectum.

Possible Curative Operation: Low Rectum (Fig. 2)

- If the cancer is small, does not deeply penetrate the tissue, and has borders that are clear of cancer, then it is reasonable not to administer any further treatment but to examine you carefully on a regular schedule.
- If the cancer in the villous adenoma is large, penetrates the deep tissue, and is too close to the sphincters or involves the sphincters of the anus, then the rectum and anus need to be removed. This means that a permanent colostomy will be necessary.
- If the cancer is large, penetrates the deep tissue, and has borders that still contain cancer, part of the rectum containing the tumor needs to be removed. The divided rectum is reconnected so that a person can have bowel movements the normal way.

Possible Operation for an Apparent Adenoma of the Colon

If the lesion in your colon cannot technically be removed safely as one piece through the anus (which is usually the case), it is better and safer if it is removed through the abdomen and as though it has cancer in it. If the removed adenoma has cancer in it, then you will have had the correct operation. If it does not have cancer in it, you will not miss the removed piece of colon and you will be rid of something that may later develop cancer in it.

This discussion describes the general principles used in deciding how to treat a lesion of the large bowel that appears to be an adenoma. Once the location of your suspicious lesion is determined, you will have a detailed explanation of your options before anything further is planned or done.

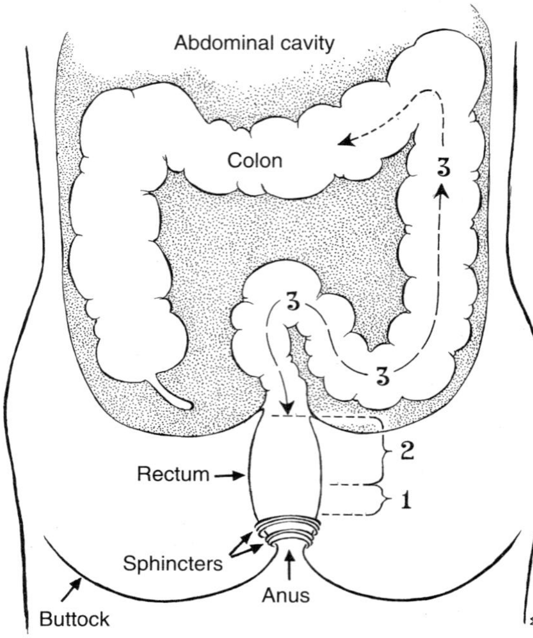

Figure 2. Colon and rectum, showing locations that may influence treatment: low rectum (1), mid and high rectum (2), and colon (3).

VILLOUS ADENOMA: High and Middle Rectum

△ GENERAL INFORMATION

Villous adenoma is a growth found in the lining of the rectum or colon. It is soft and flat, often making it difficult to feel even as the examining finger passes over it during a routine rectal examination. There can be unsuspected cancerous changes in it, or there is a risk of cancer developing in it later. The cause of villous adenoma is not known.

COMMON SIGNS AND SYMPTOMS

- Many persons have no symptoms at all.
- There may be changes in bowel habits.
- There may be some blood in the stool or just mucus.
- There may be diarrhea.

DIAGNOSIS

- About one-third of villous adenomas can be reached with the examining finger.
- About 90% can be reached with a flexible sigmoidoscope.
- They may be as small as your little fingernail to the size of your palm.
- *Flexible sigmoidoscopy*: This is done with an instrument (a flexible sigmoidoscope) that is smooth and flexible, has lenses in it and a light at its tip, and is as big around as your little finger. It can be used to inspect the inside of the lower one-fourth of your bowel. This is an office procedure.
- *Colonoscopy*: This is done with an instrument that is similar to a flexible sigmoidoscope except that it is long enough to inspect your entire colon. Also, during the colonoscopy you will be given medicine that will make you feel drowsy. The tip of the instrument will be introduced through your anus gently and then advanced up the entire bowel, which will be examined for any abnormalities.
- *Barium enema*: Liquid barium is placed in the rectum (very much like a regular enema), and x-ray pictures are taken of the barium as it flows throughout the colon. A villous adenoma can show a characteristic picture.
- *Ultrasound*: A smooth, flexible instrument as thick as your little finger (an *ultrasound probe*) is lubricated and inserted through the anus and into the rectum. From the tip of the probe, harmless, painless sound waves are aimed at the villous adenoma in the wall of the rectum. The waves bouncing back (the echoes) are seen as pictures on a screen. This can help show how deeply the adenoma (and any cancer in it) penetrates the rectal wall.
- One of the most important responsibilities with a villous adenoma is to determine whether there is cancer in it (Fig. 1). Performing the usual biopsy (taking a piece the size of a small pea, for example) can be misleading. If such a piece is negative for cancer, it does not mean that no cancer is present in a different area of the adenoma. Even several biopsies can miss a cancerous area in the adenoma. For this reason all of the adenoma must be removed so that it can be examined carefully in the pathology laboratory.

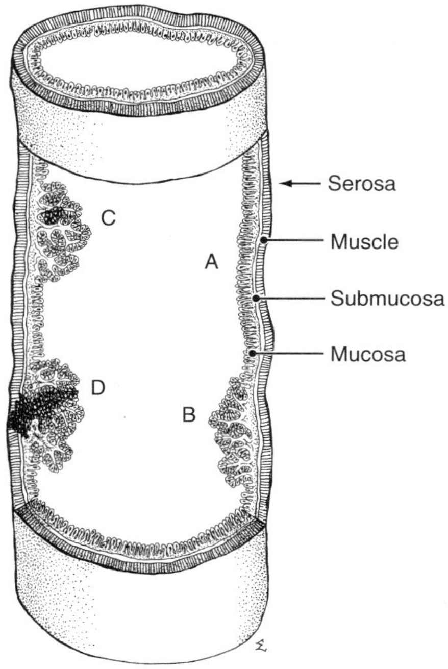

Figure 1. Segment of colon, showing normal anatomy (A); benign villous adenoma (B); villous adenoma with small, superficial cancer (C); and villous adenoma with deeply penetrating cancer (D).

○ TREATMENT

If all the villous adenoma can be removed through the anus and it is negative for cancer, then no further treatment is necessary at this time (Fig. 2).

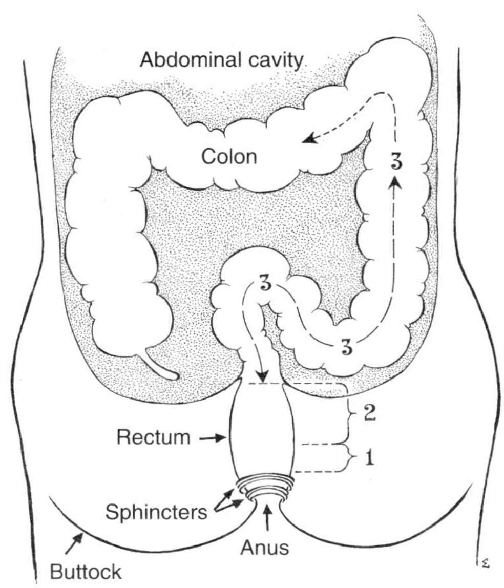

Figure 2. Colon and rectum, showing locations that may influence treatment: low rectum (1), mid and high rectum (2), and colon (3).

Many times, however, it just is not technically possible to remove completely and in one piece all of a suspicious adenoma through the anus for examination under the microscope. In such situations, it is wise to treat the adenoma as though it is cancerous even if the initial pea-sized biopsy done through the colonoscope is negative for cancer. The reasons for removing that part of the colon containing the villous adenoma are as follows:

- If cancer is later shown to be present in the removed colon, you will have had the proper treatment.
- If the removed adenoma was benign, you won't miss the extra colon.
- A lesion has been removed that could later become cancerous.

After careful consideration of all factors, the recommendation is that you have an operation to remove a portion of your rectum and to reconnect the cut ends (Figs. 3 and 4).

Note: You should know that this operation can have an important effect on your sex life. Let's discuss this further before the operation.

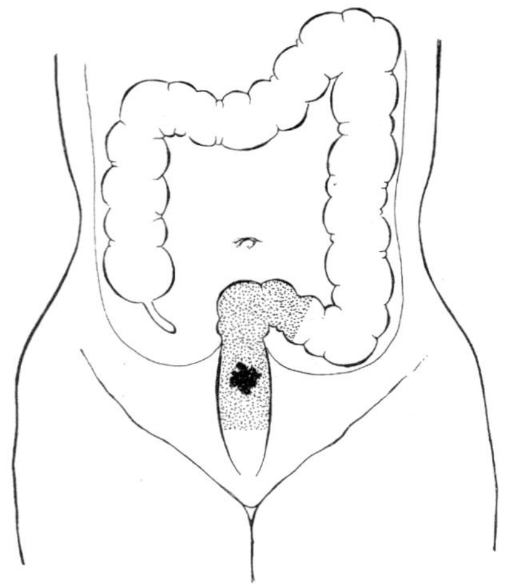

Figure 3. Possible location of the villous adenoma *(dark area)* with cancer in the high rectum. The stippled area will be resected.

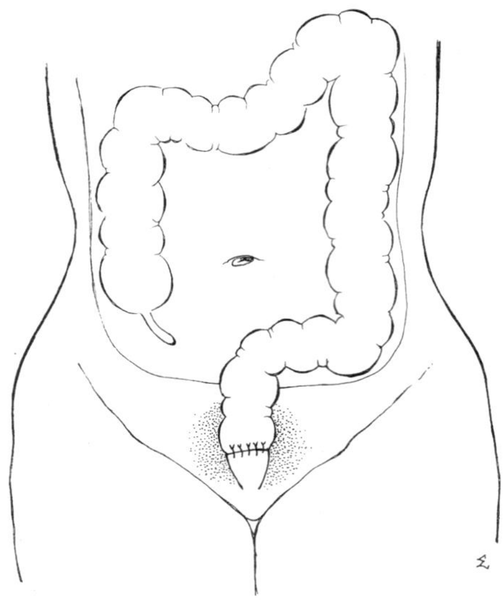

Figure 4. The divided ends of the rectum are reconnected.

PREOPERATIVE PREPARATION

- You will have an examination of your blood, urine, heart (EKG), and lungs (chest x-ray).
- You will be instructed on how to clean out your bowel.
- Do not eat or drink anything for 8 hours before the operation.

☐ OPERATION

- You will be asleep for the operation.
- The incision will be in your lower abdomen.
- The operation usually takes about 2 hours.

POSTOPERATIVE CARE

- You will be taken to a recovery room and observed. When your blood pressure, pulse, and breathing are stable, you will be taken to a regular hospital room.
- You may have a thin plastic tube in your nose for several days.
- That evening you will be helped to sit up in bed and on the next day to get out of bed.
- Pain will be controlled with medicine.
- When your bowels start working, the tube in your nose will be removed and you will be started on a liquid diet. This will be increased to more solid food as you tolerate it.
- As with any operation, complications are always possible. With this type of operation, they can include pneumonia, blood clots, leakage where the rectum was reconnected, bowel obstruction, and possibly others.
- You should be able to go home in about 5 days.
- Arrangements will be made for your medicine, follow-up office visit, and stitch removal.

✚ HOME CARE

- You may walk about as you wish, even climb stairs, but don't overdo things.
- Take medicine as prescribed for your pain.
- Unless instructed otherwise, you may shower if you wish and with any dressings on or off. After you dry yourself, replace any dressings with clean, dry ones.
- Include plenty of roughage and liquids in your diet to help prevent constipation.
- Do not drive a car unless you can move freely and without pain and are not on any medicines that decrease your alertness.
- You may return to work when you feel up to it.
- You may resume sexual activity whenever you choose.

✆ CALL OUR OFFICE IF

- The incision becomes red or swollen, or there is drainage from it.
- You develop a temperature higher than 100°F.
- You have any questions.
- You do not have a bowel movement for 36 hours.

VILLOUS ADENOMA: Low Rectum

△ GENERAL INFORMATION

Villous adenoma is a growth found in the lining of the rectum or colon. There can be unsuspected cancerous changes in it, or there is a risk of cancer developing in it later.

COMMON SIGNS AND SYMPTOMS

- Many persons have no symptoms at all.
- There may be changes in the bowel habits.
- There may be some blood in the stool or only mucus.
- There may be diarrhea.

DIAGNOSIS

- About one-third of villous adenomas can be reached with the examining finger.
- About 90% can be reached with a flexible sigmoidoscope.
- They may be as small as your little fingernail or as large as your palm.
- *Flexible sigmoidoscopy*: This is done with a flexible *sigmoidoscope* that is smooth and flexible, has lenses and a light in it, and is as big around as your little finger. It can be used to inspect the inside of the lower one-fourth of your bowel. This is an office procedure.
- *Colonoscopy*: This is done with an instrument similar to a flexible sigmoidoscope except that it is long enough to inspect your entire colon. During the colonoscopy you will be given medicine that will make you feel drowsy. The tip of the instrument will be introduced gently through your anus and then advanced up the entire bowel, which will be examined for any abnormalities.
- *Barium enema*: Liquid barium is placed in the rectum (very much like a regular enema), and x-ray pictures are taken of the barium as it flows throughout the colon to look for other abnormalities.
- *Ultrasound*: A smooth, flexible instrument as thick as your little finger (an *ultrasound probe*) is inserted through the anus and into the rectum. From the tip of the probe, harmless, painless sound waves are aimed at the villous adenoma in the wall of the rectum. The waves bouncing back (the echoes) are seen as pictures on a screen. These can show how deeply the adenoma (and any cancer in it) penetrates the rectal wall.
- It is important with a villous adenoma to determine whether there is cancer in it (Fig. 1). Performing the usual biopsy (taking a tiny piece of it) can be misleading. If such a piece is negative for cancer, it does not mean that no cancer is present in a different area of the adenoma. Even several biopsies can still miss a cancerous area in the adenoma. For this reason all of the adenoma must be removed and in one piece so that all parts of it can be examined carefully under the microscope.

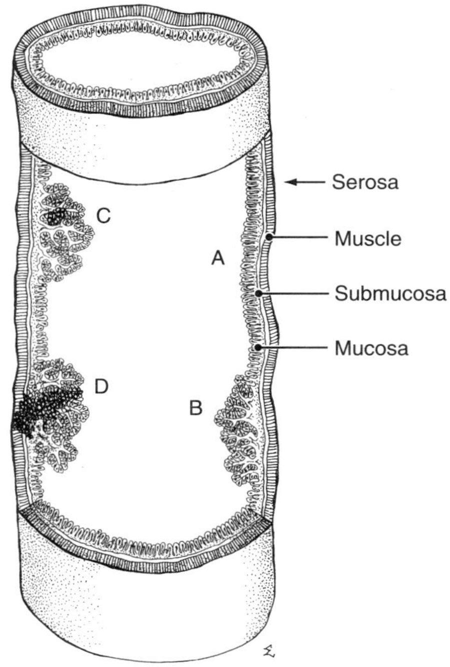

Figure 1. Segment of colon, showing normal anatomy (A); benign villous adenoma (B); villous adenoma with small, superficial cancer (C); and villous adenoma with deeply penetrating cancer (D).

○ TREATMENT

If all the villous adenoma can be removed through the anus and it is negative for cancer, then no further treatment is necessary (Fig. 2).

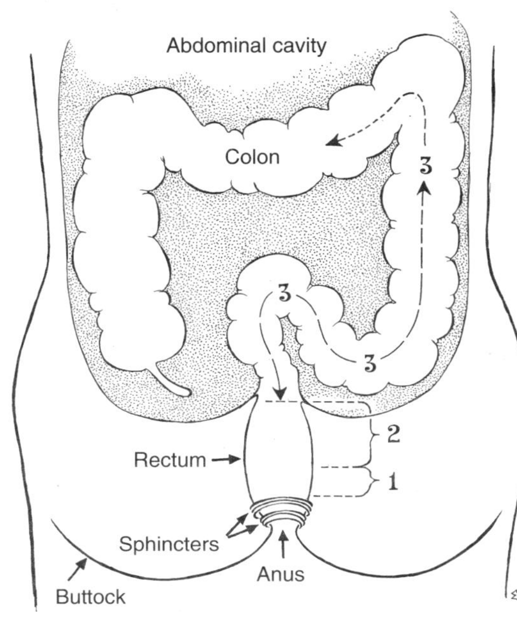

Figure 2. Colon and rectum, showing locations that may influence treatment: low rectum (1), mid and high rectum (2), and colon (3).

If it is not technically possible to remove the adenoma as described above, it is wise to treat the part of the colon with the adenoma in it as though it is cancerous. If the adenoma in the removed colon has cancer in it, then it was the proper treatment. If the removed adenoma is benign, you won't miss the extra colon and a lesion has been removed that could later become cancerous.

Your villous adenoma was in your lower rectum and anus. It has been removed and carefully examined under the microscope. There is cancer in it. Further, the cancer is penetrating the wall of the rectum and is extremely close to the muscle sphincters of your anus. It is not physically possible to do a curative operation on you without removing both your rectum and anus.

After the most careful consideration of all factors, the recommendation is that you have an operation to remove your rectum and anus with a permanent colostomy (Figs. 3 and 4). This operation will also affect your sex life.

PREOPERATIVE PREPARATION

- There will be an extensive discussion with you about the particulars of a colostomy.
- Do not eat or drink anything for 8 hours before the operation.

☐ OPERATION

- You will be asleep for the operation.
- The incision will run up and down in your lower abdomen as well as around your anal area.
- The operation usually takes about 3 hours.

POSTOPERATIVE CARE

- You will be taken to a recovery room and observed. After your blood pressure, pulse, and breathing are stable, you will be taken to a regular hospital room.
- You will have a thin plastic tube in your nose for a few days.
- Pain will be controlled with medicine.
- After the thin plastic tube that is in your nose is removed, you will be started on a liquid diet and advanced to solid food as you tolerate it.
- As with any operation, complications are always possible. With this type of operation, they can include bleeding, infection, pneumonia, blood clots, and possibly others.
- You should be able to go home in about 5 to 7 days.
- Arrangements will be made for your medicine, a visiting nurse, follow-up office visit, and stitch or clip removal.

✚ HOME CARE

- You may walk about as you wish, even climb stairs, but don't overdo things.
- You will be given a suggested diet to follow during your convalescence.
- Take the medicines as prescribed for you.
- While you are in the hospital, you will be taught by the nurse how to take care of your colostomy; it's not difficult. Even so, in the beginning there will be a visiting nurse to help you at home. Soon, you will be able to easily take care of things by yourself.

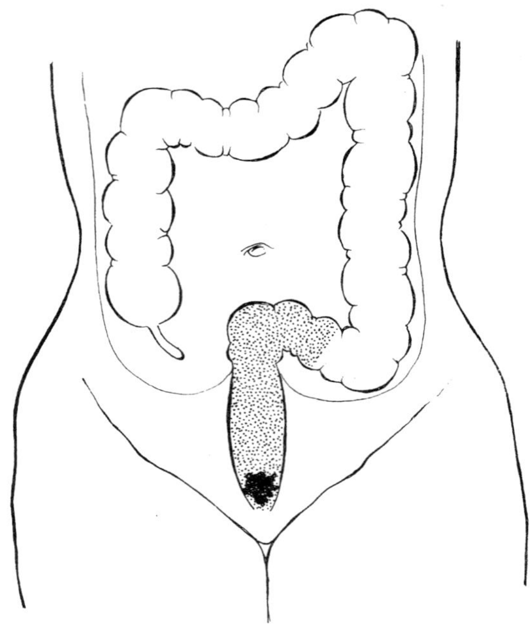

Figure 3. Villous adenoma *(dark area)* with cancer in it in the low rectum. It is penetrating the local tissue deeply and is very close to or even affecting the sphincter muscles of the anus. The stippled area needs to be removed.

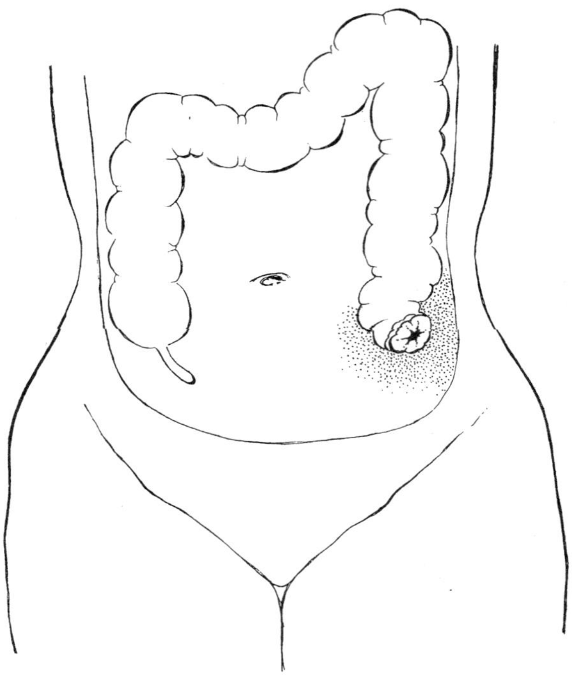

Figure 4. The rectum and anus have been removed and a permanent colostomy established.

✆ CALL OUR OFFICE IF

- The wound becomes swollen and red, or there is drainage from it.
- You develop a temperature higher than 100°F.
- You have any questions.

△ GENERAL INFORMATION

Volvulus is the twisting of the intestine on itself that causes it to become obstructed; in this instance it is the colon. Some persons have a very long colon (especially on the left side) that is not anchored too well. Because of this, it can flop around.

Rarely, a loop of this colon flips into a twist and gets stuck in that position, creating what is called a volvulus (Figs. 1 and 2). Sometimes a twisted length of colon will untwist by itself, and all is well. However, it may become twisted again. Sometimes, the volvulus won't untwist. Because the twist cuts off the blood supply to this part of the colon, gangrene can set in.

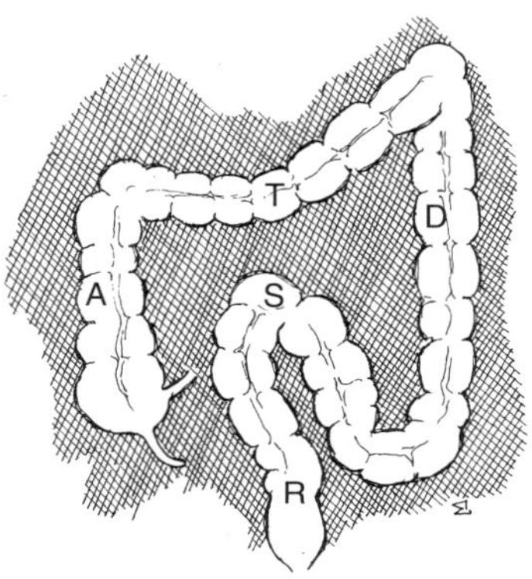

Figure 1. Normal anatomy of the large bowel. A, Ascending colon T, transverse colon; D, descending colon; S, sigmoid colon; R, rectum.

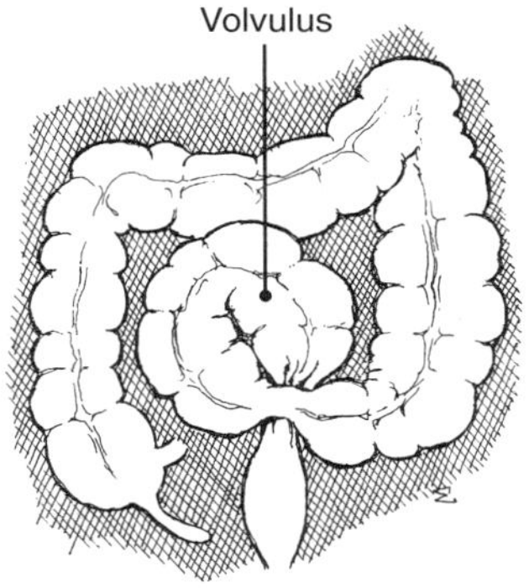

Figure 2. Volvulus occurs mostly on the left side, but it can occur on the right side. Also, the length of colon involved in the "twist" can vary considerably.

COMMON SIGNS AND SYMPTOMS

- There is abdominal distention because the twisted bowel blocks the passage of gas and stool.
- There may be cramping abdominal pain.
- A person is not able to pass gas or stool.
- There may be some fever and an elevated white blood cell count.
- If gangrene is present, then all of the above are much more intense.

DIAGNOSIS

- An x-ray of the abdomen. This may show the gas in the blocked colon and that it is caused by a volvulus.

○ TREATMENT

Nonsurgical Treatment

- Sometimes the diagnosis can be made and the treatment given at the same time without an operation. This is attempted by a specialist in radiology. Barium (it has the appearance of thick cream) is placed in the large bowel through the anus very much like a regular enema. X-ray pictures are taken of the barium as it travels up the colon. As the barium is watched under the x-ray, the pressure on the barium is very carefully and slowly increased to see whether it can force the bowel to untwist. If the bowel untwists, that's the end of the episode.

Surgical Treatment

- Sometimes, a volvulus can be corrected as described above, but it can appear again at a later time. For this reason, if the volvulus comes back (and it is corrected the same way), an operation is advised during a quiet period. It is too much to expect to be able to correct it safely without an operation each time.
- Sometimes, of course, treatment with a barium enema will not help the colon untwist. In such instances, an immediate operation is necessary to untwist the bowel before it develops gangrene.

PREOPERATIVE PREPARATION

The completeness of the preparation is influenced by how soon the operation needs to be done.

- There will be an examination of the blood, urine, heart (EKG), and lung (chest x-ray). If any abnormalities are seen, they will be corrected as much as possible before an operation.
- Do not eat or drink anything for 8 hours before the operation.
- Shower or bathe as usual on the morning of the operation.
- You may be given medicine that will make you feel drowsy before you are brought to the operating room.

□ OPERATION

- You will be asleep for the operation.

Emergency Operation

- The abdomen will be opened and the colon untwisted. If the untwisted colon looks healthy, it can be tacked down with some stitches so that it can't twist again.
- If the colon has developed gangrene, this part is removed and the ends reconnected. Sometimes, the colon is so full of feces that it is too dangerous to

reconnect it in one sitting. In such an instance, it may be necessary to do a *temporary* colostomy. A few weeks later, the colostomy will be closed, and you will have your bowel movements the normal way.

Elective Operation

- This operation is being done because of repeated episodes of volvulus. The bowel will have already been thoroughly cleansed (you will be instructed on how to do this). At the time of the operation one of two things can be done depending on the findings:
  - The bowel will be arranged in a "normal" pattern and stitched in that position so that it cannot twist again.
  - If the colon is much too long and this is the reason it flops around, some of the "extra" colon will be removed and the ends reconnected. Removing such extra colon will not affect your digestion or bowel movements.

POSTOPERATIVE CARE

- You will be taken to a recovery room and observed. When your blood pressure, pulse, and breathing are stable, you will be taken to a regular hospital room.
- You will have a thin plastic tube in your nose. It goes down to your stomach to suck up the air you swallow. It will be removed when your bowels start working.
- Pain will be controlled with medicine.
- That evening you will be helped to sit up in bed and on the next day to get out of bed.
- After the tube from your nose is removed, your diet will be as you tolerate it.
- As with any operation, complications are always possible. With this type of operation, they can include infection, pneumonia, bowel obstruction, lung or heart problems, and possibly others.
- You should be able to go home in about 1 week.
- Arrangements will be made for your medicine, follow-up office visit, and stitch or clip removal.

✚ HOME CARE

- Slowly resume your usual activities.
- Walking and otherwise moving about—in moderation—is good for your circulation, breathing, and muscle tone. Remain active as long as it doesn't hurt or tire you.
- You may eat as you did before the operation.
- You may shower or bathe as you wish, and with any dressings on or off.
  - There may be narrow strips of tape across the incision. It's all right if they get wet; they will be removed in the doctor's office.
  - After you dry yourself, replace any dressings with clean, dry ones.
- Be careful that you do not become constipated.
  - Include enough roughage and plenty of liquids in your diet.
  - You may need some help with a mild laxative (example: milk of magnesia).

✆ CALL OUR OFFICE IF

- The incision becomes red or swollen, or there is drainage from it.
- You develop a temperature higher than 100°F.
- You have any questions.

△ GENERAL INFORMATION

Vulva is the word for the outside sex organs in a woman. Cancer of the vulva occurs most commonly in older women. Also, it usually occurs on the side of the opening into the vagina (the *labia*). These cancers can spread to the lymph nodes in the groin or to the lymph nodes inside the pelvis.

COMMON SIGNS AND SYMPTOMS

The following may be present when there is a cancer in the vulva:

- A mass.
- Irritation.
- Ulceration.
- Bleeding.
- Itching.

DIAGNOSIS

Anyone with a lesion of the vulva and with the above history and findings should have that lesion examined under the microscope. This is done by using a fine, short needle to inject an anesthetic into the lesion and the surrounding tissue to make it numb. A small piece of the lesion is removed (a *biopsy*) and sent to the laboratory for examination. This is an outpatient procedure.

○ TREATMENT

The aim of treatment is to eradicate all of the cancer and any affected lymph nodes. Fortunately, surgery, x-ray treatment, or chemotherapy, either alone or together, can be effective depending on the individual circumstances.

After careful consideration of all factors, the recommendation is that you have an operation to remove this lesion. The reasons for this will have been explained to you.

PREOPERATIVE PREPARATION

- You will have an examination of your blood and urine. There will be special attention paid to the condition of your heart (EKG), lungs (chest x-ray), kidneys, and vessels to the brain and legs.
- For larger cancers, a CT scan (computed tomography scan) may be done. These are special x-rays taken by a machine that is shaped like a huge doughnut. You will lie on a table inside the "doughnut." The x-rays are taken as very thin slices through the area of your groin and pelvis. This makes it possible to look for any enlarged lymph nodes in these areas.
- You will be given instructions on how to clean out your bowel before the operation.
- Do not eat or drink anything for 8 hours before the operation.
- You may be given medicine that will make you feel drowsy before you are brought to the operating room.

□ OPERATION

- You will be asleep for the operation.
- The operation usually takes about 2 to 4 hours, depending on how much needs to be done.
- You will not receive a blood transfusion unless it is absolutely necessary.

POSTOPERATIVE CARE

- You will be taken to a recovery room and observed. When your blood pressure, pulse, and breathing are stable, you will be taken to a regular hospital room.
- There will be a small tube in your bladder for a few days so you won't have to worry about how to pass your urine during this time.
- Pain can be controlled with medicine. The nurse will give it to you, or you can give yourself a preset amount of pain medicine when you feel you need it. This is done with patient-controlled analgesia (PCA) that is connected to the tubing giving you intravenous fluids.
- That evening you will be helped to sit up in bed and on the next day to get out of bed.
- You should be able to start drinking fluids and eating a soft diet by the following morning.
- You should be able to go home in 3 to 7 days, depending on the extent of your operation.
- Arrangements will be made for your medicine, follow-up office visit, and stitch removal.
- As with any operation, complications are always possible. With this type of operation, they can include blood clots and heart or lung problems. Partial breakdown of the wound is common. This may require care by a home visiting nurse; arrangements can be made for this, if needed.

✚ HOME CARE

- You should have someone with you at home, at least for the first few days.
- You may walk as you wish, even upstairs. Do everything gradually and be careful not to tire yourself.
- You may eat as you did before the operation.
  - Include enough roughage and plenty of liquids in your diet to help avoid constipation.
  - You may need some help with a mild laxative (example: milk of magnesia).
- Take medicine as prescribed for your pain.
- You may shower if you wish. Have someone in attendance at least for the first few times.

✆ CALL OUR OFFICE IF

- The incision becomes red or swollen, or there is drainage from it.
- You develop any unusual signs or symptoms.
- You develop a temperature higher than 100°F.
- You have any questions.

△ GENERAL INFORMATION

The purpose of warm, moist packs is to make the microscopic blood vessels *(capillaries)* in an area expand. They can then bring in more blood (and the important white blood cells in it) to help fight the infection.

Warm. The heat is necessary because it stimulates capillaries to open up.

Moist. Moisture holds and transfers heat better than heat that is dry and not in close contact with the skin.

Packs. This is a convenient as well as effective way to bring warm moisture to the area.

All the above must be done correctly because too much heat can burn your skin. Also, something that is not very hot but is kept on too long can damage your skin. By contrast, something that is moist but is just at room temperature won't do much good. Unless you are positive of what you are doing, play it safe: *not* too hot; *not* too long.

There are a number of ways to apply heat to tissue. The following is one good method.

- Dissolve 1 teaspoon of ordinary table salt in 1 quart of tap water that has been made *warm, not hot*, in an ordinary clean cooking pot.
- Dip a clean face washcloth into this salt solution, lift it out, and gently squeeze the excess water from it.
- Test the moist washcloth on the back of your hand to be certain it is not too hot. Then spread it over the area to be treated.
- Over this washcloth place a piece of plastic (plastic food wrap or the plastic wrapping from the dry cleaners will do). This will prevent the warm salt solution from being absorbed into the layer over this.
- Over this plastic place a dry face cloth. This may help spread the heat more evenly.
- Over this place a heating pad set to *Low*, not medium and not high!
- Make yourself comfortable.
- It is better if you use pillows to elevate the part being treated.
- Leave the pack in position as long as you have been directed, usually for 20 to 30 minutes (Fig. 1). You don't have to do any towel changing during this session.
- Longer or more often is not necessarily better, so do it as you have been advised.
- A new moist washcloth is advisable for each new session. Just rewarm the salt solution and use the same plastic and dry washcloth.
- If possible, avoid taking your pain medicine immediately before the soaks. The medicine may keep you from properly feeling something that might be too hot.
- *Stop and remove everything if the soaks feel too warm.*
- *Do not continue with more sessions if the skin doesn't look right*, for example, if it is very red, or blotchy, or possibly with tiny blisters on it.

Using another method, you can have almost the same benefit without the plastic sheet, dry towel, and heating pad. Simply dip the washcloth in the warm salt solution, gently squeeze out the excess water, and apply the moist washcloth over the affected area.

- This method works better for some areas, such as the face.
- It can be a little sloppy.
- You need to redip the washcloth into the salt solution every few minutes as the washcloth becomes cool.
- You have to reheat the water to keep it warm. Remember, the water used for this method should *not* be hot.

✆ CALL OUR OFFICE IF

- You have any questions about any of the above.

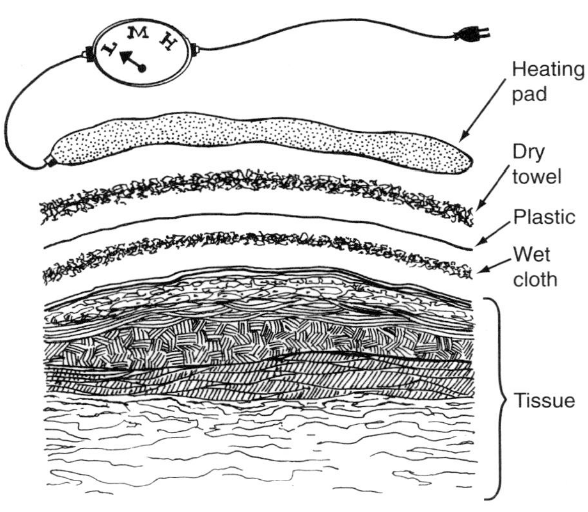

Figure 1. Although normally the various layers of warm, moist packs would lie one on top of the other, they are shown separated for the sake of clarity.

△ GENERAL INFORMATION

Many persons from the very young to old have common warts *(verruca vulgaris)*. Although warts are most often seen on the hands, they can occur on just about any part of the body. They are caused by several viruses.

This discussion concerns only warts of the hands.

COMMON SIGNS AND SYMPTOMS

- Most warts produce no symptoms at all. Sometimes, however, they may crack or be wedged right next to a fingernail and be painful to the touch. At other times, their location on the fingers interferes with work.
- Most persons are bothered by warts simply because they are unsightly.

DIAGNOSIS

- Usually, the diagnosis can be made by taking a history and doing a careful physical examination.

○ TREATMENT

- Sometimes warts will go away by themselves—either all of them or only some of them.
- There is no one treatment that is best for all warts of all sizes, or in all locations. That's why what works for one person may not work for another.
- The doctor needs to know how to perform or recommend any of several procedures.

PREPARATION

No preparation on your part is necessary for any of these procedures.

- **Freezing:** Liquid nitrogen in a special instrument is applied to the wart to freeze it to death. This is best for very new, small, and somewhat soft warts. Sometimes the area of the wart needs to be anesthetized.
- **Salicylic Acid Plaster:** This is a mild chemical, sold over the counter at drug stores, that is applied to the wart. Gradually, it burns away the wart. It is necessary to apply the chemical on the wart over a period of time. It hurts some as the base of the wart is reached. No anesthetic is necessary.
- **Excision:** If the wart is medium-sized and there's plenty of loose skin around it (example: back of the hand), it is sometimes better to remove it and to bring the skin together. This is done on an outpatient basis.

  The area of the wart is painted with an antiseptic solution and surrounded with sterile towels. A very fine short needle will be used to inject an anesthetic in the area to make it completely numb. The wart will be removed and the skin brought together with fine sutures. You should be able to be up and about right after the procedure.
- **Electrodesiccation:** This probably is the best all-around treatment. A very fine short needle is used to inject an anesthetic in the area of the wart to make it numb. A special electrical instrument with a very fine tip is used to burn the surface of the wart practically to a crisp. The burnt part of the wart is lifted off and then the base, or "core," is burned further. You will be able to leave directly after this. A sore the size of the wart remains; it heals in a week or so.

AFTERCARE

- With all the above techniques, one can return to previous activities right after the treatment.
- The hands can be washed in the usual fashion and with any bandages on or off. After you dry yourself, replace the bandages with clean, dry ones. Also, if the bandages accidentally get wet, replace them with dry ones.

✆ CALL OUR OFFICE IF

- Any treated area becomes red, more painful than before, or there is drainage from it.

△ GENERAL INFORMATION

Genital warts *(condylomata acuminata)* often have the appearance of the type of warts you see on your hands, but they are velvety and soft. They can occur just about anywhere in the external sex organs of women and men. They also can grow around and even into the anus. There may be only one or dozens of them, and they may grow so close together that they cover an entire area.

Genital warts are caused by a human papillomavirus (HPV) and are spread during sexual intercourse.

COMMON SIGNS AND SYMPTOMS

The warts themselves cause no symptoms, but because it is difficult to keep this area clean, itching and irritation are the most common symptoms.

DIAGNOSIS

- Usually, the diagnosis can be made by taking a detailed history and doing a thorough physical examination as well as removing a small piece of one of the lesions (a *biopsy*) for laboratory examination.
- Tests will need to be done to check for the possible presence of some other venereal disease.

THERAPY

The aim of treatment is to destroy the lesions by several methods. Sometimes more than one method may be used in the same area.

PREOPERATIVE PREPARATION

If there are just a few warts, they can be treated under local anesthesia. If there are many or if they are in the anus or vagina, then they are best treated under quick-acting general anesthesia.

For an operation under local anesthesia:

- Three hours before the operation, give yourself a plain Fleet enema as instructed on the package.
- Shower as usual on the morning of the operation.

For an operation under general anesthesia:

- You will have an examination of your blood, urine, and possibly of your heart (EKG) and lungs (chest x-ray).
- You may be given medicine that will make you feel drowsy before you are brought to the operating room.

□ OPERATION

The destruction of the warts can be done in several ways. Each method has its advantages and disadvantages, depending on the number of warts, their size, where they are located, and convenience to the patient.

- *Burning them with electrocautery or laser beam*: This method is simple and accurate, and there is no bleeding. It can be used for a few or for many warts.
- *Freezing them (cryosurgery)*: This method is a little more cumbersome, not as accurate, and is not too suitable when many warts need to be destroyed.
- *Applying a chemical (called podophyllum resin)*: This is more troublesome, can be somewhat untidy, is slower acting, is not too suitable when many warts are present, and often requires repeat treatments.
- *Cutting them off*: This is involved but is most suitable for individual lesions that are too large to treat by the other methods.

Local Anesthesia

- You'll be on a table lying on your side.
- The area containing the warts will be painted with an antiseptic solution.
- A short, very fine needle will be used to inject the skin containing the warts with an anesthetic. This entire skin area will become entirely numb.
- The lesions will be destroyed by one of the methods described above.
- You should be able to go home directly after the operation.

General Anesthesia

- General anesthesia is used primarily for large areas of involvement or to treat lesions inside the anus or vagina.
- You will be placed on the table and fluids started through your vein. A quick-acting general anesthesia will be given this way.
- After you are asleep, the area containing the warts will be exposed, painted with an antiseptic solution, and draped with towels.
- The warts will be destroyed in one of the ways described above.

POSTOPERATIVE CARE

- You will be taken to a recovery room and observed. When your blood pressure, pulse, and breathing are stable and you are completely alert, you should be able to go home that same day with a responsible adult.
- Arrangements will be made for medicines and follow-up office visit.
- You should know these genital warts sometimes cannot be destroyed in just one treatment session; several treatment sessions may be necessary. Also, they may be destroyed completely yet still come back.

✣ HOME CARE

- Resume your usual activities.
- You may walk about as you wish, even climb stairs.
- You may eat as you did before the operation.
- Be careful that you do not become constipated.
  - Include enough roughage and plenty of liquids in your diet.
  - You may need a mild laxative (example: milk of magnesia).
- Take medicine as prescribed for your pain.
- You may shower if you wish.
- Wearing soft cotton underwear is enough covering and also may be more comfortable.

- During the healing process, a condom should be worn during sexual intercourse.

✆ CALL OUR OFFICE IF

- You develop a temperature higher than 100°F.
- You have any questions.

FOLLOW-UP

Genital warts can be transmitted by a sex partner. It is important, therefore, that *both* partners be examined for genital warts. Also, it is most important that you and your partner and I have a conference on ways to help prevent the warts from coming back or from spreading.

WILMS' TUMOR (NEPHROBLASTOMA)

△ GENERAL INFORMATION

Wilms' tumor is a special malignant tumor of the kidney. It is special because of the following:

- It is virtually always seen in young children.
- Often it can be cured even if it is "advanced."

The exact cause of Wilms' tumor is not known, but because it sometimes is associated with several other hereditary conditions, there is a suggestion of a possible hereditary influence.

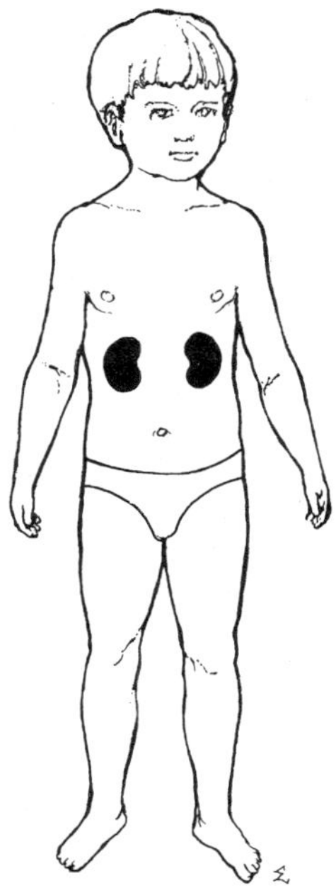

Figure 1. The kidneys *(dark areas)* are located as shown. Enlargement of one by a tumor makes it possible to feel it during a physical examination or by the mother when handling the child.

COMMON SIGNS AND SYMPTOMS

- Early, there may be no symptoms. The tumor is often discovered by the mother while bathing the child or by the pediatrician during a routine examination.
- Later, the tumor may produce a bulge on one side of the abdomen.
- Other symptoms may include abdominal pain or blood in the urine.
- There may be weight loss or a failure to thrive.

DIAGNOSIS

- A detailed history and a thorough physical examination will be done.
- It is important to know the following:
  - Whether the tumor is affecting any other organs next to it because such involvement does not mean a patient cannot be cured. Often plans can also be made to remove some (or all) of an affected neighboring organ.
  - Whether the tumor has spread to other areas in the body because this will influence what combinations of treatment should be used.
  - Whether the tumor is already in the vein draining the tumor because the surgeon can then take steps to prevent cancer cells from being squeezed out of the vein and into other areas of the body as the kidney is being handled during the operation.
- Possible tests to be done:
  - *Ultrasound*: Harmless sound waves will be aimed at the organs inside the abdomen. The sound waves bouncing back (the echoes) from this area are seen as pictures on a screen. In this way, the size and extent of the Wilms' tumor can be estimated and new growths looked for.
  - *CT (computed tomography) scan of the abdomen*: This special x-ray machine is shaped like a huge doughnut. Your child will lie on the table inside the hole in the "doughnut." The x-rays are taken as very thin slices through all of the abdomen, making it possible to see fine details in the organs and tissues in the abdomen and especially the tumor in the kidney.
  - *MRI (magnetic resonance imaging)*: No x-rays are used with this technique. Instead, it is done with harmless magnetic fields and radio waves. A computer develops the pictures to show organs from several angles. It is especially valuable for examining blood vessels and nerve tissue.

○ TREATMENT

- The treatment is an operation to either sample the tumor for identification or remove the kidney and any involved surrounding organs.
- Chemotherapy is often given following the operation.
- X-ray therapy may also be used.

PREOPERATIVE PREPARATION

- There should be no solid food for 6 hours and no liquids for 4 hours before the operation.
- Fluids will be started by vein so that the child does not become too dehydrated.
- The child will be given medicine to make her or him feel drowsy before being brought to the operating room.

□ OPERATION

- The operation will be done under general anesthesia.
- A number of wires and tubes will be connected to the child to monitor the heart, breathing, and oxygen levels in the blood as well as other important functions during sleep.
- The incision will be on the abdomen.
- No blood transfusion will be given unless it is absolutely necessary.
- The operation usually takes 2 hours or longer, depending on what may need to be removed in addition to the kidney.

POSTOPERATIVE CARE

- Your child will be taken to the Surgical Care Unit, where the doctors and nurses are very experienced at taking care of such patients.
- There will be a thin, plastic tube in the nose going down into the stomach to remove air that is swallowed. This tube will be removed as soon as the bowels start working.
- There may be a small tube in the bladder to measure accurately how much urine is made.
- Pain medicine will be given to control pain.
- As soon as the bowels start working, the tube from the nose will be removed and a liquid diet started.
- As with any operation, complications are always possible. With this type of operation, they can include bleeding, infection, bowel obstruction, and possibly others.
- Your child should be able to leave the hospital in about 1 week.
- Arrangements will be made for medicines, follow-up visit, stitch removal.

✣ HOME CARE

- Continue with the program outlined in the hospital.
- You may bathe the child as usual, but avoid any more soaking than is necessary.

✆ CALL OUR OFFICE IF

- The incision becomes red or swollen, or there is drainage from it.
- The child develops a temperature higher than 100°F.
- You have any questions.

AFTERCARE

- Wilms' tumor can be cured. An estimate of the chances can be made only after all the test results are back.
- Often the chances for cure can be improved if chemotherapy is also given. Most of the time this is the only additional therapy necessary.
- Sometimes x-ray therapy may need to be given to certain areas.
- The reason for chemotherapy and any x-ray therapy and how it is given will be explained to you in detail before anything is planned or done.

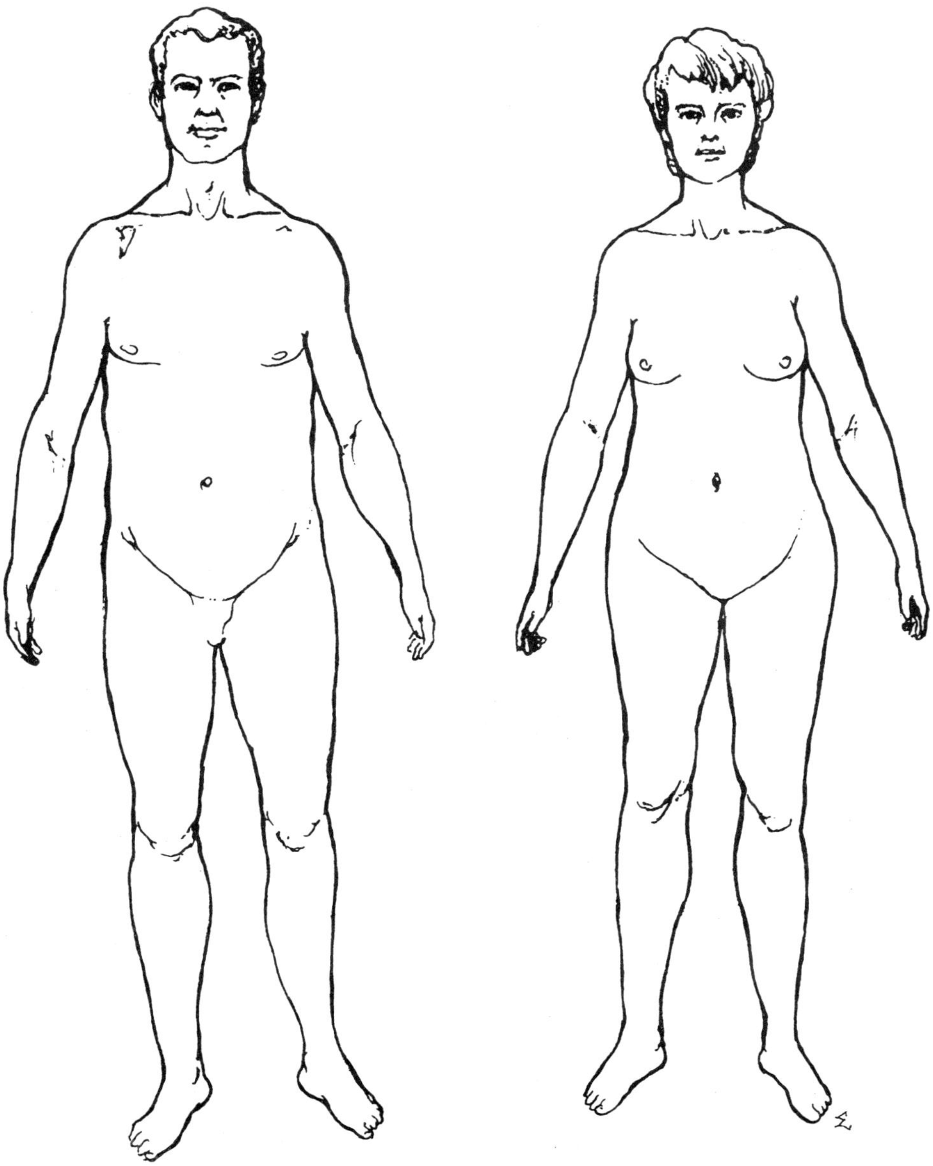

Figure 1.

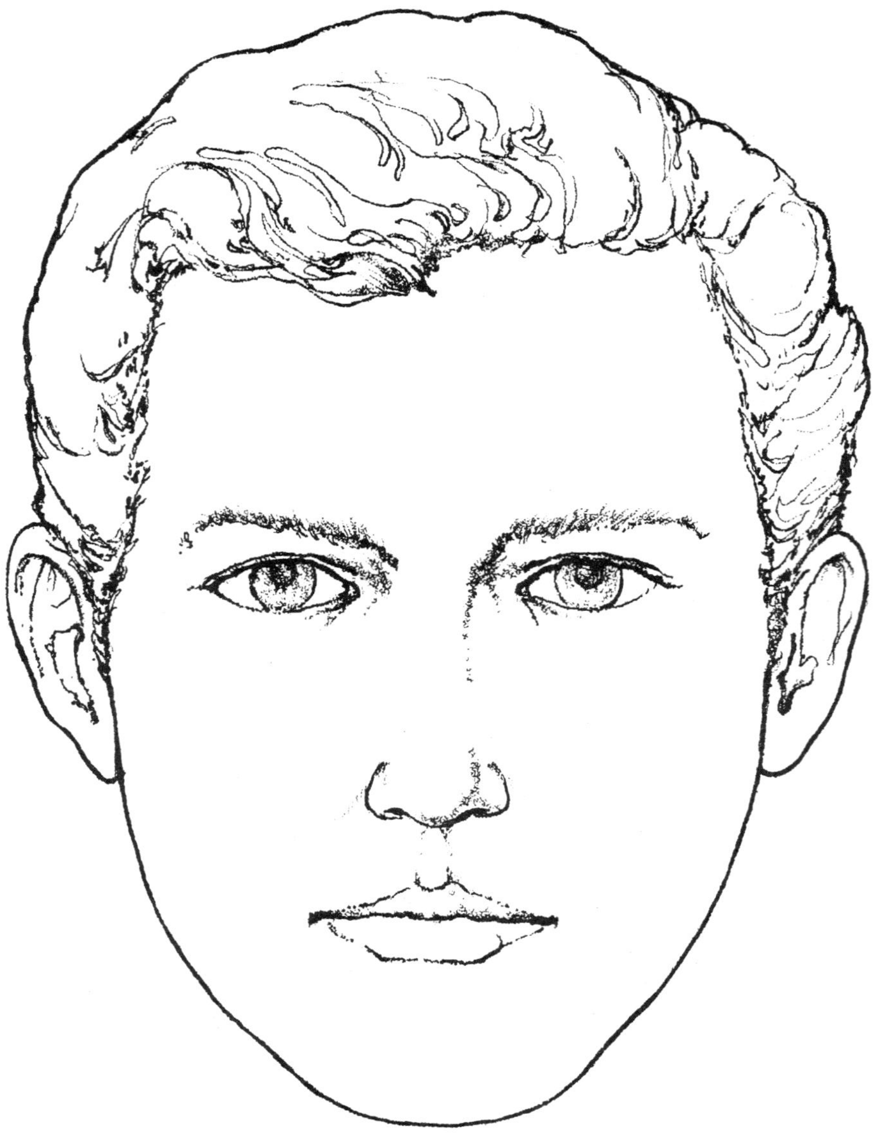

Figure 2.

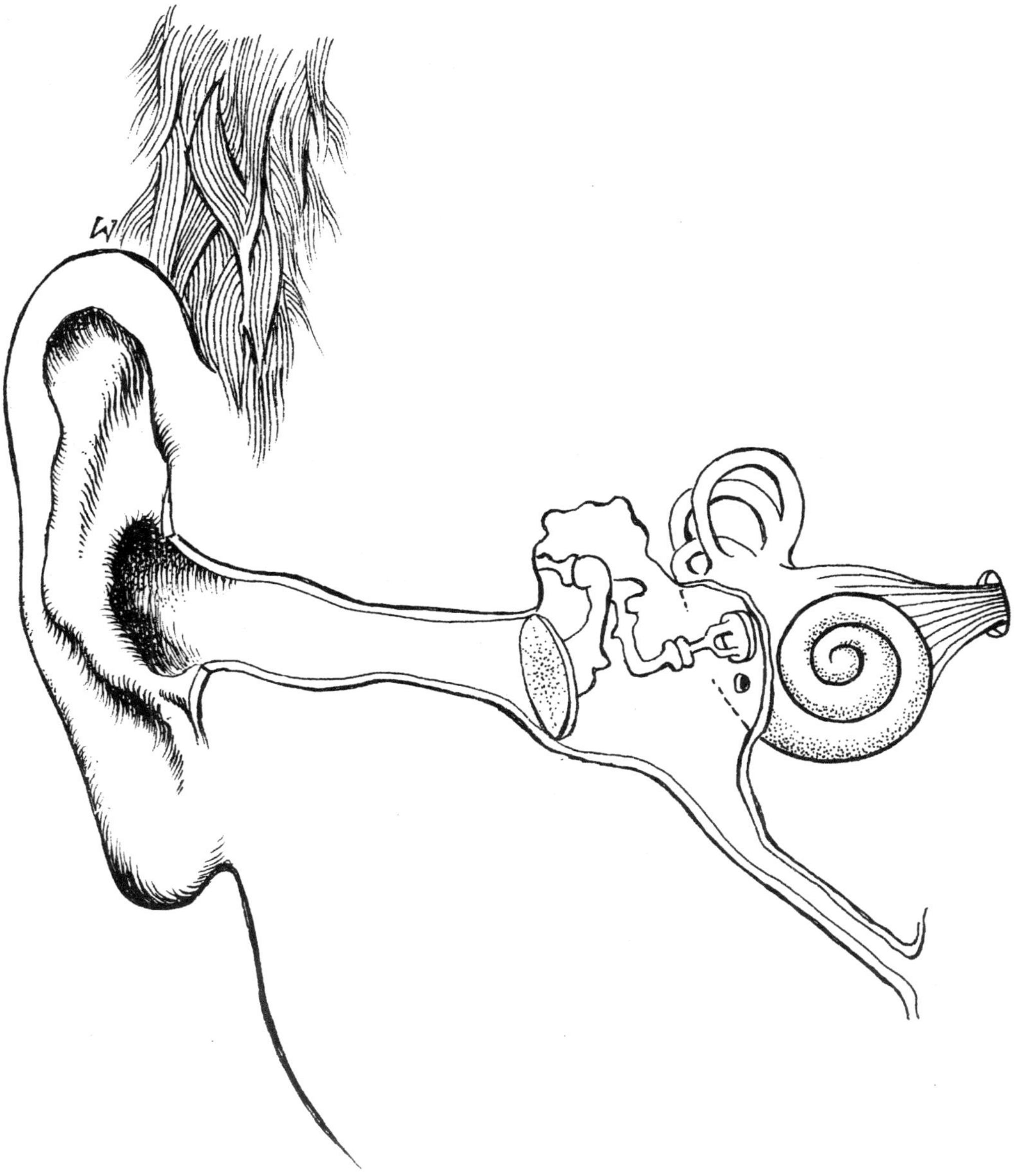

Figure 3.

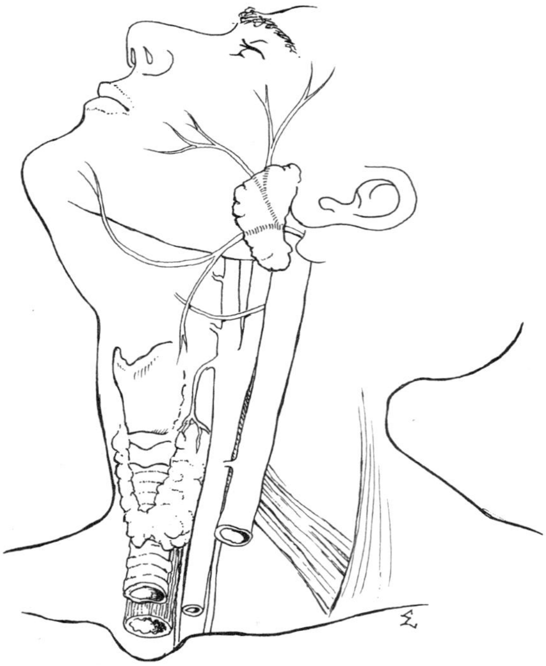

Figure 4.

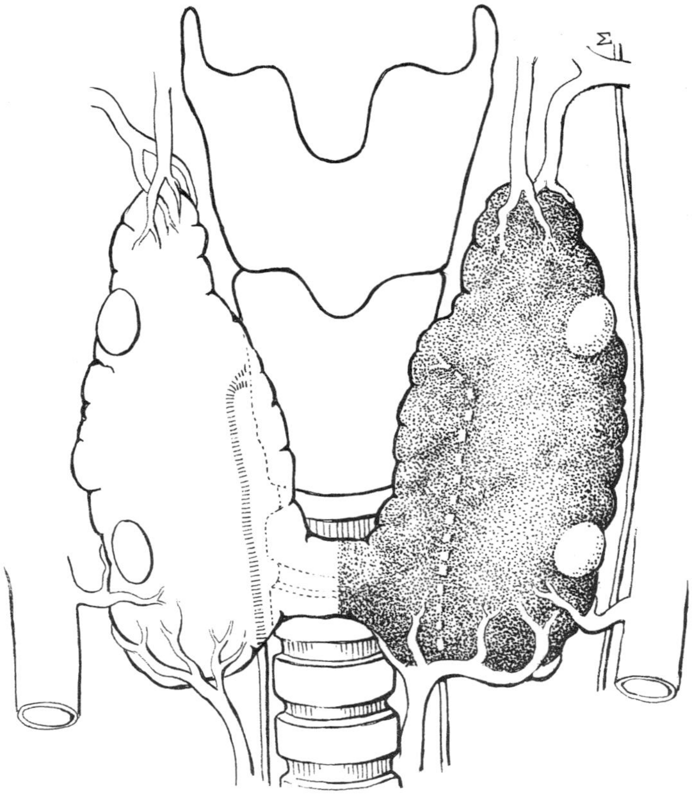

Figure 5.

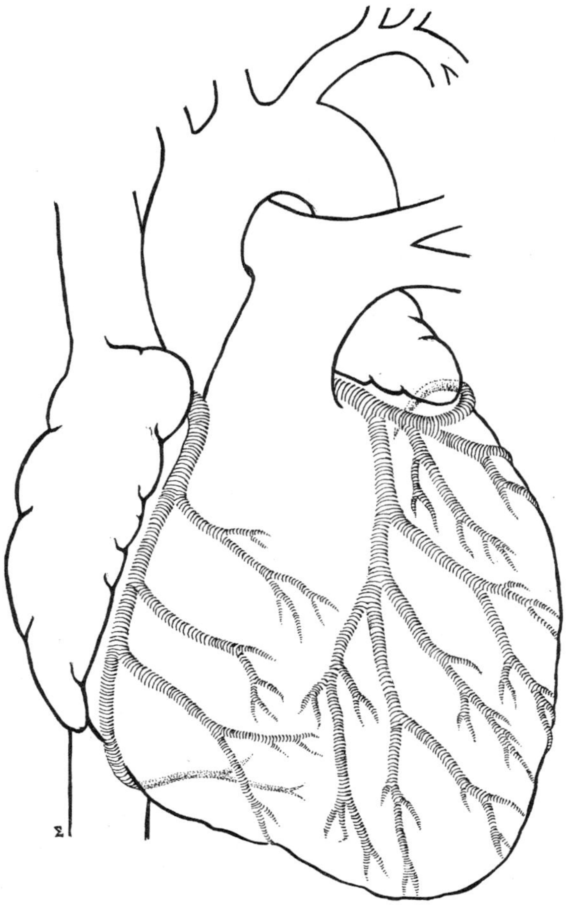

Figure 6.

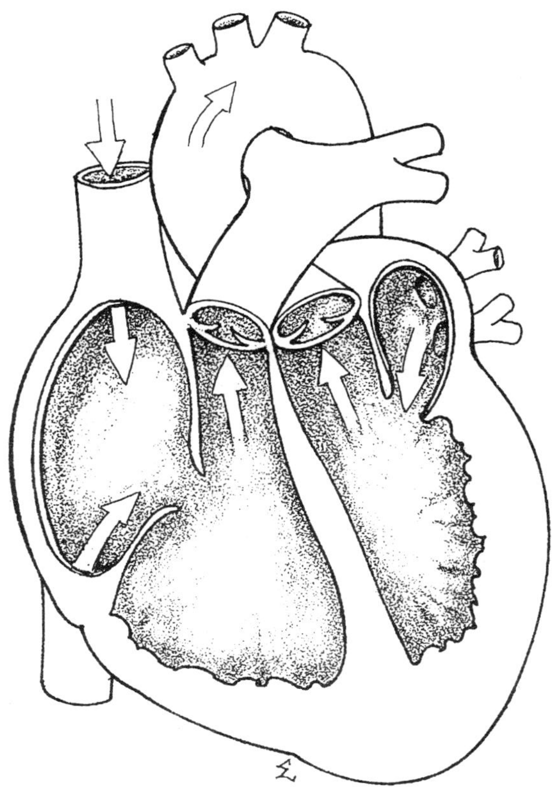

Figure 7.

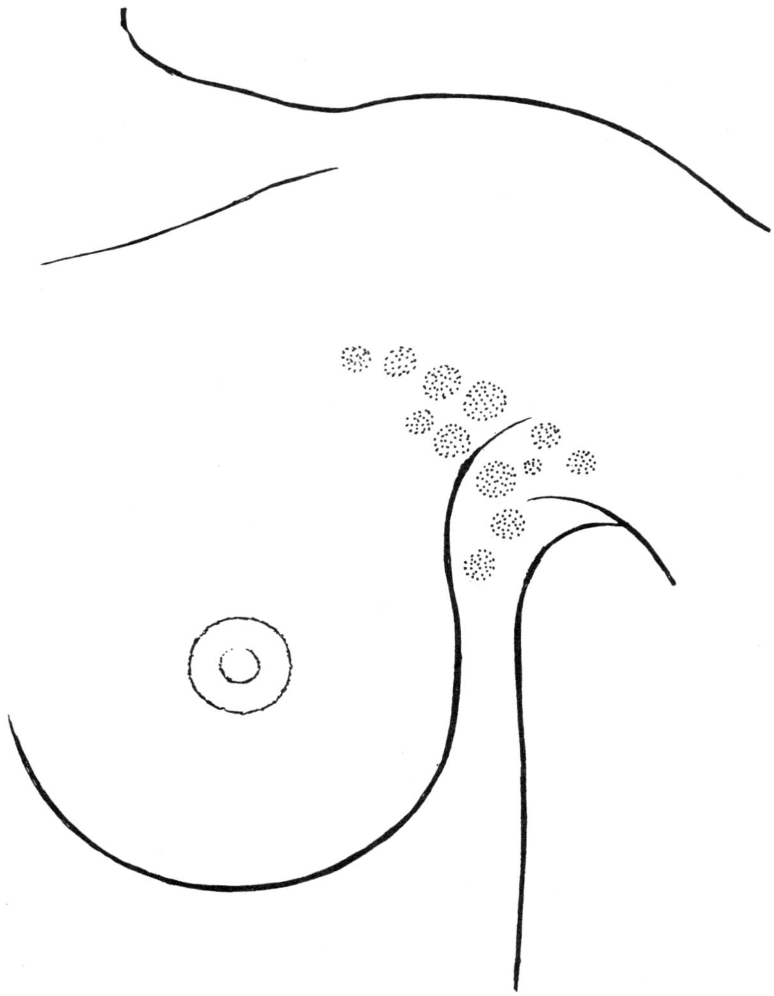

Figure 8.

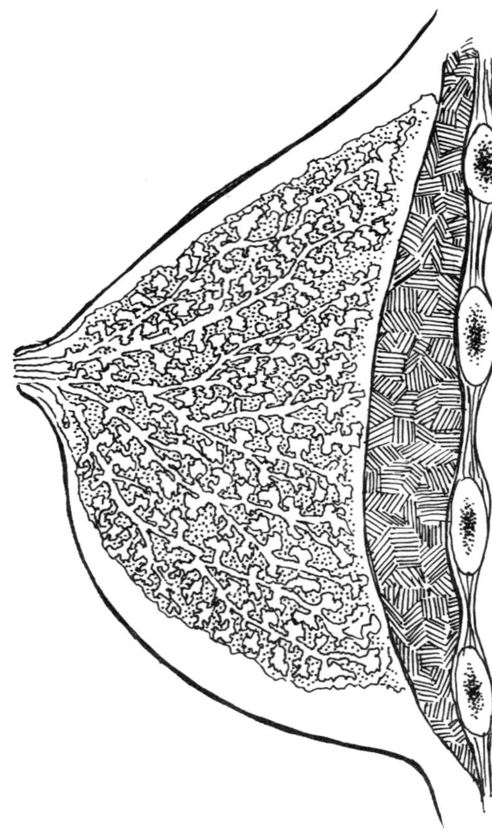

Figure 9.

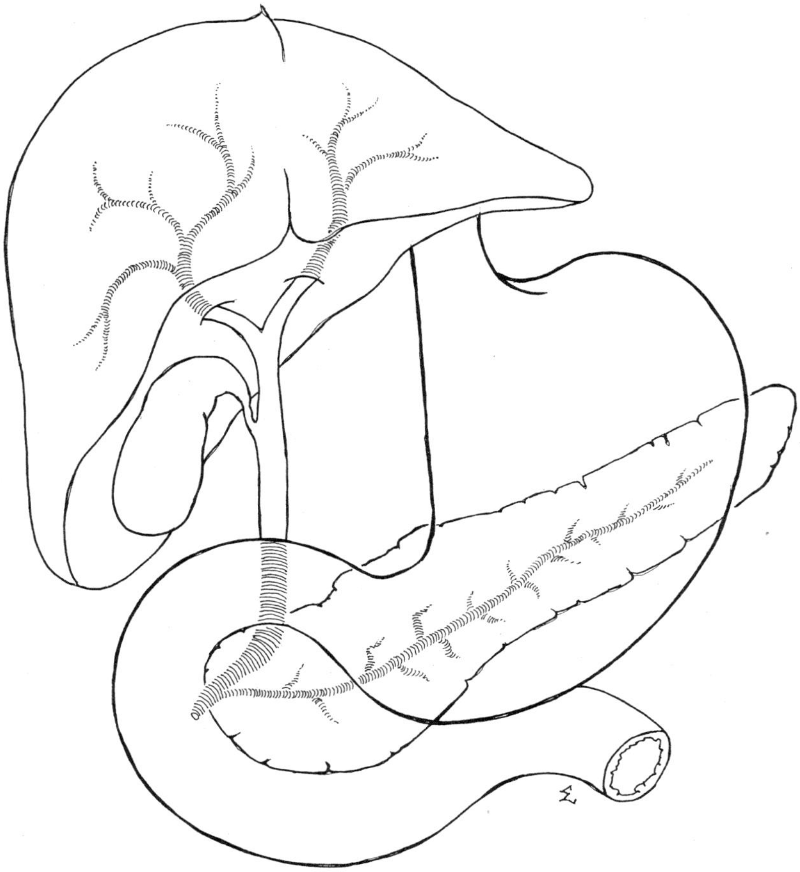

Figure 10.

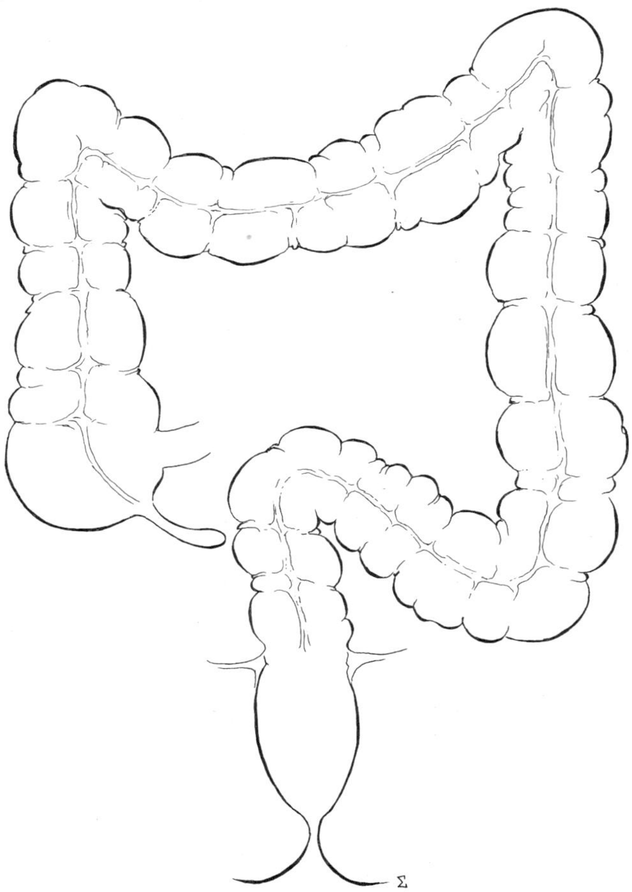

Figure 11.

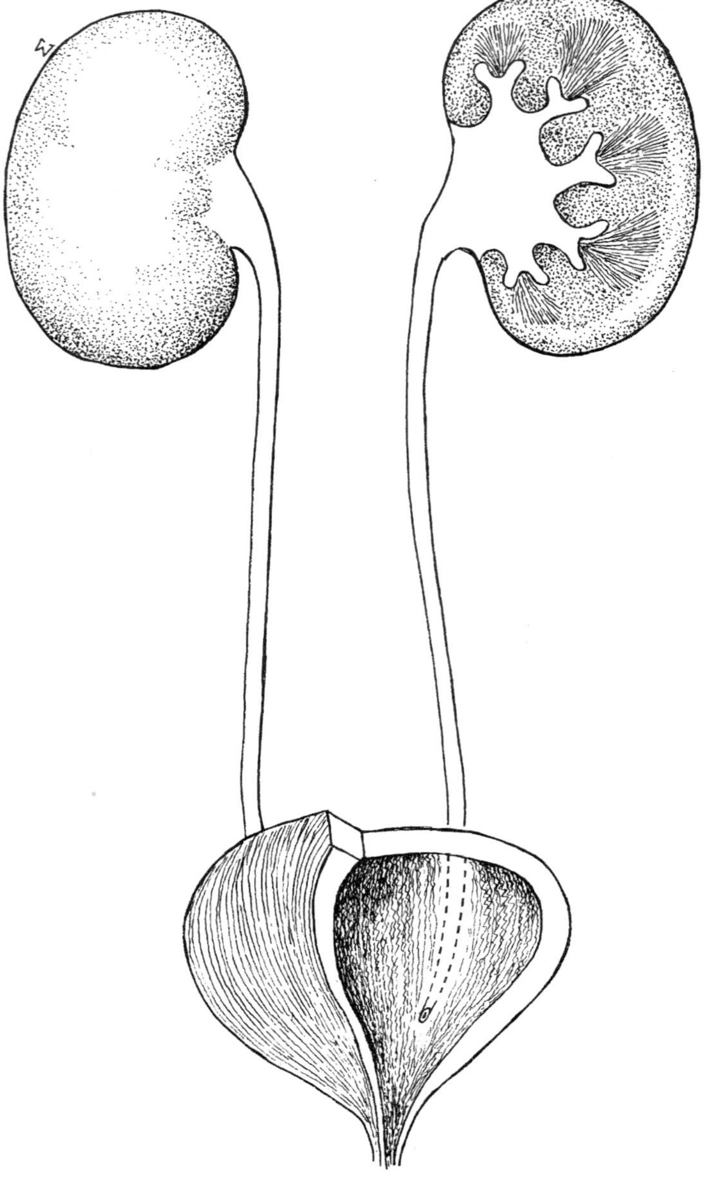

Figure 12.

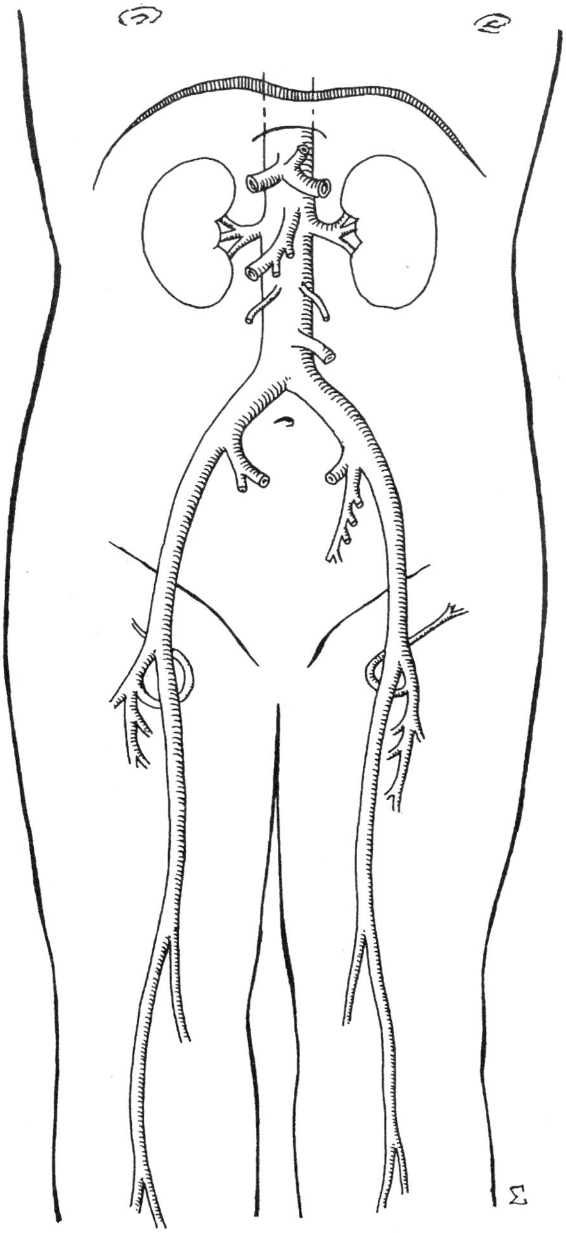

Figure 13.

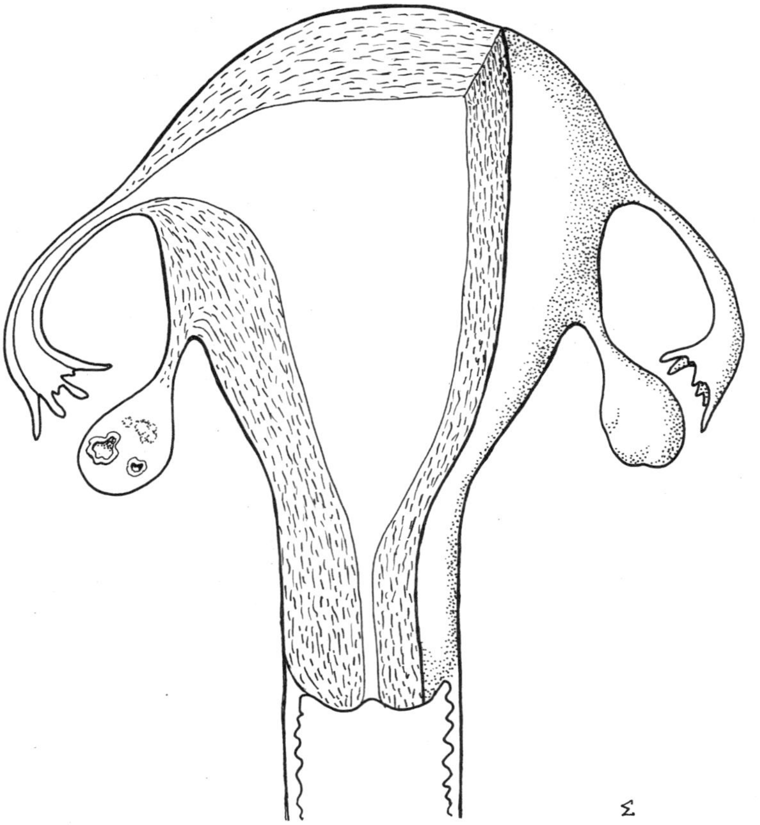

Figure 14.

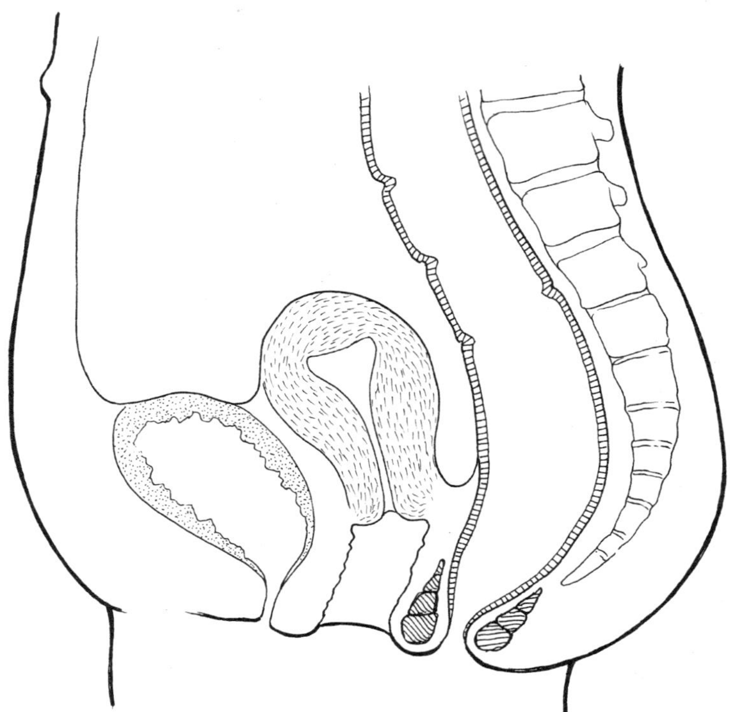

Figure 15.

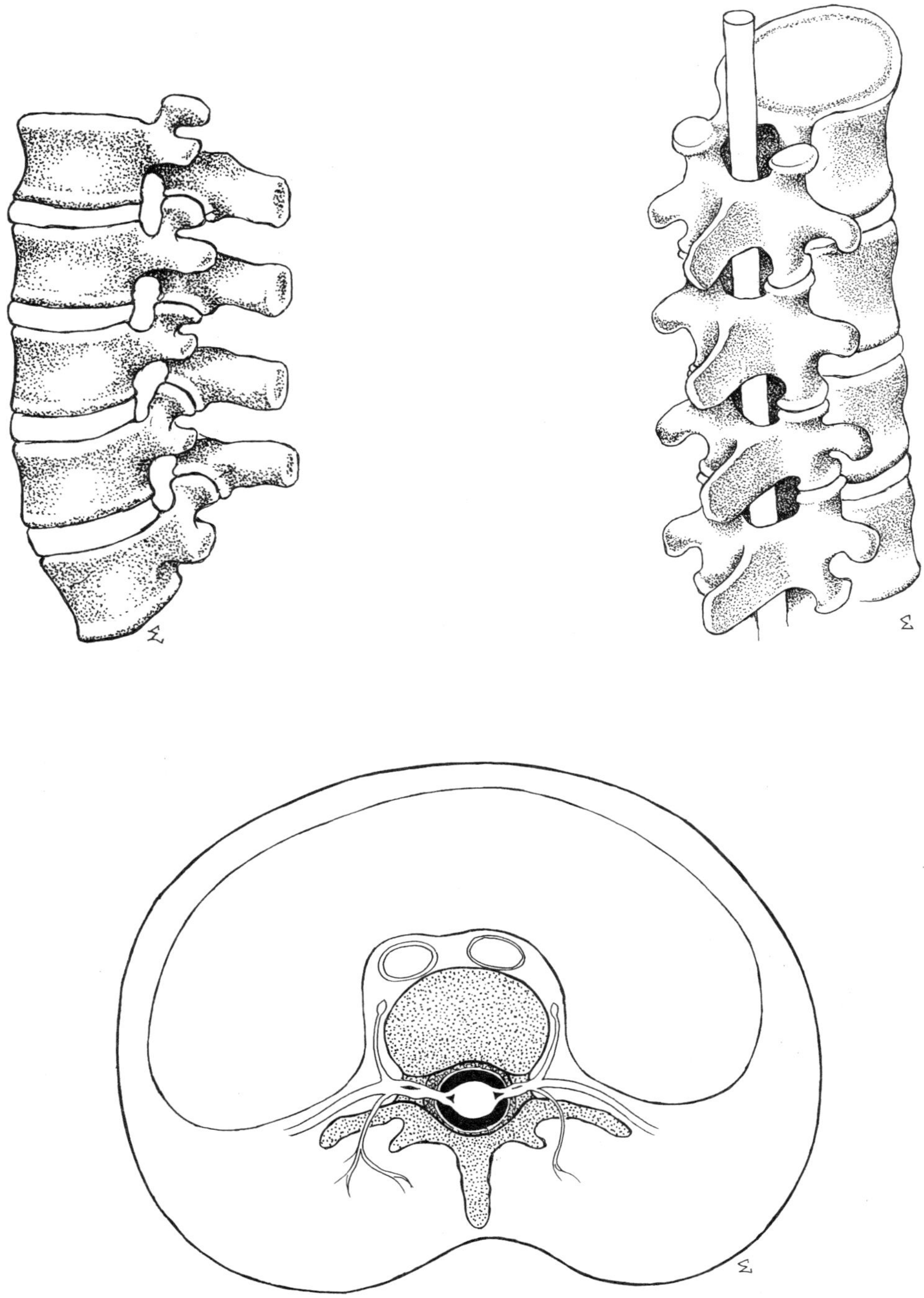

Figure 16.

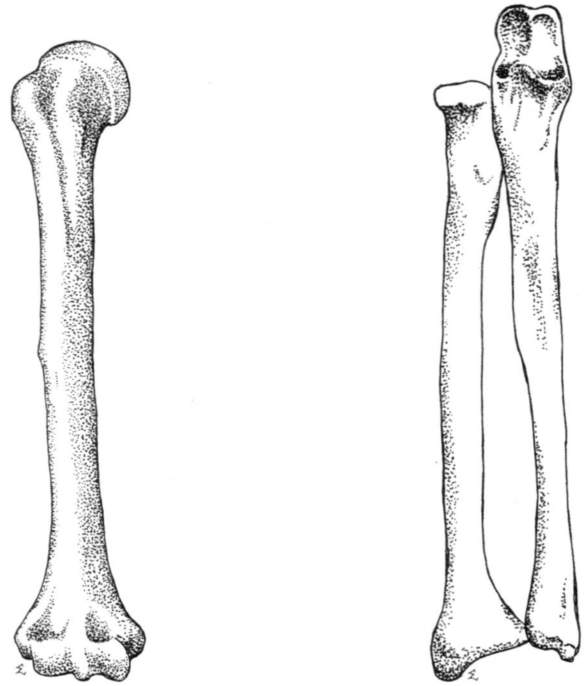

Figure 17.

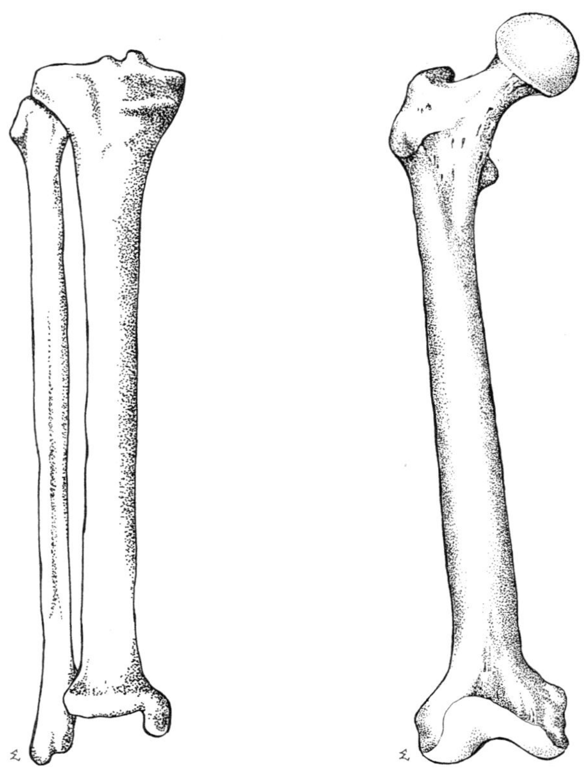

Figure 18.

INDEX

Note: Page numbers in *italics* refer to illustrations.